Applied Pharmacology
for the
Dental Hygienist

Applied
Pharmacology
for the
Dental
Hygienist

Fourth Edition

BARBARA REQUA-CLARK
Professor of Dentistry (Pharmacology)
Department of Dental Diagnostic Sciences
School of Dentistry
University of Missouri–Kansas City
Kansas City, Missouri

Fourth Editon

illustrated

Asheville-Buncombe
Technical Community College
Learning Resources Center
340 Victoria Road
Asheville, NC 28801

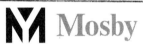 Mosby

A *Harcourt Health Sciences Company*
St. Louis   Philadelphia   London   Sydney   Toronto

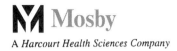

A *Harcourt Health Sciences Company*

Editor-in Chief: John A. Schrefer
Acquisition Editor: Penny Rudolph
Developmental Editor: Angela Reiner
Project Manager: John Rogers
Production Editor: Beth Hayes
Designer: Judi Lang

Fourth Edition

NOTICE

Pharmacology is an ever-changing field. Standard safety precautions must be followed, but as new research and clinical experience broaden our knowledge, changes in treatment and drug therapy may become necessary or appropriate. Readers are advised to check the most current product information provided by the manufacturer of each drug to be administered to verify the recommended dose, the method and duration of administration, and contraindications. It is the responsibility of the treating physician, relying on experience and knowledge of the patient, to determine dosages and the best treatment for each individual patient. Neither the publisher nor the editor or author assume any liability for any injury and/or damage to persons or property arising from this publication.

Mosby, Inc.
A Harcourt Health Sciences Company
11830 Westline Industrial Drive
St. Louis, Missouri 63146

Printed in the United States of America

Library of Congress Cataloging-in-Publication Data
Requa-Clark, Barbara.
    Applied pharmacology for the dental hygienist / Barbara
S. Requa-Clark.
        p.   cm.
    Includes bibliographical references and index.
    ISBN 0-8151-3630-7
    1. Clinical pharmacology   2. Dental personnel.   I. Title.
    [DNLM: 1. Dental Care.   2. Pharmacology, Clinical.   QV 50 R427ab
1999]
    RM301.28.R47   1999
    615'.1'0886176—dc21
    DNLM/DLC
                                                                99-16182

    00   01   02   03   CL/FF   9   8   7   6   5   4   3   2

Preface

The goal of this book is to produce safe and effective dental practitioners who will continue to learn for their lifetime. Learning after finishing one's formal education is critical in the area of pharmacology. New drugs are constantly being found and synthesized. New effects of old drugs are identified. New diseases and drugs for those diseases are being studied.

1. The first subgoal of *Applied Pharmacology for the Dental Hygienist* is to instill in the learner an understanding of the **need and importance of obtaining and using appropriate reference** material when needed. When confronted with a patient taking a new or unfamiliar drug, the professional will use the appropriate references to learn about the effects of the drug. Pharmacology is a field in which the turnover of new information is very fast.

2. The second subgoal is to produce professionals who will be able to **find the necessary information** about drugs with which they are not familiar. The textbook encourages the use of the current reference sources that will be available where you practice (a 1978 drug reference does not count as current!)

3. The third goal of *Applied Pharmacology for the Dental Hygienist* is for students to be able to **apply that information** to their clinical dental patients within a reasonable time.

4. In order to achieve those goals, today's student needs to be able to access new information about new drugs in the future and intelligently communicate with others (professional and patient) using the medical and unique pharmacologic vocabulary.

After using the first, second, and third editions of this textbook with several classes of dental hygiene students, and talking with others who teach pharmacology to dental hygiene students, in this edition I have attempted to add humor (a little, anyway). Just remember that Jay Leno gets paid for being funny, whereas with our lectures any humor is just an extra bonus. As with previous editions, the basic principles are the same, and you don't have to eat all the icing on the cake (other stuff)!

Because this edition jams even more facts into it, it is important to make sure that students who are using this book in conjunction with taking a class are **NOT required to learn every drug name from each class of drugs** (show this to your teacher or professor). The use of group names provides time for an in-depth consideration of properties of entire groups (see Suffixes for Drugs in Appendix E).

HOW TO USE THIS BOOK

This book is planned to include many features to assist the student with learning pharmacology. The major features are explained here so that the student can begin learning immediately. It's kind of like needing to read the directions before you put your cousin's bicycle together in time for the holidays!

- *Table of contents:* The Table of Contents lists the chapter names. The textbook's chapters are divided into sections entitled General Principles, Drugs Used in Dentistry, Drugs That May Alter Dental Treatment, and Special Situations.
- *Standardized information:* Information about each drug varies, but all drugs include a similar format so that certain sections can be easily identified. Each drug group is discussed and includes the group's indications (what it is used for), pharmacokinetics (how the body handles the drugs), pharmacologic effects (what the drug does), adverse reactions (bad things the drug does), drug interactions (how the drug reacts with other drugs in the body), and the dosage of the drug.
- *Mini table of contents:* The mini table of contents within each chapter provides page numbers. This allows the learner to look at the topics to be covered in each chapter.
- *Marginal notes:* Boxed notes are included in the page margins to identify some important concepts.
- *New vocabulary words:* Built into this textbook are two methods to attack new vocabulary words. One uses the glossary and the other uses the medical terminology process.

    Glossary words: Medical terminology words are included in the Glossary. The first time a glossary word appears in the textbook, the word is printed in **bold face.** The glossary contains definitions of many words. An example of a glossary word is **bradycardia,** which means a slow heart rate. No drug names are listed in the glossary.

    Medical terminology: Most medical terminology is comprised of parts of Greek or Latin words—prefixes, suffixes, and root words. Appendix E explains how to learn from studying the parts of a word either in the glossary or when looking up words in a medical dictionary. By writing any new words in the glossary, students expand their knowledge about medical terminology. With the example *bradycardia, brady* means slow and *cardia* refers to the heart. As new word parts are discovered, they should be added to this appendix.
- *Acronyms:* An acronym is a word formed from the initial letters or syllables of successive parts of a compound term. Many acronyms are used in medicine, and many additional acronyms are used to refer to drugs or drug groups. Some commonly used acronyms are listed in Appendix D. The student should add to these references as more acronyms are discovered. Examples of acronyms include NSAIAs, which means nonsteroidal antiinflammatory agents, and GIT, meaning gastrointestinal tract. Therefore one can say, "The NSAIAs can adversely affect the GIT."
- *Tables and boxes:* Tables and boxes provide summary information, gathering several factors together. The logos on the tables and boxes designate the type of information contained within the box.
- *Pronunciations:* For common drug names the phonetic pronunciation is included in the text. Proper pronunciation can help the student to say the drug names correctly when discussing or speaking about drugs. For example, nitroglycerin is

pronounced [nye-troe-GLI-ser-in]. The pronunciation is enclosed in squared brackets.

• *Indexes:* There are two indexes for this book. The first index helps the learner to locate different concepts. The second index contains the drug names, both generic and trade names. The reference to a word in a table or a box has a lowercase "*t*" or "*b*" printed next to the page number. Numbers for pages with illustrations are italicized. If several references are given, the primary reference is printed in **bold face,** for example, epinephrine 14, **30,** 44, *175t, 299.* Other references appear in normal text.

• *What if?* Clinical situations occur that may require relatively quick assessments and decisions. Appendix G, What if? includes summary information about drugs in pregnancy, allergy management, infective endocarditis prophylaxis, and a summary of the relationship of dental treatment, warfarin, and the International Normalized Ratio.

• *Review questions:* Review questions at the end of each chapter allow students to test their learning. They also focus on the important concepts presented in that chapter.

• *Student hints:* Students need to be informed about the names that they must be familiar with. For example, I require my students to learn the group NSAIAs and two members, ibuprofen and naproxen. Providing this information allows students to focus on the task of memorizing fewer names and gives them more time to really understand the principles associated with the drug groups. Pharmacology requires learning a lot of material that is new. Only by "keeping up" with the material can the student "keep afloat."

STUDY TIPS—HOW TO BE SUCCESSFUL IN PHARMACOLOGY

• Before the lecture, read the syllabus outline for the subject to be covered during the class period. Become familiar with the vocabulary. Guess what might be said about the various topics. Think of what has been said in pharmacology about the topic; look at your pharmacology notes to see what you already know about the topic. Skim the textbook chapter(s) assigned to identify areas to be covered.

• Attend class, take notes in your syllabus, and ask yourself questions about what was said. Compare what is said with what you previously thought about the topic.

• **Reread your lecture notes before the next day** (within 8 hours of lecture preferably). Add and complete things you remember from class. Ask fellow classmates for clarification if you have questions. Reread notes from previous classes.

• Read the textbook assignment. Note especially those areas discussed in class. Let the textbook assignment answer questions you might have had in class.

• Answer general course objectives in the front of your syllabus for the drug group covered.

• Look up words you don't know the meaning of (medical dictionary). Construct a vocabulary list for each subject. Pay attention to the derivatives of the unknown medical word—its stem, prefixes, and suffixes.

- Use active learning when studying. Be able to determine what portion of your study time is spent in active learning. Use the examples below to classify your study methods.

    Active: Write things down, make up flash cards, speak out loud, discuss the concepts with classmates, ask each other questions, give a lecture (to your parrot) without notes, make a video or audio tape recording of your performances (for your own practice), or write everything you know about a drug on an empty blackboard.

    Not active: "Looking over" notes, "reading" the book, "listening" in lecture, and "reviewing" your notes.

    Here is a questionnaire designed to check your study habits. Answer these questions honestly.

❏ Do you begin studying for the next exam the day that your next lecture is given?

❏ Do you make study aids as you go along?

❏ Do you spend time discussing pharmacology with your peers?

❏ If you have an exam on Monday, do you spend Friday night studying?

❏ If you and your friend are planning to go out dancing Friday night and your friend is late, do you use that wasted time reviewing pharmacology?

❏ If a patient cancels his or her appointment, do you use that time to study pharmacology?

❏ Did you make an audio tape of the ideas about the lecture the night of the lecture?

❏ Did you ask questions about the material before reading it?

❏ Did you read to answer those questions?

❏ Did you summarize what has been read?

❏ Did you answer the review questions? From memory? The review questions are included at the end of each chapter so the learner can check to see if the answers to these questions are known. It is a review for your benefit. The references have been all but eliminated now that access to Index to Dental Literature or Medline (through Grateful Med) is more widely available from many personal computers in libraries, schools, and offices.

❏ Did you think about what the information may mean to the dental hygienist? Trying to understand why things happen will make learning more efficient and more fun, too. What problems might be encountered when I treat this patient taking this medication? How can I minimize the chance that something untoward will happen?

❏ Did you think of examples in "real life?" By thinking of real life examples, readers can make a topic into a picture in their brain. For example, the "fight or flight" associated with the sympathetic nervous system can be visualized as a caveman being chased by hungry tiger–his eyes big and heart pounding.

Study Tips—Use of Objectives to Focus Studying

Make sure to find out what the objectives are for your pharmacology class. These are some objectives that may give you an idea about the organization of the material.

- Goals for **commonly prescribed dental drugs:**

  State the therapeutic use(s) for each drug group.

  Discuss the mechanism of action of the drug, when applicable.

  Explain the important pharmacokinetics for the drug group.

  List and describe the major pharmacologic effects associated with the drug group.

  State and discuss the important adverse reactions or side effects and their management or minimization.

  Describe any contraindications/cautions to the use of the drug group.

  Recognize clinically significant drug-drug, drug-disease, and drug-food interactions.

  Describe "patient instructions" for each drug group that could be prescribed.

- Goals for agents patients may be taking that can **alter dental treatment:**

  Determine the "dental implications" for each drug group—the dental management of dental patients taking [drug group name].

  Determine whether any dental drugs are likely to have drug interactions with these groups.

  State change(s) in the treatment plan patients taking medications would require.

Calling All Students!

And now I ask for help from the student. (Please!) You are the most important group to learn from and understand. You can help me make the book better. I encourage readers of *Applied Pharmacology for the Dental Hygienist*, whether they be students, faculty, or practitioners, to provide suggestions for improving this textbook. Your thoughts and opinions are valuable! Feel free to contact me, either through your teachers or via E-mail (clarkbr@umkc.edu). You can also find me on Mosby's dental home page (www.mosby.com/dental). You may also FAX comments or suggestions to me at (816) 235-2157.

With each edition of this book, I like to express my appreciation to the original contributors to the book from which this book evolved: Holroyd et al: *Clinical Pharmacology in Dental Practice*. Without their input, this textbook would not have been possible. My thanks go to: Ronald D. Baker, Stewart A. Bergman, William K. Bottomley, Sherry Burns, Tommy W. Gage, J. Max Goodson, Sam V. Holroyd, James L. Matheny, Norbert R. Myslinski, Barbara F. Roth-Schecter, Martha J. Somerman, Richard L. Wynn, and Samuel L. Yankel. Thanks to the support of my peers and administrators at the Dental School. Thanks to my friends, who emphatically told me never to do another edition of this textbook because it made me crazy—and they were right. But, thanks for their support anyway, especially Pamela Overman and Ann Marie Corry! My thanks also go to Dr. Terrance Harris for his diligent search for those complicated case histories that are included in the Instructor's Manual.

Barbara Requa-Clark Requa = [REEK-wah]

Contents

SECTION ONE

General Principles

CHAPTER 1

Information, Sources, and Regulatory Agencies

Pharmacology is derived from the prefix *pharmaco-*, meaning "drug" or "medicine," and the suffix *-logy*, meaning "study." Therefore pharmacology is the study of drugs. *Stedman's Medical Dictionary* defines the term **drug** as follows:

> *Therapeutic agent; any substance, other than food, used in the prevention, diagnosis, alleviation, treatment, or cure of disease.*

Others define a *drug* as any chemical substance that affects biologic systems. These defi-

nitions, however, are not complete. For example, birth control pills are indicated in the treatment of what disease? Is pregnancy a disease? Another problem with the current definition of *pharmacology* is that there is a large group of substances (drugs?) that are categorized as "dietary supplements." These agents include herbs, vitamins, **minerals,** and amino acids. Even though these substances may have pharmacologic effects on the body, they are by law *not* classified as drugs. This classification avoids the Food and Drug Administration (FDA) approval for efficacy and safety required for drugs.

3

HISTORY

In the beginning, plants found in the jungle were discovered to produce good effects.

Pharmacology had its beginning when our ancestors noticed that ingesting certain plants altered one's body functions or awareness. The first pharmacologist was a person who became more astute in observing and remembering which plant products produced predictable results. From this humble beginning, a huge industrial and academic community concerned with the study and development of drugs has evolved. Plants from the rain forest and chemicals from tar have been searched for the presence of drugs. The agents discovered and found to be useful are then prescribed and dispensed through the practice of medicine, dentistry, pharmacy, and nursing. Health care providers who can write prescriptions include physicians (for humans), veterinarians (for animals, of course), dentists (for dental problems), and optometrists (for eye problems). Physicians' assistants, nurse practitioners, and pharmacists can prescribe drugs under certain guidelines and in certain states.

PHARMACOLOGY AND THE ORAL HEALTH CARE PROVIDERS

The American Dental Association (ADA) and The American Dental Hygienists' Association (ADHA) have been analyzing tasks that oral health care providers should be able to perform during the practice of their professions. In education, these activities are termed *competencies.*

What knowledge is needed to perform the functions of a dental professional?

To perform each competency (meaning to do something), certain facts or concepts (meaning something you know) must be ac-

cessed (find it) by the dental professional. The facts or concepts needed include didactic information (something learned from a book) relative to the task being performed (a dental procedure). Decisions that surround performing the competency rely upon a body of information, termed the *foundation knowledge.* Each content area is then analyzed to determine what relationship exists between the course content, the competencies, and the appropriate foundation knowledge. Examples of questions that would need to be answered in order to perform a certain dental procedure (the foundation knowledge required to determine the pros and cons of performing a certain dental procedure on a certain patient with certain diseases) could include the questions shown in Table 1-1.

From the example in Table 1-1 it can be seen that the dental health care worker cannot practice by doing "something" to "someone" with "some problem." Thought, facts, reasoning, and problem solving are involved in making decisions about each patient seen in the dental office. Dental professionals are not robots—they use clinical judgment to make the best decisions about each patient.

Table 1-1 illustrates the relationship between the professional, the task, and the foundation knowledge. Because the dental and dental hygiene professions require knowledge and deci-

TABLE 1-1 **Relationship Between Tasks Performed in Practice and Things Learned in Pharmacology**

PROFESSIONAL	COMPETENCY (BE ABLE TO)	FOUNDATION KNOWLEDGE
Dental hygienist	Remove plaque from a patient's tooth	Does patient have a heart murmur? Does the patient need prophylactic antibiotics?
Dentist	"Restore" a carious lesion	What should be given to the patient before the dental procedure is performed?

sion making, the "explanation behind the task" is very important.

Specific topics to be covered in each discipline are determined by this process. In the best educational situation, the process would be patient specific and produce learning issues and content that cross multiple disciplines. However, in the meantime, educational experiences are still frequently organized in discipline-based units. This textbook is also arranged in that manner.

Knowledge of pharmacology is imperative in order for the dental professional to perform important functions such as the following:

- *Obtaining a health history.* To obtain a complete and useful health history, a knowledge of commonly prescribed drugs is required. Patients with systemic diseases unrelated to their dental health are often taking medication prescribed by their physician. An understanding of the actions, indications, adverse reactions, and therapeutic uses of these drugs can help determine potential effects on dental treatment. Comparing the medical conditions of the patient with the medication they are taking often raises questions in the interview.
- *Administering drugs in the office.* Because both the dentist and the dental hygienist administer certain drugs in the office, knowledge of these agents is crucial. For example, the oral health care provider commonly applies topical fluoride, and in some states both the dentist and the dental hygienist administer local anesthetics and nitrous oxide. In-depth knowledge of these agents is especially important because of their frequent use.
- *Handling emergency situations.* The ability to recognize and assist in dental emergencies requires knowledge of certain drugs. The indications for these drugs and their adverse reactions must be considered. For example, a patient having an anaphylactic reaction needs to have epinephrine administered quickly.
- *Planning appointments.* Patients taking medication for systemic diseases may require

special handling in the dental office. For example, asthmatic patients should have afternoon appointments, whereas diabetic patients usually have fewer problems with a morning appointment. Certain patients may need to take medication before their appointment. Patients with rheumatic heart disease need to be premedicated with antibiotics before some of their dental or dental hygiene appointments.

- *Choosing self-medication.* At times, the dental health care provider will self-medicate for various minor conditions. The study of pharmacology will assist the oral health care provider in an intelligent selection of an appropriate over-the-counter (OTC) product.
- *Discussing drugs.* When drugs are discussed with either the patient or another health professional, proper terminology is needed. Drugs prescribed by the dentist can cause adverse effects in the patient; patients often ask the oral health care provider questions about their medication. A knowledge of the terms used to describe adverse reactions can facilitate discussions with the patient, dentist, or physician. For example, the term allergy can refer to true allergy (e.g., **hives** from aspirin) or be used for side effects that would be expected (e.g., stomach upset). Understanding the difference between the two effects of aspirin aids in determining whether a **nonsteroidal antiinflammatory agent** (e.g., ibuprofen) can be used for dental discomfort in that particular patient. When the health history is taken and the drugs the patient is taking are listed, it is important that treatment does not begin until the drugs are checked for any problems relating to dentistry.
- *Life-long learning.* Because it is impossible to remember everything learned about current drugs and because new drugs are always being discovered and marketed, appropriate reference sources should be available and consulted. To be able to evaluate

the information retrieved from reference sources, understanding of the terminology of pharmacology and its global organization is essential.

SOURCES OF INFORMATION

One way of categorizing sources of information is by the media—books, journals, CD-ROMs, and Internet sites. Another method of classifying reference sources is by the nature of the information. For example, publications related to the subject of pharmacology can be divided into the explain-discuss type or the reference-list format.

* *Explain-Discuss Format:* Explain-discuss style publications are designed to be used to learn the overall structure of a body of information (e.g., pharmacology), as well as new things about new drugs. New concepts or discoveries, such as a new adrenergic receptor subtype or a new neurotransmitter, are included. These publications present not only facts about a drug but also the concepts behind the facts and discussion of how something produces an effect. Explain-discuss publications compare and contrast drugs within a group or between groups. In a textbook, this format would include a discussion about how aspirin produces its different effects (e.g., lowers fever) and adverse reactions (e.g., hurts stomach). Additional discussion would compare aspirin to acetaminophen (Tylenol). This reference type would also discuss the mechanism of aspirin's drug interactions.
* *Reference-List Format:* Reference-list style publications enumerate facts about drugs. They may include a limited number of drugs or most all drugs, and their lists of facts may be few or many or even all known drugs. They usually do not explain or expand the information. These publications require prior knowledge of the subject because the

vocabulary used is specific for the medical field and the facts enumerated are not discussed. Reference-list publications keep the information about each drug separate. They are often lists of pharmacologic effects, side effects, drug interactions, **contraindications,** doses, and indications.

Both explain-discuss and reference-list types of publications are often available in several different media. For example, Harrison's *Principles of Internal Medicine* is available as one giant hardback book, two smaller hardback books, a CD-ROM, or via the Internet.

Some explain-discuss publications are specific to dental patients and drugs used in dentistry. Most pharmacology books are directed toward medical education. Three textbooks that are specific to dentistry include the following:

* Requa-Clark B: *Applied Pharmacology for the Dental Hygienist,* ed 4, St Louis, 2000, Mosby. Discusses most drug groups with a slant toward use of dental drugs and the dental implications of drugs patients may be taking. Several Appendixes are included, as well as clinical decision-making charts.
* Yagiela JA, Neidle EA, Dowd, FJ: *Pharmacology and Therapeutics for Dentistry,* ed 4, St Louis, 1998, Mosby. An in-depth pharmacology textbook that includes a discussion of drugs and their dental relevance.
* Ciancio SG, ed: *ADA Guide to Dental Therapeutics,* ed 1, Chicago, 1998, ADA Publishing. Includes a very short discussion of nondental drugs with lots of tables. Dental products, not always covered by basic pharmacology books (e.g., mouthwash, antiseptics), are included.

The following are reference-list style publications that are specifically designed for dental use:

* Gage T, Pickett F: *Mosby's Dental Drug Reference,* St Louis, 1998, Mosby. Contains

concise lists of drug attributes and sections relevant to dentistry for each drug.

- Wynn RL, Meiller TF, Crossley HL: *Drug Information Handbook for Dentistry*, Hudson, Ohio, 1998, Lexicomp. Contains concise lists of drug attributes and sections relevant to dentistry for each drug. CD-ROM is available.

The following are explain-discuss style publications designed for the medical or pharmacy student:

- Goodman LS et al: *Goodman and Gilman's The Pharmacologic Basis of Therapeutics*, ed 9, New York, 1996, McGraw-Hill. Pharmacologist's standard reference book, detailed discussions on many mechanisms. Some find it difficult to read and understand; useful when studying a subject in-depth. CD ROM is available.
- Katzung BG: *Basic and Clinical Pharmacology*, ed 7, Los Altos, Calif, 1998, Appleton & Lange. Emphasizes general concepts and mechanisms and includes clinical information; good for learning the skeleton of the organization of pharmacology.
- *Mosby's GenRx 1999*, ed 9, St Louis, 1999, Mosby. Updated annually and provides valuable information about prescription drug products. Drugs are listed by generic name, and information is provided about the manufacturer, actions, usage, contraindications, precautions, warnings, and availability. On-line subscriptions are available to *Mosby's GenRx*, providing access to all drugs listed in the book, plus updates 4 times per year. Subscriptions are also available on CD-ROM, and are also updated four times per year.
- *Physician's Desk Reference* (PDR), ed 53, Montvale, NJ, 1999, Medical Economics. Most common reference book in the dental office because of its historically inexpensive price (manufacturer provided subsidies for this relatively high-priced book), not updated often, uses package insert informa-

tion approved when drug released, manufacturer purchases space for profitable products, manufacturers arranged alphabetically, drugs alphabetically listed by brand name within each manufacturer's section, no comparisons among drugs, includes color pictures of some drugs. CD-ROM is available.

The following are reference-list style publications that are general for medicine but not specifically designed for dental use:

- Olin BR, Hebel SK, Dombec CE, eds: *Drug Facts and Comparisons* (F&C), St Louis, 1999, Facts and Comparisons. Contains the most complete listing of currently available drugs, including prescription and OTC medications. It is arranged by pharmacologic class so that drugs used for the same indications are listed together. Comparisons among similar drugs are included. The index contains both generic and trade names. This is the most expensive publication listed, but student rates are available. It is available in a loose-leaf binder (updated monthly) or an annual hardback book. CD-ROM is available.
- *United States Pharmacopeia-Drug Information* (USP-DI) Volume I—*Information for the Health Care Provider*, Rockville, Md, 1999, United States Pharmacopeial Convention. This book has quarterly updates and is published every year. CD-ROM is available.
- *American Health-Systems Formulary Service— Drug information* (AHFS-DI), Bethesda, Md, 1999, American Society of Heath-Systems Pharmacists. Detailed reference source that provides an unbiased guide to all aspects of a drug's properties. Volume I is designed for the health care provider. A complex advisory panel from a cross-section of health care providers ensures that this book is unbiased. It is updated yearly, and quarterly supplements are also provided. The detail in this book is especially valuable when a specific fact on a drug is needed. CD-ROM is available.

HOW CAN A LEARNER DETERMINE WHICH LEARNING RESOURCE IS BEST TO USE?

No one but the learner can answer this question. The choice depends on why the learner is learning at this point, as well as what the learner wants or is required to know. There are many factors, such as the following:
- the nature of the pharmacology course
- the types of learning aids provided by the course
- the evaluation instruments (tests) to be used in the course
- the many specific variables of the learner

A student may study differently than a practitioner. The clinician may have a patient who has raised a question or problem in treatment, whereas the student may learn in response to test conditions.

Which learning aid to use depends on individual learning styles—alone or in a group, by reading or by visualizing, the extent of the medical vocabulary, and by the depth of the learner's background in subjects such as biology, anatomy, chemistry, physiology biochemistry, histology, calculus, and statistics.

Another factor in the choice of a learning medium is the level of detail that is desired. If one paragraph of information is sufficient, a different source would be required than if extensive details were required (e.g., two or three pages).

The following physical aspects of the resource must also be considered:
- How will the resource be used?
- Will it be at a desk?
- Do you want to be able to carry the source in your pocket?
- How heavy can the source be? (Choice of a book weighing several ounces or several pounds can make a big difference!)
- Does each learner need his or her own resource, or can resource information be shared? If active learning is to take place then sharing is not possible. With active learning, marks should be made in the book, questions should be raised by writing them, and comparisons with other written documents should be noted.
- Do you prefer to learn from a book, an audiotape, or a computer program?

How often will the source be used? And for how long will you be using it? At what level will you want to understand the material? At the lowest level of learning—list and repeat? Or at the highest level of learning—evaluating? Or somewhere in between (listing and discussing implications). Case histories give the learner practice in evaluation of a patient. Answering the questions at the end of each chapter facilitates the ability to list.

And of course budget must be considered. Pharmacology texts are available at a wide range of prices.

After you have taken all these factors into account, choose a few sources you might like. Pick two or three drugs that have some interesting dental implications (e.g., calcium channel blockers and gingival enlargement), and look them up in each potential publication. Choose one you can most easily read and understand. Sometimes the best source can only be determined after using several sources.

The following are smaller publications that that cover most drugs:

- Skidmore-Roth L: *Mosby's 2000 Nursing Drug Reference*, St Louis, 1999, Mosby.
- Ellsworth, AJ et al: *Mosby's Medical Drug Reference*, St Louis, 1999, Mosby.

The following are overviews of several drug groups. Previous knowledge of pharmacology is usually required to use this type of reference.

- Harvey RA, Champe PC: *Lippincott's Illustrated Reviews: Pharmacology*, ed 2, Philadelphia, 1997, Lippincott-Raven. (Lots of figures, simplified).
- Olson J: *Clinical Pharmacology Made Ridiculously Simple*, Med Master Series, 1997.
- Neal, MJ: *Medical Pharmacology at a Glance*, ed 3, London, 1997, Blackwell Science.

The following are lower priced paperback book references:

- *The Pill Book: The Illustrated Guide to the Most Prescribed Drugs in the USA*, ed 8, New York, 1998, Bantam.
- *About Your Medicines*, Rockville, Md, U.S. Pharmacopeial Convention.
- *Prescription Drug-Consumer Guide*,

The following references are specific for the topic of drug interactions:

- Hansten P: *The Consumer's Guide to Drug Interactions*, Collier Books, 1994.
- Tatro DS, Olin BR, Borgsdorf L: *Drug interactions: Facts—Facts and Comparisons*.

The following are medical books that are arranged by the medical conditions instead of by the drugs. They are useful when disease knowledge is required:

- *Merck Manual of Medical Information*, Merck Co., 1998. CD-ROM available.
- Fauci AS et al, eds: *Harrison's Principles of Internal Medicine*. New York, 1997, McGraw-Hill CD-ROM available.

Each publication type may be judged on its lack of bias, its currentness (How long ago was the currently available edition released?), its readability (vocabulary, simplicity of explanations, presence of visual aids), its degree of detail (all you want to know and much more, just right [like Goldilocks' porridge], or not enough to understand what is being said), and its price (Box 1-1).

Every dental office should have at least one reference book that lists the names of both prescription and OTC drugs. Further, a standard pharmacology textbook would be helpful in understanding the reference books. Because of the release of new drugs, a recent edition (not more than 1 to 2 years old) of a reference book is needed. Table 1-2 compares properties of different reference sources.

Although books serve as the usual source of information on drugs, computer software and even modem dial-up services are becoming more readily available. In addition, the practicing pharmacist can be a source of information. It is particularly important for the dental professional to establish a professional relationship with a local pharmacist, who may assist him or her in understanding the possible effects of a new drug on a patient.

DRUG NAMES

It is important for the dentist and the dental hygienist to understand the ways in which a drug can be named, because he or she must be able to discuss drugs with both the patient and the provider of the patient's care. The ability to refer to a drug's name(s) is complicated by the fact that all drugs have at least two names, and many have more.

When a particular drug is being investigated by a company, it is identified by its chemical name, which is determined by its chemical structure. If the structure is unknown at the time of investigation, a code name, usually a combina-

---

Box 1-1 EXAMPLES OF EXPLAIN-DISCUSS AND REFERENCE-LIST BASED PUBLICATIONS

Explain-discuss publications

A pharmacology textbook (or CD ROM) provides the necessary background for understanding the mechanism of action, chemistry, pharmacologic effects, adverse reactions, and therapeutic use of each group of drugs. Such a textbook can be used to prepare for a lecture or as an adjunct to the lecture when learning pharmacology. Concepts discussed in lecture may be reviewed, or more detail may be available in the book. Reading more than one author's presentation on a subject can clarify a subject for the individual reader. Some of these textbook-based publications are general, that is, they apply to all medical personnel, whereas others are addressed specifically to the dental professional.

When using the explain-discuss type of learning resource, an overview is often a good place to start. Even looking at the outline at the beginning of the chapter can be helpful. Sometimes skimming is another approach. Finally the important parts of the chapter, especially if the class lecture could not be read, should be read. But, this is not the end of the steps. Asking yourself questions about the chapters can also help. Stop reading often and state out loud what the main points of the section are to determine whether learning is going on.

This type of reference is also helpful for understanding the disease conditions that affect patients. Separating the drug facts from the disease facts is not possible because people have diseases for which they take drugs.

Reference-list publications

Reference books provide information about brand name and **generic drugs.** These books do not cover basic pharmacology or explain terms used in them, but they include the drug's mechanism of action, indications for use, contraindications, precautions, doses, and preparations available.

Reference-list publications are a starting point for determining decisions about clinical cases. Sometimes the question is whether a drug will produce a dry mouth. A list is great to answer this question (unless the source is too brief). It is important to have some global view of the drug and/or disease for which that drug is being used. Simple reference-list sources can be fleshed out using more advanced lists or even by going to the Medline looking for current journal articles via the Internet on the subject.

---

tion of letters and numbers, is assigned to the product (e.g., RU-486).

If a compound is found to be useful and it is determined that the compound will be marketed commercially, the pharmaceutical company discovering the drug gives the drug a

> Each drug has only one generic name but may have several trade names.

trade name (e.g., Coke). This name, which is capitalized, is usually chosen so that it can be easily remembered and promoted commercially. This trade name, registered as a trademark under the Federal Trade-Mark Law, is the property of the registering company. The trade name is protected by the Federal Patent Law for 17 years. Although the brand name is technically the name of the company marketing the product, it is often used interchangeably with the trade name.

TABLE 1-2 Comparisons Among Reference Sources

REFERENCE*	ORGANIZATION	BIAS	PRICE	UPDATE FREQUENCY	COMMENTS
DDR	Alphabetical by generic drug name	N	$	1/yr	Dental implications, brief
LCD	Alphabetical by generic drug name	N	$$	1/yr; CD = 4/yr	Dental implications, brief
PDR	Alphabetical by manufacturer's name; within that list by trade name	Y	$$	1/yr, 4/yr; CD = 4/yr	Package insert, not often updated, contains selected drugs
F & C	By therapeutic class	N	$$$$	1/yr; 12/yr (paper); CD = 4/yr	Has many tables, includes most all prescription and OTC drugs
NH†	Alphabetical either by generic drug name or by therapeutic class	N	$	1/yr	Nursing implications and parenteral agents included
AHFS	Alphabetical by pharmacologic class	N	$$$	1/yr; CD = 4/yr	Detailed coverage, useful to answer specific questions
USP-DI	Alphabetical by pharmacologic class	N	$$$	1/yr, 12/yr; CD = 4/yr	Extensive lists of properties of drugs

*Dental Drug Reference (DDR), Mosby; Lexi-Comp for Dentistry (LCD), Lexi-Comp; Physician's Desk Reference (PDR), Delmar; Facts and Comparisons (F & C), Facts and Comparisons; Nursing Handbook (NH), American Health System Formulary System (AHFS), United States Pharmacopeia Drug Information (USP-DI), St. Martin's.

†Examples: A-Z Nurse's Drug Reference, Therapeutic Class Drug Guide for Nurses (Delmar); Nursing Drug Handbook (Springhouse); Nurse Practitioner's Drug Handbook (Appleton Lange); Mosby's Nursing Handbook (Mosby); Nursing Drug Handbook (Saunders); Nursing Handbook (PDR).

Before any drug is marketed, it is given a generic name that becomes the "official" name of the drug. For each drug, there is only one generic name (e.g., cola) selected by the U.S. Adopted Name Council, and the name is not capitalized. This council selects a generic name that, hopefully, does not conflict with other drug names. Recently, several marketed drugs have had to have their names changed because they were confused with the name of another drug that had already been marketed.

An example of the many names a product can have is provided by lidocaine, a local anesthetic commonly used in dentistry. Figure 1-1 compares the generic and trade names of lidocaine.

After the original manufacturer's patents have expired, other companies can market the generic drug under a trade name of their choosing (e.g., Pepsi). When lidocaine first appeared on the market, it was manufactured by Astra and available only as Xylocaine, but when its patent expired, other companies started making the drug, each company giving it their own brand name (e.g., Octocaine). When a patient states an allergy to Xylocaine, the oral health care provider must be aware that lidocaine is the generic name of this drug and that the patient should not be given lidocaine under another trade name, such as Octocaine.

Drugs prescribed by physicians cause a similar problem. Patients often know these drugs by the trade name. If a patient reports an allergic reaction to Valium (the trade name), the oral health care provider must be aware that this patient should not take other brands of diazepam (the generic name).

This book uses generic names when discuss-

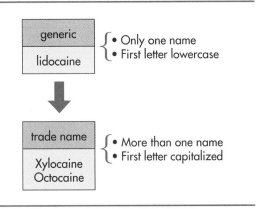

ing drugs because there is only one generic name for each drug. Trade names (also known as *proprietary* names) appear in parentheses after the generic name. Most reference books include indexes that allow a drug to be accessed using either the generic or trade name. Newer drugs are usually referred to by their trade names. Old and traditional drugs are often referred to by their generic names.

A problem occurs in naming multiple-entity drugs, that is, drugs with several ingredients. These drugs are difficult to discuss by their generic names because they contain several ingredients.

DRUG SUBSTITUTION

For dental drugs, generic substitution gives equivalent therapeutic results at a cost savings.

In the discussion of generic and trade names, the question of generic equivalence and substitution arises. Are the various different generic products equivalent? After 17 years, the patent of the original drug expires, and other companies can market the same compound under a generic name. In 1984, Congress passed the Drug Price Competition and Patent Term Restoration Act, which allowed generic drugs to receive expedited approval. The Food and Drug Administration (FDA) still requires that the active ingredient of the generic product enter the bloodstream at the same rate as the trade name product. The variation allowed for the generic name product is the same as for the reformulations of the brand name product. For the few drugs that are difficult to formulate and have narrow therapeutic indexes, no differences exist between the trade name product and the generic product—therefore generic substitution drugs give equivalent therapeutic results and provide a cost savings to the patient.

Drugs can be judged "similar" in several ways. When two formulations of a drug meet the chemical and physical standards established by the regulatory agencies, they are termed *chemically equivalent*. If the two formulations produce similar concentrations of the drug in the blood and tissues, they are termed *biologically equivalent*. If they prove to have an equal therapeutic effect in a clinical trial, they are termed *therapeutically equivalent*. A preparation can be chemically equivalent, yet not biologically or therapeutically equivalent. These products are said to differ in their bioavailability. Before generic drugs are marketed they must be shown to be biologically equivalent, which would make them therapeutically equivalent.

TOP 200 DRUGS

Appendix A lists the 200 drugs most frequently prescribed in 1998 and their pharmacologic group. In the right column of the appendix the rank order appears. This number represents the position that the drug appears in the top 200. The rank of 1 is the most frequently prescribed drug for that year. Both generic and trade names appear on the list, depending on how the prescription is written. The oral health care provider must become familiar with these names because patients may know the names of the drugs they are taking but not know how the names are spelled. By referring to the list of the top 200 drugs, the oral health care provider can check the patient's medications and spell them accurately so that they can be accessed in reference sources. This textbook discusses most of the agents included in this list.

FEDERAL REGULATORY AGENCIES

Many agencies are involved in regulating the production, marketing, advertising, labeling, and prescribing of drugs.

HARRISON NARCOTIC ACT

In 1914, the Harrison Narcotic Act established regulations governing the use of opium, opiates, and cocaine. Marijuana laws were added in 1937. Before this law, mixtures sold OTC could contain opium and cocaine. These mixtures were promoted to be effective for many "problems."

FOOD AND DRUG ADMINISTRATION

The Food and Drug Administration (FDA) of the Department of Health and Human Services grants approval so that drugs can be marketed in the United States. Before a drug can be approved by the FDA, it must be determined to be both safe and effective. The FDA requires physical and chemical standards for specific products and quality control in drug manufacturing plants. It determines what drugs may be sold by prescription and OTC and regulates the labeling and advertising of prescription drugs. Because the FDA is frequently more stringent than regulatory bodies in other countries, drugs are often marketed in Europe and South America before they are available in the United States.

FEDERAL TRADE COMMISSION

The Federal Trade Commission (FTC) regulates the trade practices of drug companies and prohibits the false advertising of foods, nonprescription (OTC) drugs, and cosmetics.

DRUG ENFORCEMENT ADMINISTRATION

The Drug Enforcement Administration (DEA) of the Department of Justice administers the Controlled Substances Act of 1970. This federal agency regulates the manufacture and distribution of substances that have a potential for abuse, including opioids (narcotics), stimulants, and sedatives.

OMNIBUS BUDGET RECONCILIATION ACT

The newest federal regulation concerning drugs is the Omnibus Budget Reconciliation Act (OBRA) of 1990. It mandates that, beginning January 1, 1993, pharmacists must provide patient counseling and a prospective drug utilization review (DUR) for Medicaid patients. Although this federal law covers only Medicaid patients, State Boards of Pharmacy are interpreting this law to apply to all patients. Dental patients who have their prescription filled at a pharmacy should receive counseling from the pharmacist about their prescriptions. It's the law!

REVIEW QUESTIONS

1. Define the term *pharmacology.*
2. Explain why the oral health care provider should have a knowledge of pharmacology.
3. Name two reference publications that are useful for looking up brand names of drugs.
4. Explain the advantages and disadvantages of these two sources.
5. State the number and type of reference books that an up-to-date dental office should have.

6. Discuss the most important features of a good reference book.
7. Define and give an example of the following terms:
   a. Chemical name
   b. Trade name
   c. Brand name
   d. Generic name
8. Explain why a list of the top 200 drugs should be available in every dental office. Explain the term *rank order*.
9. Name three federal regulatory agencies and state the major responsibility of each.

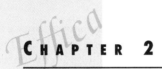

CHAPTER 2

Drug Action and Handling

To discuss the drugs used in dentistry or those that patients may be taking when they come to the dental office, the dental health care worker must be familiar with some basic principles of pharmacology. This chapter discusses the action of drugs in the body and methods of drug administration. Chapter 3 considers the problems or adverse reactions these drugs can cause. By understanding how drugs work, what effects they can have, and what problems they can cause, the dental health care worker can better communicate with the patient and other health care providers about medications the patient may be taking or may need to have prescribed for dental treatment.

Drugs are broadly defined as chemical substances used for the diagnosis, prevention, or treatment of disease or for the prevention of pregnancy. Most drugs are differentiated from inert chemicals and chemicals necessary for the maintenance of life processes (i.e., vitamins) by their ability to act selectively in biologic systems to accomplish a desired effect. Historically, drugs were discovered by randomly searching for active components among plants, animals, minerals, and the soil. Today, the search for new drugs involves a different approach—systematic screening techniques. Organic synthetic chemistry researchers continue to develop thousands of new synthetic drugs. Parent compounds that exhibit known pharmacologic activity are chemically modified to produce congeners or analogs—agents of a similar chemical structure with a similar pharmacologic effect. This technique of modifying a chemical **molecule** to provide more useful therapeutic agents has evolved from studies of the relationship between the chemical structure and the biologic activity called *structure-activity relationship* (SAR).

CHARACTERIZATION OF DRUG ACTION

Drugs can be classified based on any of the following properties:

- **Biochemical** action (e.g., hypoglycemic, or blood sugar–lowering, agents)
- **Physiologic** effects (e.g., antihypertensive, or blood pressure–lowering, agents)
- **Organ** systems involved (e.g., central nervous system stimulants, **diuretics)**

LOG DOSE–EFFECT CURVE

When a drug exerts an effect on biologic systems, the effect can be related quantitatively to the dose of the drug given. If the dose of the drug is plotted against the intensity of the effect, a curve will result (Figure 2-1). If this curve is replotted using the log of the dose (log–dose) versus the response, another curve is produced from which the potency and efficacy of a drug's action may be determined (Figure 2-2).

POTENCY

The potency of a drug is a function of the amount of drug required to produce an effect. The potency of a drug is shown by the location

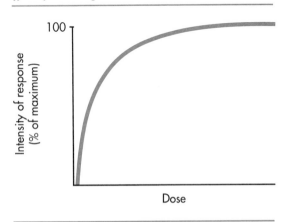

FIGURE 2-1 *Dose-effect curve. The x-axis (horizontal) is an increasing dose of the drug, and the y-axis (vertical) is an increasing effect of the drug.*

Potency—related to the **amount** of drug needed to produce effect

tency of drug *A* is greater because the dose required to produce its effect is smaller. The potency of *B* is less than *A* because *B* requires a larger dose to produce its effect.

To determine potency make a dot at the middle of the sharp upward curve. Extend a line from the dot vertically to the *x*-axis. The value on the *x*-axis is the dose that produces one half of the maximum effect. Sometimes this point used is when half of the subjects have an effect. The potency is greatest when the dose is the smallest (curve closest to the *y*-axis [darker shad-

of that drug's curve along the log-dose axis (*x*-axis). The curves in Figure 2-3 illustrate two drugs with different potencies. The po-

ing of arrow]), and it decreases as the dose increases (curve moves to the right [lighter shading of arrow]).

The potency of a drug can be expressed in terms of the median effective dose, the ED_{50}. The ED_{50} is the dose of a drug required to produce a specific effect in 50% of the subjects or the dose that produces half of the maximum effect. To determine the ED_{50} drop a vertical line from the dot in the middle of the curve to the *x*-axis (described above). The higher the potency of a drug, the lower the ED_{50} will be.

As an example of different potencies, three alcoholic beverages are compared—bourbon, beer, and wine cooler (or spritzer). One ounce of bourbon contains the same amount of alcohol as one beer (12 oz) or as one wine cooler or spritzer (16 oz [depends on dilution]). All of these drinks could equally inebriate an indi-

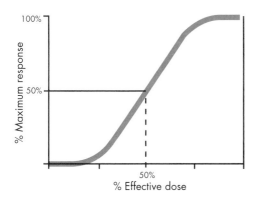

FIGURE 2-2 *Log dose–effect curve. As the dose is increased (going to the right on the* x*-axis) the effect (the* y*-axis) is zero at first, then there is a small effect, and finally the effect quickly increases. Around the dose where the line is increasing sharply is the therapeutic range of the compound. Lastly, the curve plateaus (flattens out). This is the maximum response a drug can exhibit.*

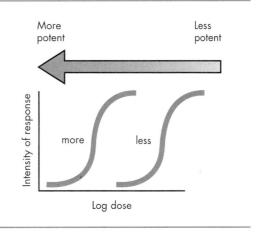

FIGURE 2-3 *Potency of agent. The arrow is shaded proportional to increasing potency.* (Dark shading, *very potent;* light shading, *low potency.*)

F I G U R E   2 - 4   *Comparison of log dose–effect curves for morphine, meperidine, and aspirin.*

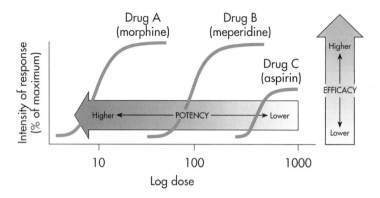

vidual (produce adverse reactions). To produce a similarly drunk individual, the same *amount* of alcohol would have to be ingested. But this amount would be contained in a different *volume* of fluid, depending on its concentration (or potency).* Therefore when someone says, "I ain't drunk 'cuz I jus' drink beer," the statement is false.

The absolute potency of a drug is immaterial as long as an appropriate dose is administered. Both meperidine and morphine have the ability to treat severe pain, but approximately 100 mg of meperidine would be required to produce the same action as 10 mg of morphine. Thus the absolute potency of morphine is 10 times that of meperidine, or meperidine is one tenth as potent as morphine, even though both agents can relieve intense pain (equal efficacy, as explained next). In Figure 2-4 the curve for drug *B* (meperidine) is to the right of the curve for drug *A* (morphine) because the dose of meperidine needed to produce pain relief is larger (10 times larger) than that for morphine. The potency of different drugs that elicit similar effects can be compared by observing the dose that produces 50% (drop

a vertical line down from the center of the curve) of the total, or maximum, effect.

EFFICACY

Efficacy is the maximum intensity of effect or response that can be produced by a drug. Administering more drug will not increase the efficacy of the drug but can often increase the probability of an adverse reaction. The efficacy of a drug increases as the height of the curve increases (Figure 2-5). The efficacy of the drugs whose curves are illustrated in Figure 2-5 are shown by the height of the curve when it plateaus (levels out horizontally). It is shaded from least (light) to most (dark) potent. In Figure 2-4, drug *A* and *B* possess equal efficacy, but unequal potency, whereas drug *C* is less efficacious. The efficacy of any drug is a major descriptive characteristic indicating its action. For example, the efficacy of drug *B* (meperidine) and drug *A* (morphine) is about the same, because both drugs relieve severe pain. But other analgesics, such as drug *C* (aspirin) are

> *Efficacy*—related to the **maximum** effect of a drug (regardless of dose)

---

*Ignoring the effect on the stomach of different nonalcoholic fluids or food ingested.

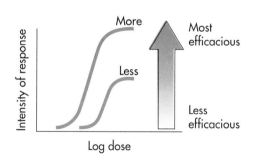

FIGURE 2-5 *Efficacy of agent.*

less efficacious because they relieve only mild to moderate pain.

If one "drink" of both bourbon (1 oz) and beer (12 oz) were ingested, they could produce equal "silliness" in an individual. If very large doses of either agent were ingested, unconsciousness could be produced. Both are equally efficacious, but they differ in their potency! *The efficacy and the potency of a drug are unrelated.* Figure 2-6 gives examples of drugs with differing potencies and efficacies.

Because death is the endpoint when measuring the lethal dose, the median lethal dose (LD_{50}) is the dose when one half of the subjects die. For obvious reasons, the LD_{50} is only determined in animals because of the scarcity of human volunteers.

CHEMICAL SIGNALING BETWEEN CELLS

For the autonomic nervous system to function, messages from the brain must be transmitted to many parts of the body commanding the parts "do something" (e.g., enlarge pupil or sweat). Complex mechanisms for transmitting these messages allow for amplification or damping of the effect, depending on a multitude of factors. The complexity allows for very fine tuning of the body's functions. Neurotransmitters are chemicals responsible for transporting a wide variety of messages across the synapse (space between **nerve** and receptor). Chemical signaling involves release of neurotransmitters, local substances, and hormone secretion.

Local. Some organs secrete chemicals that work near them. These chemicals are not released into the systemic circulation. Prostaglandins and histamine are examples. For example, a person wears a nickel-containing watch and a red spot appears on the skin beneath the watch. This localized allergic reaction is due to release of inflammatory producing substances such as histamine at that point on the skin. Because the reaction is localized, the patient's nose does not begin to run. Prostaglandins contract the uterine muscles and become important as a baby is born. When prostaglandins are released in the uterus they produce menstrual "cramps," and when released in the stomach they protect its lining.

Hormones. **Hormones** are secreted to produce effects throughout the body. Examples include insulin, thyroid hormone, and adrenocorticosteroids. These reactions are usually slower than the ones associated with the neurotransmitters.

Neurotransmitters. The messengers that move the electrical impulses from a nerve are transmitted across the synapse via **neurotransmitters.** The neurotransmitters are released and quickly travel across the synapse to the receptor (Figure 2-7). There are at least 50 different agents that transmit messages. The six most important neurotransmitters are acetylcholine, **norepinephrine**/epinephrine, dopamine, serotonin, γ-aminobutyric acid (GABA), and histamine.

MECHANISM OF ACTION OF DRUGS

After drugs have been distributed to their site of action they elicit a pharmacologic effect. The pharmacologic effect occurs because of a modulation in the function of an organism. Drugs do

F I G U R E   2 - 6   *The potency and efficacy of three drugs.*

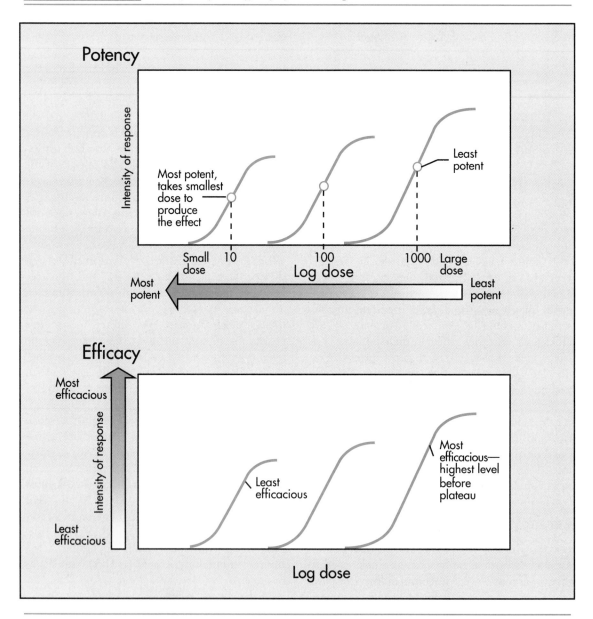

F IGURE 2 - 7 *For the neurotransmitter (or drug acting like a neurotransmitter) to complete the message it must get inside the cell. After the drug binds with its receptor the reaction often opens a channel so that the message can get inside the cell.*

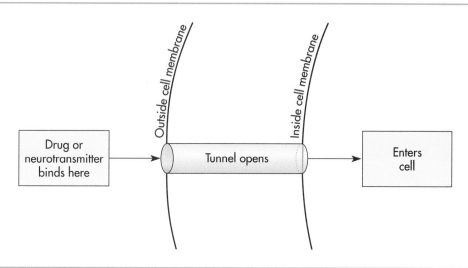

not impart a new function to the organism, they merely produce either the same action as an endogenous agent or block the action of an endogenous agent. This signaling mechanism has two functions—amplification of the signal and very flexible regulation. The presence of very fine controls to modulate the body's function allows the regulation of certain reactions, slowing or speeding them.

NERVE TRANSMISSION

Within one nerve, the transmission of impulses travels along the nerve, producing an action potential. The action potential is triggered by the neurotransmitter released at the previous synapse. Drugs that interfere with this process, such as local anesthetics (Chapter 10), block messages from being sent. The processes involved in the drug's effect begin the drug-receptor interaction. The receptors, macromolecular chemical structures, interact with both endogenous sub-

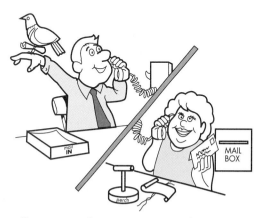

Different types of messengers are useful in different situations. (E.g., carrier pigeon = neurotransmitter, telephone = nerve action potential, letter = protein synthesis alteration [e.g., steroids].)

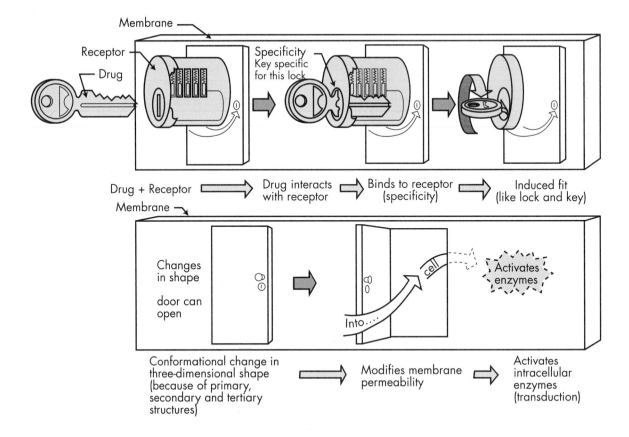

stances and drugs. This drug-receptor interaction results in a conformational (shape) change, which may allow the drug inside the cell to produce its effect or may cause the release of a second messenger, which then produces the effect. Many of the effects (see above figure) involve altering enzyme-regulated reactions or regulatory processes for protein synthesis after a series of reactions, similar to a chain reaction. These steps in the process of communicating will be briefly discussed.

RECEPTORS

There are two major molecular superfamilies of receptors. The first involves the ion channels, and the second involves interaction with a G-protein that sometimes activates a "second messenger."

- **Fast /5/ ion channel:** The fast /5/ ion channel signaling receptor consists of five transmembrane regions (can be different versions) configured around an ion channel (can be for different ions). Many copies of each receptor and many types of receptors are arranged around the ion channel. These receptors provide a mechanism by which an effect of the body will take many things into consideration (α-receptor, H-receptor, opioid receptor, glutamine, norepinephrine, acetylcholine). These reactions are faster than the G-protein–linked reactions.

FIGURE 2-8 *The neurotransmitter is transmitting the message (like electricity) across the synapse (space where nerve is absent). The neurotransmitter then interacts with the receptor (shaped to fit together), which then may signal an enzyme to be synthesized or activated.*

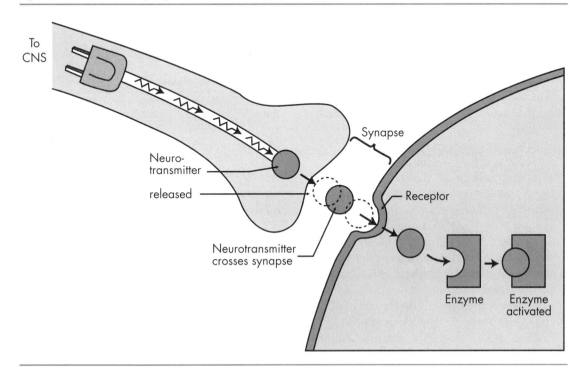

- **Slow /7/ G-protein/2nd messenger:** The slow /7/ G-protein/2nd messenger signaling receptor is made up of seven transmembrane regions that all use a G-protein and a second messenger. Within this superfamily, different neurotransmitters participate in producing the effect.

Receptor classes. All receptor types have three components—the ligand-binding domain (location where drug binds to receptor) linked by lipophilic membrane-spanning segments (opens pathway through the cell membrane) to a transmembrane or intracellular effector domain (where message is received before an effect is produced) (Figure 2-8).

ION CHANNEL RECEPTORS **Ion channel receptors** are fast-signaling receptors.

When the ion channel–linked receptors are activated, the result is an opening of the ion channel. Opening the ion channel produces a movement of ions such as sodium, **potassium,** or chloride, from areas of high concentration to areas of low concentration. This ion movement then produces an effect. There are two types of ion-channel receptors: ligand-gated and voltage-gated.

- **Ligand-gated ion-channel receptors** combine with a ligand (e.g., an endogenous substance or a drug) to produce an effect. An example of this receptor type is the nicotinic cholinergic receptor (see Chapter 5). This receptor contains four subunits: two α-, one β-, and one γ-subunit(s). These subunits are arranged in a circle, with the middle of the circle becoming a pore (hole). The nicotinic cholinergic receptor is found on the skeletal muscle cell end plate (neuromuscular junction) and in the ganglia of the automatic nervous system. Two molecules of acetylcholine bind with the α-subunits, producing a change in conformation. This change in shape induces the opening of the ion channel, increasing the permeability of the membrane to sodium and potassium. Another example of a ligand-dependent ion channel is the CNS inhibitory neurotransmitter, GABA. The benzodiazepines (drugs for anxiety, such as diazepam [Valium]) amplify the effect of the GABA receptor by augmenting the opening of Cl^- channel. Excitatory amino acids such as glycine, aspartate, and glutamate send their signals via a ligand-gated ion channel.
- **Voltage-gated ion-channel receptors** are activated by a change in the charge on the membrane or gate. This voltage change opens the voltage-dependent gate. An example of the voltage-gated ion channel is the sodium channel. Lidocaine (a local anesthetic) blocks the depolarization (change in voltage) of the nerve. Therefore the pain messages from the ends of the nerves do not continue through the nerve at the location where the lidocaine is placed. That's local **anesthesia!**

CYCLIC GUANOSINE MONOPHOSPHATE (cGMP)–LINKED RECEPTORS Cyclic guanosine monophosphate (cGMP)–linked receptors pass their message through the membrane by using a guanine nucleotide–binding regulatory protein. Named *G-protein* for short, this protein is linked to a variety of *second messengers* (actually reactions) that pass the message from the inside of the cell to the effector organ. The G-protein consists of three chains: α-, β-, and γ-. When the G-protein combines with guanosine diphosphate (GDP) it forms a helical structure that passes through the membrane 7 times (transmembrane coiling). The seven helixes arrange themselves into a circle to open and form a tunnel (see Figure 2-8). This interaction with the G-protein allows the message to pass from the outside of the cell to the inside of the cell through the tunnel formed. Once inside the cell this reaction stimulates the release of the second messengers. Chemical changes involving enzymes alter the body's function, producing an effect. In this case, the neurotransmitter would be called the *first messenger.* This system allows for amplification, as well as feedback to modulate reactions. The following are examples of second messengers:

- **Cyclic 3′,5′-adenosine monophosphate (cAMP)** is a second messenger involved in conducting the sense of smell and sight (rods and cones in the eye). When the G-protein is activated, it stimulates protein kinase A, which activates enzymes that release **glucose** or relax vascular smooth muscles. An increase in cAMP is the mechanism by which these receptors are activated: the α_2- and β-receptors, histamine, and serotonin. A decrease in cAMP is responsible for effects on the muscarinic cholinergic, opioid, and serotonin receptors.
- **Calcium/inositol phospholipid (Ca^{++}/IP_3)** is another second messenger. Acetylcholine activates the G-protein, which in turn activates the Ca^{++}/IP_3 system. This system is responsible for the action of the α_1-receptors, the muscarinic cholinergic receptors, leukotriene receptors, some $5\text{-}HT_2$ receptors, glutamate, bradykinin, and substance P receptors.

- **Diacylglycerol (DAG)** is another G-protein–linked second messenger. Activation of phospholipase C produces DAG and IP$_3$. DAG stimulates protein kinase C, and IP$_3$ releases Ca^{++}, which also activates protein kinase C.
- **Eicosanoids** are probably other second messengers. Their effect is to change phospholipase A$_2$ into arachidonic acid, which eventually is changed to the prostaglandins, thromboxanes, and leukotrienes.

ENZYME-LINKED RECEPTORS The enzyme-linked receptors have one enzymatic catalytic site on the receptor. Dimerization* of activated receptors produces a change in conformation. Protein kineses are often involved in this type of reaction. Interactions with either tyrosine kinase or guanylyl cyclase use this type of receptor. Insulin, growth factor, and cytokines activate these enzyme-linked catalytic receptors.

INTRACELLULAR RECEPTORS Lipid-soluble compounds can cross the **lipid** membrane by way of intracellular receptors and react with the receptors inside the cell. Corticosteroids, sex hormones, and thyroid hormone use this type of receptor activation. The change in confirmation induced increases the binding to specific **DNA** sequences. With binding, transcription is stimulated and protein synthesis occurs. Because DNA synthesis is involved, this receptor interaction has a delayed onset and a duration of action that outlasts the drug's presence in the body.

Two consequences of the mechanism by which hormones produce their effect are the following:
- There is a lag period of one half to several hours to produce an effect because new proteins must be synthesized (slower than enzyme-related reactions).
- Their effects persist for hours to days after the hormone has left. The reason for this effect is the slow turnover of enzymes and proteins. Receptors with tyrosine kinase activity respond to hormones such as insulin and growth factor.

Agonists/Antagonists. When a drug combines with a receptor, it alters the function of the organism. It may produce enhancement or inhibition of the function. Drugs that combine with the receptor may be classified as either agonists or antagonists (Figure 2-9).

AGONIST An agonist is a drug that: (1) has affinity for a receptor, (2) combines with that receptor, and (3) produces an effect. Naturally occurring neurotransmitters are agonists.

FIGURE 2 - 9 *Agonists and antagonists and their interactions.*

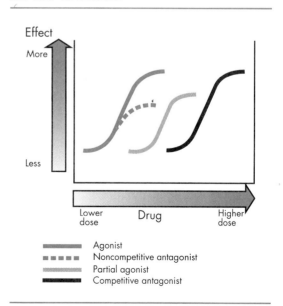

Effect

More

Less

Lower dose   Drug   Higher dose

— Agonist
- - - - Noncompetitive antagonist
▬▬▬ Partial agonist
▬▬▬ Competitive antagonist

---

*Dimerization is the production of a compound by the combination of two like molecules, usually by elimination of H$_2$O or a similar small molecule between the two or by simple noncovalent association (such as two identical protein molecules).

ANTAGONISTS An antagonist counteracts the action of the agonist. The following are three different types of antagonists:

- *Competitive antagonist:* A competitive antagonist is a drug that (1) has affinity for a receptor, (2) combines with the receptor, and (3) produces no effect. This causes a shift to the right in the dose-response curve (see Figure 2-9). The antagonist competes with the agonist for the receptor and the outcome depends on the relative affinity and concentrations of each agent. If the concentration of the agonist is increased, the competitive antagonism can be overcome and vice versa. By itself, the antagonist has no effect. It can only decrease the effect of the agonist.
- *Noncompetitive antagonist:* Noncompetitive antagonists bind to a receptor site that is different from the binding site for the agonist. This reduces the maximal response of the agonist (see Figure 2-9).
- *Physiologic antagonist:* A physiologic antagonist has affinity for a different receptor site than the agonist. This decreases the maximal response of the agonist by producing an opposite effect via different receptors.

Transport carriers are systems that are available for moving neurotransmitters or drugs into the cell. In the process of making a neurotransmitter, the precursors (chemical to make a neurotransmitter) must be taken into the cell by an active transport pump (requires ATPase). For example, the precursor for norepinephrine is tyramine, so it must be pumped into the cell. After the neurotransmitter is synthesized, it is placed in little "suitcases" called *granules*. These go to the membranes and await the signal to "dump" their contents into the synapse. After the neurotransmitter is released there are three paths that it can take. It can be broken down by enzymes designed to terminate the neurotransmitter's effect, it can migrate to the receptor and interact to produce an effect, or it can be taken up by the presynaptic nerve ending (reuptake).

Reuptake is an easy way (requires little energy) to recover the neurotransmitter for future use because it is as easy as vacuuming up dirt.

Chemical bonds. Compounds combine in the body using a variety of chemical bonds. Some are stronger than others (Figure 2-10).

IONIC BONDS Ionic bond consist of an electrostatic bond between two ions of opposite charges (e.g., Na^+/Cl^-). One ion binds with a charged group of the receptor. This is the most effective force in attracting a drug molecule to the receptor. The binding force of an ionic bond decreases with the square of the distance (r^2). These are very loose combining forces and can be "washed out" of isolated tissues, which ends the effect.

HYDROGEN BONDS The hydrogen ion (H^+) or proton is strongly electropositive. It acts as a bond for two electronegative atoms, such as O,N. This hydrogen bond is weak alone, but when the atoms are close together and several bonds are formed it produces the effect. This force varies with the fourth power of distance r^4.

VAN DER WAALS FORCES The Van der Waals forces bond is the most common bond between atoms and is referred to as *induced dipoles*. Two atoms or molecules that are close to each other have very small fluctuations in their charges. When one part becomes positively charged (+), the other becomes negative (−). The power of this bond varies with the seventh power of distance (r^7).

COVALENT BONDS The covalent bond, the most tenacious type of chemical bond, occurs when the outside electrons are shared among the elements. This is the force that holds proteins, carbohydrates, and lipids together. Because it is not rapidly reversible, it is not involved in drug receptor interactions. An example of a reaction using this bond is phase II metabolism or conjugation (e.g., glucuronidation).

FIGURE 2-10 *Two atoms combine producing different types of bonds. Some are stronger, and some are weaker.*

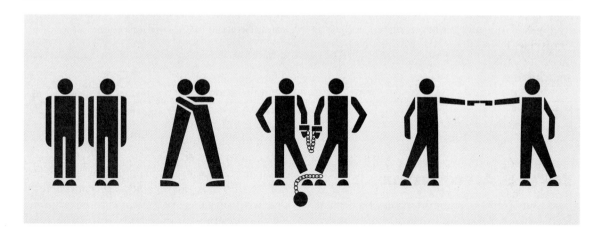

STEREOISOMERISM

Stereoisomerism occurs when a drug's structure has an asymmetric carbon atom with four different elements connected to the same carbon atom. When this occurs, the drug can exist in two different forms that are mirror images to each other. The mixture of the two forms is termed the *racemic mixture* (half in each form). The two different forms can be separated and identified using a polarizing light. When a solution of the form turns light to the right, that is termed *dextrorotatory* (*d*-). When light rotates to the left, it is termed *levorotatory* (*l*-). An analogy of stereoisomerism would be a pair of gloves. One glove fits the right (*d*-) hand, and one fits the left (*l*-) hand. The three-dimensional structure rotates the plane of polarized proteins determined by the sequence of amino acids in the deoxyribonucleic acid (DNA). An example of stereoisomerism is dextromethorphan (*d*-isomer) and levorphanol (*l*-isomer). The *d*- form, dextromethorphan, is a popular cough suppressant that does not act through opioid receptors, and the *l*- form is its isomer, levorphanol, a codeine analogue with both analgesic and addictive properties. The asymmetric carbon is referred to as a *chiral center* or a *center of chirality*. Many of these isomers exist as their racemic mixtures, even though they may have entirely different actions. Recently, more research is being performed to determine the actions of the individual isomers in hopes of obtaining more specific drug action.

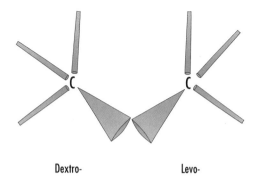

Dextro-   Levo-

The stereoisomers described above are also referred to by other names. The pair of stereoisomers can be called *enantiomers* [in-ANT-tee-o-mers], or *chirals* [KY-rals]. The corresponding processes are termed *isomerism, enantiomorphism,* and *chirality* (or *centers of chirality* [ky-RAL-uh-tee]). Therefore the following terms refer to an asymmetric carbon atom previously described: stereoisomers, enantiomers, and chirals.

ROUTES OF ADMINISTRATION AND DOSAGE FORMS

ROUTES OF ADMINISTRATION

The route [root] of administration of a drug affects both the onset and duration of response. Onset refers to the time it takes for the drug to begin to have its effect. Duration is the length of a drug's effect.

> *Route*—various ways a drug can be administered

The routes of administration can be classified as **enteral** or **parenteral.** Drugs given by the enteral route are placed directly into the gastrointestinal tract by oral or rectal administration. Parenteral administration bypasses the gastrointestinal tract and includes various injection routes, inhalation, and topical administration. In practice, the term *parenteral* usually refers to an injection.

Although oral administration is considered the safest, least expensive, and most convenient route, the parenteral route of a drug has certain advantages. The **injection** results in fast absorption, which produces a rapid onset and a more predictable response than oral administration. The parenteral route is useful for emergencies, unconsciousness, lack of cooperation, or **nausea.** Some drugs must be administered by injection to remain active. The disadvantages of the parenteral route include the facts that asepsis must be maintained to avoid **infection,** an intravascular injection can occur by accident, administration by injection is more painful, it is difficult to re-

move the drug, adverse effects may be more pronounced, and self-medication is difficult. Parenteral therapy is also more dangerous and more expensive than oral medication. Some routes of administration are shown in Figure 2-11.

Oral route

The oral route of administration is the simplest way to introduce a drug into the body. It allows the use of many dif-

> Oral—most common and most popular route

ferent dosage forms to obtain the desired results; tablets, capsules, and liquids are conveniently given. An advantage of this route is the large absorbing area present in the small **intestine.** Oral administration produces a slower onset of action than parenterally administered agents. One disadvantage of this route is that stomach and intestinal irritation may result in nausea and vomiting. Another disadvantage is that certain drugs, such as insulin, are inactivated by gastrointestinal tract acidity or enzymes.

When drugs are given orally, they initially pass through the **hepatic (liver)** portal circulation, which can inactivate some drugs. This is termed the *first-pass effect* because the drug passes through the liver first before it circulates in the systemic circulation. During the drug's first pass through the liver it is metabolized (amount metabolized varies) and the amount of drug available to produce a systemic effect is reduced. Drugs with a high first-pass effect have a larger oral to parenteral dose ratio. This means that the dose required for an equivalent effect orally is much greater that the dose needed when used parenterally. Because morphine has a high first-pass effect, the oral dose needed to produce an equivalent effect is much larger than its parenteral dose.

Blood levels obtained after oral administration are less predictable than those obtained parenterally. The presence of food in the stomach, the pathologic condition of the gastrointestinal tract, the effects of gastric acidity, and

FIGURE 2-11   *Routes of administration.* IT, *Intrathecal;* PO, *by mouth (oral);* IH, *inhalation;* IV, *intravenous;* IM, *intramuscular;* SQ, *subcutaneous;* ID, *intradermal.*

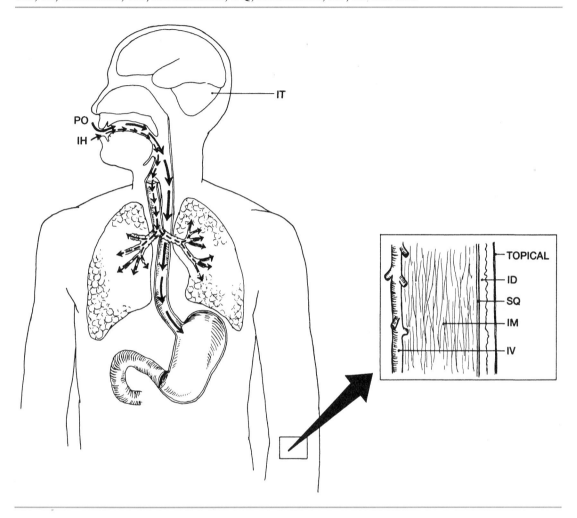

passage through the hepatic portal circulation can alter blood levels. Drug interactions can occur when two drugs are present in the stomach. The oral route necessitates greater patient cooperation.

Rectal route. Drugs may be given rectally as suppositories, creams, or enemas. Rectal administration can be used if a patient is vomiting or unconscious. This route may be used for either

a local (e.g., **hemorrhoids**) or a systemic (e.g., antiemetic) effect. Because most drugs are poorly and irregularly absorbed rectally, this route is not frequently used to achieve a systemic drug effect. Also, patient acceptance of this route is poor.

Intravenous route. Intravenous administration produces the most rapid drug response, with an almost immediate onset of action. Because the injection is made directly into the blood, the absorption phase is bypassed. Another advantage of the intravenous route is that it produces a more predictable response than oral administration because factors that affect drug absorption have been eliminated. It is also the route of choice for an emergency situation. The disadvantages of administration include phlebitis caused by local irritation, drug irretrievability (can't get it back), allergy, and side effects related to high **plasma** concentrations of the drug.

Intramuscular route. Absorption of drugs injected into the muscle occurs because of the high blood flow through skeletal muscles. Somewhat irritating drugs may be tolerated if given by the intramuscular route. This route may also be used for injection of suspensions, to provide a sustained effect. Injections are usually made in the deltoid region or gluteal mass.

Subcutaneous route. The subcutaneous route involves the injection of solutions or suspensions of drugs into the subcutaneous areolar tissue to gain access to the systemic circulation. If irritating solutions are injected, sterile abscesses may result. Insulin is commonly administered by this route.

Intradermal route. Small amounts of drugs such as local anesthetics can be injected into the epidermis of the skin to provide local anesthesia. With this type of injection, a small bump (bleb) rises as the liquid is injected just under the skin. The tuberculosis skin test is performed using the intradermal route.

Intrathecal route. Intrathecal administration involves the injection of solutions into the spinal subarachnoid space. This may be used for spinal anesthesia or for the treatment of certain forms of **meningitis.**

Intraperitoneal route. The intraperitoneal route involves placing fluid into the peritoneal cavity,

from where exchange of substances can occur. A drug may be absorbed through the mesenteric veins. This route of administration is also used for peritoneal dialysis. In this case, the substances are passing from the body to the fluid. Large volumes of fluids are slowly run into the peritoneal cavity. A waiting period of several hours allows the waste products from the body to be exchanged with the fluid in the peritoneal cavity. The fluid is removed, and the body's waste products are carried out in the fluid. This process is used as a substitute for the failing **kidney** to manage patients with renal failure.

Inhalation route. The inhalation route may be used in the administration of the gaseous, microcrystalline, liquid, or powdered form of

> Inhalation route—used for local or systemic effects. Popular for illicit drugs.

drugs. This route of administration may be used for either local or systemic effects. An example of **inhalers** being used for their local effects are those used to treat **asthma.** After inhalation, the drug is deposited on the bronchiolar endothelium and exerts its action by producing bronchodilation or reducing **inflammation.** Inhalation of aerosolized liquid in fine droplets also produces a local effect. Many commonly used inhalers contain ozone-depleting chlorofluorocarbons. Because of environmental concerns, these gases are being phased out. These propellants are being removed from the market, and inhalers containing finely powdered drugs are being substituted. The powder is inhaled into the **lungs** to produce a similar effect. One advantage of the use of the powdered form is that inhalation must continue until the visible powder is gone. General anesthetics in the form of volatile liquids such as halothane or gases such as nitrous oxide (N_2O) and **oxygen** are examples of the use of the inhalation route for systemic effects. This route of administration is popular for the abuse of many drugs (smoked or even inhaled) because of the quick onset of action and the lack of need for needles.

Topical route. Topical routes consist of application to body surfaces. Topical applications are administered to the skin, the oral mucosa, and even sublingually (under the tongue). Inhalation route could even be called topical. Drugs used topically may be intended to produce either local or systemic effects.

Because most drugs do not penetrate the intact skin, application to the skin is generally used for local effects. Corticosteroids are applied to inflamed or irritated skin. Intravaginal creams or suppositories or solutions or suspensions instilled into the eye or ear are other ways to administer topical agents to produce local effects.

Rarely, systemic side effects (unintended) can occur from the topical administration of drugs for their local effect. One example is the administration of topical corticosteroids over a large proportion of the body, resulting in symptoms of systemic toxicity (Cushing's syndrome). If an occlusive dressing (commercial plastic wrap or a plastic suit) is used or if the surface is abraded, inflamed, or sloughing, the chance of side effects increases dramatically. In the oral cavity, interruptions in the **mucous membranes** or mucosal inflammation increase the likelihood of a systemic effect. Local anesthetics sprayed into the mouth may be adsorbed and produce a blood level equivalent to that produced by intravenous administration.

Examples of drugs applied topically for a systemic effect include transdermal patches and sublingual spray or tablet administration. Drugs that frequently produce allergic reactions should not be administered topically because sensitization occurs more readily than when used orally.

SUBGINGIVAL STRIPS AND GELS A dental-specific topical application involves the placement of drug-impregnated strips or gels subgingivally. Systemic effects are minimized because small doses can be used when drugs are admin-

istered via this route. Doxycycline gel (Atridox) and a chlorhexidine-containing chip (PerioChip) are examples of agents administered into the gingival crevice.

TRANSDERMAL PATCH Transdermal drug delivery systems (drug patches) are designed to provide continuous controlled release of medication through a semipermeable membrane over a given period after application of drug to the intact skin. This eliminates the need for repeated oral dosing. Examples of patches on the market include scopolamine (Transderm-Scop), nitroglycerin (Transderm-Nitro, Nitrodisc, Nitro-Dur), clonidine (Catapres-TTS), **estrogens** (Estraderm, Climara), fentanyl (Duragesic), and nicotine transdermal patches (Nicoderm, Nicobid).

Most patches consist of several layers. Beginning with the skin, the layers are as follows: adhesive (to stick to skin), membrane (to control the rate of drug release), drug reservoir (where drug is stored), and a backing that is impenetrable to the drug (to keep drug from evaporating into the air) (Figure 2-12). Before use, the protective backing must be removed. The most common problems with transdermal patches are local irritation, erythema, and edema. This can be minimized by rotating the location

FIGURE 2-12 *Layers of transdermal patch.*

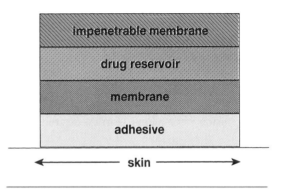

of the patch. Patches are designed to be changed daily, every few days, or weekly depending on the drug.

> *SL—"under the tongue" for systemic effects*

SUBLINGUAL AND BUCCAL ROUTES

Two ways in which drugs can be applied topically are sublingual (SL) and buccal routes. The mucous membranes of the oral cavity provide a convenient absorbing surface for the systemic administration of drugs, which can be placed under the tongue (sublingual) or on other areas of the oral mucosa (buccal pouch). Absorption of many drugs into the systemic circulation occurs rapidly. An example of this effect is the fast onset of action of nitroglycerin sublingual tablets to treat acute anginal pain. Drugs that are susceptible to degradation by the gastrointestinal tract and even the liver, such as testosterone, are safely administered as sublingual tablets because they avoid both the first-pass effect and gastrointestinal acid and enzymes.

Other routes of administration. Drugs such as progestins (Norplant) can be implanted under the skin to release a drug over a prolonged duration (5 years). Pumps that deliver drugs intravenously can be implanted in the body. When insulin pumps are used they can be programmed externally using a calculator-like keyboard.

DOSAGE FORMS

Table 2-1 lists the usual dosage forms. The most commonly used dosage forms in dentistry are the tablet and capsule given orally. Liquid solutions or suspensions are often prescribed for children. Sometimes drugs are given in solution or suspension when a liquid form is desired. Liquid forms of a drug are often used for children. For injection, the drug may be in solution, such as a local anesthetic, or it may be in a suspension, such as procaine penicillin G, when a longer duration of action is desired. Mouthwashes containing alcohol are also recommended by dental health care workers. Elixirs (contain alcohol) and syrups (contain sugar) are children's dosage forms.

PHARMACOKINETICS

Pharmacokinetics is the study of how a drug enters the body, circulates within the body, is changed by the body, and leaves the body. Factors that influence the movement of a drug are divided into four major steps: absorption, distribution, metabolism, and excretion (ADME).

PASSAGE ACROSS BODY MEMBRANES

The amount of drug passing through a cell membrane and the rate at which a drug moves are important in describing the time course of action and the variation in individual response to a drug. Before a drug is absorbed, transported, distributed to body tissues, metabolized, and subsequently eliminated from the body, it must pass through various membranes such as cellular membranes, blood capillary membranes, and intracellular membranes. Although these membranes have variable functions, they share certain physicochemical characteristics that influence the passage of drugs across their borders.

These membranes are composed of lipids (fats), proteins, and carbohydrates. The membrane lipids make the membrane relatively impermeable to ions and polar molecules. Membrane proteins function as enzymes in the transport process and also make up the structural components of the membrane. Membrane carbohydrates are combined with either proteins or lipids. The lipid molecules orient themselves so that they form a fluid bimolecular leaflet structure, with the hydrophobic (lipophilic) ends of the molecules shielded from the surrounding aqueous environment and the hydrophilic ends in contact with the water. The various proteins are embedded in and layered onto this fluid lipid

TABLE 2-1 Dosage Forms

FORM	DEFINITION	EXAMPLE
Tablet	Molded or compressed medicinal substance with inert binder included to make a hard mass	Acetaminophen tablet
Capsule	Gelatin shell that disintegrates in water to administer solids or liquids	Tetracycline capsule
Pill	Globular or ovoid dosage form made by incorporating medicinal agents with other binders to make a plastic mass; obsolete	Ferrous carbonate pill
Lozenge, troche	Flavored dosage form designed to be held in the mouth to dissolve or disintegrate slowly	Cough drop
Suppository	Single-dosage medicaton in waxy or fatty conical or ovoid shape that liberates active ingredient after insertion into the rectum or vagina for local or systemic effects	Glycerin suppository
Solution	One-phase system of two or more chemical components	Saline water
Elixir	Sweetened hydroalcoholic solution containing flavoring materials	Acetaminophen and codeine elixir; diphenhydramine
Syrup	Nearly saturated aqueous solution of sugar	Dextromethorphan syrup
Tincture	Alcholic or hydroalcoholic solution of drugs	Iodine tincture
Spirit	Solution of volatile substance in alcohol	Aromatic ammonia spirit
Lotion	Liquid suspension that can be protective	Hand lotion
Emulsion	Preparation of two immiscible liquids, usually water and oil, one dispersed as small globules in the other	Liquid petrolatum emulsion
Suspension	Dispersion containing finely divided insoluble material suspended in a liquid medium	Amoxicillin suspension
Cream	Emulsions that contain an oily and aqueous phase; external phase aqueous	Hydrocortisone cream
Ointment	Semisolid preparation for external use that is of a consistency that can be applied by rubbing; external phase oily	Hydrocortisone ointment, A and D ointment
Transdermal patch	A permeable polymer membrane backed with a drug reservoir designed to provide controlled release of medication over a given period after application to intact skin	Nitroglycerin, scopolamine, fentanyl, nicotine
Aerosol spray	Solution of volatile liquids with a propellant that delivers drugs to area	Albuterol inhaler, foot spray
Intradermal implant	Small pellets implanted under skin that allow drugs to be released slowly	Norplant
Micropump	An implanted pump that delivers drug via a needle	Insulin pump

bilayer, forming a mosaic. Studies of the ability of substances to penetrate this membrane have indicated the presence of a system of pores or holes through which lower-molecular-weight and smaller size chemicals can pass.

The physicochemical properties of drugs that influence the passage of drugs across biologic membranes are lipid solubility, degree of ionization, and molecular size and shape. The mechanisms of drug transfer across biologic membranes are passive transfer and specialized transport.

Passive transfer. Lipid-soluble substances move across the lipoprotein membrane by a passive transfer process called *simple diffusion.* This type of transfer is directly proportional to the concentration gradient (difference) of the drug across the membrane and the degree of lipid solubility. For example, a highly lipid-soluble compound will attain a higher concentration at the membrane site and will readily diffuse across the membrane into an area of lower concentration (Figure 2-13). A water-soluble agent will have difficulty passing through a membrane

Water-soluble molecules small enough to pass through the membrane pores may be carried through the pores by the bulk flow of water. This process of filtration through single-cell membranes may occur with drugs having molecular weights of 200 or less. However, drugs with molecular weights of 60,000 can "filter" through capillary membranes.

Specialized transport. Certain substances are transported across cell membranes by processes that are more complex than simple diffusion or filtration. These processes include the following:
- Active transport is a process by which a substance is transported against a concentration gradient or electrochemical gradient. This action is blocked by metabolic inhibitors. Active transport is believed to be mediated by transport "carriers" that furnish energy for the transportation of the drug.
- Facilitated diffusion does not move against a concentration gradient. This phenomenon involves the transport of some substances, such as glucose, into cells. It is also blocked by metabolic inhibitors. It has been suggested that the process of pinocytosis may explain the passage of macromolecular substances into the cells.

Figure 2-14 shows the passage of drugs across body membranes. The various aspects of this figure are discussed next, beginning with absorption.

ABSORPTION

Absorption is the process by which drug molecules are transferred from the site of administration to the circulating blood. This process requires the drug to pass through biologic membranes.

The following factors influence the rate of absorption of a drug:
- The physicochemical factors discussed previously.

FIGURE 2-13 *Passage of drug and metabolite through membranes. A, Lipid soluble, non-ionized: drug easily passes through the cell membrane from area of high to low drug concentration. B, Water soluble, ionized: drug cannot pass through the cell membrane.*

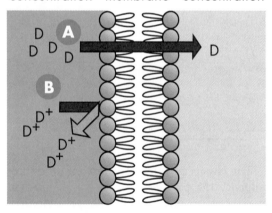

High concentration   Lipid membrane   Low concentration

- The site of absorption, which is determined by the route of administration. For example, one advantage of the oral route is the large absorbing area presented by the intestinal mucosa.
- The drug's solubility. Drugs in solution are more rapidly absorbed than insoluble drugs.

Effect of ionization. Drugs that are weak electrolytes dissociate in solution and equilibrate into a non-ionized form and an ionized form. The non-ionized, or uncharged, portion acts like a nonpolar, lipid-soluble compound that readily traverses body membranes (see Figure 2-13). The ionized portion, because it is less lipid soluble, will traverse these membranes with greater difficulty. The law of mass action determines the split between the ionized and non-ionized forms when the pH of the site is altered. Thus the more ionized the compound, the less the drug is absorbed (Figures 2-15 and 2-16).

The pH of the tissues at the site of administration and the dissociation characteristics (pK_a) of the drug will determine the amount of drug present in the ionized and non-ionized state. The proportion in each state will determine the ease with which the drug will penetrate the tissues. A review of pH is found in Figure 2-17.

WEAK ACIDS For weak acids the disassociation can be represented as follows:

$$HA \rightleftharpoons H^+ + A^-$$

When the pH at the site of absorption increases, the hydrogen ion concentration simply falls. This results in an increase in the ionized form (A^-), which cannot easily penetrate tissues.

$$\text{If pH}\uparrow \rightarrow [H^+]\downarrow \therefore [A^-]\uparrow$$

FIGURE 2-14 *Absorption and fate of a drug.*

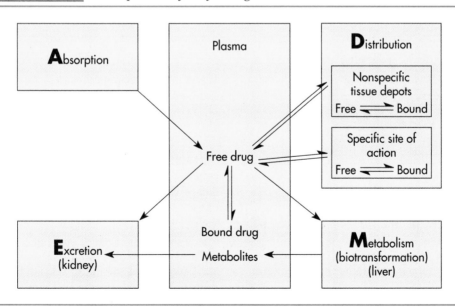

FIGURE 2-15   *Weak base.*

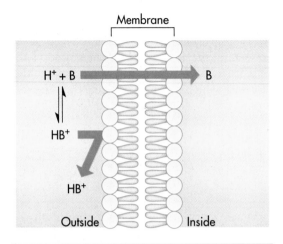

FIGURE 2-16   *Weak acid.*

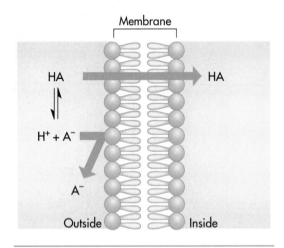

Conversely, if the pH of the site falls, the hydrogen ion concentration will rise. This results in an increase in the un-ionized form (HA), which can more easily penetrate tissues.

$$\text{If pH}\downarrow \rightarrow [H^+]\uparrow \therefore [HA]\uparrow$$

FIGURE 2-17   *Review of pH.*

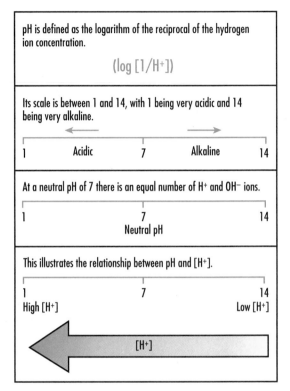

WEAK BASES For weak bases the dissociation can be represented as follows:

$$B + H^+ \rightleftharpoons BH^+$$

If the pH of the site rises, the hydrogen ion concentration will fall. This results in an increase in the un-ionized form (B), which can more easily penetrate tissues.

$$\text{If pH}\uparrow \rightarrow [H^+]\downarrow \therefore [B]\uparrow$$

Conversely, if the pH of the site falls, the hydrogen ion concentration will rise. This results in an increase in the ionized form (BH⁺), which cannot easily penetrate tissues.

F IGURE   2 - 1 8   *First order kinetics. Half-life constant throughout usual doses. Half of the dose of the drug in the body is removed with each half-life. 1. Total amount of drug in the body at any point. 2. Fraction of total drug remaining. 3. Number of half-lives that have passed.*

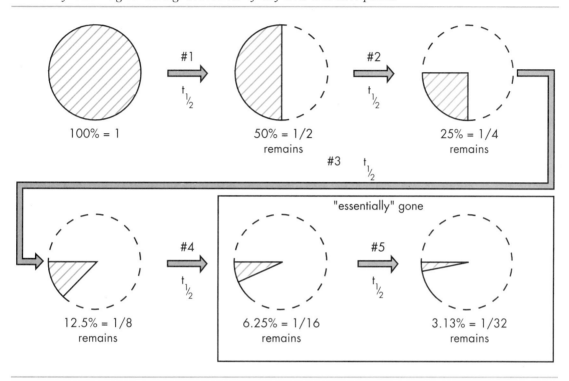

If $\downarrow$pH$\rightarrow$ [H$^+$]$\uparrow$ $\therefore$ [BH$^+$]$\uparrow$

In summary, weak *acids* are better absorbed when the pH is less than the pK$_a$, whereas weak *bases* are better absorbed when the pH$_a$ is greater than the pK$_a$ (Figure 2-18).

This dissociation also explains the fact that in the presence of infection the acidity of the tissue increases (and the pH decreases) and the effect of local anesthetics decreases. In the presence of infection, the [H$^+$] increases because of accumulating waste products in the infected area. The increase in [H$^+$] (decrease in pH) leads to an increase in ionization and a decrease in penetration of the membrane. This reduced penetration reduces the clinical effect of the local anesthetic.

Oral absorption. The dosage form of a drug is an important factor influencing absorption of drugs administered via the oral route. Unless the drug is administered as a solution, the absorption of the drug in the gastrointestinal tract involves a release from a dosage form such as a tablet or capsule. This release requires the following steps before absorption can take place:

- **Disruption:** The initial disruption of a tablet coating or capsule shell is necessary.
- **Disintegration:** The tablet or capsule contents must disintegrate (break apart).

- ***Dispersion:*** The concentrated drug particles must be dispersed (spread) throughout the stomach or intestines.
- ***Dissolution:*** The drug must be dissolved (in solution) in the gastrointestinal fluid.

A drug in solution skips these four steps, so it usually has a quicker onset of action.

Absorption from injection site. Absorption of a drug from the site of injection depends on the solubility of the drug and the blood flow at that site. For example, drugs with low water solubility, such as some penicillin salts, are absorbed very slowly after intramuscular injection. Absorption at injection sites is also affected by the dosage form. Drugs in suspension are absorbed much more slowly than those in solution. Certain insulin preparations are formulated in suspension form to decrease their absorption rate and prolong their action. Drugs that are least soluble will have the longest duration of action.

DISTRIBUTION

All drugs occur in two forms in the blood: bound to plasma proteins and as the free drug. The free drug is the form that exerts the pharmacologic effect. The bound drug is a reservoir (place to store) for the drug. The proportion of drug in each form is dependent on the properties of that specific drug (percent protein bound). Within each compartment (e.g., blood, brain) the drug is split between the bound and free drug. Only the free drug can pass across cell membranes.

Walking the pathways to the action, metabolic, and excretion site.

For a drug to exert its activity, it must be made available at its site of action in the body. The mechanism by which this is accomplished is **distribution,** which is the passage of drugs into various body fluid compartments such as plasma, interstitial fluids, and intracellular fluids. The manner in which a drug is distributed in the body will determine how rapidly it produces the desired response, the duration of that response, and, in some cases, whether a response will be elicited at all.

Drug distribution occurs when a drug moves to various sites in the body, including its site of action in specific tissues. However, drugs are also distributed to areas where no action is desired (nonspecific tissues). Some drugs, because of their characteristics, are poorly distributed to certain regions of the body. Other drugs are distributed to their site of action and then redistributed to another tissue site. The distribution of a drug is determined by several factors, such as the size of the organ, the blood flow to the organ, the solubility of the drug, the plasma protein binding capacity, and the presence of certain barriers (blood-brain barrier, **placenta).**

Distribution by plasma. After a drug is absorbed from its site of administration, it is distributed to its site of action by the blood plasma (see Figure 2-14). Therefore the biologic activity of a drug is related to the concentration of the free, or unbound, drug in the plasma. Drugs are bound reversibly to plasma proteins such as albumin and globulin. The drug that is bound to the protein does not contribute to the intensity of the drug action, because only the unbound form is biologically active. The bound drug is considered a storage site. If one drug is highly bound, another administered drug that is highly bound may displace the first drug from its plasma protein binding sites, increasing the effect of the first drug. This is one mechanism of drug interaction.

HALF-LIFE

The half-life ($t_{1/2}$) of a drug is the amount of time that passes for the concentration of a drug to fall to one half of its blood level at any time. When the half-life of a drug is short, it is quickly removed from the body and its duration of action is short. When the half-life of a drug is long, it is slowly removed from the body and its duration of action is long (Figure 2-19).

Figure 2-20 shows the percent of a drug remaining after each of four and five half-lives. Because only 3% to 6% remains after four or five half-lives, respectively, we can say that the drug is essentially gone. Conversely, it takes about four or five half-lives for a drug's level to build up to a steady state (level amount) in the body. If the half-life of a drug is 1 hour, then in 4 or 5 hours the drug would be mostly gone from the body. In 4 hours, 94% of the drug would be gone. However, if the half-life of a drug is 60 hours, then it would take 240 (10 days) to 300 hours (12 days) for that drug to be eliminated from the body. Even after discontinuing a drug with a long half-life, its effect can take several days to dissipate depending on its half-life.

BLOOD-BRAIN BARRIER

The tissue sites of distribution should be considered before administration. For example, for drugs to penetrate the central nervous system, they must cross the blood-brain barrier. The passage of a drug across this barrier is related to the drug's lipid solubility and degree of ionization. The endothelium of this barrier contains a cell layer and a basement membrane. The welding of the endothelial cells together prevents the formation of clefts, gaps, or pores that might allow the penetration of certain drugs. In order to diffuse transcellularly, the drug must penetrate the epithelial and basement membrane cells. Thiopental, a highly lipid-soluble, non-ionized drug, easily penetrates the blood-brain barrier to gain access to the **cerebrospinal fluid** and induce sleep within seconds after intravenous

F I G U R E   2 - 1 9   *The effect of pH on the dissociation of weak acids and bases.*

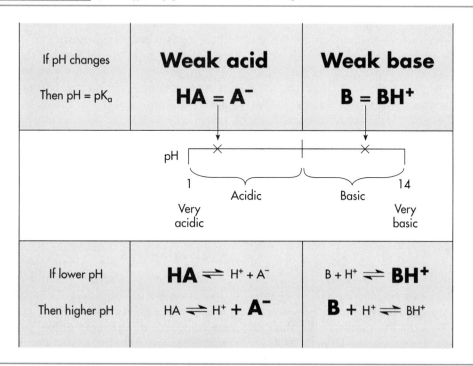

FIGURE 2-20 *Zero order kinetics;* **A,** *large dose,* **B,** *small dose; disappearance of a drug whose metabolism is saturable, with small dose* **(B)** *the drug is metabolized more quickly than when a large dose* **(A)** *is given, with large dose the metabolism cannot increase so it takes a long time for the body to clear the drug, the half-life varies with the dose of the drug.*

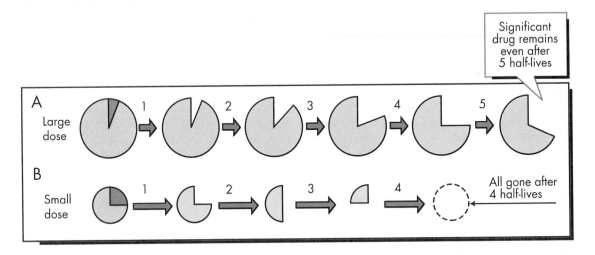

administration. In contrast, a highly ionized compound such as hexamethonium would not be likely to cross this barrier and therefore would produce few if any effects on the brain.

Placenta. The passage of drugs across the placenta involves simple diffusion in accordance with their degree of lipid solubility. Although the placenta may act as a selective barrier against a few drugs, most pass easily across the placental barrier. Lipid-soluble drugs penetrate this membrane most easily. Therefore when agents are administered to the mother they are concomitantly administered to the fetus. The term *barrier* is a misnomer.

Enterohepatic circulation. Drugs are typically absorbed via the intestines, distributed through the serum, pass to specific and nonspecific sites of action, come to the liver, and are metabolized before being excreted via the kidneys. When a drug undergoes enterohepatic circulation the process varies. The steps are the same up until the drug is metabolized. At that point, the metabolite is secreted via the bile into the intestine. The metabolite is broken down by enzymes and releases the drug. The drug is then absorbed again, and the process continues. After being taken up by the liver the second time, these drugs are again secreted into the bile. This circular pattern continues with some drug escaping with each passing. This process prolongs the effect of a drug. If enterohepatic circulation is blocked, the level of the drug in the serum will fall.

REDISTRIBUTION

Redistribution of a drug is the movement of a drug from the site of action to nonspecific sites of action. A drug's duration of action can be affected by redistribution of the drug from one organ to another. If redistribution occurs between specific sites and nonspecific sites, a drug's action will be terminated. For example, thiopental produces sleep within seconds, but the effect is terminated within a few minutes. This is because the drug is first distributed to the central nervous system (sleep), subsequently redistributed through the plasma to the muscle (action terminated), and finally reaches the fat depots of the body (no action still).

METABOLISM (BIOTRANSFORMATION)

> Drug metabolism produces compounds that are more polar (ionized) and more easily excreted.

Metabolism, which is also known as biotransformation, is the body's way of changing a drug so that it can be more easily excreted by the kidneys. Many drugs undergo metabolic transformation or change, most commonly in the liver. The **metabolite** (metabolic product) formed is usually more polar (ionized) and less lipid soluble than its parent compound. This means that renal tubular reabsorption of the metabolite will be reduced, because reabsorption favors lipid-soluble compounds. Metabolites are also less likely to bind to plasma or tissue proteins and less likely to be stored in fat tissue. Decreased renal tubular reabsorption, decreased binding to the plasma or tissue proteins, and decreased fat storage cause the metabolite to be excreted more easily. Drug metabolism is an enzyme-dependent process that has developed through evolution.

The following are mechanisms by which drugs are metabolized (Figure 2-21):

- **Active to inactive.** By metabolism, an inactive compound may be formed from an active parent drug. This is the most common type of reaction in drug biotransformation. Agents that interfere with the metabolism of certain drugs will increase the blood level of the drugs whose metabolism is inhibited. An example of this is doxycycline. Doxycycline itself is the active compound

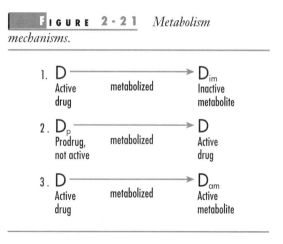

FIGURE 2-21 *Metabolism mechanisms.*

and is metabolized by the liver into a metabolite without activity. The metabolized drug is glucuronidated to become more polar and less lipid soluble.

- **Inactive to active.** An inactive parent drug may be transformed into an active compound. The inactive compound is then termed a prodrug. Interference with the metabolism of this drug will delay its onset of action because it will be harder for the active compound to be formed. For example, acyclovir is an antiviral agent. To be effective, it must be taken into the cell and phosphorylated to its active metabolite.

- **Active to active.** An active parent drug may be converted to a second active compound, which is then converted to an inactive product. The total effect of such a drug would be the addition of the effect of the parent drug plus the effect of the active drug metabolite. When an active metabolite is formed, the action of the drug is prolonged. For example, diazepam (Valium), an active antianxiety agent, is metabolized into its active metabolite, desmethyldiazepam. Diazepam's action is prolonged because of its own effect combined with that of its active metabolite.

Although the rates and pathways of drug metabolism vary among species, most studies indicate that drug biotransformation in laboratory animals is similar to that in humans. Many synthetic mechanisms of drug metabolism occur in the body to form metabolites.

First-pass effect. Metabolism of drugs may be divided into two general types: nonsynthetic (phase I) and synthetic (phase II) reactions (Figure 2-22). If a drug has no functional groups with which to combine, then the drug must undergo a phase I reaction. With this addition, the altered drug can then undergo conjugation, forming a more polar compound that can be more easily excreted.

Phase I: difficult; affected by age and drug interactions.

Phase I. In phase I reactions, lipid molecules are metabolized by the three processes of oxidation, reduction, and hydrolysis.

OXIDATION When a drug that is administered does not possess an appropriate functional group

that is suitable for combining with body acids (conjugation), the body has more difficulty detoxifying that drug. An enzyme system that is responsible for the oxidative metabolism of many drugs is located in the liver. The enzymes are located in the endoplasmic reticulum and are termed *microsomal* enzymes, because they are found in the microsomal fraction as prepared from liver homogenates. A variety of oxidative reactions, for example, as hydroxylation or the incorporation of oxygen into the substrate molecule, occur in these hepatic microsomal enzymes.

Oxidative processes involving enzymes other than those of the hepatic microsomal enzymes can take place. Some compounds are oxidatively deaminated by enzymes located in the liver, kidney, and nervous tissue. Other agents are detoxified by specific oxidative enzymes.

HYDROLYSIS Some ester compounds are metabolized by hydrolysis. Hydrolytic enzymes, found in the plasma and in a variety of tissues, break up esters and add water. The ester local anesthetics are inactivated by plasma cholinesterases.

F I G U R E   2 - 2 2   *Drug metabolism.*

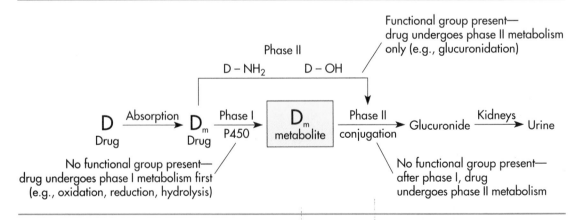

REDUCTION Many reduction reactions are mediated by the enzymes found in the hepatic microsomes.

MICROSOMAL ENZYMES Phase I reactions are carried out by the microsomal or cytochrome P-450 enzymes, which are also known as the mixed function oxidases in the liver. The concentration of these enzymes can be affected by drugs and environmental substances. Phase I metabolism may be affected by other drugs that alter microsomal enzymes—inhibition or induction.

Induction The P-450 hepatic microsomal enzymes can be induced (the amount of enzyme increased) by some drugs and by smoking tobacco. Because drugs that cause enzyme induction cause other drugs to be more quickly metabolized, the metabolized drugs will have reduced pharmacologic effects. More recent evidence has discovered that the hepatic enzymes can be divided into many categories called *isoenzymes.* Examples of isoenzymes include cytochrome P-450 2D6 and 3A4. Table 2-2 lists samples of drugs that are substrates of these enzymes, and drugs that either induce or inhibit these isoenzymes. For example, phenobarbital stimulates the production of microsomal enzymes that normally metabolize the anticoagulant warfarin. Thus, administering phenobarbi-

TABLE 2-2 Selected Cytochrome CYP-450 Isoenzymes—Substrates, Inhibitors, and Inducers

NUMBER	SUBSTRATE	INHIBITORS	INDUCERS
CYP 1A2	Antidepressants, tricyclic d-Warfarin Theophylline	Fluoroquinolones	Barbiturates Carbamazepine
CYP 2C8/9/10	Anticonvulsants NSAIAs s-Warfarin	Anticonvulsants Antidepressants, SSRI	Cimetidine Omeprazole
CYP 2C18/19	Antidepressants Naproxen Propranolol Proton pump inhibitors	Antidepressants, SSRI Imidazoles Omeprazole	Barbiturates Rifampin
CYP 2D6	Antiarrhythmics Antidepressants Antipsychotics Opioids	Antidepressants, SSRI Antipsychotics Cimetidine	Not susceptible
CYP 2E1	Alcohol	Alcohol intoxication	Alcohol, abuse (person sober)
CYP 3A3	Erythromycin	Cimetidine	
CYP 3A4	Antidepressants Benzodiazepines Calcium channel blockers Carbamazepine HMG-Co-A reductase inhibitors Imidazoles Macrolides	Antidepressants Corticosteroids Grapefruit juice Imidazoles Macrolides Omeprazole	Anticonvulsants
CYP 3A5	Lovastatin Midazolam Nifedipine		

NSAIAs, Nonsteroidal antinflammatory agents; *SSRI,* seratonin-specific reuptake inhibitor.

(Figure 2-23).

FIGURE 2-23 *Alteration of drug metabolism—induction and inhibition. Enzyme induction and inhibition alter the blood levels of drugs metabolized by the hepatic enzymes.*
A, *Normal. The liver is metabolizing drugs at the normal rate producing the normal effects.* **B,** *Induction. With enzyme induction (stimulation), increase in the enzymes causes the drug to be more quickly metabolized, and blood level of the drug and its effect are decreased (assume that metabolite is inactive). Induction = effect.* **C,** *Inhibition. With enzyme inhibition, the metabolism of drugs is slower (weaker enzymes) and the blood level of the drug that is metabolized is increased. Inhibition = effect.*

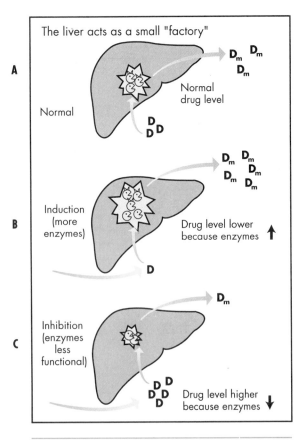

tal to a patient taking warfarin can decrease warfarin's anticoagulant response because the metabolism of the anticoagulant of the stimulation of (Figure 2-23).

Some drugs, such as valproate and carbamazepine (anticonvulsants), can also stimulate their own metabolism. The **tolerance** that patients develop to certain drugs can be explained, at least in part, by an increased ability to metabolize the drug because of stimulation of microsomal enzymes. Chapter 25 discusses these effects on microsomal enzymes in detail.

Inhibition Inhibition of the metabolism of certain drugs may occur through several mechanisms. With inhibition, the blood levels and action of the drugs metabolized by these enzymes will be increased. Examples of drugs that inhibit the metabolism of other drugs are erythromycin and cimetidine (Tagamet). Inhibiting the microsomal enzymes would result in an increase in the effect of the drugs metabolized by the liver enzymes (see Table 2-2).

Phase II. Phase II reactions involve **conjugation** with the following agents: glucuronic acid, sulfuric acid, acetic

> Phase II: easy; unaffected by age and drug interactions.

acid, or an amino acid. The most common conjugation that occurs is with glucuronic acid. This conjugation is termed *glucuronidation.* Glucuronic acid, which is a substance normally occurring in the body, may be transferred to a drug molecule that has an appropriate functional group to accept it. Functional groups that may be involved include ethers, alcohols, aromatic amines, and carboxylic acid. This mechanism, either alone or in combination with a phase I reaction, allows the body to convert a lipid-soluble drug to a more polar compound. The enzymes that mediate the conjugation are termed *transferases.*

Gate out of the body—the kidneys.

Excretion. Although drugs may be excreted by any of several routes that have direct access to the external environment, renal (kidney) excretion is the most important. Extrarenal routes include the lungs, bile, gastrointestinal tract, sweat, saliva, and milk. Drugs may be excreted unchanged or as metabolites.

KINETICS Kinetics is the mathematical representation of the way in which drugs are removed from the body. The most common mechanism is first-order kinetics.

A few drugs, such as aspirin and alcohol, exhibit zero-order kinetics. With zero-order kinetics, the rate of metabolism remains constant over time, and the same amount of drug is metabolized per unit of time regardless of dose. Zero-order kinetics occurs because the enzymes that metabolize these drugs can become saturated at usual therapeutic doses. If the dose of the drug is increased, the metabolism cannot increase above its maximum rate. With small doses, drugs with zero-order kinetics can metabolize the drug without build-up. With high doses, the metabolism of the drug cannot increase and the duration of action of the drug can be greatly prolonged (see Figure 2-20). Small changes in the dose of these drugs may produce a large change in the serum concentration, leading to unexpected toxicity.

RENAL ROUTE Elimination of substances in the kidney can occur by the following three routes:

- *Glomerular filtration:* Either the unchanged drug or its metabolites are filtered through the glomeruli and concentrated in the renal tubular fluid. This filtration process depends on the amount of plasma protein binding and the glomerular filtration rate. Bound drugs cannot be filtered and remain in the systemic circulation.

Most drugs are managed by this mechanism.

- *Active tubular secretion:* Active secretion transports the drug from the bloodstream across the renal tubular epithelial cells and into the renal tubular fluid. Glomerular filtration and active tubular secretion are relatively nonselective, and several compounds, both exogenous and endogenous (naturally occurring), can compete for transport. Secretion accounts for the less than 1 hour half-life of penicillin.* To prolong penicillin's action in the treatment of sexually transmitted diseases, probenecid is given before administering parenteral penicillin. Probenecid inhibits penicillin's secretion because both penicillin and probenecid are actively secreted (there is competition for a limited transport).

- *Passive tubular diffusion:* With most drugs, passive tubular diffusion (also termed *passive reabsorption*) plays a part in regulating the amount of drug in the tubular fluid. This process favors the reabsorption of non-ionized, lipid-soluble compounds. The more ionized, less lipid-soluble metabolites have more difficulty penetrating the cell membranes of the renal tubules, and are likely to be retained in the tubular fluid and eliminated in the urine. This process is also influenced by the urinary pH, which affects the amount of ionized and non-ionized drug in the tubular fluid. By altering the pH of the urine, drug excretion can be favored in cases of poisoning or can be inhibited when a prolongation of the drug effect is desired.

Weakly ionized acids or bases are excreted in the following fashion:

---

*That's why the urine of WW II soldiers was recycled. Shortly after its discovery, penicillin was in short supply. The penicillin recovered from the urine of one soldier could be given to another wounded soldier with an infection. (That's the ultimate in recycling!)

- *Alkaline urine:* When the tubular urinary pH is more alkaline than the plasma, weak acids are excreted more rapidly and weak bases are excreted more slowly.
- *Acid urine:* When tubular urine is more acid, weak acids are excreted more slowly and weak bases are excreted more rapidly.

EXTRARENAL ROUTES Certain drugs may be partially or completely eliminated via routes other than the kidney by the lungs. Gases used in general anesthesia are excreted across the lung tissue by a process of simple diffusion. Alcohol is also partially excreted from the lungs. (You can smell alcohol on someone's breath if they have been drinking alcohol.) This fact is used when testing a driver's breath for the presence of alcohol (Breathalyzer).

BILIARY EXCRETION Biliary excretion is the major route by which systemically absorbed drugs enter the gastrointestinal tract and are eliminated in the feces. Drugs excreted in the bile may also be reabsorbed from the intestines. Thus enterohepatic circulation, discussed earlier, prolongs a drug's action.

OTHER Two minor routes of elimination are in the milk and the sweat. The distribution of drugs in milk may be a potential source of undesirable effects for the nursing infant. Chapter 24 discusses dental drugs that can be given to nursing mothers.

SALIVA Drugs can also be excreted into the saliva. After drugs are excreted in the saliva, they are usually swallowed and their fate is the same as that of drugs ingested orally. The following drugs have been detected at significant levels in saliva after oral ingestion: aspirin, phenytoin, ampicillin, diazepam, penicillin VK, and phenobarbital. Present evidence suggests that most drugs that are secreted in the salivary **glands** enter saliva by simple diffusion, and their passage depends mainly on the lipid solubility of the drug. Thus a drug with high lipid solubility at plasma and salivary pH will readily enter saliva from plasma.

Drug levels in saliva have been studied to see if they can be used to monitor therapy with certain agents. For example, antiepileptic drug monitoring is essential for the rational treatment of **epilepsy,** and the measurement of these drugs in plasma is now routine. Assay of salivary concentrations of these drugs may become a reliable, method that is not **invasive** for predicting plasma levels. More study is needed before salivary levels can replace measuring the blood levels of the drug.

GINGIVAL CREVICULAR FLUID Drugs may also be excreted in the gingival crevicular fluid (GCF). Drugs excreted in the GCF produce a higher level of drug in the gingival crevices, which can increase their usefulness in the treatment of periodontal disease. Some drugs, for example the tetracyclines, are concentrated in the GCF. This means that the drug level of tetracycline in the GCF will be several times (4 or more times) higher than the blood level. This property makes the systemic use of a drug more effective within the gingival sulcus than one that is not concentrated.

FACTORS THAT ALTER DRUG EFFECTS

When a drug is administered, the following factors may influence or modify the drug's effect:
- *Patient compliance:* Through either lack of understanding or lack or motivation, patients often take medication incorrectly or not at all. Sometimes this may result from faulty communication, inadequate patient education, or their health belief system. Thus poor patient compliance can be an important factor in a therapeutic failure.
- *Psychologic factors:* The attitude of the prescriber and the dental staff can affect the efficacy of the drug prescribed. A **placebo** is a dosage form that looks like the active

agent but contains no active ingredients— the "sugar pill." The magnitude of the **placebo effect** depends on the patient's perception, and there is large individual variation. Health care providers can maximize the drug's effect to achieve an improved therapeutic result by talking up the drug. This may account for the popularity of herbs and plants.

- *Tolerance:* A patient may exhibit tolerance to many drugs, including the sedative-hypnotics and the opioids. Drug tolerance is defined as the need for an increasingly larger dose of the drug to obtain the same effects as the original dose, or the decreased effect produced after repeated administration of a given dose of the drug. When a patient becomes tolerant to one drug, tolerance to other drugs with similar pharmacologic actions occurs. This is termed cross-tolerance. If tolerance develops, a normal sensitivity to the drug's effect may be restored by ceasing administration of the drug. **Tachyphylaxis** is the very rapid development of tolerance, often within hours.

- *Pathologic state:* Diseased patients may respond to the administration of medication differently than other patients. For example, patients with hyperthyroidism are extremely sensitive to the toxic effects of epinephrine. Hepatic or renal disease influences the metabolism and excretion of drugs, potentially leading to an increased duration of drug action. With repeated doses in diseased patients, the serum level of a drug may become toxic.

- *Time of administration:* The time a drug is administered, especially in relation to meals, alters the response to that drug. Certain drugs with a sedative action are best administered at bedtime to minimize the sedation experienced by the patient.

- *Route of administration:* The effect of the route of administration on the onset and duration of action of a drug was discussed previously.

- *Sex:* The sex of the patient can alter a drug's effect. Women may be more sensitive than men to certain drugs, perhaps because of their smaller size or their hormones. Pregnancy alters the effect of certain drugs. Women of child-bearing age should avoid teratogenic drugs, and the oral health care provider should determine whether the patient is pregnant before administering any agent.

- *Genetic variation:* Many differences in patient response to drugs have been associated with variations in ability to metabolize certain drugs. This difference may account for the fact that certain populations have a higher incidence of adverse effects to some drugs—a genetic predisposition.

- *Drug interactions:* A drug's effect may be modified by previous or concomitant administration of another drug. There are many mechanisms by which drug interactions may modify a patient's treatment, as discussed in Chapter 25.

- *Age and weight:* The dose of a drug administered to children should be reduced from the adult dose. Age or weight has been suggested as a method of calculating a child's dose. Because of the great variability of weight in relation to age, the child's weight should be used to determine the child's dose. Because a child is not just a small adult, the manufacturer's recommendations for children's dosing would be best. The elderly may respond differently to drugs than younger patients. Whether this is solely due to changes in renal or liver function or whether being elderly patients predisposes this sensitivity is controversial.

- *Environment:* The environment contains many substances that may affect the action of drugs. Smoking induces enzymes, so higher doses of benzodiazepines are needed to produce the same effect. Some chemical contaminants such as pesticides or solvents can have an effect on a drug's action.

- **Other:** The action of drugs can be altered by the patient-provider interaction. If the patient "believes" in the substance or process (drug/herb/voodoo/incantation) being used, the patient's opinion will enhance the drug's effect. The attitude of both the patient and the provider can alter the physiology of the body. These actions may account for the positive effect of many mental exercises (e.g., meditation).

CALCULATION OF CHILDREN'S DOSAGE

The patient's weight is the usual basis for determining drug dosage, although not the ideal method. Box 2-1 lists various methods for

---

Box 2-1   CHILDREN'S DOSAGE CALCULATIONS

1. *Clark's rule:*

$$\frac{\text{Weight (lb)} \times \text{Adult dose}}{150} = \text{Infant dose}$$

2. *Fried's rule:*

$$\frac{\text{Age (mo)} \times \text{Adult dose}}{150} = \text{Infant dose}$$

3. *Young's rule:*

$$\frac{\text{Age (yr)} \times \text{Adult dose}}{\text{age (yr)} + 12} = \text{Child dose}$$

4. *Cowling's rule:*

$$\frac{\text{Age (at next birthday)} \times \text{Adult dose}}{24} = \text{Child dose}$$

5. *Surface area rule:*
   $(0.7 \times \text{Weight in lb}) + 10 = \%$ Adult dose
   $(1.5 \times \text{Weight in kg}) + 10 = \%$ Adult dose

---

determining a child's dose based on an adult dose.

Because weight may vary in children of the same age, a better method of calculating a child's or an infant's dose is based on body surface area. This method requires the use of a table or nomogram from which the body surface of the child can be determined. The child's body surface is a function of the height and weight of the child. The surface area formula is a convenient and more accurate formula than those based on the age or weight of the child.

Another method for determining the child's dose is to follow a suggested pediatric dosage schedule prepared by the manufacturer. These doses are usually given in terms of milligrams of drug per kilogram of body weight per 24 hours (occasionally dose to give every 6 hours). This is especially common for antibiotic agents. It is important to note that the 24-hour dose calculated must be divided into the number of doses to be given daily. The manufacturer's recommendations probably provide the most accurate suggestions.

Example: What is the dose of amoxicillin for rheumatic heart disease prophylaxis for a 50-lb child? (See Chapter 8.)

$$\text{Dose} = 50 \text{ mg/kg (look up)}$$

1. Change pounds to kilograms: Divide by $\cong 2$ equals 25 kg

$$\frac{2.2 \text{ lb}}{1 \text{ kg}} = \frac{50 \text{ lb}}{x \text{ kg}} \qquad x = \frac{50 \text{ kg}}{2.2} = 23 \text{ kg}$$

(child's weight in kilograms)

2. Multiply dose in milligrams per kilograms by number of kg = mg = dose

$$\frac{50 \text{ mg}}{\text{kg}} = \frac{x \text{ mg}}{23 \text{ kg}} \qquad x = (50 \times 23) \text{ mg}$$

1150 mg for RHD prophylaxis in a 50-lb child (dose [mg]/ kg × wt [kg] = dose [mg])
50 mg/kg × 25 kg = 1250 = dose

REVIEW QUESTIONS

1. Define and differentiate between the potency and efficacy of a drug.
2. Describe the dose-response curve using the terms ED_{50} (effective dose) and LD_{50} (lethal dose).
3. Define the term *pharmacokinetics*. Name the four categories involved.
4. Define the major routes of drug administration, including the following:
   a. oral
   b. intravenous
   c. inhalation
   d. topical
5. State the dosage forms most frequently used in dentistry.
6. Describe the mechanism of drug transfer across bioloDiazepamranes.
7. Explain the influence of pH on the dissociation characteristics of weak acids and weak bases.
8. Describe one dental example of each for absorption and excretion.
9. Explain each of the steps involved in oral absorption, including the following:
   a. disruption
   b. disintegration
   c. dispersion
   d. dissolution
10. Define the $t_{1/2}$, or half-life, of a drug and state its significance.
11. Define the following terms:
    a. agonist
    b. competitive antagonist
    c. physiologic antagonist
    d. isomers
    e. chirals
12. Describe the importance of the hepatic microsomal enzymes in relation to drug metabolism. Explain isoenzymes.
13. Explain the terms *first-pass effect* and *enterohepatic circulation*. State what effects these properties could have on a drug.
14. State the major route of drug excretion, and describe the three processes by which it occurs.
15. Explain how metabolism can be altered by an effect on liver microsomal enzymes.
16. If the dose of clindamycin to use before a dental procedure in a child with rheumatic heart disease is 20 mg/kg, how many milligrams should be given to a 40-lb child? A 60-lb child?

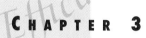

CHAPTER 3

Adverse Reactions

Although drugs may act on biologic systems to accomplish a desired effect, they lack absolute specificity in that they can act on many different organs or tissues. This lack of specificity is the reason for undesirable or adverse drug reactions. No drug is free from producing some adverse effects in a certain number of patients. It is estimated that between 5% and 10% of the patients hospitalized annually in the United States are admitted because of adverse reactions to drugs. While hospitalized, 10% to 20% of patients experience adverse reactions caused by drugs.

The dental health care worker is in a good position to observe any adverse reactions or undesirable effects caused by drugs administered in the dental office. Adverse reactions to drugs prescribed by the patient's physician can be identified in the health history. The dental health care worker should question the patient about any potential oral manifestations of drugs. For example, if the patient is taking phenytoin (Dilantin), questions about enlargement of the patient's gums should be explored. Because many drugs can produce xerostomia, complaints of dry mouth should direct the dental health care worker to examine the patient's medications. A knowledge of the typical adverse drug reactions can help dental office personnel identify, minimize, or prevent these types of reactions. Because of the rapport between a patient and the dental health care worker, the patient will often reveal important facts about the health history or ask questions concerning medications prescribed. The dental health care worker must know the terms used to describe adverse reactions in order to discuss a drug's undesirable effect accurately with other health professionals. For example, *allergy* refers to a specific type of reaction to a drug, but does not include "I've got gas!"

DEFINITIONS AND CLASSIFICATIONS

Unfortunately, every drug has more than one action. The clinically desirable actions are termed *therapeutic effects*, and the undesirable reactions are termed *adverse effects*. Dividing a drug's effects into two categories is artificial because it depends on the indication for which the drug is being used. For example, when an antihistamine used to relieve hay fever causes drowsiness, that can be considered an adverse effect. However, if the antihistamine were being used to induce sleep (**over-the-counter** [OTC] sleep aid), drowsiness would be considered the therapeutic effect.

An adverse drug reaction is a response to a drug that is not desired, is potentially harmful, and occurs at usual therapeutic doses. It may be an exaggeration of the desired response, an expected but undesired response, an allergic reaction, a cytotoxic reaction, or an effect on the fetus. Often, adverse drug reactions are divided into the following categories:

* *Toxic reaction:* This adverse drug reaction is an extension of the pharmacologic effect resulting from a drug's effect on the target organs. In this instance, the amount of the desired effect is excessive.
* *Side effect:* A side effect is a dose-related reaction that is not part of the desired therapeutic outcome. It occurs when a drug acts on nontarget organs to produce undesirable effects. The terms *side effect* and *adverse reac-*

tion often are used interchangeably. The upset stomach produced by ibuprofen is an adverse reaction when ibuprofen is given to manage pain.
* *Idiosyncratic reaction:* An idiosyncratic reaction is a genetically related abnormal drug response. Certain populations, because of their genetic constitution, are more susceptible to certain adverse reactions to specific drugs. Eskimos metabolize certain drugs faster than other populations; therefore, a larger dose of those drugs would be needed in that population (e.g., isoniazid).
* *Drug allergy:* A drug allergy is an immunologic response to a drug resulting in a reaction such as a rash or anaphylaxis. This response accounts for less than 5% of all adverse reactions. Unlike other adverse reactions, allergic reactions are neither predictable nor dose-related.
* *Interference with natural defense mechanisms:* Certain drugs, such as adrenocorticosteroids, can reduce the body's ability to fight infection. Drugs that interfere with the body's defenses cause a patient to get infections more easily and have more trouble fighting them.

The importance of distinguishing between different types of adverse effects can be seen using aspirin as an example. Aspirin can produce adverse reactions such as gastric upset or pain. At higher doses, aspirin can predictably produce toxicity such as tinnitus and hyperthermia (elevated temperature). Another type of reaction to aspirin is allergic, often involving a rash or difficulty in breathing (asthma-like reaction). These differences are significant and become pertinent when discussing an adverse reaction with another health professional. If a patient reports an adverse reaction (e.g., gastrointestinal upset) to aspirin and that is reported as an "allergy," then the patient should not be given any nonsteroidal antiinflammatory agent (e.g., ibuprofen). However, if the side effect of gastrointestinal upset is

FIGURE 3-1 *Diagram of classification of adverse drug reactions.*

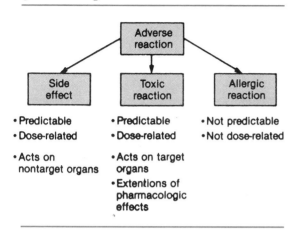

reported as a side effect, the patient may tolerate ibuprofen. It is important to describe in the patient's chart the patient's "problem" in enough detail so that the adverse reactions can be separated from the allergic reactions. Figure 3-1 describes the types of adverse reactions and notes whether they are predictable or dose dependent.

CLINICAL MANIFESTATIONS OF ADVERSE REACTIONS

Before a drug is used there must be an assessment of its risk against its benefits (risk to benefit ratio). This means that the beneficial effect of the drug must be weighed against its potential for adverse reactions. For example, one would compare the drug's therapeutic effect (e.g., growing strong fingernails) with its potential to cause an adverse reaction (e.g., irreversible baldness). In a real-life example, compare the therapeutic effect of certain drugs to produce weight loss to their potential for the serious adverse reactions of primary pulmonary hypertension (which is fatal in 50% of patients) or cardiac valvular damage.

EXAGGERATED EFFECT ON TARGET TISSUES

This type of adverse reaction causes an exaggerated effect of a drug on its target organ or tissue. This is considered to be an extension of the therapeutic effect caused by the overreaction of a sensitive patient or by using a dose that is too large. For example, a patient may experience exaggerated hypoglycemia when given a therapeutic dose of a hypoglycemic agent (pills for diabetes) for the treatment of diabetes. The patient's blood sugar may fall too low, either because of an unusual sensitivity to the drug or because the dose administered was too high for that patient. Occasionally, this type of adverse reaction may result from liver or kidney disease. Because the disease interferes with the drug's metabolism or excretion, the drug's action may be enhanced or prolonged.

EFFECT ON NONTARGET TISSUES

The effect on nontarget organs or tissues is caused by the nontherapeutic action of the drug. These reactions can occur at usual doses, but they appear more frequently at higher doses. For example, aspirin may produce gastric upset in usual therapeutic doses, but with higher doses salicylism, characterized by tinnitus, disturbances in the acid-base balance, and confusion, can result. Toxic reactions can affect many parts of the body. A reduction in the dose of a drug usually reduces these adverse reactions.

EFFECT ON FETAL DEVELOPMENT (TERATOGENIC EFFECT)

The word *teratogenic* comes from the Greek prefix *terato-*, meaning "monster" and the suffix *-genic*, meaning "producing," or "producing a malformed fetus." Since 1941, when the relationship between German **measles** and birth defects was noticed, the relationship between drugs and **congenital** abnormalities has been recognized. In 1961, thalidomide, an OTC drug marketed in Europe, was found to produce pho-comelia (short arms and legs), in the exposed fetus. In some cases only one dose of this drug produced the effect. This incident reinforced the fact that more studies were needed to determine the effect of drugs on pregnant women. For new drugs, there are many more studies on animals and their reproductive capacity before the drugs are placed on the market. Even though more information is now available about the safety of drugs in pregnant women, sufficient information is still lacking.

The Food and Drug Administration (FDA) has attempted to address the concerns about the lack of adequate knowledge of drugs by defining five FDA pregnancy categories: A, B, C, D, and X, ranked from least risky to most risky. Table 24-2 discusses the meaning of these categories. They are similar to school grades, with *A* being "best" or least teratogenic and *X* being equivalent to *F* or not ever to be used if someone might get pregnant. Some older drugs may be classified as C because there is insufficient data to place them in higher categories.

Although no drug can be considered "safe" for administration to a pregnant woman, many of the drugs used in dentistry are considered to be among the safest. These include the antibiotics penicillin and erythromycin, the pain medication acetaminophen (Tylenol), and the local anesthetic lidocaine. Even these drugs should be administered only if there is a clear need. Elective dental procedures should be conservatively addressed. Drugs that are used in dentistry that are contraindicated during pregnancy include tetracycline, nonsteroidal antiinflammatory agents, the benzodiazepines, and metronidazole. The teratogenic potential for dental drugs is discussed in Chapter 24.

Many drug manufacturers, especially those that produce some of the older drugs, continue to place in their package inserts such statements as the following:
- "There are no adequate and well-controlled studies in pregnant women."

- "Risks must be balanced against the uncontrolled disease."
- "Safety during pregnancy has not been established; use requires that potential benefits be weighed against its possible hazard to the mother and child."
- "Animal reproductive studies are not always indicative of human effects."
- "Animal reproduction studies have not been conducted with . . ."
- ". . . potential benefit must be weighed against the possible hazards to the mother and fetus."

Encouraging increases in the information provided, especially for newer agents, has resulted in more information about usage during pregnancy, such as the following statements:
- "Pregnancy category D."
- "Shown to decrease fetal birth weight when given at 50 times the dose recommended for humans."
- "No evidence of birth abnormalities or impaired fertility in doses 2 times the usual human dose."

But there are still plenty of statements such as the following:

With regard to teratogenesis, it is important to remember that the risk to the fetus must always be considered when considering the benefit to the mother. Also, dental patients do not always announce that they are pregnant, so it is important to ask any woman of child-bearing age (between 11 and 63 [a 63-year-old French woman gave birth in 1997!]), if she is pregnant. Problem drugs should be avoided as early as possible during the pregnancy. The greatest risk from exposure to drugs occurs before the pregnancy status is known.

LOCAL EFFECT

Local reactions are characterized by local tissue irritation. Occasionally, injectable drugs can produce irritation, pain, and tissue **necrosis** at the site of injection. Topically applied agents can produce irritation at the site of application. Drugs taken orally can produce gastrointestinal symptoms such as nausea or dyspepsia because of their local actions on the gastrointestinal tract.

DRUG INTERACTIONS

A drug interaction can occur when the effect of one drug is altered by another drug. These interactions may result in undesirable effects such as toxicity or lack of efficacy. Drug interactions can also produce beneficial effects. Whenever prescribing or suggesting a drug to a dental patient, the chance of drug interactions must be considered. The likelihood that a drug interaction would occur increases with the number of drugs that a patient is taking. Drug-food and drug-disease interactions may also occur. (Chapter 25 discusses drug interactions in detail.)

HYPERSENSITIVITY (ALLERGIC REACTION)

Hypersensitivity reactions occur when the **immune system** of an individual responds to the drug administered or applied. When a patient is given a drug and in several hours develops hives, this is an allergic (hypersensitivity) reaction. For a drug to produce an allergic reaction, it must act as an antigen and react with an antibody in a previously sensitized patient. This reaction is neither dose dependent nor predictable. For an allergic reaction to occur, an ingested drug may be metabolized to a reactive metabolite known as a **hapten.** This hapten can act as an antigen after combining with proteins in the body. The antigen formed then stimulates the production of an antibody. With subsequent exposure to the drug, the antibodies formed will react with the antibody (drug or metabolite) administered and elicit an antigen-antibody reaction. This reaction triggers a series of biochemical and physiologic events that can be life threatening.

Drug allergy can be divided into the following four types of reactions, depending on the type of antibody produced or the cell mediating the reaction (Table 3-1):

* *Type I* reactions are mediated by immunoglobulin E (IgE) antibodies. When a drug antigen binds to IgE antibody, histamine, leukotrienes, and prostaglandins are released, producing vasodilation, edema, and the inflammatory response. The targets of this reaction are the bronchioles, resulting in

TABLE 3-1 Hypersensitivity Reactions

Type	Mediator	Reaction	Example
I (immediate, anaphylactic)	Antibody	IgE antibody is induced by allergen and binds via its Fc receptor to mast cells and basophils. After encountering the antigen again, the fixed IgE becomes cross-linked. Inducing degranulation and release of mediators (e.g., histamine)	Anaphylaxis to penicillin
II (cytotoxic)	Antibody	Antigens on a cell surface combine with antibody; this leads to complement-mediated lysis (e.g., transfusion of Rh reactions or autoimmune hemolytic anemia	Quinine lysis platelets—thrombocytopenia
III (immune complex)	Antibody	Antigen-antibody immune complexes are deposited in tissues, complement is activated, and polymorphonuclear cells are attracted to this site causing tissue damage	Serum sickness
IV (delayed)	Cell	Helper T lymphocytes sensitized by an antigen release lymphokines upon second contact with the same antigen. The lymphokines induce inflammation and activate macrophages which, in turn, release various mediators	Poison Ivy, TB tests

From Levinson WE, Jawetz E: *Medical microbiology and immunology,* ed 2, Norwalk, Conn, Appleton & Lange.

anaphylactic shock; the respiratory system, resulting in rhinitis and asthma; and the skin, resulting in urticaria and dermatitis. Because these reactions can occur relatively quickly after drug exposure, they are known as *immediate hypersensitivity reactions.*

Anaphylaxis is an acute, life-threatening allergic reaction characterized by **hypotension, bronchospasm,** laryngeal edema, and cardiac arrhythmias that can occur within a few minutes after drug administration. Drugs used in dentistry that have produced fatal anaphylaxis include the penicillins, ester local anesthetics, and aspirin. Unexpected anaphylaxis may occur, such as after a patient has been given a dose of penicillin by injection. Oral penicillin can also produce anaphylaxis, but it is much less common.

- *Type II,* or cytotoxic/cytolytic, reactions are complement-dependent reactions involving either immunoglobulin G (IgG) or immunoglobulin M (IgM) antibodies. The antigen-antibody complex is fixed to a circulating blood cell, resulting in lysis. Examples of this reaction are penicillin-induced hemolytic anemia and methyldopa-induced autoimmune hemolytic anemia.
- *Type III,* or Arthus reactions, are mediated by IgG. In this reaction, the drug antigen-antibody complex fixes complement and deposits in the vascular endothelium. The reaction is manifested as serum sickness and includes urticarial skin eruptions, arthralgia, arthritis, lymphadenopathy, and fever. This reaction can be caused by the penicillins and sulfonamides.
- *Type IV,* or delayed-hypersensitivity, reactions are mediated by sensitized T-**lymphocytes** and macrophages. When the cells contact the antigen, an inflammatory reaction is produced by lymphokines, neutrophils, and macrophages. An example of a type IV reaction is allergic contact dermatitis caused by topical application of drugs. Both topical benzocaine and penicillin, as well as poison oak or poison ivy, can produce this type of

reaction. Reaction to "cheap" jewelry is another example.

IDIOSYNCRASY

An **idiosyncratic** reaction is a reaction that is neither the drug's side effect nor an allergic reaction. Some idiosyncrasies have been found to be genetically determined abnormal reactions, whereas others may be due to an immunologic mechanism. About 10% of black males can develop severe hemolytic anemia when given the antimalarial drug primaquine. This is due to a deficiency in an enzyme, glucose-6-phosphate dehydrogenase.

INTERFERENCE WITH NATURAL DEFENSE MECHANISMS

A drug's effect on the body's defense mechanisms can result in an adverse reaction. Long-term systemic administration of corticosteroids can result in decreased resistance to infection. Because periodontal disease involves both infection and an immune response, drugs that are immunosuppressive could exacerbate a patient's poor oral health.

TOXICOLOGIC EVALUATION OF DRUGS

Optimally, evaluations of the toxic effects of drugs are based on experiments that are performed with lower animals and clinical trials conducted in

> LD_{50}—kills ½ subjects
> ED_{50}—produces a response in ½ of the subjects

humans. Animal experiments can frequently elicit adverse reactions that could occur in humans, but unfortunately drug reactions in animals do not always predict reactions in humans. The lethal dose (LD_{50}), one measure of the toxicity of a drug, is the dose of a drug that kills 50% of the experimental animals. The median effective dose (ED_{50}) is the dose required to produce a specified intensity of effect in 50% of the animals. Figure 3-2 plots the dose of a drug against the percentage of maximum response (sleep or death) in animals. A dose-response curve is then obtained. The value on the dose axis that corresponds to the 50% intensity level on the response axis can be read directly from the curve. This figure illustrates the ED_{50} and LD_{50}.

Because all drugs are toxic at some dose, the LD_{50} is meaningless unless the ED_{50} is also known. The ratio LD_{50}/ED_{50} is the therapeutic index of a drug, or:

$$\text{Therapeutic index (TI)} = LD_{50}/ED_{50}$$

If the value of the TI is small (narrow TI), then toxicity is more likely. If the TI is large (wide TI), then the drug will be safer (Figure 3-3). A drug with a wide therapeutic index will have a large LD_{50} and a small ED_{50} (the distance between these curves is large.) A therapeutic index of greater than 10 is usually needed to produce a therapeutically useful drug. The therapeutic index is derived from animal studies determining both the LD_{50} and the ED_{50} for a variety of animals.

If a discovered or synthesized compound becomes a marketed drug, it must pass through many steps before it is approved (Figure 3-4). Animal studies begin by measuring both the acute and chronic toxicity. The LD_{50} (median lethal dose) is determined for several species of animals. Long-term animal studies continue, including searching for teratogenic effects. Toxic-

F I G U R E 3 - 2 *Dose-response curve and therapeutic index.*

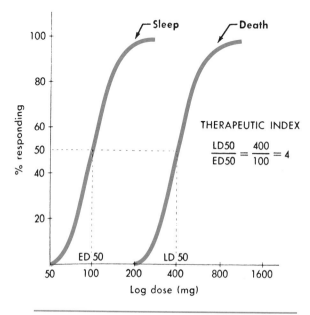

F I G U R E 3 - 3 *Difference between narrow and wide therapeutic indexes.*

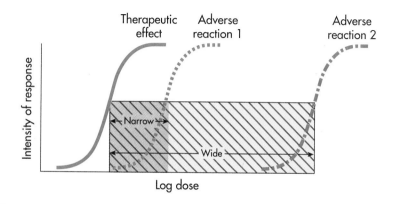

FIGURE **3 - 4**   *Developing a new drug.*

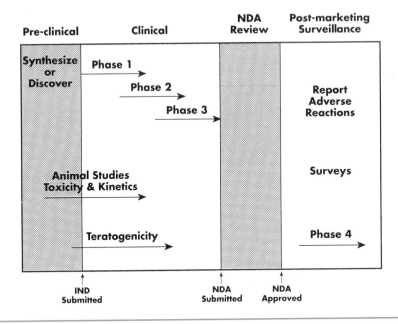

ity and pharmacokinetic properties are also noted. A new drug application (NDA) must be filed before any clinical trials can be performed. Human studies of drugs involve the following four phases:

- *Phase 1:* In phase 1, small and then increasing doses are administered to a limited number of healthy human volunteers, primarily to determine safety. This phase determines the biologic effects, metabolism, and safe dosage range in humans, as well as toxic effects of the drug.
- *Phase 2:* In phase 2, larger groups of humans are given the drug and any adverse reactions are reported to the FDA. The main purpose of phase 2 is to test effectiveness.
- *Phase 3:* In phase 3, more clinical evaluation takes place involving a large number of patients who have the condition for which the drug is indicated. During this

phase both safety and efficacy must be demonstrated. Dosage is determined during this phase too.
- *Phase 4:* Phase 4 involves postmarketing surveillance. The toxicity of the drug that occurs in patients taking the drug after it is released is recorded. Several drugs in recent years have been removed from the market only after phase 4 has shown serious toxicity.

REVIEW QUESTIONS

1. Name four classifications of adverse drug reactions.
2. Describe the problem with identifying teratogenic agents (see also Chapter 24).
3. Describe the types of adverse reactions.
4. Explain the four mechanisms by which an allergic reaction can occur.
5. Give the formula for the therapeutic index and describe its usefulness in clinical practice.

6. Describe why the importance of the risk-to-benefit ratio is helpful in deciding whether to administer a drug to a patient.

7. Explain the various stages of testing through which a drug must pass before it is marketed for the general public.

8. Describe the mechanism involved in two of the types of drug interactions that involve the liver.

9. Explain the meaning of *extension of the pharmacologic effect*. Give one example.

10. Explain what is meant by a *nontarget organ* when ibuprofen is taken to treat a toothache.

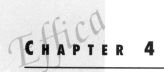

CHAPTER 4

Prescription Writing

Dental practitioners need to become familiar with the basics of prescription writing for the following reasons:

- If prescriptions are written correctly, it will save the time of the office personnel, dentist, and pharmacist who must call to clarify prescriptions.
- Prescriptions written carefully are less likely to result in mistakes.
- With extra effort when unusual prescriptions are written, the dentist can save the patient's and pharmacist's time. For example, if the unusual is explained on the prescription, problems will be minimized. Sometimes it

may be expedient to call the prescription to the pharmacy so that the unusual use can be explained and a reference given.

Historically, prescription writing was formerly a rather complex and pretentious art. Prescriptions were written in Latin and embellished by the hieroglyphics of the apothecaries' system of weights and measures. Early prescriptions were compounded from numerous constituents, and the confidence in and mystique of the prescription boosted its efficacy. In fact, it was inappropriate for the pharmacist to inform the patient what medication had been prescribed. In more recent years the following changes have simplified prescription writing:

- The pharmaceutical manufacturers provide most drugs in the dosage forms needed; therefore complicated compounding instructions can be omitted.
- Prescriptions are no longer written in Latin (although currently used abbreviations are generally derived from Latin).
- The metric system of weights and measures has nearly replaced the more confusing apothecaries' system in prescription writing.
- The use of certain abbreviations is being discouraged because of the potential for errors.

MEASUREMENT

In pharmacy, the primary measuring system is the metric system. [Please, let's use this system exclusively!] The apothecary system was commonly used in the old days, and today it is used sporadically, primarily by the old codger prescribers. Some prescribers like the idea that the apothecary system looks "cool" and is difficult for the lay public to read. Unlike the metric system, the apothecary system uses crazy conversions and weird units from history and, like the avoirdupois system, has unusual units (not based on the power of 10).

METRIC SYSTEM

Scientific calculations employ a base of 10. Consequently, the metric system, which is based on 10, is the language

> Metric system—multiples of 10.

of scientific measurement. Only metric units should be used in prescription writing.

The basic metric unit for the measurement of weight is the kilogram (kg). The basic metric unit for volume is the liter (L). One milliliter (ml), $\frac{1}{1000}$ of a liter, is exactly 1 cubic centimeter (cc). Because the various units of the metric system are based on multiples of 10, several prefixes can apply to units of both weight and volume (Table 4-1).

Solid drugs are dispensed by weight (milligrams [mg]) and liquid drugs by volume (milliliters [ml]). It is rarely necessary to use units other than the milligram or the milliliter in prescription writing (occasionally grams or micrograms are used). In addition to the milliliter, the liter is another unit used to measure volume.

Apothecary system. Although the apothecary system is cumbersome, some older practitioners continue to use it. Because the conversion between units does not involve 10 (like the convenient metric system), conversion in this system is more difficult. The units of weight include the grain (like sand) (gr), the scruple (℈), the ounce

TABLE 4-1   Metric Weight and Volume

WEIGHT		VOLUME	
1 *kilogram* (kg) =	1000 grams (g or gm)		
1 gram (g) =	10 *decigrams* (dg)	1 liter (L) =	10 *deciliters* (dl)
	100 *centigrams* (cg)		100 *centiliters* (cl)
	1000 *milligrams* (mg)		1000 *milliliters* (ml)
	1,000,000 *micrograms* (μg, mcg)		1,000,000 *microliters* (μl)

(℥), and the pound (℔). The units of volume include the dram (ʒ) and the ounce (℥). Table 4-2 shows the approximate equivalents between the metric and apothecaries' systems. Figure 4-1 shows the use of the apothecary system.

Avoirdupois system

The avoirdupois system is used in the United States in commerce. Of course, it is different than either of the other units. The product labels on food cans and quart containers of milk use this system. In this system, there are 16 oz in 1 lb.

Figure 4-2 demonstrates that 1 oz is equivalent to approximately 30 ml (1 oz) and that 1 cup equals 8 oz or 240 ml.

TABLE 4-2 Approximate Equivalents of Metric and Apothecary Systems

METRIC	APOTHECARY
WEIGHT	
60 mg	1 grain (gr)
1 gram, gm, or Gm	15 gr
30 gm	1 ounce (oz, ℥)
1 kilogram (kg)	2.2 pounds (lb)†
VOLUME	
30 ml	1 fluid ounce (fl oz, fl ℥)
500 ml	1 pint (pt)
1000 ml	1 quart (qt)

*The apothecary pound (℔) contains 12 ounces (℥)
†This unit of weight is avoirdupois, not apothecary.

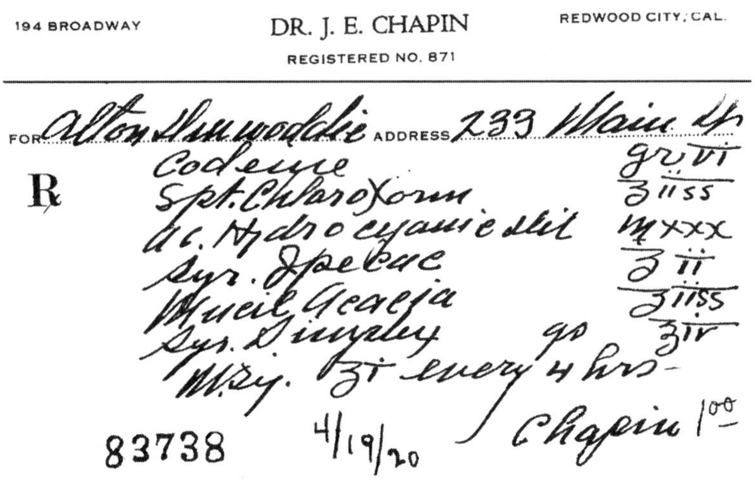

FIGURE 4-2 *Household measures. Relationship between oz and ml is illustrated.*

240 ml
8 oz
1 cup
180 ml
6 oz
3/4 cup
120 ml
4 oz
1/2 cup
60 ml
2 oz
1/4 cup

FIGURE 4-1 *Old prescription.*

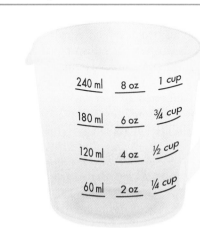

194 BROADWAY
DR. J. E. CHAPIN
REDWOOD CITY, CAL.
REGISTERED NO. 871
FOR
ADDRESS
℞
83738
4/19/20

HOUSEHOLD MEASURES

> If using available home measuring tools, use those intended for measuring indredients.

Although clinicians will direct the pharmacist to dispense a liquid preparation in milliliters, it is generally converted by the pharmacist into a convenient household unit of measurement to be included in the directions to the patient. Liquids are converted into teaspoonfuls (tsp or t; 1 tsp equals 5 ml) and tablespoonfuls (tbsp or T; 1 tbsp equals 15 ml) (Figure 4-3). When accuracy is important, such as for pediatric dosing, the pharmacist will recommend a calibrated oral syringe or dropper. These are available in 2.5-, 5-, and 10-ml volumes with milliliters marked along the length.

PRESCRIPTIONS

FORMAT

The parts of the prescription have been named and defined classically as follows:

- **Superscription:** Patient's name, address, and age; date; and the symbol ℞ (Latin for *recipe*, "[you] take" or "take thou of").
- **Inscription:** Name of drug, dose form, and amount
- **Subscription:** Directions to the pharmacist
- **Transcription (or signature):** Directions to the patient

Because the classic categorization serves no particularly useful purpose, it is more practical to consider the prescription as consisting of the heading, body, and closing (Figure 4-4).

Heading. The heading of the prescription contains the following information:

- Name,* address,* and telephone number of the prescriber (on the prescription blank)
- Name,* address,* age, and telephone number of the patient (written)
- Date of prescription* (not a legal prescription unless filled in with date); frequently missing

The name, address, and telephone number of the prescriber are important when the pharmacist must contact the prescribing clinician for verification or questions. The date is particularly important because it allows the pharmacist to intercept prescriptions that may not have been filled at the time of writing. For example, a prescription for an antibiotic written 3 months before being presented to the pharmacist might be being used for a different use than the dentist originally intended. Likewise, a prescription for a pain medication that is even a few days old requires the pharmacist to question the patient as to why the prescription is being filled so long after it was written. The age of the patient enables the pharmacist to check for the proper dose.

FIGURE 4-3 *Household measures. Use measuring devices to obtain the correct volume of liquids; if measuring devices are not available, use measuring spoons used for cooking; avoid using silverware spoons because they vary greatly in volume.*

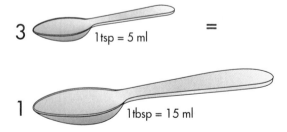

3 1 tsp = 5 ml   =

1 1 tbsp = 15 ml

---

*Required by law.

Body. The body of the prescription contains the following information:

- The symbol R*
- Name and dosage size or concentration (liquids) of the drug*
- Amount to be dispensed*
- Directions to the patient

The first entry after the R symbol is the name of the drug being prescribed. This is followed by the size (milligrams) of the tablet or capsule desired. In the case of liquids the name of the drug is followed by its concentration (milligrams per milliliter [mg/ml]). The second entry is the quantity to be dispensed, that is, the number of capsules or tablets or milliliters of liquid. This should be preceded by "Dispense:" or "Disp:" (Figures 4-5 and 4-6).

In the case of tablets and capsules, the word "Dispense" is frequently replaced with **#,** the symbol for a number. When writing prescriptions for opioids or other controlled substances, the prescriber should add in parentheses the

---

*Required by law.

number of tablets or capsules written out in Roman numerals or in longhand after the Arabic number of tablets or capsules. This reduces the possibility of an intended 8 becoming an 18 or 80 at the discretion of an enterprising patient. Directions to the patient are preceded by the abbreviation "Sig:" (Latin for *signa*, "write"). The directions to the patient must be completely clear and explicit and should include the amount of medication and the time, frequency, and route of administration. The pharmacist will transcribe Latin abbreviations (Table 4-3) into English on the label when the prescription is filled. The use of *ud* ("as directed") does not provide the proper information on the label for the patient. Often with *"ud"* prescriptions, the patient does not remember how to take the medicine. To clarify for the patient without adequate written instructions, the pharmacist must contact the prescriber for clarification (this wastes dentist, pharmacist, and patient time). After a few months the patient will forget the quick instructions given verbally in the dental office after a dental appointment. Even prescriptions for chlorhexidine should be specific for amount,

F IGURE 4 - 4   *Sample prescription label.*

Mary Smith, DDS 1234 Main St KC MO 64111   (816) 555-1234

Name _____   Date _____   ❶

Address _____   Age _____

R

Drug Name # mg tabs }   ❷

Disp: # _____   }   ❸

Sig: 1-2 tabs q 4-6 h prn pain }   ❹

Substitution Permitted   _____

          Dispense as written

DEA #   _____

          Print name

FIGURE 4 - 5 *Sample prescription for tablets.*

Name _____	Date _____
Address _____	Age _____

R̸x

Ibuprofen 400 mg
Dispense: 12 (twelve) tablets

_____   _____
Substitution Permitted   Dispense as written

DEA # _____   _____
                                                                                    Print name

FIGURE 4 - 6 *Sample prescription for liquids.*

Name _____	Date _____
Address _____	Age _____

R̸x

Penicillin VK susp. 125 mg/5 ml
Dispense 120 ml

_____   _____
Substitution Permitted   Dispense as written

DEA # _____   _____
                                                                                    Print name

time, other activities to perform, and when water can be used.

Figure 4-7 shows the body of the prescription completely written out, and Figure 4-8 shows the body of the prescription when abbreviations are used.

Closing. The closing of the prescription contains the following:
- Prescriber's signature*
- Drug Enforcement Administration (DEA) number, if required †
- Refill instructions ‡

After the body of the prescription, space is provided for the prescriber's signature. Sometimes certain states have more than one place to sign. For example, in Missouri, signing on the left agrees to substitution, whereas in Kansas the prescriber must sign on the right (Figure 4-9). Certain institutions also provide a space upon which to print the prescriber's name. This is not necessary for dentists with their own prescription blanks. If there are several dentists in one office, the names of all the dentists in the practice should be included on the prescription blanks. Then the individual dentist should check a box or circle his name so the pharmacist will know who signed the prescription.

The signature area should also include space for the DEA number. A location for refill instructions may be included, although it is not recommended. By omitting a reference to refills or leaving a space in which to put the number of refills on the prescription blank, the prescriber

---

* Required by law.
†Controlled substances. Pharmacists often need a prescriber's DEA number in order to enter a prescription into a computer, whether it is for a controlled substance or not.
‡May be included or omitted. (In general, there are few indications for providing refills on dental prescriptions. A refill on an antibiotic means that the dentist will not be examining the patient if symptoms persist (the exception is **endocarditis** prophylaxis.)

TABLE 4-3   Common Abbreviations

ABBREVIATION	ENGLISH
a or ā	before
ac	before meals
bid	twice a day
c̄	with
cap	capsule
d	day
disp	dispense
gm	gram
gr	grain
gtt	drop
h	hour
hs	at bedtime
p̄	after
pc	after meals
PO	by mouth
prn	as required, if needed
q	every
qid	4 times a day
s̄	without
sig	write (label)
s̄s̄	one-half
stat	immediately (now)
tab	tablet
tid	3 times a day
ud	as directed

---

doesn't have to remember to fill in that blank space with "0" if no refills are intended. Drugs that are not controlled substances often need a DEA number because insurance companies and computers often use that number as an identifier (this may change).

LABEL The law requires that all prescriptions must be labeled with the name of the medication and its strength. Figure 4-10 is a sample prescription label. This allows easy identification by other practitioners or quick identification in emergency situations. Note that the name, address, and telephone number of the pharmacy, the patient's and dentist's names, the directions for use, the name and strength of the medication, and the original date and the date filled (refilled) are required. The quantity of medication dispensed (number of tablets) and the number of refills remaining may be noted as well. If a ge-

FIGURE **4 - 7** *Sample prescription for tablets (abbreviated a bit).*

Name _____ Date _____
Address _____ Age _____

R𝗑 *Ibuprofen 600 mg tablets*
Dispense: 12 (twelve) tablets
(or 12 {XII} tablets)
Sig: Take 2 tablets every 4 hours if
needed for pain

Substitution Permitted _____ Dispense as written

DEA # _____ Print name

FIGURE **4 - 8** *Sample prescription for tablets (abbreviated a lot).*

Name _____ Date _____
Address _____ Age _____

R𝗑
Ibuprofen 600 mg tabs
Disp: # 12 (XII) or
 # 12 (twelve)
Sig: 2 tabs q 4 h prn pain

Substitution Permitted _____ Dispense as written

DEA # _____ Print name

F I G U R E 4 - 9 *Kansas and Missouri prescription blanks compared (determined by law). The place where the prescriber signs determines whether generic drugs are acceptable to use. Note that for each state the side differs.*

Name _____ Date _____

Address _____ Age _____

R̸

KANSAS BLANK

Sign here

Signature here allows generic substitution

_____
Dispense as written   Brand Exchange Permissible

_____
DEA #   Print name

Name _____ Date _____

Address _____ Age _____

R̸

MISSOURI BLANK

Signature here allows generic substitution

Sign here

_____
Substitution Permitted   Dispense as written

_____
Print name   DEA #

neric drug is prescribed, then the generic name of the drug and the company who manufactures it is required on the label. If the trade name is used, only the trade name is required on the label.

In most states, before a dentist can legally write a prescription for a patient, the following two criteria must be met:

- **Patient of record:** The person for whom the prescription is being written is a patient of record (no next-door neighbors or relatives, unless they are also patients of record)

FIGURE 4-10   *Typical prescription label.*

```
┌─────────────────────────────────────────┐
│ Acme Pharmacy          555-1234           │
│ 1234 Main St. Anywhere, KS 66666          │
├─────────────────────────────────────────┤
│ Rx 12345          Dr. Knowpaign           │
│ Doe, John                                 │
│ Take one tablet every four to six hours   │
│ if needed for pain.                       │
│ Acetaminophen/codeine 300 mg/30 mg        │
│ Rugby   #12   No refills 6-1-99   brc     │
└─────────────────────────────────────────┘
```

- **Dental condition:** The condition for which the prescription is being prescribed is a dental-related condition (no birth control pills or thyroid replacement drugs).

> With knowledge of a few abbreviations, you can read most prescriptions.

Abbreviations. A few abbreviation forms are used in prescription writing to save time. The abbreviations also make alteration of a prescription by the patient more difficult. In some cases they are necessary to get all the required information into the space on the prescription form. Some abbreviations that may be useful are shown in Table 4-3. If abbreviations are used on a prescription, they should be clearly written. For example, the three abbreviations *qd* (every day), *qod* (every other day), and *qid* (4 times a day) can look quite similar, but choosing the wrong one could be disastrous.

EXPLANATIONS ACCOMPANYING PRESCRIPTIONS

The dental health care worker should be able to answer the patient's questions about the prescription and should make sure that the patient knows how to take the medication prescribed (how long and when), what precautions to observe (drug interactions, possible side effects, driving limitations), and the reason for taking the medication. Information about the consequences of noncompliance should be included. By informing the patient about the medication, the likelihood that the patient will comply with the prescription instructions increases. The dental office should either keep a copy of each prescription written in the patient's record or record the medication, dose, and number prescribed. A patient should never get home and not know which drug is the antibiotic (for infection) and which is the analgesic (for pain). Side effects, such as drowsiness (for Schedule II drugs) or stomach upset, should be noted on the label.

Some drug abusers ("shoppers") search for dental offices that might provide them with prescriptions for controlled substances or prescription blanks that they can use to forge their own prescriptions. Every dental office should keep prescription blanks in a secure place. The prescriber's DEA number should not be printed on the prescription blanks, but should be written in only when needed.* The dental health care worker should watch to see that prescription blanks are not scattered around the office. If the dentist practices in a state that requires "triplicate" prescription blanks for Schedule II prescriptions, then those pads must be stored under lock and key to prevent them from being stolen.

DRUG LEGISLATION

The Food and Drug Act of 1906 was the first federal law to regulate interstate commerce in drugs.

The Harrison Narcotic Act of 1914 and its amendments provided federal control over narcotic drugs and required registration of all practitioners prescribing narcotics.

---

*Because of the use of DEA numbers to file insurance claims, there may come a time when including the DEA number on the prescription blank becomes commonplace.

▮ TABLE 4-4 Schedules of Controlled Substances

SCHEDULE	ABUSE POTENTIAL	EXAMPLES	HANDLING
I	Highest	Heroin, LSD, marijuana, hallucinogens	No accepted medical use, experimental use, only in research
II	High	Oxycodone, morphine, amphetamine, secobarbital	Written prescription with provider's signature only; no refills
III	Moderate	Codeine mixtures (e.g., Tylenol #3), hydrocodone mixtures (Vicodin)	Prescriptions may be telephoned; no more than 5 refills in less than 6 months
IV	Less	Diazepam (Valium), dextropropoxyphene forms (Darvon)	Prescriptions may be telephoned; no more than 5 refills in less than 6 months
V	Least	Some codeine-containing cough syrups	Can be bought OTC in some states

The Food and Drug Act was rewritten and became the Food, Drug and Cosmetic Act of 1938. This law and its subsequent amendments prohibit interstate commerce in drugs that have not been shown to be safe and effective. The Durham-Humphrey Law of 1952 is a particularly important amendment to the Food, Drug and Cosmetic Act because it requires that certain types of drugs be sold by prescription only. This law requires that these drugs be labeled as follows: "Caution: Federal law prohibits dispensing without prescription." This law also prohibits the refilling of a prescription unless directions to the contrary are indicated on the prescription. The Drug Amendments of 1962 (Kefauver-Harris Bill) made major changes in the Food, Drug and Cosmetic Act. Under these amendments, manufacturers were required to demonstrate the effectiveness of drugs, to follow strict rules in testing, and to submit to the FDA any reports of adverse effects from drugs already on the market. Manufacturers were also required to list drug ingredients by generic name in labeling and advertising and to state adverse effects, contraindications, and efficacy of a drug.

The Drug Abuse Control Amendments of 1965 required accounting for drugs with a potential for abuse, such as the **barbiturates** and amphetamines.

The Controlled Substance Act of 1970 replaced the Harrison Narcotic Act and the Drug Abuse Control Amendments to the Food, Drug and Cosmetic Act. The Controlled Substances Act is extremely important because it sets current requirements for writing prescriptions for drugs frequently prescribed in dental practice.

SCHEDULED DRUGS

The federal law divides controlled substances into five schedules according to their abuse potential (Table 4-4). The rules for prescribing these agents, whether prescriptions can be telephoned to the pharmacist, and whether refills are allowed differ depending on the drug's schedule. New drug entities are evaluated and added to the appropriate schedule. Drugs on the market may be moved from one schedule to another if changes in abuse patterns are discovered.

The current requirements for prescribing controlled drugs (Controlled Substance Act of 1970) are as follows:
- Any prescription for a controlled substance requires a DEA number.
- All Schedule II through IV drugs require a prescription.
- Any prescription for Schedule II drugs must be written in pen or indelible ink or typed. A designate of the dentist, such as the dental hygienist, may write the prescription, but the prescriber must personally sign the prescrip-

tion in ink and is responsible for what any designee has written.

- Schedule II prescriptions cannot be telephoned to the pharmacist (except at the discretion of the pharmacist for an emergency supply to be followed by a written prescription within 72 hours).
- Because Schedule II prescriptions cannot be refilled, the patient needs to obtain a new written prescription to obtain more medication.
- Certain states require the use of "triplicate" prescription blanks for Schedule II drugs. These blanks, provided by the state, are requested by the dentist. After a prescription is written, the dentist keeps one copy and gives two copies to the patient. The patient presents these two copies to the pharmacist, who must file one copy and send the other to the [insert state name] State Board of Pharmacy. These consecutively numbered blank prescription pads provide additional control for Schedule II drugs.
- Prescriptions for Schedule III and IV drugs may be telephoned to the pharmacist and may be refilled no more than 5 times in 6 months, if so noted on the prescription.

REVIEW QUESTIONS

1. List the information required in a prescription.
2. Perform the following conversions:
   a. Grains to milligrams and milligrams to grains (approximate). For example,
   $\frac{1}{2}$ gr equals how many milligrams?
   5 mg equals how many grains?
   b. Pounds to kilograms and kilograms to pounds. For example, if a patient weighs 55 kg, how many pounds is that?
   c. Milliliters to cubic centimeters and cubic centimeters to milliliters. For example, 15 ml equals how many cubic centimeters?
   40 cc equals how many milliliters?
   d. Teaspoonfuls to milliliters and milliliters to teaspoonfuls. For example,
   2 tsp equals how many milliliters?
   5 ml equals how many teaspoonfuls?
3. Given a prescription written using Latin abbreviations, state the directions to the patient in English. For example,
   Ibuprofen 400 mg
   Disp: 20 (twenty)
   Sig: 1-2 tabs q4h prn pain
4. Explain two precautions that should be taken in the dental office to discourage drug abusers.
5. List the components of the Controlled Substance Act, and explain how it affects the dental office.
6. Describe the difference in the rules for prescribing, providing, and refilling Schedule II and III drugs. State a difference that would change a part of your practice.
7. Describe the procedures necessary for handling controlled substances in the dental office. Explain the amount of supervision required.

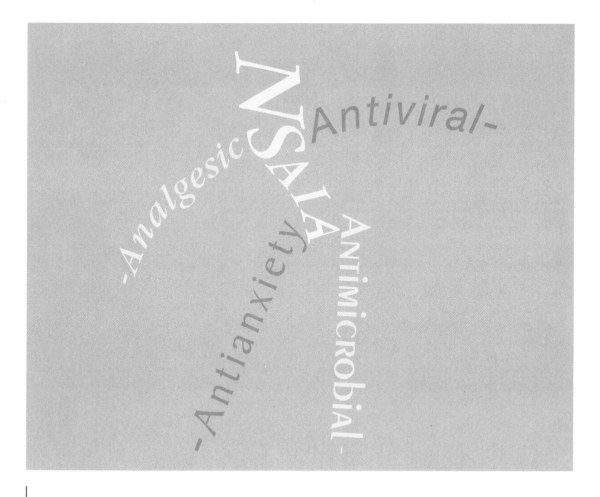

Drugs Used in Dentistry

Autonomic Drugs

The dentist and the dental hygienist should become familiar with the autonomic nervous system (ANS) drugs for three reasons. First, certain ANS drugs are used in dentistry. For example, both the vasoconstrictors added to some local anesthetic solutions and the drugs used to increase salivary flow are ANS drugs. Second, some ANS drugs produce oral adverse reactions. For example, the anticholinergics produce xerostomia. Third, members of other drug groups have effects similar to the ANS drugs. Antidepressants and antipsychotics are drug groups with autonomic side effects—specifically anticholinergic effects. An understanding of the effects of the autonomic drugs on the body will facilitate an understanding of the action of other drug groups that have autonomic effects. Before the ANS drugs can be under-

ANS drug effects are important because many other drugs have the same effects.

stood, the normal functioning of the autonomic nervous system must be reviewed. A review of the physiology of the ANS will be helpful in understanding the ANS drugs.

AUTONOMIC NERVOUS SYSTEM

The ANS functions largely as an automatic modulating system for many bodily functions, including the regulation of blood pressure and **heart rate,** gastrointestinal tract motility, salivary gland secretions, and bronchial smooth muscle. This system relies on specific neurotransmitters (chemicals that are released to send messages) and a variety of receptors to initiate functional responses in the target tissues. Before ANS pharmacology is discussed, the anatomy and physiology of this system are reviewed.

ANATOMY

The ANS has two divisions, the sympathetic autonomic nervous system (SANS) and the para-

sympathetic autonomic nervous system (PANS). Each consists of **afferent** (sensory) fibers [What's happening?], central integrating areas [Let's coordinate all this info! Hey, what did you find out?], efferent (peripheral) motor preganglionic fibers, and postganglionic motor fibers [Begin sweating! Heart begin palpitating!].

The preganglionic neuron (Figure 5-1) originates in the central nervous system (CNS) and passes out to form the ganglia at the synapse with the postganglionic neuron. The space between the preganglionic and postganglionic fibers is termed the *synapse* or *synaptic cleft.* The postganglionic neuron originates in the ganglia and innervates the effector organ or tissue.

PARASYMPATHETIC AUTONOMIC NERVOUS SYSTEM (PANS)

Cell bodies in the CNS give rise to the preganglionic fibers of the parasympathetic division. They originate in the nuclei of the third, seventh, ninth, and tenth cranial nerves (CN III, VII, IX, and X), as well as the second through the fourth **sacral** segments (S2 to S4) of the spinal cord [Sometimes referred to as the "neck and

FIGURE 5 - 1 *Typical efferent nerve. The preganglionic fiber originates in the brain. It ends at the synapse, where the neurotransmitter carries the message to the postganglionic fiber. A group of synapses make up a ganglia. The postganglionic fiber releases a neurotransmitter to send the message to effector organ.*

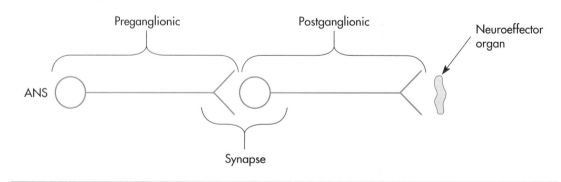

butt" distribution, but only by a verrrry few]. The preganglionic fibers of the PANS are relatively long and extend near to or into the innervated organ. The distribution is relatively simple for the third, seventh, and ninth cranial nerves, whereas the tenth or vagus nerve has a complex distribution. There usually is a low ratio of synaptic connections between preganglionic and postganglionic neurons, which leads to a discrete response when the PANS is stimulated. The postganglionic fibers, originating in the ganglia, are usually short and terminate on the innervated tissue.

SYMPATHETIC AUTONOMIC NERVOUS SYSTEM (SANS)

The cell bodies that give origin to the preganglionic fibers of the SANS span from the thoracic (T1) to the **lumbar** (L2) portion of the spinal cord [Sometimes referred to as the "in between" distribution, that is, between the two locations of the innervation of the PANS]. This produces a more diffuse effect in the SANS. The preganglionic fibers exit the cord to enter the sympathetic chain located along each side of the vertebral column. Once a part of the sympathetic chain (lumps of nerves a few inches from the vertebral column), preganglionic fibers form multiple synaptic connections (more lumps) with postganglionic cell bodies located up and down the sympathetic chain. Thus a single SANS preganglionic fiber often synapses with numerous postganglionic neurons. This produces a more diffuse effect in the SANS. The postganglionic fibers then terminate at the effector organ or tissues.

The adrenal **medulla** is also innervated by the sympathetic preganglionic fibers. It functions much like a large sympathetic ganglion, with the glands in the medulla representing the postganglionic component. When the SANS is stimulated, the adrenal medulla releases primarily epinephrine and a small amount of norepinephrine (NE) into the systemic circulation. A diffuse response is produced when the SANS is stimulated because of the high ratio of synaptic connections between the preganglionic and postganglionic fibers and because epinephrine is released by the adrenal medulla when stimulated.

FUNCTIONAL ORGANIZATION

In general the divisions of the ANS, the parasympathetic and the sympathetic, tend to act in opposite directions. The parasympathetic division of the ANS is concerned with the conservation of the body processes. Both digestion and

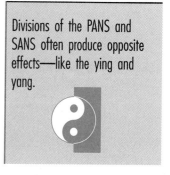

Divisions of the PANS and SANS often produce opposite effects—like the ying and yang.

intestinal tract motility are greatly influenced by the PANS. Think of PANS activation as Cleopatra lounging on a "fainting" couch (Figure 5-2). The sympathetic division is designed to cope with sudden emergencies such as the "fright or flight" or "fight or flight" situation. Imagine the effects associated with the SANS to be similar to the caveman running from a tiger (Figure 5-3). In most but not all instances the actions produced by each system are opposite—one increases the heart rate and the other decreases it, one dilates the pupils of the eye and the other constricts them. The receptors being innervated for each function may be different. For example, both the PANS and the SANS stimulate muscles in the eye that change the size of the pupil. The SANS stimulates the radial smooth muscles (out from the pupil like sun rays), producing an increase in pupil size. When the pupils are *di*lated the effect is termed my*dr*iasis (Figure 5-4). The PANS stimulates the circular smooth muscles (like a bull's-eye), producing a decrease in pupil size. When pupils are c*o*nstricted the effect is termed my*o*sis.

FIGURE 5-2 *Cleopatra on a fainting couch illustrates the action of the PANS. The functions activated are called "vegetative"—salivating, eating, increased gastrointestinal tract motility, urination, and defecation.*

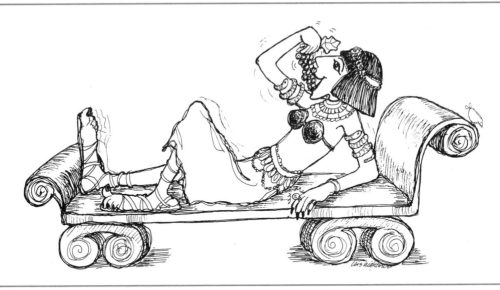

FIGURE 5-3 *A caveman running from a tiger illustrates the action of the SANS. The important functions of the SANS are called "fight or flight" and include stimulation of the heart and control of the blood vessel diameter.*

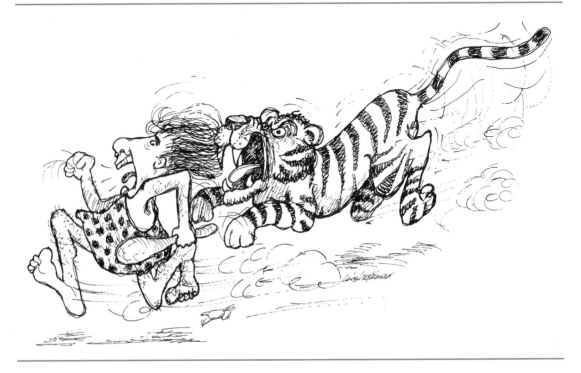

F I G U R E 5 - 4 *Terms for pupil diameter; pupil size term reminder:* my**d**riasis = *dilated, and* my**o**sis = *constricted.*

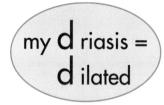

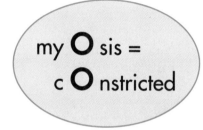

Almost all body tissues are innervated by the ANS, with many, but not all, organs receiving both parasympathetic and sympathetic **innervation.** The response of a specific tissue to stimuli at any one time will be equal to the sum of the excitatory and inhibitory influences of the two divisions of the ANS (if a tissue receives both innervations). Table 5-1 summarizes the responses of the major tissues and organ systems to the ANS. When learning the normal functions of the body, consider what would have occurred because of evolution (Box 5-1).

In addition to the dual innervation of tissues, there is another way in which the two divisions of the ANS can interact. Sensory fibers in one division can influence the motor fibers in the other. Thus, although in an isolated tissue preparation the stimulation of one of the divisions would produce a specific response, in the intact body a more complex and integrated response can be expected. The net effect would be a combination of the direct and indirect effects.

NEUROTRANSMITTERS

Communication between nerves or between nerves and effector tissue takes place by the release of chemical neurotransmitters across the synaptic cleft. **Neurotransmitters** are released in response to the nerve action potential (or pharmacologic agents in certain cases) to interact with a specific membrane component, the receptor. Receptors are usually found on the postsynaptic fiber and the effector organ but may be located on the presynaptic membrane as well (Table 5-2). The interaction between neurotransmitter and receptor is specific and is rapidly terminated by disposition of the neurotransmitter substance. There are several specific mechanisms by which the neurotransmitter produces an effect on the receptor.

> Neurotransmitters are like carrier pigeons—they carry messages.

Disposition occurs most frequently by either reuptake into the presynaptic nerve terminal, or enzymatic breakdown of the transmitter. Nerves in the ANS contain the necessary enzyme systems and other metabolic processes to synthesize, store, and release neurotransmitters. Thus drugs can modify ANS activity by altering any of the events associated with neurotransmitters: (1) synthesis, (2) storage, (3) release, (4) receptor interaction, and (5) disposition. The specificity of the neurotransmitters and receptors dictates the tissue response.

- *Between the preganglionic and postganglionic nerves:* Acetylcholine is the neurotransmitter in the synapse (ganglia) formed between the preganglionic and postganglionic nerves. Nerves that release acetylcholine are termed **cholinergic.** Because this synapse is also stimulated by nicotine, it is also termed **nicotinic** in response.
- *Between postganglionic nerves and the effector tissues:*
- *PANS:* The neurotransmitter released from the postganglionic nerve terminal is acetylcholine; as before, it is also termed *cholin-*

TABLE 5-1 Effects of the ANS on Effector Organs

Organ	Aspect	PANS		SANS		
Eye	Lens (ciliary muscle)	Contraction (near vision)	+++	β_2	Relaxation (distant vision)	+
	Iris	Contraction—miosis	+++	α_1	Contraction Radial muscle—mydriasis	++
CVS	Heart—force (inotropic)			β_1, β_2	Increase force	
	Heart, SA node—rate (chronotropic)	Decreases heart rate	+++	β_1, β_2	Increases	
Blood vessels, smooth muscles	Coronary			$\alpha_1, \beta_1, \beta_2$	Constriction (α), dilation (β)	
	Skin/mucosa			α_1, α_2	Constriction	+++
	Skeletal muscle	Dilation	+	α_1 β_2	Constriction Dilation	++
	Abdominal viscera			α_1 β_2	Constriction Dilation	
	Salivary glands	Dilation	++	α_1, α_2	Constriction	+++
Lungs	Bronchial smooth muscle	Contraction	+++	β_2	Relaxation	+
	Secretions—bronchial, nasopharyngeal		++/++ +	α_1, β_1	Secretion—increase/ decrease	
Gastrointestinal tract/genitourinary tract	Motility/tone	Contracts, increases	+++	$\alpha_1, \alpha_2,$ β_1, β_2	Relaxes	
Stomach, intestine, bladder	Sphincters	Relaxation	+/++	α_1	Contraction	
	Secretions— gastrointestinal tract	Stimulation	++/++ +	α_2	Inhibition	
	Secretion—glands; salivary	Increase—profuse and watery	+++	β	Viscous—thick	+
	Uterus	—		α_1, β_2		
Endocrine	Pancreas, acini	Secretion		α_1	Decreases secretions	
	Pancreas, islet cells	—		α_2	Decreases secretions	
	Adrenal medulla	Secretion— epinephrine/ norepinephrine				
Skin	Sweat	Secretion, generalized			Secretion, local	
	Pilomotor muscles	—		α_1	Contraction	++
Liver	Glycogen synthesis		+	α_1 β_2	Glycogenolysis Gluconeogenesis	+++
Other	Adipose tissue	—		$\alpha_2, \beta_1, \beta_2$	Lipolysis	
	Male sex organs	Erection	+++	α_1	Ejaculation	+++
	Skeletal muscle			β_2	Contraction	

BOX 5-1 EVOLUTION: WHY WE ARE THE WAY WE ARE

It would be best.

How did certain functions in our bodies become the way they are? Why are certain organs activated by certain stimuli? Let's consider the mantra, *"It would be best."* The cave human had to escape from predators in order to procreate and send genes into the next generation. So "flight or fight" served ancient humans well, that is "Let's get away from that lion!" But, what would be best for "fight or flight?"

- It would be best for the heart to beat fast, for if it did not, the human could not run and the lion would eat the human.
- It would be best if the lungs could take in lots of air; otherwise the oxygen needs of the human muscles would not be met and the lion would eat the human.
- It would be best to have the blood vessels in the skin constrict (α-receptors); otherwise when that errant lion claw scratched the human, the human would bleed and the lion would eat the human.
- It would be best if the blood vessels in the muscles were dilated (β-receptors); otherwise the oxygen supply to the muscles would be lacking and escape would be impossible and the lion would eat the human.

- It would be best for the pupil to be dilated so that the human could see the most, otherwise the human would be caught and the lion would eat the human.

If the lion ate the human, then those genes would not be passed on to the next generation. Only humans that had functions that allowed survival would pass their genes to the next generation and the next and the next. . .

It wouldn't be best . . . .

- It wouldn't be best to stop and urinate or defecate—no visits to the outhouse, otherwise the lion would eat the human.
- It wouldn't be best if the human's blood supply went to the stomach to digest food, because the lion would eat the human. It would be best to first save all the blood and send it to the muscles to make them fast and facilitate escape.
- It wouldn't be best to salivate at the sight of another animal—yum; yum isn't the best thought now, otherwise the lion would eat the human. The body has its priorities straight; it gets away from the lion chasing the human first.

TABLE 5-2 Types of Cholinergic Receptors

Receptor Site	Location	Neurotransmitter	Stimulating Agent	Blocking Agent
Muscarinic	B	Acetylcholine	Muscarine	Atropine
Nicotinic	C	Acetylcholine	Nicotine	Hexamethonium
Somatic-skeletal muscle	D	Acetycholine	Nicotine	*d*-Tubocurarine (curare)

ergic. Because the postsynaptic tissue responds to muscarine it is identified as **muscarinic.** Thus the cholinergic synapses are distinguished from one another.

- *SANS:* Norepinephrine is the transmitter substance released by the postganglionic nerves and is designated as adrenergic.
- *Neuromuscular junction:* Although not

within the ANS, the neuromuscular junction (Figure 5-5) of skeletal muscle releases the neurotransmitter acetylcholine and is termed *cholinergic.* The neuromuscular junction is part of the somatic system and is discussed in Chapters 5 and 11. The figures below and on the following page illustrates the PANS, SANS, and neuromuscular junction.

F IGURE 5 - 5   *The neuromusculor junction of skeletal muscle releases acetylcholine.*

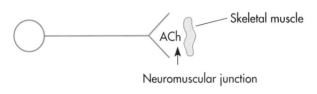

DRUG GROUPS

The four drug groups in the ANS exert their effects primarily on the organs or tissues innervated by the ANS. (They are just doing the same thing that the body would normally do when it's working.) Each of the divisions of the nervous system—the PANS and the SANS—can be affected. The action of each of the divisions of the ANS can be increased or decreased.

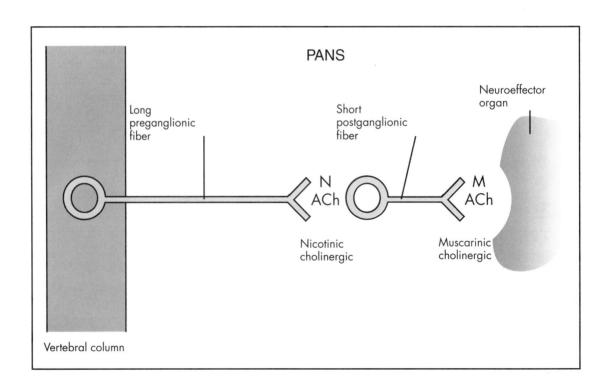

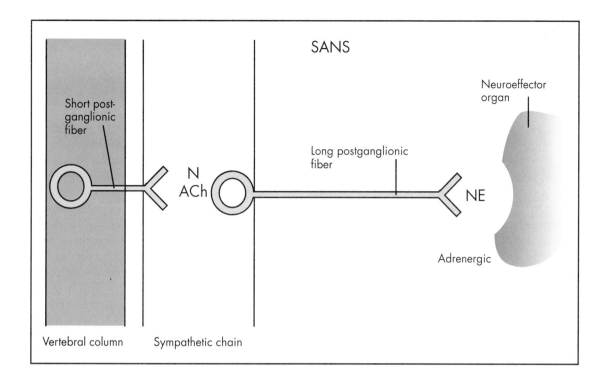

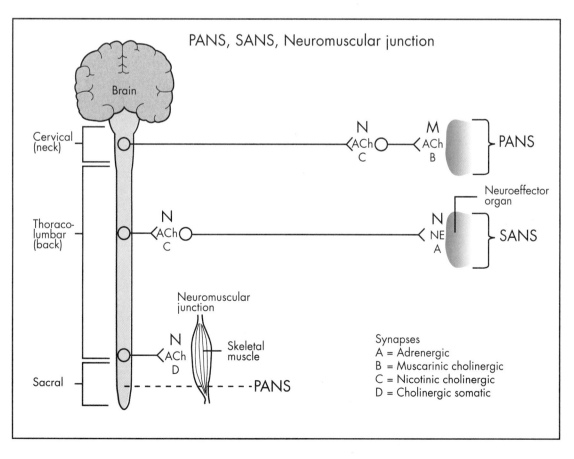

These four functions divide the ANS drugs into four groups: P+, P−, S+, and S−. Stimulation of the PANS can be abbreviated *P+*, and blocking the PANS can be abbreviated *P−*. Stimulation of the SANS can be abbreviated *S+*, and blocking the SANS can be abbreviated *S−*. These abbreviations are not routinely used in the literature, but are helpful with note taking, outlines, and discussions. The groups are named by several methods, but the basic concepts of naming include the following:

- A drug that acts at the location where acetylcholine is released as the neurotransmitter is termed *cholinergic* (from acetylcholine).
- A drug that acts at the location where norepinephrine is the neurotransmitter released is termed *adrenergic* (taken from the early trade name of epinephrine, Adrenalin).
- A drug that acts at the location where the PANS acts has the prefix *parasympatho-*.
- A drug that acts at the location where the SANS acts has the prefix *sympatho-*.
- A drug that acts at the location where a division of the ANS acts and produces the same effect as the neurotransmitter has the suffix *-mimetic* (as in *mime*, acts like). It can also be referred to as an *agonist* (see Chapter 2).
- A drug that acts at the location where a division of the ANS acts and blocks the action of the neurotransmitter has the suffix *-lytic* or *-blocker*. It can also be referred to as an *antagonist* (see Chapter 2).

Using this nomenclature, the four groups of ANS drugs can be abbreviated as P+ (cholinergics, parasympathomimetics), P− (anticholinergics, parasympatholytics, or cholinergic-blockers), S+ (sympathomimetics, adrenergics), and S− (adrenergic blockers, sympathetic blockers, sympatholytics).

PARASYMPATHETIC AUTONOMIC NERVOUS SYSTEM (PANS)

Acetylcholine has been identified as the principal mediator in the PANS. When an action potential travels along the nerve, it causes the release of the stored acetylcholine from the synaptic storage vesicles, and, if sufficient acetylcholine is released, it will initiate a response in the postsynaptic tissue. If the postsynaptic tissue is a postganglionic nerve, depolarization with generation of an action potential occurs in that neuron. In the postganglionic parasympathetic fibers, the postsynaptic tissue is an effector organ and the response will be the same as that of the neurotransmitter. The action of the released acetylcholine is terminated by hydrolysis by acetylcholinesterase to yield the inactive metabolites choline and acetic acid (see diagram below).

Some of the postsynaptic tissues respond to acetylcholine because of an interaction between acetylcholine and these tissues. In order to be an effective mediator, acetylcholine must fit both physically and chemically at the receptor. It has been shown that atropine [A-troe-peen] can block the action of acetylcholine at the postganglionic endings in the PANS, but not at the neuromuscular junction. In contrast, curare blocks the response of skeletal muscle to acetylcholine, but does not block its effect on tissues such as the salivary gland. Hexamethonium blocks the action of acetylcholine at the ganglia. From these observations, one can infer that there are differences among receptors that have acetylcholine as a

> **3 ACh receptors**
> **1.** PANS
> **2.** Ganglionic
> **3.** Neuromuscular junction

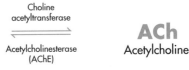

A + **Ch** ⇌ **ACh**
Acetyl   Choline   Acetylcholine
(CoA)

Choline acetyltransferase
Acetylcholinesterase (AChE)

	CLASSIFICATION	DRUG NAME	THERAPEUTIC USE
TABLE 5-3 — **Cholinergic (Parasympathomimetic) Agents**			
Direct–acting	Choline esters	Bethanechol (Urecholine)	Urinary retention
	Other	Pilocarpine (Isopto Carpine)	Glaucoma
	Other	Pilocarpine (Salagen)	Xerostomia
Indirect–acting	Reversible agents	Physostigmine	Some drug overdoses
		Neostigmine (Prostigmin)	Myasthenia gravis, reversible
		Pyridostigmine (Mestinon)	nondepolarizing **muscle relaxants**
	Irreversible organophosphates	Malathion, Parathion	Agricultural insecticides
		Sarin (GB)	"Nerve gases," chemical
		Tabun	warfare

neurotransmitter—subtypes of acetylcholine-innervated receptors that are located in anatomically different synapses. Other factors such as the amount of acetylcholine released, the size of the synaptic cleft, and the tissue penetration of a drug may also account for differences in the response of the receptor to drugs at each acetylcholine-mediated junction.

CHOLINERGIC (PARASYMPATHOMIMETIC) AGENTS

Depending on their mechanism of action (Table 5-3) the **cholinergic (parasympathomimetic)** agents are classified as direct (acts on receptor) acting, or indirect (causes release of neurotransmitter). The direct acting agents (Figure 5-6) include the choline derivatives and pilocarpine. The choline derivatives include both acetylcholine and other, more stable choline derivatives. These derivatives of acetylcholine possess activity similar to PANS stimulation but have a longer duration of action and are more selective.

The indirect-acting (see Figure 5-6) parasympathomimetic agents or cholinesterase inhibitors act by inhibiting the enzyme cholinesterase.

When the enzyme that normally destroys acetylcholine is inhibited, the concentration of

FIGURE 5-6 *Mechanism of action of cholinergic (P+) agents: direct- and indirect-acting.*

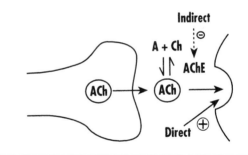

acetylcholine builds up (it is not being destroyed), resulting in PANS stimulation.

Pharmacologic effects

CARDIOVASCULAR The cardiovascular effects associated with the cholinergic agents are the result of both direct and indirect actions. The direct effect on the heart produces a negative chronotropic and negative inotropic action. A decrease in cardiac output is associated with these agents.

The cholinergic agents' effects on the smooth muscles around the blood vessels results in relaxation and vasodilation, producing a decrease in total peripheral resistance. The indirect effect of these agents is an increase in heart rate and cardiac output. Because the direct and indirect effects of these agents on the heart rate and cardiac output are opposite, the resulting effect will depend on the concentration of the drug present. Generally, there is **bradycardia** and a decrease in blood pressure and cardiac output.

GASTROINTESTINAL The cholinergic agents excite the smooth muscle of the gastrointestinal tract, producing an increase in activity, motility, and secretion.

EYE The cholinergic agents produce miosis and cause cycloplegia. Cycloplegia is a spasm of accommodation, so that the eye becomes focused for near vision. Because intraocular pressure is also decreased, these agents are useful in the treatment of glaucoma.

Salivation
Lacrimation
Urination
Defecation

Adverse reactions. The adverse reactions that are associated with the administration of the cholinergic agents are essentially extensions of their pharmacologic effects. When large doses of these agents are ingested, the resultant toxic effects are described by the acronym *SLUD*: salivation, lacrimation, urination, and defecation. With even larger doses, neuromuscular **paralysis** can occur as a result of the effect on the neuromuscular junction. Central nervous system (CNS) effects such as confusion can be seen if toxic doses are administered.

The treatment of an **overdose** of cholinesterase inhibitors such as the insecticides or organophosphates (parathion) includes a combination of pralidoxime [pra-li-DOX-eem] (2-PAM, Protopam) and atropine. Pralidoxime regenerates the irreversibly bound acetylcholine receptor sites that are bound by the inhibitors [knocks

them off like a prize fighter], and atropine blocks [competitively] the muscarinic effects of the excess acetylcholine present.

Contraindications. The relative contraindications to or cautions with the use of the cholinergic agents stem from these agents' pharmacologic effects and adverse reactions. They include the following:
- *Bronchial asthma:* Cholinergic agents may cause bronchospasms or precipitate an asthmatic attack.
- *Hyperthyroidism:* **Hypothyroidism** may cause an increased risk of **atrial fibrillation.**
- *Gastrointestinal tract or urinary tract obstruction:* If either the gastrointestinal tract or urinary tract is obstructed and a cholinergic agent is given, an increase in secretions and motility could cause pressure and the system could "back up."
- *Severe cardiac disease:* The reflex **tachycardia** that can result from administering anticholinergic agents may exacerbate a severe cardiac condition.
- *Myasthenia gravis treated with neostigmine:* Patients with **myasthenia gravis** should not be given irreversible cholinesterase inhibitors because neostigmine would be occupying the enzyme and the irreversible agent would not function.
- *Peptic ulcer:* Anticholinergic agents stimulate gastric acid secretion and increase gastric motility. This action could exacerbate an ulcer.

Uses. The direct-acting agents are used primarily in the treatment of glaucoma, a condition in which the intraocular pressure is elevated. Occasionally, they are used to treat myasthenia gravis, a disease resulting in muscle weakness from an autoimmune reaction that reduces the effect of acetylcholine on the voluntary muscles. The urinary retention that occurs after surgery is also treated with the choline esters (see Table 5-3).

Pilocarpine [pye-loe-KAR-peen] (Salagen), a naturally occurring cholinergic agent, is used in the treatment of xerostomia, but its success may be limited because of the myriad of potential side effects. Common side effects from pilocarpine include perspiration (sweating), nausea, rhinitis, chills, and flushing. Pilocarpine is available in 5-mg tablets. The usual dose of pilocarpine is 5 mg tid. This can be obtained by giving one 5-mg tablet tid (cost for a month's supply is $100). Pilocarpine is also available as ophthalmic solution in strengths ranging from 0.5% to 10%. It is used topically in the eye to treat glaucoma. Several strengths (e.g., 2%) are available as generic preparations. By taking the ophthalmic solution orally (units are drops), the patient can obtain the usual dose. The usual dose of pilocarpine (5 mg) is contained in 5 drops of 2% pilocarpine ophthalmic solution. The starting dose for pilocarpine for xerostomia using the pilocarpine ophthalmic solution is 5 drops tid (one month's supply is $12).

The indirect-acting cholinergic agents, the cholinesterase inhibitors, are divided into groups based on the degree of reversibility with which they are bound to the enzyme. Edrophonium is rapidly reversible, whereas physostigmine and neostigmine are slowly reversible. These agents are used to treat glaucoma and myasthenia gravis.

Physostigmine [fi-zoe-STIG-meen] (Antilirium) has been used to treat reactions caused by several different kinds of drugs. Acute toxicity from the anticholinergic agents (such as atropine), as well as other agents that have anticholinergic action (such as the phenothiazines, tricyclic antidepressants, and antihistamines), has been treated with physostigmine.

The cholinesterase inhibitors developed for use as insecticides and chemical warfare agents are essentially irreversible; and what do you think they are called?—the *irreversible* cholinesterase inhibitors. Members of this group include parathion, malathion, and sarin [used on a subway in Japan to poison riders].

ANTICHOLINERGIC (PARASYMPATHOLYTIC) AGENTS

The anticholinergic agents prevent the action of acetylcholine at the postganglionic parasympathetic endings. The release of acetylcholine is not prevented, but the receptor site is competitively blocked by the anticholinergics. Thus the anticholinergic drugs block the action of acetylcholine on smooth muscles (e.g., intestines), glandular tissue (e.g., salivary glands), and the heart. These agents are called antimuscarinic agents because they block the muscarinic receptors and not the nicotinic receptors.

Pharmacologic effects

CENTRAL NERVOUS SYSTEM EFFECTS
Depending on the dose administered, the anticholinergics can produce CNS stimulation or depression. For example, usual therapeutic doses of scopolamine more frequently cause sedation, whereas atropine in high doses can cause stimulation. Atropine and scopolamine are tertiary agents, and propantheline [proe-PAN-the-leen] (Pro-Banthine) and glycopyrrolate (Robinul) are quaternary agents (Figure 5-7). Because of their water solubility, quaternary agents do not penetrate the CNS well. The tertiary agents are lipid soluble, and they can easily penetrate the brain. The quaternary agents have fewer CNS adverse reactions because they are less likely to enter the brain.

EFFECTS ON EXOCRINE GLANDS
The anticholinergics affect the exocrine glands by reducing the flow and the volume of their secretions. These glands are located in the respiratory, gastrointestinal, and genitourinary tracts. This effect is used therapeutically in dentistry to decrease salivation and create a dry field for certain dental procedures such as obtaining a difficult impression.

EFFECTS ON SMOOTH MUSCLE
Anticholinergics relax the smooth muscle in the respiratory and gastrointestinal tracts. Ipratropium is an an-

FIGURE 5-7 *Anticholinergics, brain penetration. Quaternary amines are charged and hydrophilic (water soluble) so they cannot easily penetrate the brain. Tertiary amines are uncharged and lipophilic (lipid soluble) so they easily penetrate the brain.*

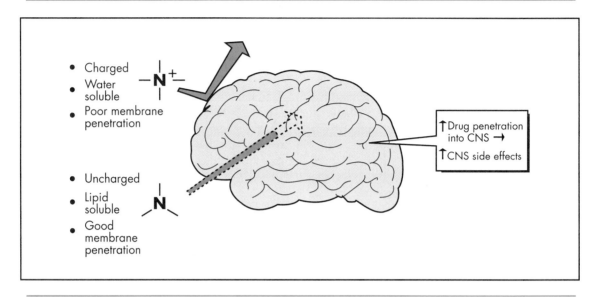

- Charged
- Water soluble
- Poor membrane penetration

−N+−

- Uncharged
- Lipid soluble
- Good membrane penetration

−N−

↑Drug penetration into CNS →
↑CNS side effects

ticholinergic inhaler used to treat asthma. This effect on gastrointestinal motility has given rise to the name *spasmolytic agents*. If these drugs are used repeatedly, constipation can result. By delaying gastric emptying and by decreasing esophageal and gastric motility, the anticholinergics may exacerbate the condition. The smooth muscle in the respiratory tract is relaxed by the anticholinergic agents, causing bronchial dilation. This effect is used to treat asthma.

EFFECTS ON THE EYE The parasympatholytics have two effects on the eye, *mydriasis* and *cycloplegia*. Cycloplegia refers to paralysis of accommodation so that the lens is focused for distance vision and near vision is blurred. The effects of cycloplegia and mydriasis are useful to prepare the eye for ophthalmologic examinations. For eye examinations, the **mydriasis** dilates the pupil so that the retina can be exam-

ined, and the cycloplegia allows for proper measurements to make glasses. These effects occur when the drug is given topically or systemically.

CARDIOVASCULAR EFFECTS With large therapeutic doses, the anticholinergic agents can produce vagal blockade, resulting in tachycardia. This effect has been used therapeutically to prevent cardiac slowing during general anesthesia. With small doses, bradycardia predominates. This variable response in the heart rate occurs because heart rate is a function of both direct (increased heart rate) and indirect (decreased heart rate) effects.

Adverse reactions. The adverse reactions associated with the anticholinergics are essentially extensions of their pharmacologic effects. These can include xerostomia (see Appendix H for a discussion of drugs that cause **xerostomia** and a discussion of artificial salivas), blurred vision, **photophobia,** tachycardia, fever, and urinary and gastrointestinal stasis. Hyperpyrexia (elevated temperature) and hot, dry, flushed skin caused by a lack of sweating are also seen. Hyperpyrexia is treated symptomatically.

Anticholinergic toxicity can cause signs of CNS excitation including delirium, **hallucinations,** convulsions, and respiratory depression.

Contraindications. Specific contraindications or cautions to the use of the anticholinergic agents include the following.

GLAUCOMA Anticholinergics are the only ANS drug group that can cause an acute rise in intraocular pressure in patients with narrow-angle (angle closure) glaucoma. Glaucoma is divided into narrow-angle (5% of glaucoma cases) and open-angle glaucoma (95% of glaucoma cases); cases of narrow-angle glaucoma are uncommon. Anticholinergic drugs can precipitate an acute attack in unrecognized cases of this rare condition. If narrow-angle glaucoma is diagnosed, emergency ophthalmic surgery must be immediately performed to relieve the eye pressure. In contrast, the patient with wide-angle glaucoma who is currently receiving treatment with eyedrops (many types) can be given a few doses of anticholinergic agents with impunity.

PROSTATIC HYPERTROPHY Because the anticholinergic agents can exacerbate urinary retention, older men with prostatic hypertrophy (many men over 50 years old) who are already have difficulty urinating should be given these agents only with great caution. Acute urinary retention that may require catheterization can occur.

INTESTINAL OR URINARY OBSTRUCTION OR RETENTION Constipation or acute urinary retention can be precipitated by the use of these agents in susceptible patients. Constipation can

be exacerbated, especially in patients with chronic constipation. [Give them an opioid {narcotic} for pain control to "cinch" the situation!]

CARDIOVASCULAR DISEASE Because anticholinergic agents have the ability to block the vagus nerve, resulting in tachycardia, patients with cardiovascular disease should be given these agents cautiously.

Use

PREOPERATIVE MEDICATION The anticholinergic agents are used preoperatively for two reasons. First, they inhibit the secretions of saliva and bronchial **mucus** that can be stimulated by general anesthesia. Second, they have the ability to block the vagal slowing of the heart that results from general anesthesia.

TREATMENT OF GASTROINTESTINAL DISORDERS Many types of gastrointestinal disorders associated with increased motility or acid secretion have been treated with anticholinergic agents. For example, patients with gastric ulcers are sometimes treated with the anticholinergic agents, even though there is little proof of their effectiveness. Both nonspecific diarrhea and hypermotility of the colon have also been treated with these agents. In the doses used, it is difficult to prove that the anticholinergic agents are effective for these purposes.

OPHTHALMOLOGIC EXAMINATION Because of the ability of anticholinergic agents to cause mydriasis and cycloplegia, they are commonly used topically before examinations of the eye. Producing mydriasis allows the full visualization of the retina. Cycloplegia is useful to relax the lens so that the proper prescription for eyeglasses may be determined.

REDUCTION OF PARKINSON-LIKE MOVEMENTS Before the advent of levodopa, anticholinergic agents were commonly used to reduce the tremors and rigidity associated with **Parkin-**

son's disease. Patients treated with these agents predictably experienced the side effects of dry mouth and blurred vision. At present, anticholinergic agents are only occasionally used in combination with levodopa for the treatment of Parkinson's disease.

The phenothiazines, used to treat psychoses, can produce extrapyramidal (Parkinson-like) side effects. These include abnormal mouth and tongue movements, rigidity, tremor, and restlessness. Anticholinergic agents such as trihexyphenidyl [trye-hex-ee-FEN-I-dill] (Artane) and benztropine [BENZ-troe-peen] (Cogentin) are often administered concurrently with the phenothiazines to reduce rigidity and tremor.

MOTION SICKNESS Scopolamine, because of its CNS depressant action, is used to treat motion sickness. Transdermal scopolamine is applied behind the ear to prevent motion sickness before boating trips.

DENTISTRY Anticholinergic agents can be used to produce a dry field before some dental procedures. The most commonly used agents, atropine, methantheline, and propantheline, as well as others, are listed in Table 5-4 with their usual oral doses. This dose should be administered between 1 and 2 hours before the dental appointment. Often it takes even longer to achieve the maximum effect because as it begins to work it relaxes the gastrointestinal tract and inhibits its own absorption. The dose may be repeated if no results are obtained within 1 hour. Given in appropriate oral doses (e.g., 0.5 mg atropine or 1 to 2 mg glycopyrrolate [glye-koe-PYE-roe-late] [Robinul]) these agents produce approximately equivalent results.

Drug interactions. The most important drug interaction associated with the anticholinergic agents is an additive anticholinergic effect. Other agents that have anticholinergic effects, such as the phenothiazines, antihistamines, and tricyclic antidepressants, can be additive with the parasympatholytics. Mixing more than one drug group possessing anticholinergic effects can lead to symptoms of anticholinergic toxicity, including urinary retention, blurred vision, acute **glaucoma,** and even paralytic ileus. Dental office personnel must pay careful attention to the medications the patient is taking in order to

TABLE 5-4	Anticholinergic (Parasympatholytic) Agents		
CATEGORY	AGENT	PO DOSE (MG)*	ROUTE OF ADMINISTRATION
TERTIARY			
Natural alkaloids	Atropine	0.4-0.6	PO, P, ophth
	L-Hyoscyamine (hyoscyamine) (Levsin), Anaspaz	0.125	PO, inj
	Scopolamine (hyoscine) (Transderm-Scop)	0.4-0.6	P, ophth
Synthetic esters	Cyclopentolate (Cyclogyl)	—	Ophth
	Dicyclomine (Bentyl)	20	PO, P
QUATERNARY			
Esters	Glycopyrrolate (Robinul)	1-2	PO, P
	Ipratropium (Atrovent)		Inhalation
	Propantheline (Pro-Banthine)	7.5-15	PO

*Usual oral dose (mg).
PO, Oral; *P,* parenteral (injection), *ophth*, ophthalmic.

rule out excessive anticholinergic effects. Patients receiving methotrimeprazine [meth-oh-trye-MEP-ra-zine] (Levoprome) concurrently with scopolamine have reported extrapyramidal (Parkinson-like) symptoms. If a patient is taking a cholinesterase inhibitor, particularly neostigmine, atropine could interfere with its cholinergic effect.

NICOTINIC AGONISTS AND ANTAGONISTS

Nicotine, which is present in cigarettes, is so toxic that one drop on the skin is rapidly fatal. In low doses, it produces stimulation because of depolarization. At high doses it produces paralysis of the ganglia, resulting in respiratory paralysis. Peripherally, it increases blood pressure and heart rate and increases gastrointestinal motility and secretions. Nicotine constricts the blood vessels and reduces blood flow to the extremities. Nicotine is addicting, and withdrawal can occur. It is used as an insecticide.

SYMPATHETIC NERVOUS SYSTEM

The major neurotransmitters in the SANS include norepinephrine and epinephrine. They are synthesized in the neural tissues and stored in synaptic vesicles. Norepinephrine is the major neurotransmitter released at the terminal nerve endings of the SANS. With stimulation, epinephrine is released from the adrenal medulla and distributed throughout the body via the blood. Dopamine receptors are important in the brain and splanchnic and renal vasculature. There are currently several dopamine receptor subtypes (D_1 to D_5). They are divided into two groups: one group is D_1 and D_5 and the other group is D_2, D_3, and D_4. Each of these receptor subtypes may be further divided into A and B, for example, D_{1A} and D_{1B}.

The term catecholamine is made up of two terms that relate to their structure. *Catechol* refers to 1,2-dihydroxybenzene. *Amine* refers to the chemical structure $-NH_2$. Norepinephrine, epinephrine, and dopamine are endogenous sympathetic neurotransmitters that are catecholamines. Isoproterenol (Isuprel) is an exogenous catecholamine. This term is used to refer to the epinephrine contained in a lidocaine with epinephrine solution.

The adrenergic drugs can be classified by their mechanism of action (Figure 5-8) as follows:

- **Direct action:** Epinephrine, norepinephrine, and isoproterenol produce their effects directly on the receptor site by stimulating the receptor.
- **Indirect action:** These agents, such as amphetamine, release endogenous norepinephrine, which then produces a response. Depletion of the endogenous norepinephrine with reserpine diminishes the response to these agents.
- **Mixed action:** These agents, such as ephedrine, can either stimulate the receptor directly or release endogenous norepinephrine to cause a response.

Norepinephrine's action is terminated primarily by reuptake into the presynaptic nerve terminal by an amine-specific pump. The norepinephrine taken up in this manner is stored for reuse. In addition, two enzyme systems, monoamine oxidase (MAO) and catechol-O-

F IGURE 5 - 8 *SANS: direct-, mixed-, and indirect-acting adrenergic agents.*

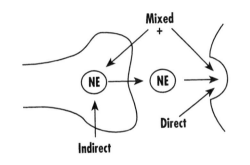

methyltransferase (COMT), are involved in the metabolism of a portion of both epinephrine and norepinephrine.

SYMPATHETIC NERVOUS SYSTEM RECEPTORS

As early as 1948, the existence of at least two types of adrenergic receptors, termed alpha (α) and beta (β), was recognized. The activation of α-receptors causes a different response than the activation of β-receptors. More subreceptor types are now known.

α-Receptors. The stimulation of the α-receptors results in smooth-muscle excitation or contraction, which then causes vasoconstriction. Because α-receptors are located in the skin and skeletal muscle, vasoconstriction of the skin and skeletal muscle follows stimulation. Drugs that block the action of neurotransmitters on the α-receptors are referred to as *α-adrenergic blocking agents.*

β-Receptors. There are at least two types of β-receptors, β_1 and β_2. β_1-Receptor excitation causes stimulation of the heart muscle, resulting in a positive chronotropic effect (increased rate) and a positive inotropic effect (increased strength). There are at least two types of β-receptors, β_1 and β_2. β_1-Receptor excitation causes stimulation of the heart muscle, resulting in a positive chronotropic effect (increased rate) and a positive inotropic effect (increased strength). The β_1-receptor controls the heart, and we have only one heart (Figure 5-9). Other actions thought to be associated primarily with β_1-receptor stimulation include metabolic effects on glycogen formation (glycogenolysis).

The stimulation of the β_2-receptors results in smooth-muscle inhibition or relaxation. Because the blood vessels of the skeletal muscle are innervated by β_2-receptors, stimulation causes vasodilation. Relaxation of the smooth

muscles of the bronchioles, also containing β_2-receptors, results in bronchodilation. β_2-Receptor stimulation produces bronchodilation in the lungs, and we have two lungs (see Figure 5-9). Drugs with this effect have been used in the treatment of asthma. The type of receptor found in a given tissue determines the effect adrenergic agents will produce on that tissue (see Table 5-1).

Agents that block β-receptor effects are called *β-adrenergic blocking agents.* Some (such as propranolol) are nonspecific, blocking both β_1-receptors and β_2-receptors, whereas others are more selective, blocking primarily β_2-receptors.

FIGURE 5-9 *β-Receptors: β_1 and β_2.*

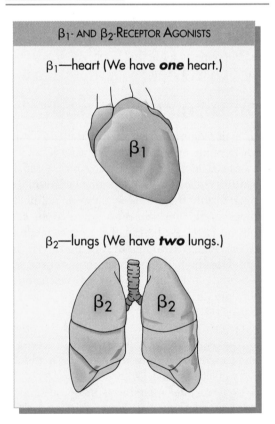

ADRENERGIC (SYMPATHOMIMETIC) AGENTS

Adrenergic agents play an important part in the treatment of anaphylaxis and asthma and are added to local anesthetic solutions (vasoconstrictors) to prolong their action. Table 5-5 lists some adrenergic agents.

Pharmacologic effects. When discussing the pharmacologic effects associated with the adrenergic drugs, it is important to note the proportion of α-receptor and β-receptor activity each possesses. For example, epinephrine has both α-receptor and β-receptor activity, norepinephrine and phenylephrine stimulate primarily

TABLE 5-5 Adrenergic Receptor Agonists (Sympathomimetic Adrenergic Agonists)

	DRUG	RECEPTORS	INDICATIONS
Endogenous catecholamines	Epinephrine (Adrenalin) (Primatine)	α/β	Anaphylaxis, asthma
	Norepineprine (Levophed)		
	Dopamine (Intropin)	$\alpha/\beta/D_{1\,\&\,2}$	Shock, vasopressor, cardiac stimulant
α_1-Selective	Phenylephrine (Neo-Synephrine)	α_1	Decongestant
	Methoxamine (Vasoxyl)		
	Midodrine (ProAmatine)		
	Naphazoline (Privine, Naphcon)	α	"Get the red out!" ophthalmic drops
	Tetrahydrozoline (Tyzine, Visine)		
	Oxymetazoline (Afrin, Neo-Synephrine 12 hour, Ocuclear)		
	Xylometazoline (Otrivin, Neo-Synephrine Long-acting, Cholorohist LA)		
α_2-Selective	Clonidine (Catapres)	α_2	Antihypertensives
	Methyldopa (Aldomet)		
	Guanfacine (Tenex)		
	Guanabenz (Wytensin)		
β-Nonselective	Isoproterenol (Isuprel)	β	Bradycardia
β_1-Selective	Dobutamine (Dobutrex)	$\beta_1>\beta_2$	Cardiac decompensation
β_2-Selective	Albuterol (Proventil, Ventolin)	$\beta_2>\beta_1$	Asthma
	Metaproterenol (Alupent)		
	Salmeterol (Serevent)		
	Ritodrine (Yutopar)	$\beta_2>\beta_1$	Uterine relaxation
	Terbutaline (Brethine)		
	Metaraminol (Aramine)		
Miscellaneous indirect-acting	Amphetamine	CNS/α/β	Attention deficit disorder (ADD)
	Dextroamphetamine (Dexedrine)		
	Amphetamine aspartate, sulfate, saccharate, and sulfate (Adderall)		
	Methamphetamine (Desoxyn)		
	Methylphenidate (Ritalin)		
	Pemoline (Cylert)		
	Ephedrine		Methamphetamine precursor
	Pseudoephedrine (Sudafed)		Decongestant
	Phendimetrazine		Decongestant, diet
	Phenmetrazine (Preludin)		
	Phenteramine (Ionamin)		
	Phenylpropanolamine ([PPA], Progest, in Entex-LA)		

α-receptors, and isoproterenol acts mainly on β-receptors. Although the effects of these agents depend on their ability to stimulate various receptors, the general actions of the adrenergic agents are discussed with specific reference to α-receptor or β-receptor effects as applicable.

CENTRAL NERVOUS SYSTEM The sympathomimetic agents such as amphetamine produce CNS excitation, or alertness. With higher doses, anxiety, apprehension, restlessness, and even tremors can occur.

CARDIOVASCULAR

Heart The general effect of the sympathomimetics such as epinephrine on the heart is to increase its force and strength of contraction. The final effect on blood pressure is a combination of the *direct* and the *indirect* effects. Norepinephrine, primarily an α-agonist, produces vasoconstriction that increases peripheral resistance, resulting in an increase in blood pressure. With an increase in blood pressure, the vagal reflex decreases the heart rate. Epinephrine, an α- and β-agonist, constricts the α-receptors and dilates the β-receptors. This produces a widening of the **pulse** pressure (systolic blood pressure–diastolic blood pressure) with an increase in systolic and a decrease in diastolic blood pressures. Isoproterenol, primarily a β-agonist, produces vasodilation (lowers peripheral resistance) that triggers an increase in heart rate (vagal reflex). Figure 5-10 illustrates the effects of the adrenergic agents on pulse rate, blood pressure, and peripheral resistance.

Vessels The vascular responses observed with the sympathomimetics depend on the location of the vessels and whether they are innervated by α-receptors or β-receptors or both. Agents with α-receptor effects will produce vasoconstriction primarily in the skin and mucosa (innervated with α-receptor fibers), whereas agents with β-receptor effects will produce vasodilation

of the skeletal muscle (innervated with β-receptor fibers). The resultant effect on the total peripheral resistance is an increase with an α-receptor agent and a reduction with a β-receptor agent.

Blood pressure The sympathomimetic effect on the blood pressure is generally an increase. With epinephrine, which has both α-receptor–stimulating and β-receptor–stimulating properties, there is a rise in systolic pressure and a decrease in diastolic pressure. With norepinephrine there is a rise in both systolic and diastolic pressures. With isoproterenol there is little change in systolic pressure, but a decrease in diastolic pressure occurs.

EFFECTS ON THE EYE The sympathomimetic agents have at least two effects on the eye: a decrease in intraocular pressure, which makes them useful in the treatment of glaucoma, and mydriasis.

EFFECTS ON THE RESPIRATORY SYSTEM These agents cause a relaxation of the bronchiole smooth muscle because of their β-adrenergic effect. This has made them useful in the treatment of asthma and anaphylaxis.

METABOLIC EFFECTS The hyperglycemia resulting from β-receptor stimulation can be explained on the basis of increased glycogenolysis and decreased insulin release. Fatty acid mobilization, lipolysis, and gluconeogenesis are stimulated, and the basal metabolic rate is increased.

EFFECTS ON THE SALIVARY GLANDS The mucus-secreting cells of the submaxillary glands and sublingual glands are stimulated by the sympathomimetic agents to release a small amount of thick, viscous saliva. Because the parotid gland has no sympathetic innervation (only parasympathetic) and the sympathomimetics

FIGURE 5 - 1 0   *The effects of norepinephrine, epinephrine, and isoproterenol on the heart rate, blood pressure, and peripheral resistance.*

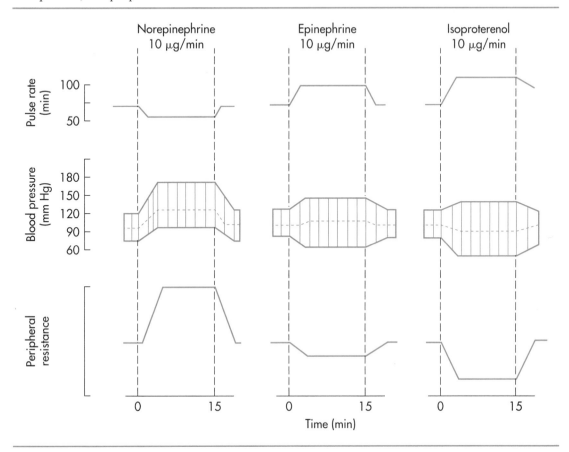

produce vasoconstriction, the flow of saliva is often reduced, resulting in xerostomia.

Adverse reactions. The adverse reactions associated with the adrenergic drugs are extensions of their pharmacologic effects. Anxiety and tremors may occur, and the patient may have palpitations. Serious arrhythmias can result. Agents with an α-adrenergic action can also cause a dramatic rise in blood pressure. The sympathomimetic agents should be used with caution

in patients with angina, hypertension, or **hyperthyroidism.**

Uses

VASOCONSTRICTION

Prolonged action The sympathomimetic agents are used in dentistry primarily because of their vasoconstrictive action on the blood vessels. Agents with an α effect (vasoconstriction) are frequently added to local anesthetic solutions.

These vasoconstrictors prolong the action of the local anesthetics and reduce their potential for systemic toxicity.

Hemostasis The adrenergic agents have been used in dentistry to produce hemostasis. Epinephrine can be applied topically or infiltrated locally around the bleeding area. Epinephrine-containing retraction cord, used to stop bleeding and to retract the gingiva before taking an impression, can produce problems such as systemic toxicity. Epinephrine is quickly absorbed after topical application if the tissue is injured. The total amount of epinephrine given by all routes must be noted to prevent an overdose.

Decongestion Sympathomimetic agents are often incorporated into nose drops or sprays (see Table 5-5) to treat nasal congestion. These agents provide symptomatic relief by constricting the vessels and reducing the swelling of the mucous membranes of the nose. Within a short time the congestion can return, a condition called rebound congestion. With repeated local use, systemic absorption can cause problems even greater than rebound congestion. Systemic decongestants or topical intranasal steroids are now preferred.

CARDIAC EFFECTS
Treatment of shock The value of the adrenergic agents in the treatment of shock is controversial. These drugs will elevate a lowered blood pressure, but correcting the cause of shock is more important. Some agents with both α effects and β effects (such as dopamine) are used.

Treatment of cardiac arrest The sympathomimetic agents, especially epinephrine, are used to treat **cardiac arrest.**

BRONCHODILATION The use of the sympathomimetic agents in the treatment of respiratory disease stems from their action as **bronchodilators.** Patients with asthma or **emphysema** are frequently treated with adrenergic agents to provide bronchodilation. In the treatment of anaphylaxis, when bronchoconstriction is predominant, epinephrine is the drug of choice.

CENTRAL NERVOUS SYSTEM STIMULATION Amphetamine-like agents have been used and abused as "diet pills." They are indicated for the treatment of **attention deficit disorder** (ADD) and **narcolepsy.**

Specific adrenergic agents

EPINEPHRINE The drug of choice for acute asthmatic attacks and anaphylaxis, epinephrine (Epi) [ep-i-NEF-rin] (Adrenalin), may be administered by both the intravenous and subcutaneous routes. It is also used in patients with cardiac arrest. It is added to local anesthetic solutions to delay absorption and reduce systemic toxicity (see Chapter 10). Epinephrine should be stored in amber-colored containers and placed out of the reach of sunlight, because light causes deterioration. As it deteriorates, epinephrine first turns pink, then brown, and finally precipitates. Solutions of epinephrine with any discoloration or precipitate should be discarded immediately. [Might want to check that expiration date, too!]

PHENYLEPHRINE Phenylephrine [fen-ill-EF-rin] (Neo-Synephrine) causes primarily α-receptor stimulation, which produces vasoconstriction in the cutaneous vessels. This leads to an increase in total peripheral resistance and systolic and diastolic pressures. A reflex vagal bradycardia also results. Phenylephrine is used as a mydriatic and in nose sprays (Neo-Synephrine) or drops to relieve congestion.

LEVONORDEFRIN Levonordefrin [lee-voe-nor-DEF-rin] (Neo-Cobefrin), a derivative of norepinephrine, is a vasoconstrictor frequently added to local anesthetic solutions. Although claims made for this drug include less CNS excitation and cardiac stimulation, the dosage required to produce vasoconstriction equal to that caused by epinephrine is higher. Therefore it is difficult to distinguish levonordefrin's effects from those of other vasoconstrictors. Its effects resemble those of α-receptor stimulation.

ISOPROTERENOL Isoproterenol [eye-soe-proe-TER-e-nole] (Isuprel) is a synthetic catecholamine whose action is limited to the β-receptors. Because it is a nonspecific β-agonist, its use in the treatment of bronchial asthma is outdated. It was used in the past to treat asthma, but specific β-agonists (e.g., albuterol; see Table 5-5) have supplanted its use. The β-blocking agents (e.g., propranolol) interfere with the action of isoproterenol.

EPHEDRINE AND PSEUDOEPHEDRINE In contrast to the catecholamines, ephedrine and pseudoephedrine (Sudafed) [soo-doe-e-FED-rin] are effective when taken orally and have a longer duration of action. They have both α- and β-receptor activity. Their mechanism of action is mixed; that is, they have both direct and indirect action. They are often used in combination with other agents for patients with asthma. They are also present in over-the-counter (OTC) products designed for the treatment of the common cold or allergies, such as pseudoephedrine (Sudafed). Phenylpropanolamine is also used for nasal congestion. Its central effects make it a staple in OTC diet pills, and **insomnia** and nervousness can result. The newest use of these agents is to "cook" them to produce methamphetamine, which is used illicitly.

DOPAMINE Dopamine [DOE-pa-meen] (Intropin) is a neurotransmitter in parts of the CNS. It is both an α-agonist and a β-agonist and is employed primarily in the treatment of shock. It is a precursor of norepinephrine and epinephrine synthesis, as shown in Figure 5-11. Dopamine first acts on the β-receptors of the heart, producing a positive chronotropic and inotropic effect. In higher doses it stimulates the α-receptors, producing vasoconstriction. How-

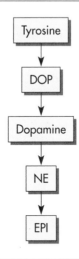

FIGURE 5 - 1 1 *Synthesis of epinephrine from tyrosine, including the intermediate steps involving dopamine.*

ever, it exerts an unusual vasodilating effect in certain vessels and produces an increase in blood flow to the renal, splanchnic, cerebral, and coronary vessels. Ventricular arrhythmias and hypotension can occur.

DIPIVEFRIN Dipivefrin [dye-PIV-e-frin] (Propine) and epinephrine are sympathomimetic ophthalmics that are used to treat glaucoma. They decrease the production of aqueous humor (β-receptor effect), increase its outflow (β-effect), and produce mydriasis (primarily α-effect). Dipivefrin, a prodrug, is metabolized in vivo to epinephrine. It may produce fewer side effects than epinephrine because it penetrates into the eye better and is used to treat chronic open-angle glaucoma.

Central nervous system stimulation. Adrenergic agonists with some specificity for CNS stimulation are used for both legitimate and illegitimate purposes.

Methylphenidate [meth-ill-FEN-I-date] (Ritalin), pemoline [PEM-oh-leen] (Cylert), and dextroamphetamine [dex-troe-am-FET-a-meen] (Dexedrine), are adrenergic agents used to treat ADD in both children and adults. These agents, given to hyperactive children and adults, reduce impulsivity and increase attention span. Some children with ADD will exhibit excessive motor activity—turn around in chair, stand up from chair, grab dental instruments, squirt the water, and ask about everything. Side effects exhibited with this use include insomnia and anorexia. ADD has also been known as *attention deficit hyperactivity disorder* (ADHD) and *minimal brain dysfunction* (MBD) and children with the disorder have been referred to as *hyperkinetic* children.

Adrenergics that are used as "diet pills" include phentermine* [FEN-ter-meen] (Fastin, Lonamin), phendimetrazine* [fen-dye-ME-tra-zeen] (Plegine), diethylpropion [dye-eth-il-PROE-pee-on] (Tenuate), fenfluramine* [fen-FLU-ra-meen] (Pondimin), and dexfenfluramine, [deks-fen-FLU-ra-meen] (Redux). OTC diet pills contain phenylpropanolamine [feen-il-PRO-pa-nol-a-meen] (Dexatrim), which is also used as a decongestant. Weight loss, to produce euphoria, and "staying awake" are not legitimate medical uses for adrenergic agents. Truck drivers have used these agents to keep them awake for very long hours. Hallucinations and **psychosis** made these truck drivers dangerous.

Narcolepsy, a disease in which spontaneous deep sleep can occur at any time, is treated with the sympathomimetic amines. Tolerance to the effect does not seem to occur. Amphetamines may have a supplementary use in the treatment of parkinsonism because they cause the release of dopamine and can counteract the sedative effects of the mainstay drugs.

ADRENERGIC BLOCKING AGENTS

Adrenergic blocking agents can block all the adrenergic receptors (α- and β-blockers), just the α-receptors (α-blockers), just the β-receptors (β-blockers), or just α₁-receptors (α₁-blockers),

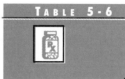

TABLE 5-6	Adrenergic Receptor Antagonists (Sympatholytics, Adrenergic Blockers)

α-ADRENERGIC RECEPTOR ANTAGONISTS	
RECEPTOR	EXAMPLES
α	Phentolamine (Regitine)
	Tolazoline (Priscoline)
$\alpha_1 > \alpha_2$	Phenoxybenzamine (Dibenzyline)
$\alpha_1 >>> \alpha_2$	Prazosin (Minipress)
	Terazosin (Hytrin)
	Doxazosin (Cardura)
α_2	Yohimbine
α Partial agonist and antagonist	Ergot

β-ADRENERGIC RECEPTOR ANTAGONISTS (L = LOW, I = INTERMEDIATE, H = HIGH ISA*)	
Nonspecific (nonselective) β	Carteolol (Cartrol)
	Carvedilol (Coreg)
	Levobunolol (Betagan)
	Metipranolol
	Nadolol (Corgard)
	Oxprenolol (Trasicor)
	Penbutolol (Levatol)
	Pendolol (Visken)
	Propranolol (Inderal)
	Timolol (Timoptic, Blocadren)
Specific (selective) $\beta_1 > \beta_2$	Acebutolol (Sectral)
	Atenolol (Tenormin)
	Betaxolol (Kerlone)
	Bisoprolol (Zebeta)
	Esmolol (Brevibloc)
	Metoprolol (Lopressor, Toprol)

α AND β-ADRENERGIC ANTAGONISTS	
α, β	Labetalol (Normodyne)

α₂-receptors, β₁-receptors (β₁-blockers), or β₂-receptors (β₂-blockers) (Table 5-6).

α-Adrenergic blocking agents. The α-adrenergic blocking agents competitively inhibit the vasoconstricting effects (α-receptor effects) of the adrenergic agents. This reduces the sympathetic tone in the blood vessels, producing a decrease in the total peripheral resistance. The resulting

*Removed from market.

decrease in blood pressure stimulates the vagus, thereby producing a reflex tachycardia. Patients who are pretreated with α-blocking agents and given epinephrine exhibit a predominance of β-effects (vasodilation), which lowers blood pressure. This effect is termed **epinephrine** reversal because the blood pressure goes down instead of going up. The α-adrenergic blockers also block the mydriasis that these agents normally cause.

The agents phenoxybenzamine [fen-ox-ee-BEN-za-meen] (Dibenzyline) and phentolamine [fen-TOLE-a-meen] (Regitine) are α-blockers. They are used in the treatment of peripheral vascular disease when vascular spasm is a common feature (such as Raynaud's syndrome) and in the diagnosis and treatment of pheochromocytoma, a catecholamine-secreting tumor of the adrenal medulla.

Other examples of a_1-adrenergic blocking agents are, tolazoline [toe-LAZ-a-zeen] (Priscoline), prazosin [PRA-zoe-sin] (Minipress), terazosin [ter-AY-zoe-sin] (Hytrin), and doxazosin [dox-AY-zoe-sin] (Cardura), are competitive blockers of the α-receptor. They are effective in the treatment of hypertension and are discussed in the chapter on cardiovascular drugs (Chapter 15). These agents are also indicated in the management of Raynaud's vasospasm and in the treatment of benign prostatic hypertrophy (to increase ease of urination).

β-Adrenergic blocking drugs. The β-blocking drugs competitively block the β-receptors in the adrenergic nervous system. Their generic names end in *–olol,* so they can be easily recognized. Because β-receptor stimulation produces vasodilation, bronchodilation, and tachycardia, β-blockers would block these effects, producing bradycardia and, in asthmatics, possible bronchoconstriction. Their exact effect is determined by the tone in the sympathetic nervous system. The β-blockers may be either nonspecific (nonselective), such as propranolol [proe-PRAN-oh-lole] (Inderal), or specific (selective), such as atenolol [a-TEN-oh-lole] (Tenormin). The spe-

cific β-blockers have more activity on the heart and blood vessels (β-receptors) than on the lungs (β-receptors). This specificity, or selectivity, produces fewer side effects. The selective β-blockers also have a lower chance of causing drug interactions.

Propranolol (Inderal) is a β-blocker that depresses the heart (negative chronotropic and inotropic effect), produces bronchoconstriction, and can cause hypoglycemia. It is used in the treatment of arrhythmias (for its quinidine-like effect), angina, hypertension, and migraine headache prophylaxis. Diseases in which tachycardia occurs, such as hyperthyroidism and pheochromocytoma, can be symptomatically treated with propranolol. The β-blockers are discussed in Chapter 15. Figure 5-12 shows a drug interaction between epinephrine and propranolol. The patient, a 55-year-old female, is taking 40 mg of propranolol bid for migraine headache prophylaxis. She is given 12 ml of lidocaine 1% with 1:100,000 epinephrine.

α- And β-blocking agents. Labetalol [la-BET-a-lole] (Normodyne, Trandate) has both α- and β-blocking action. Because the β-blockers are designated using the suffix *-olol,* this α- and β-blocker uses the suffix *-alol.* It is a selective α-blocker and nonselective β-blocker. It is indicated for the treatment of hypertension and produces a fall in blood pressure without reflex tachycardia.

NEUROMUSCULAR BLOCKING DRUGS

The neuromuscular blocking drugs are agents that affect transmission between the motor nerve endings and the nicotinic receptors on the skeletal muscle. These blocking agents act either as antagonists (nondepolarizing) or agonists (depolarizing).

Nondepolarizing (competitive) blockers. Indigenous people living along the Amazon have used poison arrows when hunting animals. The poison is the neuromuscular blocking drug curare,

FIGURE 5-12 *Effect of epinephrine given to a patient already taking nonspecific β-blockers. X-axis (arrow), 0.12 mg (12 ml, 1:100,000) epinephrine administered. BP, Blood pressure; HR, heart rate.*

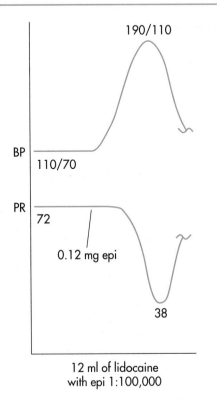

12 ml of lidocaine
with epi 1:100,000

most primitive—diaphragmatic breathing. Nature has planned that loss of function is in the order of least important to most important (the diaphragm). Curare's duration of action is between 20 minutes and 2 hours, depending on the dose.

Depolarizing agents. Depolarizing agents such as succinylcholine [suk-sin-ill-KOE-leen] attach to the nicotinic receptor and, like acetylcholine, result in depolarization. The constant stimulation of the receptor causes the sodium channel to open, producing depolarization (phase I). Transient fasciculations of the muscles result. With time, the receptor cannot transmit any further impulses and repolarization occurs as the sodium channel closes (phase II). A flaccid paralysis is produced by resistance to depolarization.

Succinylcholine produces muscle fasciculations followed by paralysis. The paralysis lasts only a few minutes because it is broken down by plasma cholinesterase.

Succinylcholine can produce cardiac arrhythmias, hyperkalemia, and increased intraocular pressure. When it has been used in general anesthesia in conjunction with halothane, succinylcholine has precipitated malignant hyperthermia in susceptible patients (heredity). The drug of choice for **malignant** hyperthermia is dantrolene (Dantrium). Sometimes a small dose of curare is administered before the administration of succinylcholine to block the fasciculations of the succinylcholine. This reduces the postoperative muscle pain.

or *d*-tubocurarine. This nondepolarizing blocker combines with the nicotinic receptor and blocks the action of acetylcholine. The depolarization of the membrane is inhibited and muscle contraction is blocked. These competitive blockers can be overcome by the administration of cholinesterase inhibitors such as neostigmine.

Paralysis of the small facial muscles is followed by paralysis of the fingers, limbs, extremities, and trunk. The function of the muscles involved in respiration is lost, beginning with the intercostal muscles. The last function lost is the

REVIEW QUESTIONS

1. Compare and contrast the anatomic and functional organization of the parasympathetic and sympathetic nervous systems.
2. State the responses of the major tissues and organ systems to the adrenergic (sympathetic) and cholinergic (parasympathetic) nervous systems.

3. State the location(s) of acetylcholine and norepinephrine, the two major neurotransmitter substances.

4. Describe the major methods by which the actions of acetylcholine and norepinephrine are terminated.

5. State the sites of the muscarinic and nicotinic receptors and describe an agent that blocks each of these sites.

6. Explain the difference in mechanism of action between the direct-acting and indirect-acting cholinergic agents.

7. Describe the pharmacologic effects of the cholinergic agents on the heart, gastrointestinal tract, and eye.

8. State two major uses of the cholinergic agents.

9. Describe a unique dental use for pilocarpine.

10. State a use for physostigmine in the treatment of an overdose.

11. Describe the pharmacologic effects of the anticholinergic agents on the exocrine glands, smooth muscle, and eye.

12. Explain the adverse reactions associated with the anticholinergic agents.

13. State the contraindications and cautions to the use of anticholinergic agents and explain their relationship to the pharmacologic effects of these agents.

14. State the major therapeutic uses of the anticholinergics.

15. Discuss the relative α-receptor and β-receptor effects possessed by epinephrine, norepinephrine, and isoproterenol. Include the effects of these agents on the blood pressure, heart rate, and blood vessels.

16. State the pharmacologic effect of the adrenergic agents on the eye, bronchioles, and salivary glands.

17. State the therapeutic uses of the adrenergic agents, especially the uses these agents have in dentistry.

18. Explain the limits to the accepted medical uses of the amphetamine-like agents. Explain why ephedrine tablets are bought by the case by some individuals.

19. Name the pharmacologic class to which propranolol (Inderal) belongs. Describe the effects that make it useful in the treatment of arrhythmias, angina, and hypertension.

20. Differentiate between "selective" and "nonselective" β-blockers. Name a difference important to the dental health team (drug interaction).

21. Describe the mechanism by which epinephrine reversal occurs.

Nonopioid (Nonnarcotic) Analgesics

Pain control is of great importance in dental practice. It is often pain that brings the patient to the dental office. Conversely, pain can be the factor that keeps the patient from seeking dental care at the appropriate time. Thus dental treatment is often rendered on the inflamed, hypersensitive tissues of a patient who suffers from mental fatigue after long endurance of pain.

The dental health care provider must be able to recognize and evaluate a patient's need for medication to control pain. Because pain is such a complex phenomenon, the entire patient must be considered before the type of medication that may be needed is determined.

PAIN

The sensation of pain is the means by which the body is made urgently aware of the presence of tissue damage. Pain represents a protective reflex for self-preservation. Just as the hand is quickly removed from a hot object, a painful dental abscess brings the patient to the dental office seeking professional assistance for its resolution. Pain is a diagnostic symptom of an underlying pathologic condition. Although the relief of pain is an immediate objective, only by treatment of the underlying cause is the ultimate resolution achieved.

The two components of pain are perception and reaction. Perception is the physical component of pain and involves the message of pain that is carried through the nerves eventually to the cortex. Reaction is the psychological component of pain and involves the patient's emotional response to the pain. Although individuals are surprisingly uniform in their perception of pain, they vary greatly in their reaction to it (Figure 6-1). A decrease in the pain threshold (a greater reaction to pain) has been said to be associated with emotional instability, anxiety, fatigue, youth, certain nationalities, women, and fear and apprehension. The pain threshold is raised by sleep, sympathy, activities, and analgesics (Figure 6-2). As a result, analgesic therapy must be selected for the individual (Figure 6-3).

FIGURE 6-2 *Factors that alter the pain threshold. Sleep raises the threshold and fear lowers it.*

FIGURE 6-1 *Effect of analgesics on perception and reaction. NSAIAs affect the perception of pain (peripherally), and the opioids affect the reaction of the brain (cognitive interpretation).*

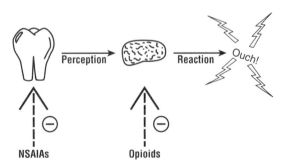

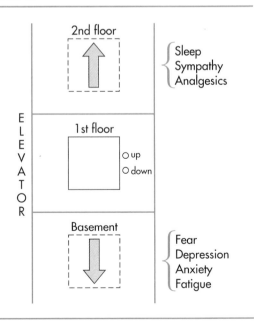

A level of discomfort that may not require drug treatment in one person may demand extreme therapy in another. Although some patients undergoing routine exodontia require no postoperative medication, even the strongest analgesics will not completely control postoperative extraction pain in other persons. Because many patients respond when given a placebo, the inclusion of a placebo is required for any acceptable analgesic clinical trials. A placebo is an inert substance made to look similar to the study medicine. In clinical trials neither the investigator nor the patient can know whether or not the placebo was used in each patient (double-blind study). The investigator only decodes the patients, their treatment groups, and their results after all the data have been collected. The confidence in the drug must be conveyed to the patient by the dental health care worker in order to elicit the most positive response for patients. We are still searching for the mechanism by which the placebo response occurs.

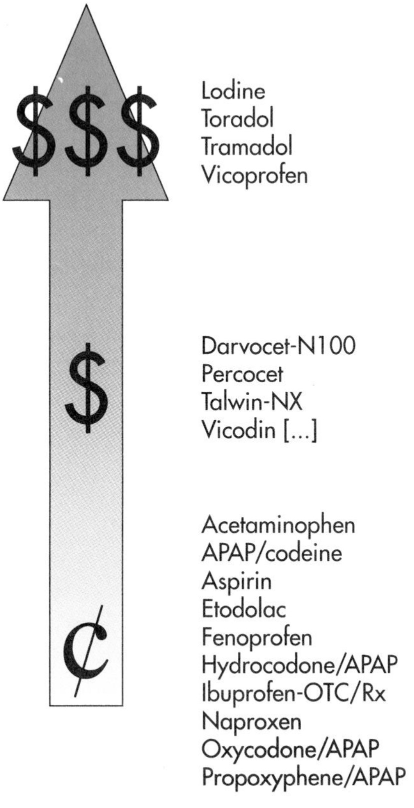

One difficulty encountered when evaluating an analgesic is related to the design of clinical trials. Reliable results are difficult to produce when measuring and comparing the analgesic potency of various agents, because the pain threshold is altered by many factors. Because experimentally induced pain does not produce reliable results, most modern studies on analgesics are done on "real" pain. The dental extraction presents an ideal pain model for testing analgesic efficacy.

FIGURE 6-3 *Comparison of the relative price of analgesics. Drugs within each price category are arranged alphabetically.*

Lodine
Toradol
Tramadol
Vicoprofen

Darvocet-N100
Percocet
Talwin-NX
Vicodin [...]

Acetaminophen
APAP/codeine
Aspirin
Etodolac
Fenoprofen
Hydrocodone/APAP
Ibuprofen-OTC/Rx
Naproxen
Oxycodone/APAP
Propoxyphene/APAP

CLASSIFICATION

The analgesic agents can be divided into two groups, the nonopioids, also called the *nonnarcotic, peripheral, mild,* and antipyretic analgesics, and the opioids, also called the *narcotic, central,* or *strong* group (Figure 6-4).

An important difference between the nonopioid and the opioid analgesics is their sites of action. Nonopioid analgesics act primarily at the peripheral nerve endings, although their antipyretic effect is mediated centrally. Opioids act primarily within the central nervous system (CNS).

Another difference between the opioids and the nonopioid analgesic agents is their mechanism of action. The action of the nonopioid analgesic agents is related to their ability to inhibit prostaglandin synthesis. The opioids affect the response to pain by depressing the CNS (the reaction). The side effect profiles of the two groups also differ.

The nonopioids can be divided into the **salicylates** (aspirin-like group), acetaminophen,

F IGURE 6 - 4   *Categories of analgesics.*

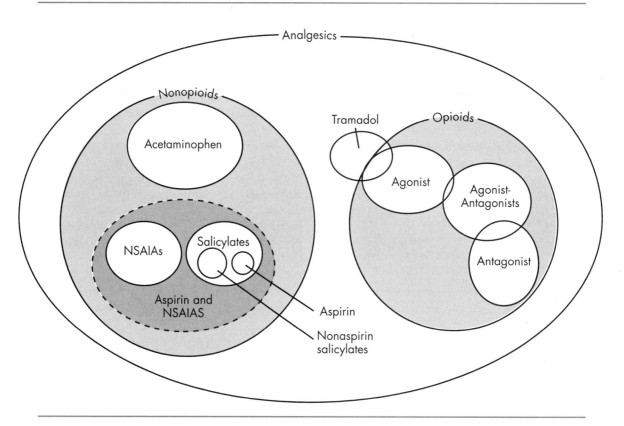

and the nonsteroidal antiinflammatory agents or drugs (NSAIAs/NSAIDs) (Box 6-1). Aspirin, a member of the salicylates, will be discussed first.

SALICYLATES

Since antiquity, extracts of willow bark containing salicin have been used to reduce fever. Since that time, many other salicylates [sa-LI-si-lates] have been synthesized, but aspirin is the most useful salicylate for analgesia. Box 6-2 lists some analgesic and some topical salicylates. Because aspirin is the prototype salicylate, it will be discussed.

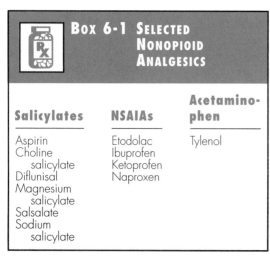

BOX 6-1 SELECTED NONOPIOID ANALGESICS

Salicylates	NSAIAs	Acetamino-phen
Aspirin	Etodolac	Tylenol
Choline	Ibuprofen	
salicylate	Ketoprofen	
Diflunisal	Naproxen	
Magnesium		
salicylate		
Salsalate		
Sodium		
salicylate		

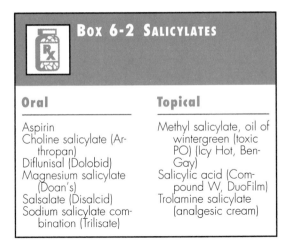

BOX 6-2 SALICYLATES

Oral	Topical
Aspirin	Methyl salicylate, oil of
Choline salicylate (Ar-	wintergreen (toxic
thropan)	PO) (Icy Hot, Ben-
Diflunisal (Dolobid)	Gay)
Magnesium salicylate	Salicylic acid (Com-
(Doan's)	pound W, DuoFilm)
Salsalate (Disalcid)	Trolamine salicylate
Sodium salicylate com-	(analgesic cream)
bination (Trilisate)	

ACETYLSALICYLIC ACID

Chemistry. Acetylsalicylic acid (aspirin, ASA) is broken down into acetic acid (HA) and salicylic acid (SA).

$$\text{ASA} \longrightarrow \text{HA} + \text{SA}$$

Aspirin   Acetic   Salicylic
               acid   acid

Acetic acid imparts the characteristic vinegar odor to a bottle of aspirin. Therefore the degree of breakdown of aspirin can be roughly determined by smelling a bottle of aspirin tablets. (If you think "phew" when you open an aspirin bottle, it's time to purchase a new bottle!) Also, salicylic acid is a strong keratolytic agent (used to remove plantar warts from the bottom of feet) and may cause additional adverse gastrointestinal effects if degraded aspirin is administered orally.

Mechanism of action. The mechanism of aspirin's analgesic, antipyretic, antiinflammatory, and anti-platelet effects is related to its ability to in-

hibit prostaglandin synthesis. Aspirin inhibits the enzyme cyclooxygenase (COX, prostaglandin synthase) by acetylating serine, which results in inhibition of the production of prostaglandins. Figure 6-5 shows the synthesis of the prostaglandins and leukotrienes from arachidonic acid. Prostaglandins, lipids that are synthesized locally by inflammatory stimuli, can sensitize the pain receptors to substances such as bradykinin. Therefore a reduction in prostaglandins results in a reduction in pain. Because aspirin blocks the synthesis of prostaglandins, it is more effective if given before the painful stimuli are experienced. Because of this mechanism, aspirin is more effective against "throbbing" pain (caused by inflammation, and common in dentistry) than against "stabbing" pain (direct effect on nerve endings).

Pharmacokinetics. Aspirin is rapidly and almost completely absorbed from the stomach and small intestine, producing its peak effect on an empty stomach in 30 minutes (90 minutes for salicylate). The buffered tablet reaches its peak in about 20 minutes (salicylate). Before a tablet of aspirin can be absorbed it must be dispersed and dissolved. Addition of a buffer to the tablet facilitates this process. This is borne out by the somewhat quicker peak of action and higher blood levels attained with buffered aspirin preparations. Buffered aspirin has a higher proportion of the aspirin in the ionized form, which should make absorption slower, but this is offset by the increase in the rate of dissolution, which is facilitated. This difference in absorption has not been shown to translate into a clinically significant quicker effect.

Aspirin may be administered rectally as suppositories if vomiting is present. Because this route is more erratic and unpredictable it should only be used when the oral route is not feasible. An aspirin tablet should never be applied topically to the oral mucosa to treat a toothache. A painful ulceration can occur. Any benefit from

FIGURE **6 - 5** *Synthesis of prostaglandins and leukotrienes, site of action of aspirin and NSAIAs (interfere with prostaglandin synthesis).*

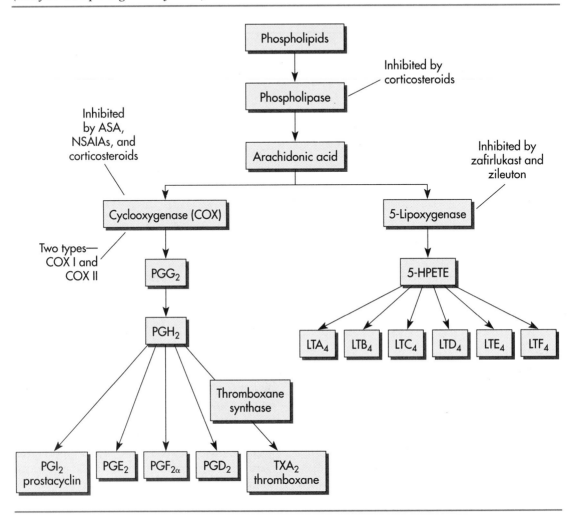

this practice would come from inadvertent swallowing of the aspirin or local damage to nerve endings.

Aspirin is widely distributed into most body tissues and fluids. It is poorly bound to plasma proteins. It is hydrolyzed to salicylate in the mucosa of the gastrointestinal tract and on first pass through the liver. The half-life of unhydrolyzed aspirin is about 15 minutes. Aspirin is hydro-

lyzed to salicylate, which is conjugated with glycine and glucuronic acid by the liver microsomal enzymes. Salicylate is excreted by a capacity-limited process. For this reason, the half-life is dose dependent. With small doses the half-life is 2 to 3 hours; with higher doses a half-life of 15 to 30 hours can be attained. The half-life varies with the dose because a constant *amount* rather than a constant *percentage* of the drug is metabolized per hour. This type of metabolism is called *zero-order kinetics.* In a poisoning situation, the excretion of aspirin can be increased by alkalinization of the urine with sodium bicarbonate. This increases the proportion of the aspirin that is in the ionized form and is therefore excreted.

Pharmacologic effects

ANALGESIC Aspirin's analgesic effect has been repeatedly demonstrated in many clinical trials. In fact, new drugs are often compared in analgesic strength to aspirin. Aspirin typically relieves mild to moderate pain such as a headache or toothache. For more intense pain the agents or stronger opioids are required because the analgesic potency of aspirin is weaker than the other agents mentioned. Because of its easy accessibility and long history of use, aspirin's worth as an analgesic is often unrecognized by the lay public. Figure 6-6 shows a dose-response curve for aspirin versus placebo.

ANTIPYRETIC The ability of aspirin to reduce fever (antipyretic effect) results from its inhibition of prostaglandin synthesis in the hypothalamus. Hypothalamic prostaglandin synthesis is caused by elevated blood levels of **leukocyte** *pyrogens* induced by inflammation. Increased hypothalamic prostaglandin levels produce increased body temperature. Therefore the inhibition of hypothalamic prostaglandin synthesis results in a return to more normal body temperature. Aspirin reduces fever by inducing peripheral vasodilation and sweating. Although it reduces an elevated temperature, it has no effect on normal body temperature. In fact, in toxic doses it produces hyperthermia (see the section on adverse reactions).

ANTIINFLAMMATORY Aspirin's antiinflammatory effect is derived from its ability to inhibit prostaglandin synthesis. The prostaglandins are potent vasodilating agents that also increase capillary permeability. Therefore aspirin causes decreased **erythema** and swelling of the inflamed

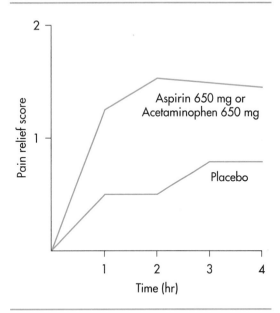

FIGURE 6-6 *Analgesic efficacy over time of aspirin versus placebo.*

area. This antiinflammatory action is useful in dental patients because inflammation is a significant part of most dental pain. Patients with arthritis may be given large doses of aspirin to provide symptomatic relief of pain and inflammation in the joints.

URICOSURIC Even though large doses (greater than 3 gm/day) of aspirin can produce a uricosuric effect, small doses (less than 1 gm/day) produce uric acid retention (Figure 6-7). Aspirin can also counteract the uricosuric effect of probenecid [proe-BEN-e-sid] (Benemid), which is used to treat gout. Aspirin is no longer used as a uricosuric agent because more effective agents are available to treat gout.

ANTIPLATELET Aspirin irreversibly binds to **platelets.** Its antiplatelet effect has been shown to be clinically effective for secondary myocardial infarction prevention in adults. The effect of aspirin on platelets depends on the dose taken. Aspirin has (+/−) an effect on two substances involved in **blood clotting**—thromboxane A₂ and prostocycline. Depending on the dose, aspirin can either inhibit prostacyclin (inhibits aggregation) or thromboxane A₂ (stimulates aggregation). Figure 6-8 demonstrates that inhibition of thromboxane A₂ would prevent clotting because thromboxane A₂ promotes clotting. Further studies are needed to determine aspirin's usefulness and dose in preventing clotting events in different patient populations. Low-dose aspirin has been shown to be effective not only for prevention of myocardial infarction, but it is now recommended for both men and women over the age of 50. Other recommendations include taking an aspirin if a **heart attack** is suspected. Aspirin's effects by dose are illustrated in Figure 6-9.

F I G U R E 6 - 7   *Relative analgesic efficacy of commonly used dental analgesics versus placebo over 4 hours.*

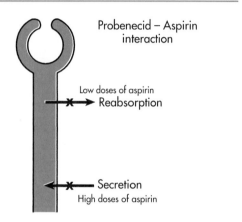

F I G U R E 6 - 9   *Effect of thromboxanes and prostacyclins on platelet aggregation.*

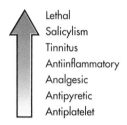

F I G U R E 6 - 8   *Low doses of both aspirin and probenecid block reabsorption; high doses of both block secretion of agents.*

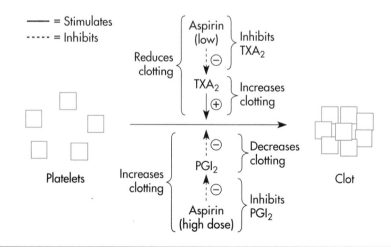

Adverse reactions. In sufficiently high doses, aspirin can produce a variety of undesirable effects. Some of aspirin's side effects can be minimized, but not eliminated. Precautions and contraindications for the administration of aspirin are listed in Table 6-1.

Gastric effects are common.

GASTROINTESTINAL EFFECTS Aspirin's most frequent side effect is related to the gastrointestinal tract. It may be simple dyspepsia, nausea, vomiting, or gastric bleeding. These adverse effects result from direct gastric irritation and from inhibition of prostaglandins. Because prostaglandins are responsible for inhibition of gastric acid secretion and stimulation of the cytoprotective mucus in the stomach, aspirin counteracts these effects. In high doses, aspirin's stimulation of the chemoreceptor trigger zone in the CNS can also produce nausea and vomiting. Salicylate-induced gastric bleeding is painless and in most instances does not significantly affect a patient's health. However, salicylates may exacerbate preexisting ulcers, **gastritis,** or hiatal **hernia.**

BLEEDING At usual therapeutic doses, aspirin irreversibly interferes with the clotting mechanism by reducing platelet adhesiveness (stickiness or aggregation) caused by interfering with adenosine diphosphate (ADP) release. The bleeding time is prolonged and each platelet is affected until new platelets are formed (4 to 7 days). Replacement of all of the affected platelets is not required to produce normal clotting. After about 20% of the platelets have been replaced with newly formed platelets, clotting will return to normal by about 36 hours. Therefore, with lower doses of aspirin, 1½ days should elapse to obtain normal clotting. With large doses of aspirin, the half-life is prolonged. Aspirin inhibits the production of prothrombin, resulting in

TABLE 6-1 **Precautions and Contraindications for the Administration of Aspirin**

DISEASE OR CONDITION	DRUG USED	COMMENTS
Myocardial infarct, atrial fibrillation, valve replacement	Warfarin (Coumadin)	Increases anticoagulant effect of warfarin
Peptic ulcer (heartburn), gastroesophageal reflux disease (GERD)	H_2-Blockers (e.g., cimetidine)	Gastric irritant effect
Pregnancy	Proton pump inhibitors (e.g., omeprazole)	Possible alteration of labor and delivery
Gout	Probenecid (Benemid)	Antagonizes uricosuric effect of probenecid
Arthritis, cancer, psoriasis	Methotrexate	Increases toxicity of methotrexate
Rheumatic fever, arthritis	Large doses of aspirin	Do not add more aspirin if patient taking large doses already
Hemophilia	Factor VIII	Gastric bleeding
Hypoprothrombinemia		Bleeding
Vitamin K deficiency, alcoholism		Bleeding
Glucose-6-phosphate dehydrogenase deficiency		Hemolysis
Diabetes	Oral hypoglycemics	Hypoglycemics

hypoprothrombinemia. Three other mechanisms—the local irritant effects on the stomach, the decrease in platelet stickiness, and the loss of protective mucosa magnify adverse effects on the stomach. Salicylate-induced gastric bleeding is painless. With a small loss of blood, aspirin does not produce significant bleeding. Salicylates may exacerbate preexisting conditions such as ulcers, gastritis, hiatal hernia, or gastrointestinal esophageal reflux disease (GERD).

REYE'S SYNDROME In children and adolescents with either chickenpox or **influenza,** the use of aspirin has been epidemiologically associated with Reye's [rize] syndrome. In place of aspirin, acetaminophen is used in pediatrics for both its analgesic and antipyretic action. Reye's syndrome is associated with hepatotoxicity and encephalopathy, commonly fatal.

HEPATIC AND RENAL EFFECTS Rarely, aspirin can produce hepatotoxicity. Renal papillary necrosis and interstitial **nephritis** leading to dialysis is associated with certain analgesic use. It may be caused by intake of aspirin concomitantly with the coal tar derivatives (acetaminophen).

PREGNANCY AND NURSING Even though animal studies have shown that aspirin can produce birth defects, human studies have demonstrated only a slight positive correlation between chronic aspirin ingestion and congenital abnormalities. With aspirin abuse, increased risk of stillbirth, or neonatal death, as well as decreased birth weight, have been shown to occur. With near-term, high-dose administration of aspirin, gestation can be prolonged, parturition delayed, and risk of hemorrhage increased in the newborn and mother. Even mature closure of the patent ductus arteriosus (hole in fetal heart) has been reported. Prostaglandins produce uterine contractions, useful in childbirth but not during menstruation. Although salicylates are excreted in the breast milk, usual occasional therapeutic doses of aspirin do not present a problem for the healthy nursing infant.

HYPERSENSITIVITY (ALLERGY) The incidence of true aspirin allergy is less than 1% (0.2% to 0.4%). Many patients with "allergy to aspirin" in their charts, upon questioning, actually have stomach problems rather than a true allergy. In the patient's chart, it is important to differentiate aspirin's adverse reactions from its hypersensitivity reactions. Adequate questioning of patients who "claim" to be allergic to aspirin is needed because patients with true aspirin hypersensitivity cannot be given any of the NSAIAs because of some cross-hypersensitivity. Allergic reactions can vary from rash, wheezing, urticaria, and angioneurotic edema to anaphylactic shock. When a true aspirin allergy exists, any aspirin-containing products or NSAIAs should be avoided.

> True aspirin allergy is uncommon.

Asthmatics are more likely to have a hypersensitivity reaction to aspirin, with the incidence ranging from 5% to 15%. The aspirin hypersensitivity triad—*aspirin hypersensitivity*, *asthma*, and *nasal* **polyps**—often occur together. This reaction is thought to be due to the shunting of the products of arachidonic acid from the production of prostaglandins to the leukotrienes and is thought to be a potential mechanism for this hypersensitivity. These patients exhibit cross-hypersensitivity between aspirin and other agents, including the nonsteroidal antiinflammatory agents, and they should not be given any NSAIAs.

Toxicity. An overdose of aspirin can produce harmful effects and even death.

SYMPTOMS When the blood level of salicylates reaches a certain level, a toxic reaction, referred to as **salicylism,** occurs. It is characterized by tinnitus, headache, nausea, vomiting, dizziness, and dimness of vision. Hyperthermia and electrolyte imbalance can also occur. With higher levels, stimulation of respiration leads to hyperventilation, which produces respiratory alkalosis. Compensatory alkalosis results in renal loss of bicarbonate, sodium, and potassium. Both respiratory and metabolic acidosis ensue. The cause of death from aspirin poisoning is usually acidosis and electrolyte imbalance.

> Toxicity prevention involves childproof containers.

Prevention. Children are the primary victims of accidental poisoning. The lethal dose of aspirin for a child is 4 gm, and the lethal dose of aspirin for an adult is 10 to 30 gm. Education of the parents regarding the potential for poisoning and proper storage, as well as childproof containers for over-the-counter (OTC) aspirin, have significantly reduced accidental poisonings in children.

Treatment. Treatment of aspirin poisoning includes removing excess drug in the stomach by inducing emesis or administering activated charcoal to adsorb the aspirin. Other symptoms are treated symptomatically. For example, hypothermia is treated with cooling baths or "blankets,"

acidosis with sodium bicarbonate, hypokalemia with potassium, and hypoglycemia with intravenous glucose.

Drug interactions. The drug interactions of aspirin are listed in Table 6-2 and in Table 25-1. Some of the more notable are briefly discussed.

- **Warfarin.** The drug interaction between aspirin and warfarin can result in bleeding. Warfarin [WAR-far-in], an oral anticoagulant, is highly protein bound to plasma protein–binding sites. If aspirin is administered to a patient taking warfarin, it can displace the warfarin from its binding sites, increasing its anticoagulant effect. Also, aspirin affects both platelets and the gastrointestinal tract. Bleeding and hemorrhage may result from these interactions.

- **Probenecid.** Aspirin interferes with probenecid's [proe-BEN-e-sid] uricosuric effect. Aspirin has been reported to have precipitated an acute attack of gout. Avoid using aspirin in patients taking probenecid.

- **Methotrexate.** Methotrexate [meth-oh-TREX-ate] (MTX) is an antineoplastic drug used to treat certain kinds of **cancer** and autoimmune diseases (arthritis, **psoriasis**). Aspirin can displace MTX from its protein-binding sites and can also interfere with its clearance. This results in an increased serum

TABLE 6-2 Selected* Drug Interactions of Aspirin

Medical Drug Group	Example	Potential Outcome
Oral anticoagulants	Warfarin (Coumadin)	Hemorrhage/bleeding
Uricosurics	Probenecid (Benemid)	ASA interferes with uricosuric effect
Sulfonylureas	Tolbutamide (Orinase); chlorpropamide (Diabinese)	Decreases blood sugar (hypoglycemia)
Antimetabolites	Methotrexate (MTX)	Increases MTX toxicity

*For a more complete listing see Table 25-1.

concentration and MTX toxicity, such as bone marrow depression.

- **Sulfonylureas.** Higher doses of salicylates (more than 2 gm) may produce a hypoglycemic effect. One proposed mechanism involves the displacement of the sulfonylureas from their plasma protein–binding sites by aspirin. This hypoglycemia effect can also be observed with insulin.
- **Antihypertensives.** Aspirin reduces the antihypertensive effect of many hypertensives including angiotensin-converting enzyme (ACE) inhibitors, β-blockers, and thiazide and loop diuretics. This requires several doses of aspirin over a few days. Aspirin's effect on the renal function, resulting in water and sodium retention, may contribute to this effect.

Uses. One use of aspirin is to provide analgesia for mild to moderate pain. It is the analgesic against which new analgesics are measured for efficacy. Its antipyretic effect is useful in the control of fever, but should be avoided in children (Reye's syndrome). Its antiinflammatory action is employed in the treatment of inflammatory conditions such as rheumatic fever and arthritis. Because of its effect on platelet aggregation (inhibition), aspirin is used to prevent unwanted clotting (more than 50 years old or previous myocardial infarction). In some patients the incidence of myocardial infarction has decreased, but the overall **mortality** remained the same.

Dosage and preparations. The usual adult dosage of aspirin for the treatment of pain or fever is 650 mg (two 5-gr tablets) every 4 hours. The dose for arthritis is between 3 and 6 gm/day. For prevention of myocardial infarction, the dose is less than 300 mg/day (sometimes 160 mg/day or 325 mg every other day). The dosage for children is 60 to 80 mg/kg/24 hours (maximum 3.6 gm/24 hr) divided into four to six doses or 5 mg/lb (see Table 6-10).

Many types of preparations containing aspirin are available by prescription and OTC (Table 6-3). Some of these types are as follows.

REGULAR ASPIRIN A single-entity form of aspirin includes the commonly used 325-mg (5-gr) tablet and 81-mg flavored children's tablet. Many brand and generic-products are available in all strengths.

ENTERIC-COATED ASPIRIN Aspirin can be formulated with a coating that dissolves in the intestine rather than the stomach. The advantage of enteric-coated aspirin is that gastric symptoms are reduced. The disadvantage is that these products can give erratic absorption and unreliable blood levels. The onset of action is too long to make them useful for acute dental pain. They have limited use in treatment of chronic arthritis when gastric irritation is a problem. They can be used when daily aspirin is used for clot prevention.

COMBINATIONS

With buffer Buffered tableted preparations, although claimed to produce fewer gastrointestinal side effects, have never been shown to do so. They are absorbed at a slightly quicker rate. The liquid buffered preparations do produce less gastrointestinal irritation, but they contain sodium, which is relatively contraindicated in high blood pressure.

With another analgesic Aspirin is often combined with acetaminophen or an opioid such as codeine. Although these combinations are additive, mixing aspirin with acetaminophen may increase the chance of renal toxicity. Mixing aspirin with an opioid can allow a decrease in the amount of the opioid in the product and therefore reduce its side effects.

With sedatives Adding a sedative to aspirin can make it more effective if anxiety is a substantial

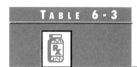

TABLE 6-3	Selected OTC Aspirin-Containing Products

ASPIRIN		INGREDIENTS		
TYPE OF ASPIRIN	SELECTED BRAND NAMES	AMOUNT OF ASPIRIN (mg)	OTHER	APPROXIMATE AMOUNT (mg)
Regular	Bayer	500, 325	None	
	Empirin	325		
	St. Joseph	325		
	Bayer, low dose	81		
Enteric coated	Ecotrin	500, 325	None	
	Ecotrin, low dose	81		
Buffered tablets	Bufferin	324	Magnesium carbonate	100
			Aluminum glycinate	50
	Ascriptin	325	Magnesium-aluminum hydroxide	150
Buffered solutions	Alka-Seltzer	324	Sodium bicarbonate	2000
			Citric acid	1000
Combinations	Various	250	Acetaminophen	150
			(Salicylamide)	150
	Excedrin tablets	250	Caffeine	65
			Acetaminophen	250
	Anacin	400	Caffeine	32
	Fiorinal*	325	Butalbital	50
			Caffeine	40

*By prescription only.

component of the pain. Prescribing a separate antianxiety agent would give the prescriber more control and is preferred.

With caffeine Caffeine potentiates the analgesic effect of aspirin and other analgesics. The addition of 130 mg of caffeine is equivalent to increasing the dose of the analgesic by between one third or more. Most proprietary preparations contain about one-half this much caffeine. (But you can always take two tablets of most analgesics.)

OTHER SALICYLATES

Sodium, choline, **magnesium** salicylate and salicylamide, and salsalate are other salicylates. These agents claim to have fewer gastrointestinal side effects, but this claim has little docu-

mentation. Their efficacy as analgesic agents and the appropriate doses for analgesia need to be determined. Two advantages of these agents are that *they are thought to have no effect on platelets and no cross-hypersensitivity with aspirin.* Magnesium is contraindicated in renal disease and sodium in cardiovascular disease. Salicylamide is a very weak analgesic. Salsalate is made up of the combination of two salicylic acids.

Diflunisal. Diflunisal [dye-FLOO-ni-sal] (Dolobid) is a salicylate classified as an NSAIA. Its peak action occurs 2 to 3 hours after ingestion, and its half-life is 8 to 12 hours in the normal patient. It is as effective as the other NSAIAs in the treatment of pain. Like other NSAIAs, diflunisal can be administered before a dental procedure to delay the onset of postsurgical pain. Because of its long half-life, it is dosed only 2 or

3 times daily. The general comments relating to the NSAIAs also apply to diflunisal. Its antipyretic effect is not clinically useful.

NONSTEROIDAL ANTIINFLAMMATORY AGENTS (NSAIAs) OR DRUGS (NSAIDs)

> Kissin' cousins of aspirin.

The NSAIA analgesics are a rapidly growing group that have important application in dentistry. Their mechanism of action and many of their pharmacologic effects and adverse reactions resemble those of aspirin. Many authors agree that the NSAIAs are the most useful drug group for the treatment of dental pain. They currently make up only a small percentage of our analgesic prescriptions. The availability of OTC NSAIAs gives the dental health care worker several products that can be recommended for purchase. Whether a prescription should be written for an NSAIA or an OTC NSAIA recommended depends on appraisal of the patient's attitudes.

CHEMICAL CLASSIFICATION

NSAIAs are divided into several chemical derivatives: the propionic acids, acetic acids, fenamates, pyrazolones, oxicams, and others. Table 6-4 lists the NSAIAs by chemical classification, pharmacokinetic parameters, analgesic dose, and dosing interval. Most members of the propionic acid derivative group, along with mefenamic acid and diflunisal, are approved for use for the management of pain.

MECHANISM OF ACTION

Like aspirin, NSAIAs inhibit the enzyme cyclooxygenase (prostaglandin synthase), resulting in a reduction in the formation of prostaglandin precursors and thromboxanes from arachidonic acid (see Figure 6-5). Many of the actions, as well as the adverse reactions, of the NSAIAs result from their inhibition of prostaglandin synthesis.

PHARMACOKINETICS

Most NSAIAs peak in about 1 to 2 hours (see Table 6-4). The effect of food on absorption of the NSAIAs approved to treat pain is to reduce the rate but not the extent of absorption of ibuprofen, the naproxens, and diflunisal. There is no effect on absorption of the NSAIAs with oral **antacids,** except for diflunisal (antacids reduce absorption). They are metabolized in the liver and excreted by the kidney. The half-lives of the individual agents are listed in Table 6-4. Biliary or fecal excretion occurs with the fenamates, piroxicam, sulindac, and tolmetin.

PHARMACOLOGIC EFFECTS

The analgesic, antipyretic, and antiinflammatory actions of the NSAIAs result from the same

> The Three A's

mechanism as aspirin—inhibition of prostaglandin synthesis by inhibiting cyclooxygenase. In the treatment of gout the action of the NSAIAs is related to their analgesic and antiinflammatory actions but is independent of their effect on serum uric acid. NSAIAs are useful for treating dysmenorrhea, or painful **menstruation,** because an excess of prostaglandins in the uterine wall produces painful contractions.

ADVERSE REACTIONS

Gastrointestinal effects. Gastrointestinal irritation, pain, and bleeding problems leading to tarry stools can occur with all the NSAIAs. The prostaglandins stimulate the production of cytoprotective mucus and stimulate gastric acid secretion. Prostaglandin inhibitors, such as

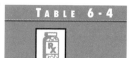

TABLE 6-4   Nonsteroidal Antiinflammatory Agents [NSAIAs], Peak, Half-life, and Analgesic and Maximm Dose (3/99)

DRUG NAME		PEAK (hr)	HALF-LIFE (hr)	ANALGESIC DOSE (mg) AND INTERVAL q (hr)	MAXIMUM DAILY DOSE (mg)
PROPIONIC ACID DERIVATIVES					
Ibuprofen[a] (Motrin, Rufen)		1-2	1.8-2.5	400 q4-6	3200
Flurbiprofen[b] (Ansaid-PO, Ocufen-ophth)		1.5	5.7	50 q4-6	300
				Ophthalmic solution to prevent inhibition of intraoperative miosis	
Fenoprofen (Nalfon)		1-2	2-3	200 q4-6	3200
Naproxen (Naprosyn)		2-4	12-15	500 stat; 250 q6-8	1500
Naproxen sodium[c] (Anaprox)		1-2	12-13	550 stat; 275 q6-8	1375
Ketoprofen (Orudis)[d]	I[e]	0.5-2	2-4	25-50 q6-8	300
Suprofen (Profenal)				Ophthalmic solution to prevent inhibition of intraoperative miosis	
Ketoprofen (Oruvail)	SR[f]	None	2-4	—[g]	300
Oxaprozin (Daypro)		3-5	42-50	1200 mg/24h	1800
ACETIC ACID DERIVATIVES					
Indomethacin (Indocin)	I[e]	1-2	4.5	25 mg q8-12h	200
Indomethacin SR (Indocin SR)	SR[f]	2-4	4.5-6	75 mg q12-24h	150
Sulindac (Clinoril)[h]		2-4	(8-16)[i]	150-200 mg q12h	400
Tolmetin (Tolectin)		0.5-1	1-1.5	400 mg q8h	2000
Diclofenac (Cataflam)	I[e]	1	1-3	50 q6-8	150
Diclofenac (Voltaren)	SR[f]	2-3	1-2	—[g]	200
Etodolac (Lodine)	I[e]	1-2	7.3	2-400 q6-8	1200
Etodolac (Lodine-XL)	SR[f]	None	7.3		1200
Ketoprofen (Orudis)	I[e]	0.5-2	2-4	25-50 q6-8	300
Ketoprofen (Oruvail)	SR[f]	None	2-4	—[g]	300
Ketorolac (Toradol)[j]		0.5-1	2.4-8.6	10 q4-6	40
NONACIDIC AGENT					
Nabumetone[k] (Relafen)		2.5-4	(22.5-30)[l]	800 mg/24h	2000
FENAMIC ACID DERIVATIVES					
Meclofenamate (Meclomen)		0.5-1	2-3	50 q4-6	400
Mefenamic acid[b] (Ponstel)		2-4	2-4	500 stat; 250 q6	1000
SALICYLATES					
Diflunisal (Dolobid)[m]		2-3	8-12	1000 stat; 500 q8-12	1500
OXICAMS					
Piroxicam (Feldene)[n]		3-5	30-86	20 mg/24h	20

NOTE: NSAIAs marketed and subsequently removed from market, often within months: Suprofen (Suprol) PO, zomepirac (Zomax),[o] carprofen (Rimadyl), benoxaprofen (Oraflex), bromfenac (Duract)[p].
[a]OTC as Ibuprofen, Motrin-IB, Advil, Haltran, Medipren.
[b]Therapy not usually to exceed 1 week.
[c]OTC as Aleve.
[d]OTC as Orudis-KT.
[e]*I*, immediate action.
[f]*SR*, sustained release action.
[g]Not approved for use as simple analgesic.
[h]Prodrug converted in liver to active sulfide metabolite.
[i]Half-life of metabolite.
[j]For short-term (<5 days) treatment following the use of the parenteral form.
[k]Prodrug converted to active metabolite.
[l]Half-life with chronic use in parenthesis ( ).
[m]Salicylate.
[n]qd dosing for arthritis, very long-acting.
[o]Fatal hypersensitivity reactions.
[p]Hepatic toxicity.

NSAIAs, can interfere with the normal protective mechanisms in the stomach and increase acid secretion, causing symptoms or even an ulceration or perforation. A prostaglandin, misoprostol [mye-soe-PROST-ole] (Cytotec) (PGE_2), is available to prevent NSAIA-induced ulcers.

Central nervous system effects.
The dose-dependent CNS side effects include sedation, dizziness, confusion, mental depression, headache, vertigo, and convulsions. Because of the CNS effects of the NSAIAs, patients taking them should be cautioned about driving an automobile. These agents are not addicting, tolerance does not develop, and no withdrawal syndrome can be induced.

Blood clotting.
The NSAIAs *reversibly* inhibit platelet aggregation because they inhibit thromboxane A_2 production. In contrast to aspirin, their effect remains only as long as the drug is present in the blood—1 day for ibuprofen, 4 days for naproxen, and 2 weeks for oxaprozin.

Renal effects.
Renal effects of the NSAIAs include renal failure, cystitis, and an increased incidence of urinary tract infections. The NSAIAs have little effect on the patient with normal kidney function; however, with disease, decreases in both renal blood flow and glomerular filtration rate can occur. NSAIAs have precipitated renal insufficiency. With decreased renal function, peripheral edema with fluid retention has been noted.

Other effects.
Other adverse effects associated with the NSAIAs are muscle weakness, ringing in the ears, hepatitis, hematologic problems, and blurred vision.

Oral effects.
Oral manifestations reported include ulcerative stomatitis, gingival ulcerations, and dry mouth.

Hypersensitivity reactions.
Like aspirin, the NSAIAs can induce a wide range of hypersensitivity reactions, including hives or itching, angioneurotic edema, chills and fever, Stevens-Johnson syndrome, exfoliative dermatitis, and epidermal necrolysis. Anaphylactoid reactions including bronchospasm (wheezing) have been reported.

Zomepirac (Zomax) is an example of an NSAIA that was removed from the market in response to a few fatal reactions. Zomepirac produced hypersensitivity reactions. Some of the patients who died should never have been given zomepirac because of their positive history of aspirin hypersensitivity. Benoxaprofen and suprofen, two propionic acid derivatives, were also marketed and then removed from the market because of toxicity. The lesson that these products teach us is that a new drug may cause previously undiscovered adverse reactions and should not be used without a clear advantage over available drugs. Also, any drug that is contraindicated in a certain situation should not be used in that situation. (Zomepirac was contraindicated in aspirin-sensitive patients, but was prescribed for them anyway!)

Pregnancy and nursing.
Like aspirin, the NSAIAs given late in pregnancy can

> Contraindicated in pregnancy

prolong gestation, delay parturition, and produce **dystocia** or premature closure of the ductus arteriosus. The uterine prostaglandins are responsible for parturition and closure of the ductus arteriosus. Fenoprofen, ibuprofen, and naproxen have not been shown to be teratogenic in animal studies (FDA pregnancy category B). Diflunisal, tolmetin, and mefenamic acid have been shown to be teratogenic in animals (FDA pregnancy category C).

Ibuprofen has not been detected in breast milk, whereas fenoprofen and mefenamic acid are present in very small quantities. Small amounts of both naproxen (1% of serum) and diflunisal (5% of serum) are excreted in breast milk. Ibuprofen is the drug of choice for treating a nursing woman.

Drug interactions. The drug interactions of the NSAIAs are summarized in Table 6-5. Interactions continue to be under investigation for their clinical significance and presence with each NSAIA. Lithium toxicity has been produced in those patients taking lithium for bipolar **affective disorders.** NSAIAs may increase the effect of digoxin, a drug used for congestive **heart failure.** Digoxin's narrow therapeutic index is one reason for caution. NSAIAs have been shown to reduce the effect of agents used as antihypertensives, such as diuretics, **ACE inhibitors,** and β-blockers. Probenecid can increase the serum levels of the NSAIAs. NSAIAs can increase the toxicity of cyclosporin and MTX. Before patients are given NSAIAs the drug interactions should be checked.

CONTRAINDICATIONS AND CAUTIONS

The contraindications and cautions for using an NSAIA (Table 6-6) are related to their adverse reactions. Patients with asthma, cardiovascular or renal diseases with fluid retention, coagulopathies, peptic ulcer, and ulcerative **colitis** should be given NSAIAs cautiously, if at all.

Patients also at higher risk for adverse reactions include those with renal function impairment or a history of previous hypersensitivity to aspirin or other NSAIAs, and geriatric patients, who are more prone to adverse hepatic or renal reactions (Box 6-3 lists the patient instructions for NSAIAs). NSAIAs are contraindicated during all trimesters of pregnancy.

THERAPEUTIC USES

Medical. Depending on the specific NSAIA and the clinical trials that have been conducted, medical use of NSAIAs may include many conditions. **Osteoarthritis,** rheumatoid arthritis, gouty arthritis, fever, dysmenorrhea, and pain are indications for the NSAIAs. Accepted unlabeled indications for which NSAIAs are frequently prescribed include bursitis and tendonitis.

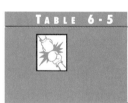

TABLE 6-5	Selected* Drug Interactions of the Nonsteroidal Antiinflammatory Agents (NSAIAs)

DRUG	POTENTIAL OUTCOME
Lithium	Increased effect of lithium
Methotrexate (MTX)	Increased effect of MTX leads to bone marrow toxicity
Diuretics	Reduced antihypertensive effect
ACE† inhibitors	Reduced hypertensive effect
β-Blockers	Reduced hypertensive effect
Digoxin	Increased digoxin effect

*For a more complete listing see Table 25-2.
†ACE, Angiotensin converting enzyme.

Box 6-3 PATIENT INSTRUCTIONS FOR USE OF NONSTEROIDAL ANTIINFLAMMATORY AGENTS

- Take with a full glass of water.
- Take with food to minimize gastrointestinal irritation.
- Use caution with driving because of possible drowsiness or dizziness.
- Do not use aspirin concurrently.
- If pain does not subside within a few days, call the dentist.
- Do not take OTC analgesics with prescription NSAIAs.

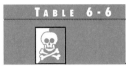

TABLE 6-6	**Contraindications and Cautions to Use of Aspirin (ASA) and Nonsteroidal Antiinflammatory Agents (NSAIAs)**	

DRUGS	DISEASE	COMMENTS
Aspirin Small doses	Prevent clotting, heart disease	May use NSAIAs, continue aspirin
High doses	Rheumatic fever	Aspirin lowers blood level of NSAIAs
Lithium	Bipolar (manic) disorder	NSAIAs reduce lithium clearance—potential lithium toxicity
H₂-Blockers Proton pump inhibitors	Peptic ulcer, gastroesophageal reflux disease	Gastric bleeding, esophagitis
Methotrexate (MTX)	Rheumatoid arthritis, psoriasis, cancer	Potentiates methotrexate toxicity—bone marrow suppression*
Vitamin K deficiency	Alcoholism, liver disease	Bleeding
Warfarin	Myocardial infarction, atrial fibrillation, prosthetic heart valve	Aspirin contraindicated—bleeding, use NSAIAs with caution
Factor VIII	**Hemophilia**	
Probenecid*	Gout	Probenecid inhibits excretion of NSAIAs
Colchicine	Gout	More GI adverse reactions
Allopurinol	Gout	No contraindications
None	Pregnancy	Contraindicated throughout pregnancy
None	Glucose-6-phosphate dehydrogenase deficiency	**Hemolysis**
None	Hypoprothrombinemia	Bleeding

*Once-a-week dosing as for autoimmune diseases can be used with caution.

Dental. The NSAIAs are useful in the management of dental pain. Many studies that have compared the analgesic efficacy of the NSAIAs with that of the opioid analgesics find that they are equivalent in many clinical situations. For example, usual analgesic doses of NSAIAs have been shown to be as effective as 650 mg of aspirin or acetaminophen plus 60 mg of codeine, and even as effective as the intermediate-strength opioid combinations (oxycodone plus aspirin or acetaminophen). In usual prescription doses, NSAIAs can be shown to be statistically significantly better than codeine alone, aspirin, acetaminophen, or placebo. It is difficult to understand why the dental use of the NSAIAs has decreased. All NSAIAs are equally efficacious at equi-analgesic doses. Figure 6-10 shows the pain relief over time of several commonly used analgesics. Their relative effectiveness will be discussed in the following paragraphs.

SPECIFIC NONSTEROIDAL ANTIINFLAMMATORY AGENTS

Ibuprofen. Ibuprofen [eye-byoo-PRO-fen] (Advil, Motrin), the oldest member of the NSAIAs, has the most clinical experience. It is rapidly absorbed orally, and food decreases its rate but not its extent of absorption; antacids have no effect. The half-life is about 2 hours. Its onset of action is about half an hour, and its duration of action is 4 to 6 hours. It undergoes hepatic metabolism and is excreted by the kidney. It is an effective analgesic and has been studied in many dental

FIGURE 6-10 *Time-effect curves for placebo, codeine, aspirin, aspirin plus codeine, and ibuprofen. The mean pain relief scores are plotted against time in hours. (From Cooper SA, et al: Pain relief over time for placebo, codeine, aspirin, aspirin plus codeine, and ibuprofen.* Pharmacotherapy, 2:162-167, 1982.)

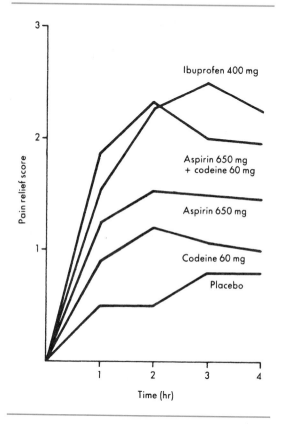

650 mg of aspirin, 600 mg of acetaminophen, and both aspirin and acetaminophen when combined with 60 mg of codeine (see Figure 6-10). A shallow dose-response curve for ibuprofen has been demonstrated, with some finding no difference between the 200-mg and 300-mg doses and others finding no difference between the 400-mg and 800-mg doses. The 200-mg (OTC) dose of ibuprofen has been shown to be as effective as two 325-mg doses of acetaminophen or aspirin. The 400-mg to 600-mg doses produce about the same degree of effectiveness, but the higher doses produce a longer duration of action (drug level stays above an analgesic dose longer because the blood level is higher).

The usual analgesic dose of ibuprofen is 400 to 800 mg every 4 to 6 hours. The higher range of dose may produce more antiinflammatory effects. Most studies can easily demonstrate that 400 mg of ibuprofen is better than any usual therapeutic doses of codeine.

Ibuprofen is available over the counter in 200-mg tablets and by prescription in 400-, 600-, and 800-mg tablets. Side effects such as CNS effects are dose dependent, so they occur more frequently at the higher end of the dosage range. Ibuprofen is also available in suspension form for pediatric use over the counter and is often used as an antipyretic. (See Table 6-11 for patient instructions for the use of NSAIAs.)

Naproxen and naproxen sodium. Naproxen [na-PROX-en] (Naprosyn) and naproxen sodium (Anaprox) are propionic acid NSAIAs that have slightly longer half-lives than ibuprofen and can be dosed on an 8- to 12-hour schedule. They should also be given with a loading dose (see Table 6-4). Their pharmacologic effects, adverse reactions, and efficacy are similar to those of ibuprofen. In addition to tablets, this product is available in suspension form. Figure 6-11 shows data for a patient taking lithium who begins taking naproxen. Note that naproxen lev-

| Longer acting |

situations. Ibuprofen is the drug of choice for treatment of dental pain when an NSAIA is indicated. Only in rare cases or if new information becomes available are other NSAIAs indicated. When a longer-acting agent is desired for patient convenience, the naproxens can be used.

Clinical trials in dental pain management testify to ibuprofen's effectiveness. A dose of 400 mg of ibuprofen is usually more effective than

FIGURE 6-11 *Change in serum lithium levels in patients given naproxen (N = 7). Results are expressed as mean ± standard error.*

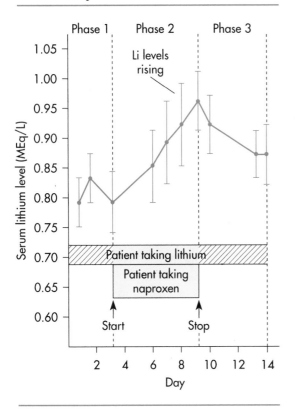

els rise when naproxen is given because it inhibits lithium clearance.

Other nonsteroidal antiinflammatory agents. Other NSAIAs (see Table 6-4) such as fenoprofen, ketorolac, or diflunisal (discussed previously) may be used for patients who do not respond to either ibuprofen or naproxen (sodium). Certain patients need an agent with which they are not familiar. "Shoppers" looking for scheduled drugs respond better to an unknown drug's name. Prescribing one of the new NSAIAs whose name has not yet become familiar may be effective.

Ketorolac [kee-TOE-role-ak] (Toradol) is a newer NSAIA. The use of this agent had increased because it was being heavily advertised to dental professionals. It is equivalent in efficacy to the other NSAIAs; however, unlike other NSAIAs, it is available parenterally. Make sure that before a new agent is prescribed it has some *documented* clinical advantage.

Ketorolac is an NSAIA indicated for the short-term (up to 5 days) management of moderately severe acute pain that requires analgesia at the opioid level. It is contraindicated as a prophylactic analgesic before any major surgery when hemostasis is critical because of the increased risk of bleeding. Oral ketorolac is indicated only as continuation therapy to intravenous or intramuscular ketorolac (must use injectable before prescribing the tablets).

Bromfenac (Duracet), a new NSAIA, is a relative of diclofenac [dye-KLOE-fen-ak]. (Note similarity in the name.) Bromfenac has now been removed from the market because of severe hepatic toxicity with fatalities. This illustrates the reason for not using the "newest" NSAIA, using your patients as "guinea pigs." When a new drug is on the market, wait for about a year before prescribing it, to be sure that it does not have negative side effects not described in the accompanying literature.

COX II–specific agents. All of the currently available NSAIAs inhibit both cyclooxygenase (COX) I and COX II. COX I is a widely distributed, constitutive (present at all times) enzyme responsible for the adverse reactions of the NSAIAs—such as stomach problems, reduced renal function, fluid retention, and reduced platelet adhesiveness. COX II is an inducible enzyme that is synthesized only when inflammation occurs.

COX II–specific inhibitors, because they inhibit COX II (good) much more than COX I (bad), should have much fewer adverse reactions than the former NSAIAs. Celecoxib (Celebrax), a COX II–specific inhibitor, has recently been

▮ **TABLE 6-7**	Cyclooxygenase (COX) Receptors—COX-1 and COX-2		
COX RECEPTORS	ENZYME	EFFECTS	EXAMPLES
COX I-II	Both		Ibuprofen Naproxen Meclofenamate
COX-I–specific	Constitutive, always present, wide distribution	Side effects seen in renal blood flow, fluid and electrolytes, stomach mucosal integrity, and vasomotor tone, uterus	Indomethacin Sulindac
COX-II–specific COX II >> I	Inducible, expression variable	Antiinflammatory	Celecoxib (Celebra), rofecoxib (Vioxx)

released and is indicated for arthritis. In prerelease studies, fewer side effects were noted with celecoxib than with the usual NSAIAs. Celecoxib has not been proved to be a very effective analgesic, but other agents with similar action will be developed and may be better analgesics. Table 6-7 lists some NSAIAs grouped by COX inhibition.

ACETAMINOPHEN

Acetaminophen [a-seet-a-MEE-noe-fen] (paracetamol, *N*-acetyl *p*-aminophenol; Tylenol) is the only member of the *p*-aminophenols currently available for clinical use. Acetanilid, the parent compound, was introduced in 1886 and rapidly shown to be too toxic. Phenacetin, removed from the market in 1983, was more toxic than acetaminophen. Acetaminophen is used as an analgesic and antipyretic in children and in adults when aspirin is contraindicated.

PHARMACOKINETICS

Acetaminophen is rapidly and completely absorbed from the gastrointestinal tract, achieving a peak plasma level in 1 to 3 hours. After therapeutic doses, it is excreted with a half-life of 1 to 4 hours. Acetaminophen is metabolized by the liver microsomal enzymes to the glucuronide conjugate, the sulfuric acid conjugate, and cysteine. When large doses are ingested, an intermediate metabolite is produced that is thought to be hepatotoxic and possibly nephrotoxic. Acetaminophen and aspirin are equally efficacious (kills the same degree of pain) and equally potent (same dose in milligrams needed for effect) as analgesics and antipyretics.

PHARMACOLOGIC EFFECTS

The analgesic and antipyretic effects of acetaminophen are approximately the same potency (on a milligram for milligram basis) as aspirin (see Figure 6-6). This means that acetaminophen and aspirin are equally efficacious, and, because virtually the same doses are used for each agent, they are equally potent. However, acetaminophen does not possess any clinically significant antiinflammatory effect. Therefore it is less useful in the treatment of arthritis. Differences in degree of prostaglandin synthesis inhibition at different sites may account for this difference in action.

Therapeutic doses of acetaminophen have no effect on the cardiovascular or respiratory system. In contrast to aspirin, acetaminophen does not produce gastric bleeding or affect platelet adhesiveness or uric acid excretion.

> Alcoholics should avoid acetaminophen.

ADVERSE EFFECTS

The principal toxic effects of acetaminophen are hepatic necrosis and nephrotoxicity.

Hepatic effects. The toxic metabolite of acetaminophen that contributes to hepatic necrosis is N-acetyl-*p*-benzoquinonamine. Hepatic necrosis may occur in adults after the acute ingestion of a single dose of 20 to 25 gm of acetaminophen; 25 gm or more is potentially fatal. Symptoms during the first 2 days after intoxication are minor. Nausea, vomiting, anorexia, and abdominal pain may occur. Liver injury becomes manifest on the second to third day, with alterations in plasma enzyme levels (elevated transaminase and lactic hydrogenase), elevated bilirubin levels, and prolongation of **prothrombin time.** Hepatotoxicity may progress to encephalopathy, coma, and death. If the patient recovers, no residual hepatic abnormalities persist. Patients with hepatic disease, such as those with a history of hepatitis, should avoid acetaminophen.

Alcohol stimulates the oxidizing enzymes that metabolize acetaminophen to its toxic metabolite. Depending on the amount of alcoholic beverages ingested, the maximum dose of acetaminophen varies. The normal maximum dose of acetaminophen (4 gm) may be used in patients who usually do not drink. The dose should be restricted to 2 gm if a patient is a moderate drinker (less than three alcohol beverages daily). Alcoholics or patients who normally ingest three or more alcohol beverages daily should avoid acetaminophen completely (Table 6-8).

Treatment of toxicity. The treatment of overdose toxicity should begin with gastric lavage if a drug has recently been ingested. The administration of activated charcoal and magnesium or sodium sulfate solution should follow. The administration of sulfhydryl groups in the form of oral N-acetylcysteine reduces or even prevents liver damage if given soon enough after ingestion.

TABLE 6-8 **Maximum Acetaminophen (NAPAP) Dose Related to Alcohol Use**

CHRONIC ALCOHOL CONSUMED	MAXIMUM DAILY DOSE OF NAPAP (gm)
None	4 for a short period; 2.6 for chronic use
Moderate drinking (less than three drinks per day)	2
Alcoholic and three or more drinks per day	None

NAPAP, N-Acetyl-*p*-aminophenol (acetaminophen).

Nephrotoxicity. Nephrotoxicity has been associated with long-term consumption. The primary lesion appears to be a papillary necrosis with secondary interstitial nephritis. Although no single agent can be identified, prolonged consumption of analgesics can lead to kidney disease. Because analgesics are used in dental practice on a short-term basis, the possibility of nephrotoxicity does not present a significant problem in dental therapy. Concurrent chronic use of the combination of acetaminophen and aspirin or NSAIAs increases the risk of analgesic nephropathy, renal papillary necrosis, endstage renal disease, and cancer of the kidney or urinary **bladder.**

DRUG INTERACTIONS

Acetaminophen is remarkably free of drug interactions at its usual therapeutic doses. The hepato-

> DI = Essentially nonexistent

toxicity of acetaminophen can be potentiated by administration of agents that induce hepatic microsomal enzymes such as barbiturates, carbamazepine, phenytoin, and rifampin. Chronic large doses of alcohol can increase the toxicity of acetaminophen.

TABLE 6-9 Acetaminophen Dosing Chart (mg)

Weight (lbs)	Age	mg	Liquid/Elixir* 160 mg/5 ml (# tsp)
24	<2	Consult	Consult
25-35	2-3	160	1
36-47	4-5	240	1.5
48-59	6-8	320	2
60-71	9-10	400	2.5
72-95	11	480	3

NOTE: Obtain the child's weight in pounds; check weight column and determine applicable row; read the dose (mg) column to determine dose; identify preparation parent has or will purchase; determine the volume or number of tablets needed for the dose and product.
*Caution: Preparations with different concentrations available, number of teaspoonfuls only for this concentration; infants' concentrated drops uses much less volume.

USES

Acetaminophen is employed as an analgesic and antipyretic. It is especially useful in patients who have aspirin hypersensitivity or in whom aspirin-induced gastric irritation would present a problem. In young children its use as an antipyretic has replaced aspirin because of aspirin's association with Reye's syndrome. It is not known to what degree the long-term use of therapeutic doses of acetaminophen might produce renal lesions. It has a greater propensity for producing hepatic necrosis when a large acute dose (overdose) is ingested.

DOSAGE AND PREPARATIONS

Acetaminophen is available in many combinations and elixirs (Tylenol, Tempra). The usual adult dose is 1 (325 or 500 mg) or 2 tablets or capsules. Not more than 4 gm in 24 hours should be ingested by adults. Various elixirs, drops, and chewable tablets that are convenient for administration to children are available. The concentration of the elixir is 120 mg/5 ml (1 teaspoonful) or 160 mg/5 ml; the drops contain 60 mg/0.6 ml.

TABLE 6-10 Analgesic Dosing by mg/lb

Drug	Dose in mg/lb
Acetaminophen	5
Aspirin	5
Ibuprofen	5
Naproxen	2.5

Acetaminophen should not be administered to children less than 3 years old or for more than 10 days except on a prescriber's advice. The dosing of acetaminophen in children can be determined using Table 6-9. Table 6-10 gives the dose of acetaminophen, aspirin, ibuprofen, and naproxen on a milligram per pound basis.

DRUGS USED TO TREAT GOUT

Gout is an inherited disease occurring primarily in men, with an onset that usually involves one joint, often the big toe or knee. Both hyperuricemia and urate crystals, or tophi, may be found in the joints or other tissues. The excess uric acid may be due to excessive production or reduced excretion of uric acid (two types of gout). The disease responds to colchicine.

Both the NSAIAs and colchicine are used to treat acute attacks of gout. Other agents, such as probenecid and allopurinol [al-oh-PURE-i-nole], are available to prevent gout. These are briefly mentioned here, although they are not analgesics per se.

COLCHICINE

Colchicine [KOL-chi-seen] has only one indication—the treatment of an acute attack of gout. It is so specific in its action on gouty attacks that it is sometimes used to diagnose the disease. Colchicine is taken hourly at the onset of the attack or until side effects, such as nausea and vomiting, are intolerable. Its mechanism is complex, but it appears to inhibit the chemotactic property of leukocytosis and interfere with the inflammatory response to urate crystals. Colchicine possesses many side effects, but gastrointestinal toxicity, including nausea, vomiting, and diarrhea, occurs frequently (up to 80%). Bone marrow depression and hypersensitivity have also been reported.

ALLOPURINOL

Allopurinol (Zyloprim) is a xanthine oxidase inhibitor that inhibits the synthesis of uric acid. It is used to prevent excessive uric acid from forming. It is also used in patients receiving either **chemotherapy** or irradiation for malignancy because the death of many cells causes a release of large amounts of uric acid precursors. The side effects associated with allopurinol include hepatotoxicity of a hypersensitivity type. If a pruritic rash should occur, the drug should be promptly discontinued because fatalities have been reported. This drug is not indicated for asymptomatic hyperuricemia.

PROBENECID

The other approach to prevention of gout is to increase the excretion of uric acid by the administration of a uricosuric agent such as probenecid (Benemid) (see Figure 6-8). Probenecid, by blocking the tubular reabsorption of filtered urate, prevents new tophi and mobilizes those present. Increasing frequency or severity of acute gouty attacks is an indication for uricosuric administration.

Gastrointestinal side effects and hypersensitivity may occur with probenecid use. Headaches and sore gums have also been reported. Concurrent administration of aspirin can interfere with the uricosuric action of probenecid. Diabetic tests using the copper sulfate urine test (Clinitest) may have false-positive results. Occasionally probenecid and colchicine are combined, with the colchicine preventing acute attacks and the probenecid enhancing the excretion of uric acid. Probably a more rational approach is to administer each drug separately as needed. Maintenance of adequate urinary output (at least 2 L) is important to minimize the precipitation of uric acid in the urinary tract.

Probenecid increases the level of the NSAIAs and penicillin. In the latter case this effect can be used therapeutically (see discussion of penicillin in Chapter 8). For prevention of acute gout either probenecid or allopurinol can be used. The treatment of acute gout normally employs NSAIAs and colchicine.

For mild to moderate pain the drug of choice is either acetaminophen or aspirin in adults. Aspirin provides an antiinflammatory effect but is contraindicated in children and adolescents. If both aspirin and acetaminophen provide inadequate pain relief, then ibuprofen can be used. Its analgesic efficacy parallels that of many products combining nonopioids with opioids, such as aspirin with codeine (Empirin #3).

REVIEW QUESTIONS

1. Name the two components of pain, and state which one varies and which one is constant among patients.
2. List four factors that lower the patient's pain threshold and two that raise it.
3. Describe the placebo effect and discuss its place in the clinical studies of dental analgesics.
4. Compare and contrast the nonopioid and opioid analgesics with respect to the following:
   a. site of action
   b. mechanism of action
   c. efficacy
   d. addiction and tolerance
   e. toxicity
5. Compare the mechanism of action of aspirin and the NSAIAs.

6. State and describe three major effects and four other effects of aspirin.
7. Name the toxic reaction to the salicylates and describe its symptoms.
8. Describe the nature and extent of the most serious drug interaction with aspirin. Explain the other drug interactions of aspirin.
9. Name disease states contraindicating the use of aspirin.
10. Explain the contrast between the uricosuric effect of aspirin alone and its interaction with probenecid.
11. Name the therapeutic uses of aspirin.
12. State some other agents that are commonly combined with aspirin, and describe the rationale, if any, of the combinations.
13. List the various dosage forms of aspirin and their purported and proved advantages, if any.
14. Compare and contrast the pharmacologic effects of aspirin and acetaminophen. Efficacy? Potency?

15. List an adverse effect of acetaminophen and describe its symptoms and treatment.
16. Explain two uses of acetaminophen.
17. Explain the role of acetaminophen in the treatment of dental pain.
18. Explain the role of the NSAIAs for the treatment of dental pain.
19. Name the major adverse reaction of the NSAIAs.
20. State three NSAIAs useful as analgesics. Describe one difference among them.
21. State three contraindications to the use of the NSAIAs. Compare these with those of aspirin.
22. Compare the mechanisms of action between allopurinol and probenecid.
23. State which agents are used to treat an acute attack of gout and which are used prophylactically.

Opioid (Narcotic) Analgesics and Antagonists

The opioid analgesics are frequently used to manage dental pain in patients in whom nonsteroidal antiinflammatory agents (NSAIAs) are contraindicated. The dental hygienist and the dentist should be aware of the opioid groups, side effects, relative potency, and proper place in the management of dental pain.

HISTORY

Opium is the dried juice from the unripe seed capsules of the opium poppy. As early as 4000 BC, many cultures had recognized the euphoric effect of the poppy plant. In the early 1800s, morphine and codeine were isolated from opium. Until about 1920, patent medicines containing opium were promoted for numerous uses. When these agents, used orally, became unlawful, narcotic (opioid) abuse by injection began and has continued until the present.

TERMINOLOGY

| Narcotic = Opioid |

The terms used to refer to this drug group have changed over the years. *Narcotics*, the original name for this group of drugs, is derived from the Greek word that means "stupor." At first, the term *narcotics* was used to refer to drugs that are derivatives of opium poppy. Drugs in different pharmacologic classes with central nervous system (CNS) depressant effects also began to be lumped into the narcotic group because they caused stupor. This designation then became confusing because the drugs in it had different properties. *Opiates* was the next term that was used. It refers to drugs that are derived from the substances in the opioid poppy. Other chemical agents that produced opiate effects but did not have a structure like the opiates were synthesized but were not opiate like. To be more inclusive, another name for this group was adopted—*opioids*. The term *opioids* was then used to include not only the former opiates but also former opiates, other structurally different agents, their antagonists, and the receptors stimulated by the opioids. The old term *narcotic* is still used in older publications or by older practitioners.

CLASSIFICATION

The clinically useful opioids may be divided in several different ways. One way to divide these agents is by their mechanism of action at the receptor sites: agonists, mixed opioids, and antagonists. Table 7-1 shows the classifications.

TABLE 7-1 Classification of the Opioids by Receptor Action

GROUP	SUBGROUP	EXAMPLE
Opioid agonists		Morphine, codeine
Mixed opioids	Agonist–antagonists	Pentazocine
	Partial agonists	Buprenorphine
Antagonists		Naloxone

The opioids may also be classified by their chemical structure (Box 7-1). Structural classification is useful when the patient has a history of an allergy. Agents with the most similar chemical structure are more likely to be cross-allergenic; conversely, those with very different structures are much less likely to exhibit cross-allergenicity. The chemical structure groups include morphine/codeine, methadone, morphinan, eperidine, and others. The largest group is the morphine/codeine group, of which codeine is a member. A patient with a true allergy to codeine should be given an analgesic *not* in that group.

| Structure related to cross-allergenicity |

Opioids may be classified by their efficacy (Table 7-2). Efficacy classification assists in selection of the proper opioid based on the amount of pain relief needed. The amount of pain experienced is usually related to the individual patient and his or her reaction to the dental procedure as well as the specific dental procedure being performed. Although "bigger" procedures may elicit more pain, the characteristics of the patient play a more important role.

MECHANISM OF ACTION

The opioids bind to receptors located in both the CNS and the spinal cord, producing an

BOX 7-1 OPIOID ANALGESIC AGENTS BY STRUCTURE GROUP

Morphine and codeine

Hydromorphone (Dilaudid)
Hydrocodone (in Vicodin)
Dihydrocodeine (in Synalgos-DC)
Oxycodone (in Percadon, Percocet, Tylox)

Methadone

Methadone (Dolophine)
Propoxyphene (Darvon)

Morphinan

Butorphanol (Stadol)
Pentazocine (in Talwin-Nx)

Meperidine

Meperidine (Demerol)
Fentanyl (Sublimaze)
Diphenoxylate (in Lomotil)
Loperamide (Imodium)—OTC

Other

Buprenorphine (Buprenex)

altered perception of reaction to pain (see Figure 6-1).

Receptors that mediate specific pharmacologic effects and adverse reactions are stimulated to varying degrees by individual opioids.

Important receptors include μ, κ, and δ.

The discovery of three groups of endogenous substances with opioid-like action—the enkephalins, **endorphins,** and dynorphins—has helped explain the presence of these receptors. These naturally occurring peptides all possess analgesic action and have addiction potential. They probably function as neurotransmitters, but their exact function has not been elucidated. They may be involved in the analgesic action of a placebo and the enhancement of well-being that occurs with running (an increase in β-endorphins).

Table 7-3 describes the pharmacologic effects of selected opioid receptors and effect of some opioids on these receptors. Opioids may be complete agonists, partial agonists, agonist-antagonists, or antagonists. The three opioid receptors that have been characterized in more detail and that are stimulated by the opioids are the mu (μ), kappa (κ), and delta (δ) receptors. Differences in affinity for and action of by different opioids in tolerance to pain might even be due to variations in the endogenous levels of the neurotransmitters. Differences in affinity for and action of different opioids at these and other specific receptors explain some of the differences among the different opioids' adverse reactions (Figure 7-1). For example, the κ-receptor is responsible for dysphoria. Pentazocine, a κ-receptor agonist, produces dysphoria; morphine has no effect on the κ-receptor and produces much less dysphoria. Naloxone is an antagonist at the three receptor sites. More opioid receptors are sure to be identified and characterized. As more subreceptor types are elucidated, it will be possible to further separate beneficial (analgesic) effects of the opioids from their side effects (e.g., respiratory depression, constipation, drug dependence).

PHARMACOKINETICS

ADME, an acronym of the first letters of each component of drug handling, refers to absorption, distribution, metabolism, and excretion.

- **Absorption:** Most opioid analgesic agents are absorbed well when taken orally; absorp-

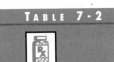

| **TABLE 7-2** | **Selected Opioid Analgesics by Efficacy, Dosing Interval, Usual Doses, and Schedule** |

Drug Name	Dosing Interval (hr)	Usual Dose (mg)*	Comments	Schedule for Controlled Substances
Strongest				
Morphine	4-6	IM: 10	Standard agent; prototype	II
Methadone (Dolophine)	4-6†	IM: 10 PO: 10	Used PO for "methadone maintenance"	II
Meperidine (Demerol)	3-4	IM: 100 PO: 50	Abused by professionals	II
Hydromorphone (Dilaudid)	4-6	PO: 2	Most potent on a mg for mg basis	II
Intermediate				
Oxycodone (in Percodan, Percocet, Tylox, Roxiprin, Roxicet)	4-6	PO: 5	Popular with addicts "shopping" for opioids	II
Pentazocine (in Talwin NX)	4-6	PO: 50	Has antagonist properties	IV
Weakest				
Hydrocodone (in Vicodin, Lortab, Lorcet)	4-6	PO: 5		III
Codeine (in Tylenol #3, Empirin #3)	4-6	PO: 30	#2 = 15 mg; #3 = 30 mg; #4 = 60 mg	III
Dihydrocodeine (in Synalgos-DC)	4-6	PO: 30	16 mg per dose	III
Propoxyphene (in Darvocet-N 100)	4-6	PO: 65 (HCl) or 100 (N)	65 mg HCl = 100 mg napsylate	IV

*Average dose.
†Dosing interval in methadone maintenance 24 hours.
HCl, Hydrochloride; *IM,* intramuscularly; *N,* napsylate; *PO,* orally.

FIGURE 7-1   *Effects of morphine, pentazocine, and naloxone at the μ, κ, and δ receptors.*

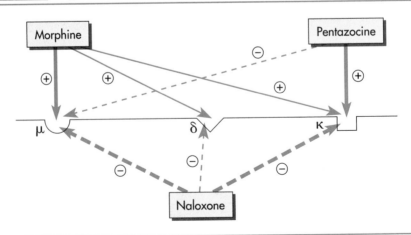

TABLE 7-3 Opioid Receptors, Effects, and Stimulation by Various Opioids

	μ (MU)		δ (DELTA)		SIGMA (σ)	EPSILON (ε)	κ (KAPPA)		
Effects	Supraspinal analgesia, sedation, miosis (pruritus)	Spinal analgesia, respiratory depression, euphoria, physical dependence, constipation	???Analgesia (?emotion, seizures)		Autonomic stimulation, dysphoria, hallucinations, nightmares, anxiety, ?antianalgesic	Analgesia	Analgesia (1 = spinal, 3 = supraspinal, sedation, myosis (?micturition, diuresis) ?dysphoria		
	μ1	μ2	δ1	δ2	σ	ε	κ1	κ2	κ3
ENDOGENOUS OPIOIDS									
Enkephalins	Ag		Ag						
β-Endorphins	Ag		Ag						
Dynorphin	Wk Ag						Ag		
OPIOID AGONISTS									
Morphine	Ag		Wk Ag				Wk Ag		
Codeine	Wk Ag		Wk Ag						
Fentanyl	Ag		Ag				Ag		
MIXED OPIOIDS									
Pentazocine	[Wk] Ant, [pAg]						Ag		
Buprenorphine	p Ag						Ant		
Butorphanol	Wk-p Ag						Ag		
Nalbuphine	Antagonist						Agonist		
Dezocine	p-Ant						Ag		
OPIOID ANTAGONISTS									
Naloxone	Ant		[Wk] Ant				Ant		
Nalmefene	Ant		?Ant				?Ant		
Naltrexone	Ant		?Ant				?Ant		

*Ag, Agonist; pAg, partial agonist; wk-Ag, weak agonist; Ant, competitive antagonist; pAnt, partial antagonist; O, no effect; ?, unknown.
NOTE: Opioids affect pain by these mechanisms: central, spinal, supraspinal, and peripheral mechanisms.
Nocio—peripheral, central.
Neurotransmitters—via norepinephrine, seratonin, epidural α-agonist potentiates.
Opioids, decrease Ca influx through Ca channels, enhance K conductance (open channels)—hyperpolarization.
Naloxone attenuates analgesic effects of acupuncture and placebo after minor surgery, but hyperalgesic after major surgery.

tion occurs from the lungs and from the nasal and oral mucosa. Absorption occurs through the mucous membranes of the nose and the intact skin. A nasal spray for one opioid, butorphanol (Stadol NS) is available. Absorption through the skin is used to advantage with transdermal patches of fentanyl (Duragesic).

> First-pass metabolism reduces bioavailability.

- **Distribution:** After absorption, the opioids undergo variable first-pass metabolism in the liver or intestinal cell wall, which reduces their bioavailability. The oral to parenteral ratio determines the difference in bioavailability between an opioid administered orally and one given parenterally. For example, the ratio is 0.2 to 0.3 for morphine, 0.25 to 0.7 for meperidine, and 0.4 to 0.7 for codeine. Therefore about two thirds of codeine administered orally reaches the systemic circulation, whereas only about one fourth of morphine does. The opioids are bound to plasma proteins to varying degrees (morphine 35%, meperidine 60%). The opioids are also distributed to the fetus in pregnant women, accounting for the respiratory depression produced in the fetus when the mother is given opioids near term.
- **Metabolism:** The major route of metabolism for the opioids is conjugation with glucuronic acid in the liver. Given orally, most opioids have a similar duration of action for analgesia—4 to 6 hours.
- **Excretion:** Metabolized opioids are excreted by glomerular filtration as their metabolites. The metabolites and the unchanged drug are excreted in the urine.

The dosing interval and usual dose of some opioids are listed in Table 7-2. In general, their onset is within 1 hour and their duration necessitates dosing every 4 to 6 hours.

PHARMACOLOGIC EFFECTS

Although the pharmacologic effects and the adverse reactions of the opioids are closely related, they are discussed separately. A pharmacologic effect may also be an adverse reaction, depending on the clinical use of the agent. In general, *the severity of the side effects is proportional to the agent's efficacy (strength)*.

Analgesia. The opioid analgesics provide varying degrees of analgesia, depending on the

> Efficacy is variable among opioids.

strength of the agent. Figure 7-2 shows the relative analgesic efficacy of selected opioids. Morphine is the opioid agonist by which other opioids are measured. The strongest opioids can reduce even the most severe pain; the weaker agents mixed with nonopioids are equivalent to the NSAIAs in their ability to relieve pain; the analgesic potency of the weakest agent (codeine) is low.

Codeine raises the pain threshold and affects the cerebral cortex to depress the reaction to pain. Both μ-receptors and κ-receptors are involved in producing analgesia. The opioids alter the patient's reaction to painful stimuli, possibly by altering the release of certain central neurotransmitters.

F IGURE　7 - 2　*Comparing strengths of opioids. Opioids vary in efficacy (maximal effect attained) from codeine (low) to morphine (high).*

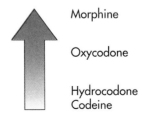

Sedation and euphoria. In the usual therapeutic doses the opioid analgesics generally produce sedation by κ-receptor stimulation. This may potentiate their analgesic effect and relieve anxiety. This effect is additive with other CNS depressants, such as alcohol. With larger doses, or if the pain is suddenly removed, euphoria can result. CNS excitation rarely occurs.

Cough suppression. The opioids exert their antitussive action by depressing the cough center, located in the medulla. The dose that produces the antitussive effect is much lower than that required for analgesia, so the least potent agents are effective (such as codeine). Related compounds, such as dextromethorphan, are often used as antitussives.

Gastrointestinal effects. The opioids increase the smooth muscle tone of the intestinal tract and markedly decrease its propulsive contractions and motility. This effect has made opioids useful in the symptomatic treatment of diarrhea. Opioid-like agents without analgesic properties, such as diphenoxylate (in Lomotil), are used for this effect to treat diarrhea.

ADVERSE REACTIONS

Unlike many other drugs, the adverse reactions of the opioids are not related to a direct damaging effect on hepatic, renal, or hematologic tissues but rather are an extension of their pharmacologic effects. Like the pharmacologic effects, the adverse reactions of the opioid analgesics are proportional to their analgesic strength. Table 7-4 lists contraindications and cautions for the use of opioids.

Not a problem with usual doses in normal patients.

Respiratory depression. The opioid analgesic agonists depress the respiratory center in a dose-related manner. This is usually the cause of death with an overdose. The depression is related to a decrease in the sensitivity of the brainstem to carbon dioxide. Both the rate and depth of breathing are reduced. In elderly or debilitated patients, the usual therapeutic dose of morphine can produce a significant decrease in pulmonary ventilation. Reduced ventilation produces vasodilation, which results in an increase in intracranial pressure. Opioids should not be used in patients with head injuries. Opioids may also mask CNS diagnostic symptoms. Patients with hyperthyroidism are more tolerant to the depression, whereas patients with myxedema are more sensitive.

Nausea and emesis. Analgesic doses of opioid analgesics often produce nausea and vomiting. This is due to their direct stimulation of the chemoreceptor trigger zone (CTZ), located in the medulla. This side effect is reduced by discouraging ambulation. Administration of repeated, regular doses of an opioid can prevent vomiting by depressing the vomiting center (VC), another area in the CNS distinct from the chemoreceptor trigger zone.

Constipation. The opioids produce constipation by producing a tonic contraction of the gastro-

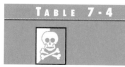

TABLE 7-4	Contraindications and Cautions to the Use of Opioids
CONDITION	COMMENT
Alcoholic or addict	Greater potential for abuse
Head injury	Can increase intracranial pressure
Chronic pain (e.g., TMD)	Addiction potential limits duration
Respiratory disease	Respiratory depression can occur
Pregnancy	Respiratory depression near-term (fetus)
Nursing	No problem: watch infant
Nausea	Additive nausea
Constipation	Exacerbates or produces constipation

intestinal tract. Small doses of even weak opioids frequently have this effect, and their duration outlasts their analgesic effect. Even with continued administration, tolerance does not develop to this effect.

Myosis. The opioid analgesics cause myosis, an important sign (pinpoint pupils) in diagnosing an opioid overdose or identifying an addict. Tolerance does not develop to this effect.

Urinary retention. The opioids increase the smooth muscle tone in the urinary tract, thereby causing urinary retention. They also produce an antidiuretic effect by stimulating the release of antidiuretic hormone (ADH) from the **pituitary gland.** This reaction may pose a problem in patients with prostatic hypertrophy.

Central nervous system effects. Occasionally, opioids may produce CNS stimulation, exhibited by anxiety, restlessness, or nervousness. Dysphoria can also occur from the opioids.

Cardiovascular effects. The opioids may depress the vasomotor center and stimulate the vagus nerve. With high doses, **postural hypotension,** bradycardia, and even syncope may result.

Biliary tract constriction. In high doses, the opioids may constrict the biliary duct, resulting in biliary colic. This effect is important in patients passing gallstones who are being treated with opioids.

Histamine release. Because the opioids can stimulate the release of histamine, itching and urticaria can result from their administration. This effect can occur at the site of intramuscular injection or at remote sites (e.g., itchy nose).

Pregnancy and nursing. Opioids have not been shown to be teratogenic, although they may prolong labor or depress fetal respiration if given near term. Infants born to mothers using high-dose opioids, as in an addict, can have marked depressed respiration and experience withdrawal symptoms. The amount of opioid excreted in the mother's milk when therapeutic doses are given to the mother would pose no problem to the normal infant. Morphine and codeine are classified as Food and Drug Administration (FDA) pregnancy category C. Acetaminophen is a category B drug.

Drug interactions. Some of the drug interactions of the opioids are listed in Table 7-5. A more de-

TABLE 7-5 Drug Interactions of the Opioids

	MEDICAL DRUG	POTENTIAL OUTCOME
GENERAL OPIOIDS	Alcohol	Additive CNS depression
	Barbiturates	
SPECIFIC OPIOIDS		
Propoxyphene	Carbamazepine	Carbamazepine toxicity
Meperidine	Barbiturates	↑ Toxicity of meperidine
	Chlorpromazine, neuroleptics	↓ BP → CNS depression
	Monoamine oxidase inhibitors	Severe reactions, excitation, rigidity, ↑ BP
Methadone	Barbiturates	↓ Methadone levels
	Phenytoin	↓ Methadone levels; withdrawal
	Rifampin	

tailed table is available in Chapter 25 (see Table 25-3). The most common outcome is sedation.

ADDICTION

The degree of **addiction** potential of opioids is proportional to their analgesic strength. This fact limits the usefulness of the strongest of these agents. Because the duration of use in dentistry is usually short, addiction does not often pose a problem for the dentist. NSAIAs should be used to control dental pain in the addict. An addict will develop tolerance to the effects of the opioids, except for **myosis** and constipation. The rate of development of tolerance is related to the strength of the opioid and its frequency of use.

Overdose. The major symptom of opioid overdose is respiratory depression. In addition to pinpoint pupils and coma, this symptom is pathognomonic for opioid overdose. Opioid overdose is treated with an antagonist, naloxone, discussed later in this chapter.

Withdrawal. After abruptly discontinuing the opioids a withdrawal syndrome occurs. The symptoms include yawning, lacrimation, perspiration, rhinorrhea, gooseflesh ("cold turkey"), irritability, nausea, vomiting, tachycardia, tremors, and chills. The name "cold turkey" comes from the symptom of piloerection (like when you're cold). This reminded addicts of the way a turkey looks (little bumps).

Identification of addict. "Shoppers" are addicts who try to find a physician or dentist who will prescribe their drug of choice. There have even been organized groups of "shoppers" headed by an individual. The members of the groups are directed to physicians and dentists with complaints whose symptoms are taught to them. Prescriptions for controlled substances that are given to these "patients" are returned to the leader and the "patients" are paid for their time. New dentist offices are often targets for "shop-

ping." If a prescription for a controlled substance is obtained, more addicts will be contacting the office. This is *not* the type of "practice builder" that any dental office needs. Dental practitioners should become suspicious if any of the following "shopper" symptoms are present:

- Requests a certain drug and says it's better; he or she may stumble over the name
- Claims many allergies and says lots of pain medications do not work
- Cancels dental appointments because he or she claims to be going out of town on business
- Experiences pain for days after scaling and root planing
- Moves from dental office to dental office because "others do not understand"
- Claims a "low pain threshold"
- Needs refills several days after a dental procedure without complications

Treatment. The following four general methods are used for treating opioid addiction. One method

> Methadone maintenance one way

involves substituting the equivalent amount of an oral opioid (usually methadone) for the injectable form that the addict had been using (e.g., heroin) and then gradually withdrawing that oral form. Another method involves going "cold turkey" by abruptly withdrawing the opioid and using adjunctive medication to alleviate the symptoms of withdrawal, such as phenothiazines, clonidine, or benzodiazepines. A third method involves maintaining a patient on high doses of methadone, termed methadone maintenance. With this method, the patient takes supervised large oral doses of methadone on a daily basis. Because the patient develops a tolerance for the effects of the opioids, a block is produced that prevents heroin-like agents from producing the "rush" feeling after injecting. The last method involves administering an orally effective, long-acting antagonist, naltrexone (Trexan). Naltrexone blocks the action of usual doses of opioid administered illicitly. No treatment for opioid addiction is successful in all patients.

ALLERGIC REACTIONS

True opioid allergy is very uncommon.

The most common type of true allergic reactions to the opioids is dermatologic in nature, including skin rashes and urticaria. Reports of gastrointestinal side effects are frequently reported as allergies but are side effects of the opioids. Contact dermatitis can occur with topical exposure. These allergic reactions have to be differentiated from the symptoms related to the histamine-releasing properties of the opioids. If a patient gives a history of a *true* allergic reaction to an opioid, an opioid from a different chemical class should be chosen (see Box 7-1). Figure 7-3 shows choices of analgesics for the patient allergic to codeine. Some brands of opioid analgesic combinations are formulated with sodium bisulfite. In patients with sulfite hypersensitivity, reference sources should be consulted to determine which brand contains sulfites.

DRUG INTERACTIONS

Additive CNS depression is a common problem.

The respiratory depression produced by the opioids is additive with that produced by other CNS depressants. Alcohol or sedative-hypnotic agents can potentiate the opioids' respiratory depressant effect. When promethazine or hydroxyzine (antihistamines) is added to an opioid regimen, the opioid dose should be reduced.

Meperidine, but not the other opioids, can interact with the **monoamine oxidase inhibitors,** a group of drugs used, rarely, to treat hypertension or depression. CNS excitation, hypertension, and hypotension have been reported to oc-

cur. The accumulation of a metabolite of meperidine, normeperidine, may be responsible for the increased effect of meperidine in the presence of the antipsychotic agents such as chlorpromazine.

SPECIFIC OPIOIDS

OPIOID AGONISTS

The analgesic action of the most commonly used opioids (agonists) is related to their action on the μ-receptors and κ-receptors (see Table 7-3 and Figure 7-1, morphine). These agonist opioids are discussed first.

Morphine. Morphine [more-FEEN] is considered to be the prototype opioid agonist against which other opioids are measured. An equivalent number of milligrams of each opioid is compared with 10 mg of morphine. Morphine is used parenterally to control postoperative pain in hospitalized patients. It is also used orally, primarily in the treatment of terminal illnesses. Sustained release morphine tablets are the most commonly used form of morphine for outpatient use in the terminally ill. Few, if any, sustained release analgesics are useful in dentistry because the patient needs immediate relief, not future relief. The usual oral dosing interval and route of administration are listed in Table 7-2.

Oxycodone. Oxycodone [ox-i-KOE-done] is used alone or combined with either aspirin (in Percodan) or acetaminophen (in Percocet, Tylox) (Table 7-6) to provide relief of moderate to severe pain. Combining an opioid with a nonopioid analgesic produces an additive analgesic effect with fewer adverse reactions. Oxycodone retains about two thirds of its action when given orally. It bridges the gap between codeine and morphine in terms of strength of analgesic action.

Hydrocodone. There are many combinations of hydrocodone [hye-droe-KOE-done] and acet-

FIGURE **7-3** *Codeine allergy decision tree. Use this decision tree to choose an analgesic for patients with a history of codeine allergy.* NSAIA, *Nonsteroidal antiinflammatory agents;* APAP, *acetaminophen;* NX, *naloxone.*

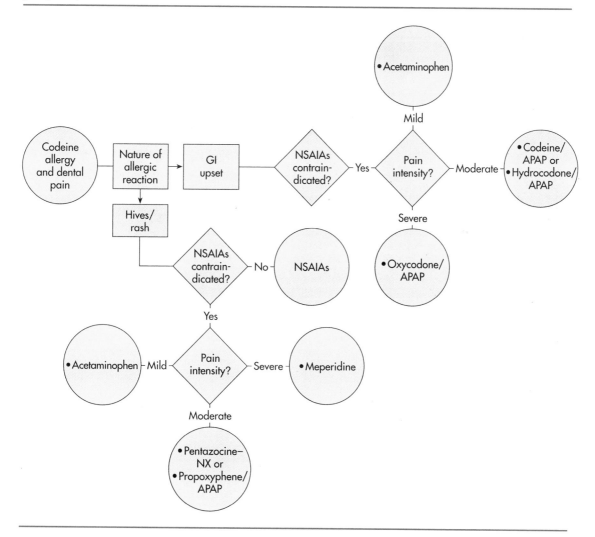

aminophen including the original, which contains 5 mg of hydrocodone and 500 mg of acetaminophen (5/500). Various combinations of the two ingredients, hydrocodone and acetaminophen, include ranges of 5 to 10 mg of hydrocodone and 500 to 750 mg of acetaminophen. The companies offering brand name combinations seem to manufacture new combinations to thwart the development of generic equivalents. The original product combination (hydrocodone/APAP; 5/500) is recommended for the majority of dental patients with pain. To change the dose of this drug combination, the number of tablets per dose can be altered (from

TABLE 7-6   Constituents of Common Opioid Analgesic Products

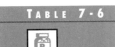

TRADE NAME	OPIOID (mg)	EFFICACY (+ TO ++++)	OTHER INGREDIENTS (mg)
Propxyphene (Darvon) compound-65	Propoxyphene HCl (65)	+	Aspirin (389) Caffeine (32.4)
Darvocet*,† N-100	Propoxyphene napsylate (100)	+	Acetaminophen (650)
Tylenol #1-4*	Codeine #1 (7.5) #3 (30) #2 (15) #4 (60)	++	Acetaminophen (300) Sodium metabisulfite (trade name); generic also available
Tylenol with codeine elixir	Codeine (12 mg/5 ml)	++	Alcohol (7%) Sucrose
Phenaphen #2-4	Codeine (15, 30, 60)	++	Acetaminophen (325)
Empirin #2-4	Codeine (15, 30, 60)	++	Aspirin (325)
Fiorinal #3	Codeine (30)	++	Aspirin (325) Butalbital (50) Caffeine (40)
Fioricet with codeine	Codeine (30)	++	Acetaminophen (325) Butalbital (50) Caffeine (40)
Talwin NX*	Pentazocine (50)	+++	Naloxone (0.5)
Vicodin, Lortab, Lorcet	Hydrocodone (5-10)	++	Acetaminophen (500-700)
Vicoprofen	Hydrocodone (7.5)	++	Ibuprofen (200)
Percodan, Roxiprin, Endodan*	Oxycodone (~5)	+++	Aspirin (325)
Percocet, Roxicet, Endocet, Oxyco-cet	Oxycodone (5)	+++	Acetaminophen (325)
Tylox	Oxycodone (5)	+++	Acetaminophen (500)
OxyContin‡	Oxycodone (10, 20, 40, 80)	+++	None
Oxycodone liquid	Oxycodone 20 mg/ml, 5 mg/5ml	+++	
Demerol	Meperidine (50, 100)	+++	None
Demerol APAP	Meperidine (50, 100)	+++	Acetaminophen (300)
Mepergan Fortis	Meperidine (50)	+++	Promethazine (25)
Dilaudid	Hydromorphone (1, 2, 3, 4, 8)	++++	None

*Most commonly prescribed.
†Suffix of "-cet" shows contains acetaminophen.
‡Sustained-release product; not for acute pain.

one half to 2 tablets). This strength is available generically and is inexpensive. As with any opioid product containing acetaminophen, the total dose of acetaminophen should not exceed 4 gm (Chapter 6, p 124). Upper limits for the total daily dose per day must not be exceeded. With combination products, the maximum daily dose (for a person who drinks less than 3 drinks per day) is 6 tablets for products containing 650 mg and 5 tablets for those with 750 mg per dosage form.

Codeine. Codeine [KOE-deen] is the most commonly used opioid in dentistry, and it is combined with aspirin (Empirin #3) or acetaminophen (Tylenol #3) for oral administration. Other constituents including caffeine and aluminum/magnesium hydroxides (antacid) are often included in these analgesic combinations. Codeine has a relatively weak analgesic action compared with morphine, hydromorphone, hydrocodone, or even oxycodone. Some commonly used analgesic combinations are listed in Table 7-6. Evidence for hydrocodone's efficacy being more than that of codeine is lacking because hydrocodone was previously used (and therefore tested) as an antitussive.

For some combinations the amount of codeine in a product is designated by #1 (7.5 mg; ⅛ gr), #2 (15 mg; ¼ gr), #3 (30 mg; ½ gr) and #4 (60 mg; 1 gr). Generally, doses greater than 30 to 60 mg of codeine are poorly tolerated by the patient (too much nausea). In pain studies it is difficult to show that 30 mg of codeine is any better than a placebo; and 60 mg of codeine has an analgesic strength about the same as 650 mg of aspirin or acetaminophen or 200 mg of ibuprofen. Because of codeine's weak analgesic efficacy, prescription doses of nonsteroidal anti-inflammatory agents often produce better results in the management of dental pain. When codeine is combined with nonopioid analgesics, there is additive analgesic activity. In the combination products, lower doses of each analgesic may be used and there is a potential for a reduction in adverse reactions.

> Popularity is unrelated to analgesic efficacy.

Propoxyphene. An opioid that is synthetic and is chemically similar to methadone is the drug propoxyphene [proe-POX-i-feen] (which is in Darvocet N-100). Its analgesic efficacy has been questioned (see Table 7-6), but it is certainly no more efficacious than 2 tablets of aspirin or acetaminophen. It is available combined with aspirin and caffeine or acetaminophen, which adds to its puny efficacy. Its adverse effects include nausea, vomiting, dizziness, and physical dependence. Hundreds of deaths have been associated with its overdose, often in combination with alcohol. With the availability of other agents, it is difficult to justify the use of propoxyphene. However, propoxyphene is very commonly prescribed in medicine. The reason for this is that it acts as the bridge (in the provider's perception) when "waffling" on whether or not to give an opioid. [There must be lots of "wafflers."]

Meperidine. The favorite drug of abuse of medical personnel is meperidine [me-PAIR-i-deen] (Demerol). It requires 100 mg to equal about 10 mg of morphine. The drug interactions between meperidine and both the monoamine oxidase inhibitors and phenothiazines must be considered before using meperidine. Meperidine is a poor choice for oral use because it has a high first-pass effect, a shorter duration of action, and more drug interactions. It may be useful as an ingredient in an anxiolytic "medley" given as an oral preoperative. Although occasionally used in outpatient dentistry, it has little if any use.

Hydromorphone. An orally effective opioid, hydromorphone [hye-droe-MORE-fone] (Dilaudid) is reserved for the management of severe pain. It is more potent than morphine and better absorbed orally, but it tends to produce similar adverse reactions. Its use in dentistry should be limited to rare situations, limited numbers, and careful monitoring. It is a favorite of the addict because of its strength (see Table 7-6).

Methadone. Methadone [METH-e-done] (Dolophine) is used primarily in the treatment of opioid addicts. It is used either to withdraw the patient gradually or for methadone maintenance. Because it has a longer duration of action, withdrawal from methadone is easier than from heroin.

Fentanyl family—Al, Sue, and the kids—zero and remy. Fentanyl [FEN-ta-nil] (Duragesic, Sublimaze), sufentanil [sue-FEN-ta-nil] (Sufenta), and alfentanil [al-FEN-ta-nil] (Alfenta) are short-acting parenterally administered agonist opioid analgesics that are used perioperatively or during general anesthesia. They provide analgesia during and immediately following general anesthesia. Fentanyl is used in combination with droperidol [droe-PER-i-dol] (Inapsine) to induce or supplement general or regional anesthesia and to produce general anesthesia. Postoperative ventilation and observation are needed when these agents are used. Fentanyl is also available as a patch (Fentanyl [Duragesic] Transdermal System) for application to the skin every 3 days. The patches provide constant pain relief for the terminally ill. Sometimes oral morphine is used concomitantly as needed to control "breakthrough" pain.

MIXED OPIOIDS

Mixed opioids include the agonist-antagonist opioid analgesics and the partial agonists. The only mixed opioid available for oral use is the agonist-antagonist pentazocine. Butorphanol (Stadol), available as a nasal spray, is also in this group. This group is ripe for research to develop opioids with adequate analgesic potency and fewer side effects, such as respiratory depression and addiction potential, than the agonist opioids. At the present time, their place in dental therapeutics is unclear.

Agonist-antagonist opioids

PENTAZOCINE The only agonist-antagonist opioid available in oral form is pentazocine [pen-TAZ-oh-seen] (Talwin). It produces CNS effects not unlike the opioid agonists, including analgesia, sedation, and respiratory depression. The type of analgesia it produces is somewhat different from that produced by the agonist opioids. This may be due to its agonist action at the

κ-receptors and δ-receptors and its antagonist action at the μ-receptor (see Figure 7-1). (References differ in attributing the dysphoric and psychomimetic adverse reactions—some say δ, and others say σ.)

The adverse reactions of pentazocine include sedation, dizziness, nausea, vomiting, and headache. Opioid-like effects on the gastrointestinal tract occur with pentazocine. Psychomimetic effects, including nightmares, hallucinations, and dysphoria, have been reported. With high doses, respiratory depression can occur. Unlike the agonist opioids, increasing the dose of pentazocine does not result in a commensurate increase in respiratory depression; that is, respiratory depression is nonlinear. Unlike the opioid agonists, pentazocine can increase both the blood pressure and heart rate. This may be related to its catecholamine-releasing properties.

The drug of choice to treat pentazocine overdose is naloxone. With abuse, repeated injections in the same location can result in severe sclerosis, fibrosis, and ulceration. Because pentazocine was initially thought not to have abuse potential, many pentazocine abusers have been produced. A popular mixture termed "Ts and Blues" is a combination of pentazocine (Talwin) and pyribenzamine (blue-colored tablet), an antihistamine. Because of its weak antagonist property, it may precipitate withdrawal in the addict.

Pentazocine is available as tablets containing 50 mg of pentazocine and 0.5 mg of naloxone, a pure opioid antagonist (Talwin-NX). Naloxone, a Schedule IV opioid, was added to pentazocine to reduce its addiction potential. How does it do this? First, naloxone, a pure agonist, is effective parenterally but not orally because it is inactivated. Second, if the tablet is taken by the intended oral route, the naloxone will not affect its analgesic potency because it is rapidly inactivated when taken orally. Third, if the contents of the tablet are injected parenterally, the active naloxone will counteract the action of pentazocine, reducing its positive effects. This combination tablet has resulted in a tablet that is more difficult to abuse and whose street value was cut in half. [Don't say drug addicts don't know their pharmacology.]

Parenterally available agonist-antagonists include dezocine [DEZ-oh-seen] (Dalgan), nalbuphine [NAL-byoo-feen] (Nubain), and butorphanol [byoo-TOR-fa-nol] (Stadol). Dezocine has agonist action at the κ-receptor and antagonist action at the μ-receptor. Its analgesic strength is comparable to morphine at usual therapeutic doses. Like pentazocine, these other agonist-antagonists demonstrate nonlinear respiratory depression. Sedation, nausea, vomiting, xerostomia, and headache are side effects of these drugs. These agents produce fewer psychomimetic effects than pentazocine, but more than the agonists.

When originally marketed, these agonist-antagonists were said to have much less addiction potential or even none at all. They were not placed on any narcotic schedule by the Drug Enforcement Administration (DEA). Butorphanol, available as a nasal spray, has been marketed for some time. Because of the nature of the patient use of this agent in clinical practice, most pharmacists consider this product to be "addicting." The current literature and clinical practice has determined that these agents do, in fact, have addiction potential. If they are added to the list it would not be surprising. [Act on an opioid receptor, but are not addicting. Hum . . ., am I surprised that they might have addiction potential? Remember, walks like a duck, sounds like a duck, looks like a duck—I wonder what it could be?]

Partial agonists.

The first and only available partial agonist is buprenorphine [byoo-pre-NOR-feen] (Buprenex). It is a partial μ-receptor agonist, but has no δ-receptor action. In abstinent morphine-dependent patients, buprenorphine suppresses withdrawal; in stabilized opioid-dependent patients it precipitates withdrawal. Its abuse potential seems to be low, and it is classified as a Schedule V drug. Buprenorphine is currently available only for parenteral use, but alternative dosage forms such as sublingual or nasal spray are being investigated.

Opioid Antagonists

NALOXONE Naloxone [nal-OX-zone] (Narcan) is an essentially pure opioid antagonist that is active parenterally. It antagonizes the μ-receptors, κ-receptors, and δ-receptors. When given alone, it produces few pharmacologic effects in the usual therapeutic doses. Naloxone is the drug of choice for treating agonist or mixed opioid overdoses. It will reverse opioid-induced respiratory depression. If another agent, for example, a barbiturate, is responsible for the depression, naloxone does not add to the respiratory depression. If administered to an addict who has taken an overdose of an opioid, small doses must be carefully titrated or opioid withdrawal may be produced. Naloxone is now marketed for the management of alcoholism. It also serves as a useful tool in research to determine the role of the opioid receptors in hypnosis, acupuncture, and the placebo effect.

> Naloxone reverses opioid.

Naloxone is given intravenously or intramuscularly with an average adult dose of 2 mg and a range of doses between 0.4 and 10 mg. Doses should be repeated if the duration of action of the opioid is longer than that of naloxone.

Effects should occur within 1 to 2 minutes. Doses may be repeated at 2- to 3-minute intervals. If no response occurs after 10 mg is administered, the diagnosis of opioid overdose must be questioned. If any opioid is used in the dental office, the dental office emergency kit should contain naloxone.

NALMEFENE Nalmefene [NAL-me-

> Nalmefene reverses opioid overdose.

feen] (Revex) is another parenteral opioid antagonist used to reverse opioid overdose.

NALTREXONE   A long-acting, orally effective opioid antagonist, naltrexone [nal-TREKS-zone] (ReVia) is indicated for the maintenance of the opioid-free state in detoxified, formerly opioid-dependent patients. It should not be administered until the patient has remained opioid free for at least 1 week and has had a negative naloxone challenge. It is also used in the management of alcohol abstinence. Its adverse reactions include insomnia, nervousness, headache, abdominal cramping, nausea, vomiting, and arthralgia. Acute **hepatitis** and **liver failure** have been associated with naltrexone. It is administered daily or in some instances 3 times weekly. Patients on naltrexone should not be given opioid analgesic agents for management of dental pain.

> Naltrexone is used to prevent opioid and alcohol use in addicts.

TRAMADOL

Tramadol (Ultram) is a new, unique analgesic with an interesting mechanism of action. It has μ-opioid agonist action and inhibits the reuptake of norepinephrine and serotonin (modifies the ascending pain pathways). It has some of the properties of an opioid (like codeine and hydrocodone) because of its μ-agonist activity, but not all the properties because it does not affect the other two opioid receptors—the κ and δ receptors. Tramadol's other mechanism involves the inhibition of reuptake of norepinephrine and serotonin, similar to the mechanism of the antidepressants.

Adverse reactions of tramadol include CNS effects, such as dizziness, somnolence, headache, and stimulation. Gastrointestinal tract side effects include nausea, diarrhea, constipation, and vomiting. Palpitations, diaphoresis, and seizures have been reported in patients taking tramadol. Watch for signs of addiction [again not scheduled—but we shall see].

Tramadol's analgesic efficacy is difficult to assess because most studies are unpublished and therefore cannot be judged; studies comparing tramadol with nonsteroidal agents or stronger opioids have not been done. Tramadol efficacy is stated in Table 7-7.

> Analgesic efficacy unimpressive; lack of addiction potential questioned.

The usual adult dose is 50 to 100 mg every 4 to 6 hours, not to exceed 400 mg/day.

Because of its weak analgesic activity and its exorbitant cost compared with established analgesics, its use is difficult to justify. [Of interest, it is moving up the top 200 list of most commonly prescribed drugs—suggesting even more wafflers.]

DENTAL USE OF OPIOIDS

The advent of the NSAIAs has produced a change in the use of the opioids in dental prac-

TABLE 7-7 Relative Efficacy of Tramadol (Ultram)

Tramadol Dose (mg)	Compared with Codeine (mg)	Comparison with Combinations
50	=60	<#2 ASA #3 codeine (total = 650/60)
75		≥APAP/propoxyphene 650/100
100	>60	<#2 ASA/ codeine #3 (total = 650/60)
150	>60	≥APA/propoxyphene 650/100
5 TIMES A DAY 50		= #1 tablet acetaminophen 300/codeine 30 mg = #1 tablet of aspirin 300/ codeine 30 mg

tice. Most dental pain can be better managed by the use of NSAIAs. In the patient in whom NSAIAs are contraindicated, the dentist has a wide range of opioids from which to choose. By beginning with codeine or hydrocodone combinations and progressing to oxycodone combinations, almost all dental pain can be managed. Only in rare cases and for very short periods (1 to 2 days) should stronger opioids be prescribed for outpatient dental pain.

Patients with chronic pain should be managed with nonopioid therapies and referred to appropriate specialists depending on the nature of their chronic pain. In the treatment of chronic pain, opioids are not indicated. New patients with a complaint of pain should be seen in the dental office and definitive treatment rendered. Opioid prescriptions should be given only for small amounts, without refills, and only if the patient has dental treatment performed. If dental pain persists, the patient should be seen in the dental office for evaluation and local treatment. If the patient demands opioids repeatedly, the patient should be referred to a pain clinic for evaluation. Temporomandibular disease (TMD), formerly called TMJ (joint), often produces chronic pain. When pain becomes chronic, the mechanisms producing the pain differ from that of acute pain. Treatment of TMD should include NSAIAs, and possibly muscle relaxants, and tricyclic antidepressants.

REVIEW QUESTIONS

1. Name the two ways in which opioid analgesic agents may be grouped, and state a reason for each system.
2. State three receptor types and explain how agonist and antagonist actions at these sites can explain the difference in action among the opioids.
3. Describe how the pharmacologic effects and adverse reactions of the opioids are related in contrast to the pharmacologic

effects and adverse reactions of other groups of drugs.
4. Name four pharmacologic effects of the opioids.
5. Describe the two adverse reactions of the opioids to which tolerance does not develop.
6. Describe the two most common adverse reactions associated with the opioids and explain their management in the patient.
7. Define the following terms:
   a. Physical dependence
   b. Withdrawal
   c. Tolerance
8. Discuss three conditions in which opioids would be contraindicated or in which they should be used with caution.
9. Explain the additive respiratory depression with the opioid analgesic agents, and state the other drug with which they are additive.
10. Describe the four major therapeutic uses of the opioids.
11. State the ways in which the opioids differ from one another.
12. State the most potent orally effective opioid.
13. Describe the major use of methadone at the present time.
14. Explain the place for the use of meperidine in dentistry. State the major mistake that is made in prescribing meperidine (check dose and duration).
15. Describe two major disadvantages to the use of pentazocine.
16. Explain the agonist and antagonist properties of pentazocine, and describe how this can produce two problems in an opioid addict.
17. Explain why pentazocine is combined with naloxone in Talwin NX.
18. Describe the use of the most frequently employed opioid in dental practice.
19. Explain the use of propoxyphene in dentistry, and state the degree of its proven clinical effectiveness.

20. Explain the use of naloxone for an emergency situation. State the situations in which it would be indicated and contraindicated. List two mistakes that could be made.
21. Discuss the disease states in which a particular analgesic drug should be avoided, and select an alternative choice.
22. Describe two methods of treating opioid addicts.
23. State the relative strengths of codeine, oxycodone, and morphine.
24. Describe the "warning signs" that may tip off the presence of a "shopper."
25. State the indications for the use of naltrexone.
26. Explain the advantages, if any, of using tramadol for dental pain.

Antiinfective Agents

Antiinfective agents play an important role in dentistry because infection, after pain management, is the dental problem for which drugs are most frequently prescribed. As our knowledge about the etiology of dental diseases is continually increasing and the involvement of microorganisms becoming better understood, dental health care workers continue to better understand the proper place of antibiotics and their effect on **microorganisms.** Another important piece of the puzzle of infection is the immunologic response of the host. This puzzle piece has not yet led to therapeutic intervention strategies, but in the future, "Who knows?"

Dental infections can be divided into several types as follows:

- **Caries:** Caries, produced by *Streptococcus mutans*, is the first important dental infection that the newly erupting teeth of the young patient face. At present, traditional antiinfective agents have not been useful for this problem in the general population. The treatments of choice involve the use of fluoridated water, local physical removal of bacterial plaque from teeth on a regular basis (good oral hygiene, dental prophylaxis), and appropriately placed sealants.

- **Periodontal disease:** In the adult patient, the dental health care team's biggest dental problem is periodontal disease. With an increase in knowledge about antiinfective agents, dental teams will be better able to understand and properly administer new treatments for this disease, such as tetracycline fibers. Because it is now known that microorganisms such as *Actinobacillus actinomycetemcomitans*, black-pigmented bacteroides, motile rods, and spirochetes are involved in periodontal disease, development of a more rational approach to treatment of periodontal disease may be possible. Table 8-1 lists the common organisms that are involved in periodontal infections and the sensitivity or resistance to the antibiotics tested. Treatments that use localized methods of drug delivery (e.g., tetracycline fibers) hold promise for the future management of periodontal disease.

- **Localized dental infections:** Most localized dental infections are extensions that arise from either periodontic- or endodontic-related sources. For most localized dental infections, if adequate drainage can be obtained, antiinfective agents are not indicated

TABLE 8-1 **Periodontal Microbes, Their Presence and In Vitro Susceptibility to Certain Antimicrobial Agents**

Organisms	LJP	AP	R	PEN	AMX	TET	DOX	CLN	MET	CIP
Actinobacillus actinomycetem-comitans	+	+	+	1-16	1-16	2-8	6	R	32	<1
Porphyromonas gingivalis (Bacteroides gingivalis)	−	+	+	<1	ND	2	1	<1	4	<1-2
Prevotella intermedia (Bacteroides intermedius)	+	+	+	5	ND	6	3	<1	2	<1
Eikenella corrodens	+	+	+	8-9	8	3-32	6	R	R	<1
Fusobacterium spp.	+	+	+	2-5	2	2	2	<1	1	3
Campylobacter rectus (Wolinella recta)	−	+	+	1	1	2	1	1	2	R

Modified from Slots J, Rams TE: Antibiotics in periodontal therapy: advantages and disadvantages, *J Clin Periodontol* 17:479-493, 1990.
LJP, Localized juvenile periodontitis; *AP*, adult periodontitis; *R*, "refractory" adult periodontitis; +, elevated proportions of bacteria; −, regular proportions or not detected or studied; *PEN*, penicillin G; *AMX*, amoxicillin; *TET*, tetracycline; *DOX*, doxycycline; *CLN*, clindamycin; *MET*, metronidazole; *CIP*, ciprofloxacin; *MIC*, minimal inhibitory concentrations for 90% of strains (μg/m), except penicillin G, which is U/ml; *ND*, not determined.

unless the patient is immunocompromised (Box 8-1). In the occasional situation in which antibiotics are indicated, the antibiotic of choice is determined by the organisms likely to be present.

- **Systemic infections:** Systemic dental infections can be identified because they produce systemic symptoms such as fever, malaise, and tachycardia. Lesions associated with infections producing these types of symptoms should be drained, but if this is not possible, antibiotics should be given. The duration of therapy should include the number of days for the signs and symptoms to be totally gone plus 2 or 3 days [that will be easy to predict!]. If the dental infection has systemic symptoms, the use of antiinfective agents is indicated and may even be critical.

DENTAL INFECTION "EVOLUTION"

Dental infections often follow similar pathways of "evolution" from their beginning to their end. In the beginning, the organisms responsible for a dental infection are primarily gram-positive cocci, such as *Streptococci viridans* or α-hemolytic streptococci. After a short time, the gram-positive infection begins to include a variety of both gram-positive and gram-negative anaerobic organisms, such as *Peptostreptococcus* (peptococcus) and *Bacteroides* (*Porphyromonas* and *Prevotella* species). At this point the infection is termed a *mixed* infection. Over time, the proportion of organisms that are anaerobic increases. With additional time and no treatment, the infection progresses until it consists of predominantly anaerobic flora. At this point, the anaerobic organisms coalesce into an abscess, often visible on radiograph (x-ray).

The choice of antibiotics for a dental patient's infection depends on where it is in its evolution. If the infection is just beginning, the organisms most likely to be present are gram-positive cocci. Penicillin VK is the drug of choice, unless the patient has a penicillin allergy. In patients allergic to penicillin, alternatives might include erythromycin or clindamycin. When the infection is at the mixed stage, agents effective against either gram-positive organisms or anaerobic organisms may be successful. Treating gram-

---

BOX 8-1 DISEASES, CONDITIONS, AND DRUGS THAT DECREASE RESISTANCE TO INFECTION

Diseases

Addison's disease
AIDS-related complex
Human immunodeficiency virus (HIV)
Alcoholism
Blood dyscrasias
Cancer
Cirrhosis of the liver
Diabetes mellitus
Down syndrome
Immunoglobulin deficiency
Leukemia
Malnutrition
Splenectomy

Drugs

Immunosuppressive drugs such as:
  Azathioprine (Imuran)
  Cyclophosphamide (Cytoxan)
  Cyclosporin (Sandimmune)
  Methotrexate (Rheumatrex)
  Adrenocorticosteroids

---

positive organisms is easier, and the drug of choice is penicillin VK or, with a penicillin allergy, erythromycin. For anaerobic organisms, metronidazole is effective. By eradicating one group of organisms, the balance between the two types of organisms is altered and the body can then resolve the infection. Clindamycin affects both gram-positive cocci and gram-positive and gram-negative anaerobes. Historically, oral surgeons have been comfortable using clindamycin, but other dentists have avoided it because of the association with pseudomembranous colitis.

To treat a dental infection, it is critical to know what organism(s) is likely to be involved and the sensitivity of those organisms to antibiotics. No small task! But decisions are based on the *likelihood* of certain infections and their *likely* sensitivities. [It's called an educated guess!]

HISTORY

In 1932, Gerhard Domagk of Germany observed that Prontosil protected mice against infection by streptococcal bacteria. This milestone

in medical history led to the development of the sulfonamides and marked the beginning of systemic antimicrobial therapy.

In 1940, Chain and Florey of England observed that interest had been focused on the sulfonamides and that other possibilities, notably those connected with naturally occurring substances, should be considered.

In 1928, Fleming of England (certainly a poor housekeeper who did not wash his Petri dishes) observed that a mold, *Penicillium notatum*, produced a substance that inhibited the growth of certain bacteria. He named this substance "penicillin" and suggested that it might be useful for application to infected wounds. In their classic paper, Chain and co-workers reported the low toxicity and systemic antibacterial effectiveness of penicillin. The excitement that began with the sulfonamides was transferred to the penicillins. As each new antibiotic is marketed, this excitement is transferred to the newest antibiotic developed. For years, scientists have been concerned about the indiscriminate use of antibiotics. Recent developments, such as totally resistant strains of bacteria, have made this concern even more important. Patients go to the doctor with health conditions and demand antibiotics. Doctors often provide antibiotics, even though the infection is most likely viral. The antibiotics will not improve the condition and may even make the patient resistant to the antibiotic. Unfortunately, however, it takes less time to write a prescription for an antibiotic than to explain the rationale for not using antibiotics to a potentially angry patient.

DEFINITIONS

A discussion of individual antimicrobial agents is preceded by definitions of the following terms:

- **antiinfective agents:** Substances that act against or destroy infections.
- **antibacterial agents:** Substances that destroy or suppress the growth or multiplication of bacteria.
- **antibiotic agents:** Chemical substances produced by microorganisms that have the capacity, in dilute solutions, to destroy or suppress the growth or multiplication of organisms or prevent their action. The difference between the terms *antibiotic*, *antiinfective*, and *antibacterial* is that antibiotics are produced by microorganisms, whereas the other agents may be developed in a chemistry laboratory (not from a living organism). *Antibacterial* refers to a substance from any source that inhibits or kills bacteria. The term *antiinfective* refers to a substance from any source that inhibits or kills organisms that can produce infection, such as bacteria, protozoa, viruses, and so forth. This difference is largely ignored in general conversation, and antiinfectives are often referred to as "antibiotics."
- **antimicrobial agents:** Substances that destroy or suppress the growth or multiplication of microorganisms.
- **antifungal agents:** Substances that destroy or suppress the growth or multiplication of fungi.

- **antiviral agents:** Substances that destroy or suppress the growth or multiplication of viruses.

The following are definitions of commonly used terms:
- **bactericidal:** The ability to kill bacteria. This effect is irreversible; that is, if the bacteria are removed from the drug, they do not live.
- **bacteriostatic:** The ability to inhibit or retard the multiplication or growth of bacteria. This is a reversible process because if the bacteria are removed from the agent, they are able to grow and multiply.

Whether an antibacterial agent is labeled *bactericidal* or *bacteriostatic* depends on variables such as the dose used or the organism being treated. Box 8-2 lists the most common antimicrobial agents and classifies them as bacteriostatic or bactericidal.

BOX 8-2 CLASSIFICATION OF ANTIINFECTIVE AGENTS—BACTERICIDAL OR BACTERIOSTATIC

Bactericidal	Bacteriostatic
Aminoglycosides	Chloramphenicol
Bacitracin	Clindamycin*
Cephalosporins	Macrolides*
Metronidazole	Spectinomycin
Macrolides*	Sulfonamides
Penicillins	Tetracyclines
Polymyxin	Trimethoprim
Quinolones	
Rifampin	
Vancomycin	

*May be bactericidal against some organisms at higher blood levels.

- **blood (serum) level:** Concentration of the antiinfective agent present in the blood or serum. The importance of the serum level is that certain levels of an antibiotic are required to produce an effect on various types of organisms. For an antibiotic to be effective the dose given must produce this concentration in the blood.
- **infection:** Infection is not only an invasion of the body by pathogenic microorganisms but also a reaction of the tissues to their presence. The presence of a **pathogen** does not constitute "invasion." In fact, many potential oral pathogens are part of the normal floral in the mouth, but they only cause infection if their relative numbers rise. The factors that determine the likelihood of a microorganism causing an infection are the following:
  - disease-producing power of the microorganism (virulence)
  - number of organisms present (inoculum)
  - resistance of the host (immunologic response)

Host resistance should be considered as having both local and systemic components. Systemically, both drugs (steroids and antineoplastic agents) and diseases (acquired immunodeficiency syndrome [AIDS] and insulin-dependent diabetes mellitus [IDDM]) may reduce a patient's **immunity** (see Box 8-1) and increase the chance of an infection. Sleep deprivation and anxiety can also reduce a patient's immunologic response to infection.

- **minimum inhibitory concentration (MIC):** Lowest concentration needed to inhibit visible growth of an organism on media after 18 to 24 hours of **incubation.** This in vitro test is more reliable and quantitative than the disk tests.
- **resistance:** Resistance (related to antibiotics) is the natural or acquired ability of an organism to be immune to or to resist the effects of an antiinfective agent. *Natural* resistance occurs when an organism has always been resistant to an antimicrobial agent because of the bacteria's normal properties such as lipid structures in the cell wall. *Acquired* resistance occurs when an organism that was previously sensitive to an antimicrobial agent develops resistance. This can occur by natural selection of a spontaneous mutation ("survival of the fittest"). An increase in the use of an antibiotic in a given population (e.g., a hospital) increases the proportion of resistant organisms in that population. Conversely, a decrease in the use of an antibiotic decreases the proportion of organisms resistant to that antibiotic in that given population.

Another method by which resistance develops is by the transfer of DNA genetic material from one organism to another via transduction, transformation, or bacterial conjugation. The first organism, which is resistant to one or more antibiotics, transfers its genetic material to a second organism. The second organism, which was not previously resistant, thus becomes resistant to the same antibiotic as the first organism without ever having been exposed to that antibiotic. This transfer of genetic material from one organism to another may occur among very different microorganisms, including transfer from a nonpathogenic bacteria to a pathogenic bacteria. The three most common mechanisms of acquired resistance are a decrease in bacterial permeability, the production of bacterial enzymes, and an alteration in the target site.

- **spectrum:** Range of activity of a drug. The spectrum of activity of an antibacterial agent may be narrow, intermediate, or broad. A narrow-spectrum agent acts primarily against a smaller group of bacteria such as gram-positive cocci, gram-negative rods, gram-positive or gram-negative anaerobes, or viruses.
- **superinfection, suprainfection:** Infection caused by the proliferation of microorgan-

isms different from those causing the original infection. When antiinfectives disturb the normal flora of the body, the emergence of organisms unaffected by or resistant to the antibiotic used can occur. Superinfection is more often caused by broad-spectrum antibiotics such as tetracycline, and increases when taken for a longer period of time. In this case, a reduction in the number of gram-positive and gram-negative bacteria allows the overgrowth of the **fungus,** *Candida albicans.* The pathogenic organisms emerging in a superinfection generally are more difficult to eradicate than the original organism and are more likely to exhibit resistance. The fact that the practitioner can *cause* as well as *eliminate* infections emphasizes the importance of determining a definite need before these drugs are used. [Let's stamp out, or at least reduce, **iatrogenic** infections!]

- **synergism:** Synergism occurs when the combination of two antibiotics produces more effect than would be expected if their individual effects were added. In other words, $1 + 1 > 2$. Combinations of antibiotics that are bactericidal are generally synergistic. Combinations of those that are bacteriostatic are merely additive ($1 + 1 = 2$).
- **antagonism:** Antagonism occurs when a combination of two agents produces less effect than either agent alone. A combination of a bactericidal agent and a bacteriostatic agent is often poorer than either alone. In other words, $1 + 1 < 2$ (see Box 8-2).

CULTURE AND SENSITIVITY

Ideally, all infections requiring antimicrobial therapy would be cultured and sensitivity tests performed. Culturing involves growing the bacteria from a sample of infective exudate, and sensitivity testing involves exposing the organism to certain test antibiotics and determining whether the organism is sensitive or resistant. Today, in part at least because of the inappropriate use of antiinfective agents, organisms are more quickly becoming resistant to antibiotics. Figure 8-1 illustrates the antimicrobial spectrum of some antibiotics.

Culture and sensitivity is the only way to be sure that a drug will kill or inhibit the growth of the infecting microorganisms in a patient-specific infection. In practice, this is often difficult. In dentistry, the need for anaerobic culturing makes obtaining a sample and culturing it more difficult. Another problem is that many dental infections are often of mixed origin so that the results of the cultures are difficult to interpret. In cases of a serious infection, an infection in a compromised patient, or an infection that is not responding to treatment, it is imperative that a culture be taken.

CULTURE

When a culture is taken, proper collection materials (tubes or vials with the correct media) and methods must be used to obtain reliable results. Dental professionals need to communicate to the laboratory personnel the nature of the appropriate cultures to be taken. The laboratory personnel should perform a Gram's stain so that they may report all of the bacteria present in high numbers. Both obligate and facultative anaerobes should be preserved

Depending on the site, the collection method varies. Examples of methods include: for an **abscess,** aspiration with a needle; for a draining lesion, a swab from an anaerobic pack; and for endodontic treatment, properly handled absorbent points. Collection methods should be adapted in order to keep the anaerobes alive. For the periodontal pocket, the sterile paper point or the explorer can be used to sample the pocket.

Care must be taken not to contaminate the sample with supragingival plaque, which has a different microbial constitution. In at-risk patients, a culture should be taken before antibiotics are administered because antibiotics can alter the nature of the microbes so that identification

FIGURE 8-1 *Visual representation of a dental spectrum of action for dentally useful antiinfective agents.*

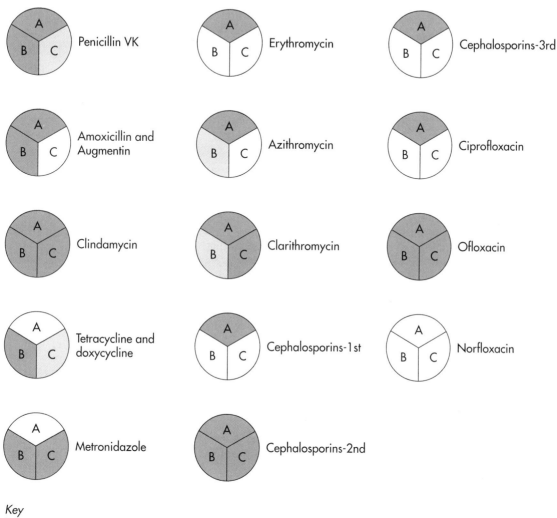

Key

A = Aerobic gram-positive
B = Anaerobic gram-positive
C = Anaerobic gram-negative

is more difficult. Infections in problem sites and in problem patients should be cultured.

SENSITIVITY

After the organism is identified, it is grown on culture medium (Figure 8-2). Observing whether the organisms are sensitive or resistant to certain test antibiotics assists in determining which antibiotic to use in difficult infections. One to two days are required before the results of this test are available. Although therapy is begun before this time, it may be changed after the results are available. If clinical response has been adequate, often the original antibiotic is continued despite sensitivity results. Figure 8-1 provides a visual representation of the spectrum of action of dentally useful antiinfective agents against the most common organisms associated with dental infections—gram-positive aerobes, gram-positive anaerobes, and gram-negative anaerobes.

INDICATIONS FOR ANTIMICROBIAL AGENTS

Considerable controversy exists regarding the need for antimicrobial agents in various situations. The two categories of indications are prophylactic and therapeutic.

THERAPEUTIC INDICATIONS

Although there is no simple rule to determine whether antimicrobial therapy is needed in dentistry, many infections do not require it. Most patients without immune function deficiencies, in whom drainage can be obtained, need no antibiotics to manage their dental infections. [Would you give an antibiotic every time a "zit" was pinched in a patient with acne?] Table 8-2 lists the indications for treatment of dental infections and the antibiotics of choice and their alternatives. If local resistance patterns vary from those found in the table, antibiotic choice

FIGURE 8-2   *Culture and sensitivity. Antibiotic (Ab) disc with clear zone shows sensitivity. Disc with no clear zone shows resistance.*

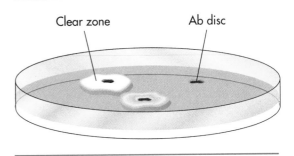

should be based upon that information. However, before a decision is made there are several factors that must be considered.

The patient. The best defense against a pathogen is the host response. A properly functioning defense mechanism is of primary importance. When this defense is lacking, the need for antimicrobial agents is more pressing.

The infection. The virulence and invasiveness of the microorganism are important in deciding the acuteness, severity, and spreading tendency of an infection. An acute, severe, rapidly spreading infection should generally be treated with antimicrobial agents, whereas a mild, localized infection in which drainage can be established need not be treated. If the periodontal pocket (site) remains active despite repeated root planing, then the use of antibiotics to alter the flora may be considered.

When antimicrobial agents are to be used in the treatment of dental infections, the organisms likely to produce the infection and their susceptibility to antimicrobial agents must be considered. Table 8-2 lists the antimicrobials of choice for various dental situations (when culture and sensitivity tests are unavailable) and alternatives if the drugs of choice cannot be used. When two antimicrobial agents have approximately the

TABLE 8-2 Antimicrobial Use in Dentistry*

INFECTION SITUATION	DRUG(S) OF CHOICE	ALTERNATIVE DRUG(S)
PERIODONTAL DISEASE		
Acute necrotizing ulcerative gingivitis†	Penicillin VK	Metronidazole
	Amoxicillin	Tetracycline
Abscess (perio)	Penicillin VK	Tetracycline
Localized juvenile periodontitis (LJP)	Doxycycline	Amoxicillin + metronidazole
	Tetracycline	Augmentin (amoxicillin + clavulanate)
Adult periodontitis†	Not usually treated with drugs	Clindamycin
Rapid advancing periodontitis (RAP)	Doxycycline	Amoxicillin + metronidazole
	Tetracycline	
	Metronidazole	
ORAL INFECTIONS		
Soft tissue infections (abscess, cellulitis, postsurgical, periocoronitis)	Penicillin VK	Doxycycline
	Amoxicillin	Clindamycin
		Cephalosporin
		Tetracycline
Osteomyelitis	Penicillin VK	Clindamycin
	Amoxicillin	Cephalosporin
MIXED INFECTIONS INSENSITIVE TO PENICILLIN		
Aerobes	Amoxicillin	Cephalosporin
		Sulfonamides
		Tetracycline
Anaerobes and chronic infections	Metronidazole	Cephalosporin
	Clindamycin	Augmentin
		Tetracycline
		Metronidazole + penicillin
PROPHYLAXIS FOR INFECTIVE ENDOCARDITIS		
Rheumatic heart disease and prosthetic heart valve‡	**No penicillin allergy:**	Clarithromycin
	Amoxicillin§	Azithromycin
	Penicillin allergy:	Clindamycin
Patient with LJP	Doxycycline for 3 wk followed by usual regimen (see above)	

*Clinical conditions may alter drug therapy.
†No antimicrobial agents are usually required for these conditions.
‡See Table 8-5.
§See Table 8-3.
LJP, Localized juvenile periodontitis.

same therapeutic effect and their cost to the patient is very different, the cost of therapy is another consideration.

To answer the question as to whether an antibiotic is effective in a certain dental infection, one needs many patients with similar infections in which half are given active antibiotics and half are given placebo antibiotics. This study would help to define the proper use of antibiotics in dental infections. This slow testing has begun, using antibiotics in periodontal situations, but there is still much to discover.

PROPHYLACTIC INDICATIONS

Few situations arise for which a definite indication for prophylactic antibiotic coverage exists. One clear-cut use of antibiotics for prophylaxis before a dental procedure (recommended by the American Heart Association and the American Dental Association) is a history of rheumatic or congenital heart disease or the presence of a **heart valve** prosthesis. The reason that this is a clear-cut indication for prophylactic antibiotics is *not* due to a predominance of evidence of effectiveness but rather because of the publishing of the guidelines. The principle behind these guidelines is that dental procedures *may* produce **bacteremia** and that those bacteria may lodge in previously rough areas in and around the valves. Prophylactic antibiotics are given in the "hope" (often misplaced) that they will kill the bacteria before or soon after they "settle" in the heart, and prevent the bacteria from growing and causing an episode of infective endocarditis which can produce more valvular damage.

A few other prophylactic uses of antimicrobial agents are discussed at the end of this chapter. An example is in cases of compound mandibular fracture, in which the use of prophylactic antimicrobial agents has reduced the rate of infection.

Although dental studies concerning the value of prophylactic antibiotics are controversial, the *failure* of prophylactic antibiotic coverage to prevent postsurgical infections is well documented in the medical literature. When the dentist gives an antibiotic to a patient to prevent a potential infection, the risk-to-benefit ratio must be considered. On the positive side (benefit), the administration of an antibiotic might prevent an infection if the correct antibiotic to treat the yet-to-be infection is chosen. On the negative side (risk), the administration of prophylactic antibiotics might result in an adverse effect such as nausea, suprainfection, allergy, or resistance. If a sufficient number of well-controlled studies were available, the solutions to such dilemmas might be better defined.

GENERAL ADVERSE REACTIONS ASSOCIATED WITH ANTIINFECTIVE AGENTS

SUPERINFECTION (SUPRAINFECTION)

All antiinfective agents can produce an overgrowth of an organism that is different from the original infection and that is resistant to the agent being used. The wider the spectrum of the antiinfective agent and the longer the agent is administered, the greater the chance of superinfection occurring (Box 8-3). This side effect can be minimized by use of the most specific antiinfective agent, the shortest effective course of therapy, and adequate doses.

ALLERGIC REACTIONS

All antiinfective agents, just like all drugs, have the potential to produce a variety of allergic reactions, ranging from a mild rash to fatal anaphylaxis. Some antiinfective agents, such as the penicillins and the cephalosporins, are more allergenic than other agents. Many antiinfective agents, such as erythromycin and clindamycin, have a low allergenic potential.

DRUG INTERACTIONS

Antiinfective agents can interact with **oral contraceptives,** oral anticoagulants, and other antiinfectives (**bacteriostatic agent** interferes with bactericidal agent).

BOX 8-3 THE GARDEN

The normal oral flora is like a healthy, green, lush lawn. Because the lawn is dense and healthy it shades the ground so that weeds cannot grow. Because the lawn is well it competes well with the weeds. In this situation there are few weeds germinating and few full grown weeds in the lawn. Then a drought develops, and some sections of the lawn become thin and bare spots appear. In this case, small weeds can germinate and begin to grow in the bare or sparse spots. Because the sun can now reach the ground, these weeds are nourished. The small weeds become larger and begin to invade the lawn. These larger weeds are like a "suprainfection" in that now the lawn has a different plant growing than it originally had.

Oral contraceptives. Although the occurrence is extremely rare, most antiinfective agents have been implicated in a drug interaction with the oral contraceptives—that is, reducing their effectiveness. Antiinfective agents are variable in the possibility of interacting with birth control pills, but data concerning a ranking of these agents are limited. The steps in handling of the oral contraceptive by the body are thought to be as follows:

1. *Absorption into circulation.* When a patient ingests an oral contraceptive, it is absorbed from the intestine into the systemic circulation.
2. *Conjugation in the liver.* In its pass through the liver, the birth control pill is conjugated so that its excretion will be facilitated (more polar and more water soluble).
3. *From the liver via bile to the intestine.* The conjugate is then excreted via the bile into the intestinal tract.
4. *Cleavage of the conjugate.* In the intestine, the estrogen conjugate is hydrolyzed (broken down) by the bacteria in the intestines, releasing the free estrogen.
5. *Reabsorption.* The free estrogen is then reabsorbed into the blood stream, where the process begins again. This enterohepatic circulation produces certain blood levels of estrogen in women taking birth control pills. Interference with this process might be responsible for potential drug interactions between estrogens and antibiotics.

When a woman taking an oral contraceptive is given an antibiotic the above process may be slightly changed as follows:

1. to 3. Same.
4. *Cleavage of conjugate.* When antibiotics are given, the number of bacteria in the intestine falls. Hydrolysis of the estrogen conjugate does not occur.
5. *Reabsorption.* Because the estrogen remains conjugated, it will not be reabsorbed because the conjugate has low lipid solubility. The absorption of estrogen decreases

and its blood level falls. Evidence of a lowered estrogen level may be inferred by reports of menstrual irregularities (breakthrough bleeding) in women on oral contraceptives given antibiotics. But this is not the case. A recent thorough review of the literature has concluded that "the alleged ability of commonly employed antibiotics to reduce the effectiveness of oral contraceptive agents is not adequately supported by clinical research."[1] Considering the number of women-years of oral contraceptive use and the paucity of documented birth control failures, this conclusion fits with the facts.

This drug interaction, although unlikely, should be discussed with the patient whenever a patient using oral contraceptives receives a prescription for an antibiotic. Of those antibiotics used in dentistry, ampicillin and the tetracyclines are the most likely to produce this effect. In certain patients, alternative birth control measures should be used during antibiotic administration.

Oral anticoagulants. Antiinfective agents can potentiate the effect of oral anticoagulants. Oral anticoagulants are vitamin K inhibitors, so interfering with the production of vitamin K could increase the anticoagulant effect. Bacterial flora in the intestine produce most of the vitamin K in our bodies. Antiinfective agents (e.g., tetracycline) reduce the bacterial flora that produce vitamin K. With the vitamin K reduced, the oral anticoagulant's effect is increased. Erythromycin inhibits the enzymes that metabolize warfarin, leading to an increase in warfarin levels. Prolongation of the **International Normalized Ratio (INR)** leading to bleeding or hemorrhage may result. INR should be monitored more closely in patients on antiinfective therapy. Antiinfective agents interact to varying degrees depending on the antibiotic (Table 8-3).

Other antiinfectives. Antibiotics that act at the same receptor may compete for that receptor and should not be given together (e.g., erythromycin and clindamycin). An antibiotic that has bacteriostatic properties stops the bacteria from growing, thereby inhibiting the action of a bactericidal agent (requires growing and actively dividing cells to work). Except in a few unusual, nondental cases, one antibiotic should be chosen and used alone.

GASTROINTESTINAL COMPLAINTS

All antiinfective drugs can produce a variety of gastrointestinal complaints. The complaints include stomach pain, increased motility, and diarrhea. The incidence varies greatly, depending on the particular agent employed, the dose of that agent, and whether the patient takes the drug with food. Erythromycin has the highest incidence of gastrointestinal complaints of any of the antibiotics. More serious gastrointestinal complaints, such as pseudomembranous colitis, which has been historically linked with clindamycin, are now known to occur not only with a wide variety of antiinfective agents (cephalosporins, amoxicillin) but also in the absence of any antimicrobial agents.

PREGNANCY

The antimicrobial agents that can be used during pregnancy to treat infections are limited. Although the risk-to-benefit ratio must be considered whenever pregnant women are given any medications, penicillin and erythromycin have not been associated with **teratogenicity** and are frequently used. The use of clindamycin is probably also acceptable, but before any antibiotics are used in the pregnant dental patient the patient's obstetrician should be contacted (this procedure also helps prevent medical-legal problems). Metronidazole is not usually used during pregnancy, but exceptions exist. The tetracyclines are contraindicated during pregnancy because of their effect on developing teeth and skeleton.

DOSAGE FORMS

Adult dosage forms of antibiotics are commonly tablets and capsules. Children's dosage forms, including liquid and chewable antibiotic dosage forms, contain sugar as their sweetening agent. After the dentition has erupted, the dental health care worker should encourage the parent or child to brush the child's teeth after the use of these agents. The chewable tablets can stick to the teeth, especially in the pits. Long-term administration of antibiotics could increase the child's caries rate.

COST

Cost is an important factor in choosing an antibiotic for a patient. If the perfect antibiotic is chosen and prescribed but the patient does not purchase the medication because it is too expensive, then poor results are likely. The best inexpensive antibiotic that can be taken will be more effective than an expensive one that cannot be purchased. Figure 8-3 compares the cost of various antiinfective agents.

PENICILLINS

The penicillins [pen-i-SILL-ins] can be divided into four major groups (Table 8-3). The first group contains penicillin G and V, the second group is composed of the penicillinase-resistant penicillins, the third group contains amoxicillin, and the fourth group consists of extended-spectrum penicillins. Because the penicillins have many properties in common, their similarities are discussed first. In dentistry, the first and third groups are commonly used.

SOURCE AND CHEMISTRY

The mold *Penicillium notatum* and related species produce the naturally occurring penicillins. The semisynthetic penicillins are produced by chemically altering the naturally produced penicillins. The penicillin structure includes a

FIGURE 8-3 *Relative cost of dentally useful antifungal agents.*

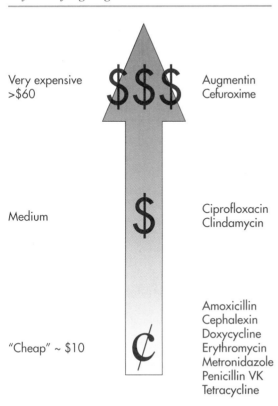

Very expensive >$60

Augmentin
Cefuroxime

Medium

Ciprofloxacin
Clindamycin

"Cheap" ~ $10

Amoxicillin
Cephalexin
Doxycycline
Erythromycin
Metronidazole
Penicillin VK
Tetracycline

β-lactam ring fused to a five-member, S-containing thiazolidine ring. Neither of these rings has much antimicrobial action alone. Active penicillins are produced by adding different functional groups to position 6. Cleaving these functional groups from their two-ring structure results in a loss of antimicrobial activity. When the β-lactam ring is broken, such as in the presence of penicillinase, the antimicrobial activity of the compound is lost (see equation, p. 163).

The addition of organic groups at the R position confers antibacterial activity to the compounds formed from 6-aminopenicillanic acid. These R groups create the various penicillins that were originally designated with letters, for example, penicillin G and penicillin V. The penicillins can be inactivated by any reaction that removes the R group or, in the case of penicillinase, breaks the β-lactam ring *(B)*. Salts of the penicillins are made by reactions at the thiazolidine *(T)* carboxyl (−COOH) group.

Although many naturally occurring penicillins have been produced, only penicillin G (Na^+/K^+ penicillin) is of use today. The various semisynthetic penicillins are formed by substituting other groups at the R position.

PHARMACOKINETICS

Penicillin can be administered either orally or parenterally but should not be applied topically because its allergenicity is greatest by that route. When penicillin is administered orally, the amount absorbed depends on the type of penicillin. The percentage can vary from 0% to more than 90% (see Table 8-3). When the percentage absorbed is too low, as with methicillin, the penicillin is available only for injection. Penicillin V is better absorbed orally than penicillin G, so penicillin V is used for administration of oral penicillin

The oral route provides the advantages of convenience and less likelihood of a life-threatening allergic reaction. The disadvantages of using the oral rather than the parenteral route are that the blood levels rise slower, the blood levels are less predictable because of variable absorption or lack of patient compliance (biggest problem), and some penicillins are degraded by gastric acid. The highest blood levels are obtained if the patient takes the penicillin orally at least 1 hour before or 2 hours after meals, but penicillin V and amoxicillin can be taken without regard to meals.

After absorption, penicillin is distributed throughout the body, with the exception of cerebrospinal fluid, bone, and abscesses. This includes the tissue, saliva, and kidneys. Penicillin crosses the placenta and appears in breast milk.

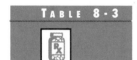

TABLE 8-3   Penicillins

Drug Name	Routes	Penicillinase Resistant	Acid Stable	Absorbed Orally (%)	Protein Bound (%)
PENICILLIN G AND V					
Penicillin G (Pentids)	PO, IM, IV*	No	No	15–30	60
Penicillin G procaine (Crysticillin)	IM	No	No	—	
Penicillin G benzathine (Bicillin L-A)	IM	No	No	—	60
Penicillin V (Pen-Vee K, V-Cillin K)	PO	No	Yes	60–75	75–80
PENICILLINASE-RESISTANT					
Methicillin (Staphcillin)	IM, IV	Yes	No	0	30-45
Nafcillin (Unipen, Nafcil)	PO, IM, IV	Yes	Yes	10–15	90
Oxacillin (Prostaphilin, Bactocill)	PO, IM, IV	Yes	Yes	20–30	95
Cloxacillin (Tegopen, Cloxapen)	PO	Yes	Yes	40–60	95
Dicloxacillin (Dynapen, Dycill)	PO	Yes	Yes	40–60	98
AMPICILLINS					
Ampicillin (Polycillin, Omnipen)	PO, IM, IV	No	Yes	30–40	20
Bacampicillin (Spectrobid)	PO	No	Yes	Very good	20
Amoxicillin (Amoxil, Larotid)	PO	No	Yes	75–90	20
Amoxicillin + clavulanate (Augmentin)	PO	Yes	Yes	Very good	20
EXTENDED SPECTRUM					
Carbenicillin indanyl (Geocillin)	PO	No	Yes	80	50
Carbenicillin (Geopen, Pyopen)	IM, IV	No	—	—	50
Ticarcillin (Ticar)	IM, IV	No	—	—	45
Mezlocillin (Mezlin)	IM, IV	No	—	—	16–42
Piperacillin (Pipracil)	IM, IV	No	—	—	16

*PO, orally; IM, intramuscularly; IV, intravenously. Bold type indicates drugs most used in dentistry.

> Penicillin—tubular secretion in the kidney; half-life = ½ hour.

Penicillin is metabolized by hydrolysis in the liver and undergoes tubular secretion in the kidney. The elimination half-life for both penicillin G and penicillin V is about 0.5 hour. In five half-lives, about 2.5 hours, these penicillins are virtually eliminated from the body. Probenecid, a uricosuric agent, interferes with penicillin's secretion and therefore produces higher blood levels and prolongs its action. This may be used to therapeutic benefit treating sexually transmitted diseases in one office visit.

MECHANISM OF ACTION

Penicillin is a very potent bactericidal agent that attaches to penicillin-binding proteins (PBPs) on the bacterial cell membrane. The PBPs are enzymes that are involved in the synthesis of the cell wall and the maintenance of the cell's structural integrity. Penicillin acts as the structural analogue of acyl-D-alanyl-D-alanine, inhibiting the formation of cross-linkages (transpeptidases). This destroys cell wall integrity and leads to lysis. The penicillins are more effective against rapidly growing organisms.

SPECTRUM

Penicillin G and V's narrow spectrum of activity includes gram-positive cocci such as *Staphylococcus aureus, Staphylococcus pneumoniae, Streptococcus pyogenes, Streptococcus viridans,* and certain gram-negative cocci such as *Neisseria gonorrhoeae* (produces gonorrhea) and *Neisseria meningitidis.* Penicillin is also effective against spirochetes and anaerobes such as *Actinomyces, Peptococcus, Pep-*

tostreptococcus, *Bacteroides*, *Corynebacterium*, and *Clostridium* species. The spectrum of action of the penicillins matches the microbes responsible for many periodontal conditions (Table 8-4). The other penicillins have a somewhat different spectrum that is discussed in each section.

The antibacterial activity of penicillin is standardized in international units (IU). One international unit has the activity of 0.6 μg of the master standard of sodium penicillin G, so 1 mg of pure sodium penicillin G equals 1667 IU. About 400,000 IU of penicillin V is equivalent to 250 mg. Penicillin G is usually measured in international units, whereas other penicillins are expressed in milligrams.

RESISTANCE

Resistance to penicillin can occur by several different mechanisms. Penicillinase-producing staphylococci are resistant because their enzymes destroy some penicillins. These penicillinases inactivate the penicillin moiety by cleaving the β-lactam ring.

6-aminopenicillanic acid

In hospital environments, more than 95% of the population of staphylococci are penicillinase-producing organisms. Clavulanic acid serves as a substrate, which allows the use of amoxicillin to treat penicillinase-producing organisms. Certain bacteria have an outer cell membrane that prevents penicillin from reaching the PBPs.

Although most oral strains of *S. viridans* are sensitive to penicillin, an increasing number of strains are becoming resistant. The amount of bacterial resistance is proportional to the clinical use of the antibiotic—frequent use leads to increased resistance (and vice versa).

T ABLE 8 - 4 Periodontal Microbes and Their In Vitro Susceptibility to Penicillin and Amoxicillin

ORGANISMS	PENICILLIN G	AMOXICILLIN
Actinobacillus actinomycetemcomitans	1–16	1–16
Porphyromonas gingivalis (Bacteroides gingivalis)	<1	Not determined
Prevotella intermedia (Bacteroides intermedius)	5	Not determined
Eikenella corrodens	8–9	8
Fusobacterium spp.	2–5	2
Campylobacter rectus (Wolinella recta)	1	1

Modified from Slots J, Rams TE: Antibiotics in periodontal therapy: advantages and disadvantages, *J Clin Periodontol* 17:479-493, 1990.

ADVERSE REACTIONS

The untoward reactions to the penicillins can be divided into toxic reactions and allergic or hypersensitivity reactions. The penicillins are the most common cause of drug allergies.

Toxicity. Because penicillin's toxicity is almost nonexistent, large doses have been tolerated without adverse effects. For this reason there is a large margin of safety when penicillin is administered. With massive intravenous doses, direct central nervous system (CNS) irritation can result in convulsions. Large doses of penicillin G have been associated with renal damage manifested as fever, eosinophilia, rashes, albuminuria, and a rise in blood urea nitrogen (BUN). Hemolytic anemia and bone marrow depression have also been produced by penicillin. The penicillinase-resistant penicillins are significantly more toxic than penicillin G. Gastrointestinal irritation can manifest itself as nausea with or without vomiting. The irritation caused by injection of penicillin can produce sterile abscesses if given intramuscularly or **thrombophlebitis** if given intravenously.

ALLERGY AND HYPERSENSITIVITY

The penicillins are one of the most allergenic groups of drugs. Allergic reactions to penicillin is the greatest danger associated with their use. These reactions include all types of hypersensitivity reactions, type I through type IV (see Table 3-1) and varying degrees of severity. The following are types of allergic reactions associated with the penicillins:

- *Anaphylactic reactions:* Anaphylactic shock, an acute allergic reaction, occurs within minutes after the administration of penicillin and presents the most serious danger to patients. It is characterized by smooth muscle contraction (e.g., bronchoconstriction), capillary dilation (shock), and urticaria caused by the release of histamine and bradykinin. If treatment does not begin immediately, death can result. The treatment of anaphylaxis is the immediate administration of parenteral epinephrine.
- **Rash:** All types of skin rashes have been reported in association with the administration of penicillin. This type of reaction accounts for 80% to 90% of allergic reactions to the penicillins. These rashes are usually mild and self-limiting but can occasionally be severe. Even contact dermatitis has occurred as a result of topical exposure, for example, while preparing an injectable solution (type IV).
- *Delayed serum sickness:* Serum sickness is manifested as fever, skin rash, and eosinophilia or severely as arthritis, purpura, lymphadenopathy, splenomegaly, mental changes, an abnormal electrocardiogram, and edema. It usually takes at least 6 days to develop and can occur during treatment or up to 2 weeks after treatment has ceased.
- *Oral lesions:* Delayed reactions to penicillin can exhibit themselves in the oral cavity. These include severe stomatitis, furred tongue, black tongue, acute glossitis, and cheilosis. These oral lesions can occur most commonly with topical application but have been reported from other routes.
- *Other reactions:* Interstitial nephritis, hemolytic anemia, and eosinophilia are types of allergic reactions occasionally reported during penicillin therapy.

Allergic reactions to penicillin always should be considered when penicillin is prescribed. Some studies indicate that 5% to 10% of patients receiving penicillin will have a reaction. Allergic reactions to oral penicillin are less common than with parenteral penicillin. Anaphylactic reactions are more frequent in patients pretreated with β-blockers and subsequently given oral penicillin. Anaphylactic reactions in these patients have been reported to be difficult to treat.

When reactions to penicillin occur, the consequences are often serious. It is estimated that an anaphylactic reaction occurs in up to 0.05% of penicillin-treated patients, with a mortality of 5% to 10%. It is estimated that 100 to 300 deaths occur annually in the United States because of an allergic reaction to penicillin. Although the chance of a serious allergic reaction to penicillin is greater after parenteral administration, anaphylactic shock and death after oral use have also been reported. Patients who have a history of any allergy are more likely to be allergic to penicillin.

Allergic reactions to penicillin of any type may be followed by more serious allergic reactions on subsequent exposure. Any history of an allergic reaction to penicillin contraindicates its use, and another antibiotic should be substituted. However, a negative history does not guarantee the lack of a penicillin allergy. If a penicillin is prescribed and any question of a reaction remains, make sure that the patient is somewhere where help can be summoned if necessary after the first dose is taken.

Testing. In certain clinical cases when the use of penicillin is critical, testing for penicillin allergy can be done. Because the testing itself may precipitate an anaphylactic reaction, it should only be undertaken in a situation in which life support equipment, drugs, and personnel are immediately available. It should *never* be done in an outpatient dental office.

Penicillin itself does not act as a hapten, but it is metabolized to a hapten. Allergic reactions from penicillin can be in response to the *major* determinant, resulting in a skin reaction, or to the *minor* determinant, producing anaphylaxis. The major determinant, termed *major* because of the frequency rather than the severity of the reaction, is produced by a reaction to penicillenic acid producing the penicilloyl determinant. The *minor determinant* (MDM), so termed because it happens less often, is produced by either penicilloic acid or penicillin itself. Both penicilloyl-polylysine (PPL, Pre-Pen), the major determinant, and penicillin itself or the minor determinant mixture (MDM) must be used to test for penicillin allergy. Both false-positive and false-negative reactions may occur, but when both of these determinants are negative the administration of penicillin is probably safe. These tests are only sensitive to type I allergic reactions.

Uses

Penicillin is an important antibiotic in medical and dental practice. Its use in dentistry results from its bactericidal potency, lack of toxicity, and spectrum of action, which includes many oral flora. It is often employed for the treatment of dental infections. Table 8-2 demonstrates the dental infections for which penicillin is the drug of choice if patients are not allergic to it. Amoxicillin, a close penicillin relative, is also used for specific prophylactic indications. It is the agent of choice for the prophylaxis of infective endocarditis in nonallergic patients who have a history of rheumatic heart disease or valve damage (see the discussion on antibiotic prophylaxis of infective endocarditis at the end of this chapter). Penicillin's effectiveness in the treatment dental infections is explained by its effectiveness versus many aerobic and anaerobic bacteria.

SPECIFIC PENICILLINS

Penicillin G. Penicillin G, the prototype penicillin, is available as sodium, potassium, procaine, or benzathine salts. These salts differ in their onset and duration of action and the plasma levels attained. Figure 8-4 compares the blood levels attained by the intravenous administration of the potassium salt and the intramuscular administration of the potassium, procaine, and benzathine salts. Note that the potassium salt given intravenously produces the most rapid and highest blood level, whereas the benzathine salt given intramuscularly produces the lowest and most sustained blood level. The potassium and procaine salts, given intramuscularly, produce intermediate blood levels and durations of action. The penicillins' duration of action is inversely proportional to the solubility of the penicillin form—least soluble is longest-acting.

The sodium salts of penicillin should be avoided in patients with a limited sodium intake such as cardiovascular patients. Renal patients should not be given potassium salts, which can result in hyperkalemia. Patients may be allergic to the procaine moiety in procaine penicillin G. Both procaine and benzathine penicillins are suspensions given intramuscularly, from which the penicillin is slowly released. The benzathine form is given once monthly to patients with a history of rheumatic heart disease for prophylaxis.

Penicillin V. Penicillin V has a spectrum of action very similar to that of penicillin G. Given orally, penicillin V produces higher blood levels than an equivalent amount of penicillin G. Penicillin V has never been proved to be of greater therapeutic value than penicillin G given in higher doses. Because of the higher blood levels, penicillin V is used almost exclusively in the treatment of many common dental infections. The potassium salt of penicillin V (K penicillin V or penicillin VK) is more soluble than the free acid and therefore is better absorbed when taken orally. Table 8-2 lists some situations in which

F IGURE 8 - 4   *Comparative blood levels of penicillin G salts.*

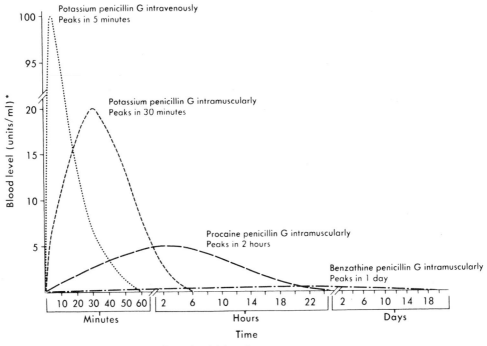

*Blood level attained when 1 million units administered.

penicillin is the drug of first choice if the patient is not allergic to it. The usual adult dose is 500 mg qid for treatment of an infection for a minimum of 5 and preferably 7 to 10 days.

Penicillinase-resistant penicillins. Penicillinase resistant penicillans should be reserved for use against only penicillinase-producing staphylococci. Compared with penicillin G, the penicillinase-resistant penicillins are less effective against penicillin G–sensitive organisms. They also produce more side effects such as gastrointestinal discomfort, bone marrow depression, and abnormal renal and hepatic function. Patients allergic to penicillin are also allergic to the penicillinase-resistant penicillins.

Because cloxacillin and dicloxacillin are better absorbed than the other penicillinase-resistant penicillins, they are the drugs of choice.

Ampicillins. Ampicillin [am-pi-SILL-in] and amoxicillin [a-mox-i-SILL-in] are frequently used in medicine. These penicillinase-susceptible penicillins have a spectrum of action that includes gram-positive cocci, *Hemophilus influenzae*, and enterococci such as *Escherichia coli*, *Proteus mirabilis*, and *Salmonella* and *Shigella* species. Ampicillin is usually used to treat gonococcal infections, either alone or with probenecid as a single oral dose (3.5 gm).

Amoxicillin, a relative of ampicillin, is preferred for most other indications because it pro-

TABLE 8-5	**Macrolides**		

DRUG	FOOD	METABOLISM/EXCRETION	DOSE
Erythromycin	MT*	Hepatic, in bile	250–500 mg q6h
Base (E-Mycin, Ery-Tab, Eryc, PCE, various)			
Stearate (Erythrocin, Erypar)			
Estolate (Ilosone)	OK*	Hepatic, in bile	250–500 mg q6h
Ethyl succinate (EES, Pediamycin)			400–800 mg q6h
Azithromycin (Zithromax)	MT	Unchanged in bile	500 mg stat, then 250 mg qd
Clarithromycin (Biaxin)	OK	Metabolized to active; renal	500 mg bid

*MT, Take on an empty stomach (1 hour before or 2 hours after); OK, may take without regard to meals.

duces higher blood levels, is better absorbed, requires less frequent dosing (3 times daily versus 4 times daily for penicillin VK or ampicillin), and its absorption is not impaired by food. Amoxicillin is the drug of choice for prophylaxis of rheumatic heart disease before a dental procedure. Amoxicillin is used to treat upper respiratory tract infections *(H. influenzae)*, urinary tract infection *(E. coli)*, and meningitis *(H. influenzae)*. **Otitis media** in children is often treated with amoxicillin. Amoxicillin is also available mixed with clavulanic acid, a β-lactamase inhibitor (Augmentin). Clavulanic acid combines with and inhibits the β-lactamases produced by bacteria. Therefore the amoxicillin is protected from enzymatic inactivation. This combination can be used with penicillin-producing organisms. It has had some use in the management of certain periodontal conditions (see Table 8-2).

Both ampicillin and amoxicillin can produce a variety of allergic reactions. Ampicillin is much more likely to produce rashes than other penicillins. Most agree that the ampicillin rash is not of an allergic or immunologic nature. This unusual ampicillin-related rash is much more common in patients with mononucleosis (almost 100%) or those taking allopurinol. Cross-allergenicity between penicillin VK, amoxicillin, and ampicillin is complete [omitting the "weird" ampicillin rash].

Extended-spectrum penicillins. Carbenicillin [kar-ben-i-SILL-in] has a wider spectrum of action than penicillin G, with special activity against *P. aeruginosa* and some strains of *Proteus*. It is not penicillinase-resistant and is available parenterally to treat systemic infections.

MACROLIDES

The macrolide antibiotics consist of erythromycin, clarithromycin, and azithromycin (Table 8-5).

ERYTHROMYCIN

Erythromycin [er-ith-roe-MYE-sin], a high-molecular-weight organic base, has a spectrum of action against gram-positive organisms that is similar to that of penicillin V. It is active against most gram-positive aerobes (*Staphylococcus* and *Streptococcus* organisms) and gram-negative aerobes (*Moraxella, Bordetella, Legionella, Campylobacter, and Neisseria* organisms). It is ineffective against the typical anaerobes found in dental infections, such as *Bacteroides, Peptococcus,* and *Peptostreptococcus* organisms. It is also active against *Chlamydia trachomatis, Mycoplasma pneumoniae, Treponema pallidum,* and *Entamoeba histolytica*. It was isolated from the bacterial strain *Streptomyces erythraeus* in 1952.

Pharmacokinetics. Erythromycin is administered orally as tablets, capsules, or oral suspensions, and in intravenous and intramuscular forms. Because erythromycin is broken down in the gastric fluid, it is formulated as an enteric-coated tablet, capsule, or insoluble ester to reduce degradation by stomach acid. It should be administered 2 hours before or 2 hours after meals (see Table 8-5). The peak blood level varies between 1 and 6 hours. Although food reduces the absorption of erythromycin, it may be necessary to administer it with food to minimize its adverse gastrointestinal effects. Its half-life is 2 hours. No therapeutic difference has been demonstrated among the different erythromycin products (see Table 8-5). Erythromycin is distributed to most body tissues, excreted in the bile, partially reabsorbed through enterohepatic circulation, and excreted in the urine and feces.

Mechanism and spectrum. Erythromycin is usually bacteriostatic and interferes with protein synthesis by inhibiting the enzyme peptidyl transferase at the P site of the 50S ribosomal subunit. Its spectrum of action closely resembles that of penicillin against gram-positive bacteria. It is also the drug of choice for *Bordetella*, *Legionella*, and *Actinomyces* organisms, *Mycoplasma pneumoniae*, *Entamoeba histolytica*, some *Chlamydia* species, and diphtheria. It is also indicated for streptococcal and staphylococcal infections, syphilis, and gonorrhea. Bacterial resistance can occur as a result of demethylation of an adenine residue in the 23S ribosomal ribonucleic acid. Cross-resistance has been reported between erythromycin and clindamycin. About half of hospital staphylococcal infections are resistant to erythromycin.

Erythromycin is not effective against many infections caused by obligate anaerobes involved in some dental infections, and therefore it is a poor second choice to penicillin to treat anaerobic dental infections. If the infection is serious, erythromycin should not be used unless culture and sensitivity tests are available. If the causative agent is a gram-positive agent, erythromycin may be effective. The therapeutic effectiveness of erythromycin to treat dental infections may be the result of local intervention measures such as debridement and drainage.

Adverse reactions. With usual therapeutic doses of erythromycin, side effects other than gastrointestinal are usually minimal. Allergic reactions to erythromycin are uncommon.

GASTROINTESTI-
NAL EFFECTS The side effects most often associated with erythromycin admin-

> Gastrointestinal complaints common, many stop taking.

istration are gastrointestinal and include stomatitis, abdominal cramps, nausea, vomiting, and diarrhea. These effects occur more frequently in 4 times daily versus twice daily dosing and with higher (2 gm/day) versus lower (1 gm/day) doses. In one study, at least one gastrointestinal side effect occurred in an average of about 50% of patients, with about 20% discontinuing their medication because of side effects.

CHOLESTATIC JAUNDICE Cholestatic **jaundice** has been reported primarily with the estolate form, but has also been reported with the ethylsuccinate form. Erythromycin base has not been associated with this reaction. Symptoms include nausea, vomiting, and abdominal cramps followed by jaundice and elevated liver enzyme levels. Patients with a history of hepatitis should be given erythromycin base or stearate. The mechanism of this adverse effect is believed to be a hypersensitivity reaction.

Drug interactions. Erythromycin can increase the serum concentrations of theophylline, digoxin, triazolam, warfarin, carbamazepine, and cyclosporine. This effect may produce toxicity, depending on the doses of each drug. The mechanism by which erythromycin produces these drug interactions may involve inhibition of hepatic metabolism of these drugs. Table 8-6 lists some drug interactions of the macrolides. Table 25-4 lists other erythromycin drug interactions.

Uses. Because erythromycin is active against essentially the same aerobic microorganisms as penicillin, it is the drug of first choice against these infections in penicillin-allergic patients. Erythromycin is not effective against the anaerobic *Bacteroides* species implicated in many dental infections. A major difference between penicillin and erythromycin is that erythromycin

is bacteriostatic rather than bactericidal. This may be a factor in treating a compromised patient (see Box 8-1). The various preparations of erythromycin are shown in Table 8-7.

The usual dose of erythromycin is 250 or 500 mg qid. This would be equivalent to 400 or 800 mg of erythromycin ethyl succinate. The higher the dose, the more poorly erythromycin is tolerated by the patient. Avoid giving a "loading dose" because of the chance of producing gastrointestinal distress that would discourage the patient from continuing the erythromycin.

TABLE 8-6   Erythromycin Drug Interactions

DRUG INTERACTING	MECHANISM	MANAGEMENT
Antibiotics—clindamycin, penicillin	Interferes with action of other antibiotics	Choose one antibiotic for both purposes; stop one while administering the other
Carbamazepine (Tegretol)	Increased serum levels of carbamazepine	
Antihistamines, some nonsedating—terfenidine (Seldane) and astemizole (Hismanal)	OK to use with loratidine (Claritin)	OK for 2 doses
Oral contraceptives (OC); birth control pills (BCP)	Decreased effectiveness of OC	Use alternative method (e.g., condoms) until end of that cycle (rest of the month)
Warfarin (Coumadin)	Increased warfarin effect	Bleeding increased
Theophylline (Theodur, Slo-bid)	Increased theophylline toxicity	OK to give 2 doses

TABLE 8-7   Macrolide Pharmacokinetics

MACROLIDE	$T_{1/2}$ (HR)	PEACK (HR)	METABOLISM	ELIMINATION
Erythromycin	1.4-2	2-4	Metab >90%	Biliary
Azithromycin (Zithromax)	34-57	2-3		> 50% bile
Clarithromycin (Biaxin)	5-7; 7*	2-3	Hepatic	Renal 20%-40%, Metabolized 15%
Dirithromycin (Dynabac)	30-50	4-5	Nonenzymatic hydrolysis during absorption	All bile

*All macrolides are concentrated in tissues such as macrophages and phagocytes between 20 to 100 times over the serum level.

AZITHROMYCIN AND CLARITHROMYCIN

Both azithromycin [ay-ZITH-roe-my-sin] (Zithromax, Z-pak) and clarithromycin [klare-ITH-roe-my-sin] (Biaxin) are newer macrolide antibiotics like erythromycin. They inhibit RNA-dependent protein synthesis by binding to the 50S ribosomal subunit, resulting in blockage of transpeptidation. They have activity against aerobic gram-positive cocci such as *Staphylococcus* and *Streptococcus* organisms and gram-negative aerobes. In contrast to erythromycin, azithromycin and clarithromycin have variable action against some anaerobes. They are bacteriostatic and can be taken without regard to meals.

Although much less frequent than with erythromycin (1:3), adverse reactions relate to the gastrointestinal tract (1:7), including dyspepsia, diarrhea, nausea, and abdominal pain. Azithromycin has been reported to elevate liver function tests (LFTs) and should be used with caution in patients with hepatic impairment. Clarithromycin can produce an abnormal taste.

Several drug interactions can occur with both agents because of their reduction in the metabolism of certain drugs metabolized in the liver. Azithromycin can increase the levels of astemizole, loratadine, carbamazepine, digoxin, and triazolam but does not affect either warfarin or theophylline. The peak of azithromycin is reduced by cations such as magnesium and aluminum, but the total drug absorbed is not affected. Clarithromycin increase the levels of drugs metabolized in liver, such as theophylline, carbamazepine, digoxin, omeprazole, and astemizole. Like the other macrolides, clarithromycin inhibits the 3A4 isoenzyme of the cytochrome P-450 (see discussion of cytochromes in Chapter 25) liver microsomal enzymes. With patients taking cisapride who are given clarithromycin, an increase in the levels of cisapride leading to serious cardiac arrhythmias has been reported.

Azithromycin and clarithromycin are indicated as alternative antibiotics in the treatment of common orofacial infections caused by aerobic gram-positive cocci and susceptible anaer-obes. The dose for azithromycin consists of 5 days of therapy: first day, 250 mg bid, and then 250 mg/day for 4 more days; for clarithromycin it is 500 mg bid for 7 to 10 days. When amoxicillin and clindamycin cannot be used for the prophylaxis of endocarditis and prosthetic joint infections, these macrolides can be used as alternative antibiotics. The dose for prevention of bacterial endocarditis or joint prosthesis is 500 mg 1 hour before the dental procedure.

TETRACYCLINES

The tetracyclines [te-tra-SYE-kleens] are broad-spectrum antibiotics affecting a wide range of microorganisms (Table 8-8). Their adverse effects on developing teeth are well known.

The first tetracycline was isolated from a *Streptomyces* strain in 1948. Since then, other tetracyclines have been derived from different species of *Streptomyces*, and the rest have been produced semisynthetically. The tetracyclines are closely related chemically as well as clinically.

PHARMACOKINETICS

The tetracyclines are most commonly given by mouth. Absorption following oral administration varies but is fairly rapid. There is wide tissue distribution, and tetracyclines are secreted in the saliva and in the milk of lactating mothers (one-half plasma concentration). Tetracyclines are concentrated by the liver and excreted into the intestines via the bile. Enterohepatic circulation prolongs the action of the tetracyclines after they have been discontinued. The tetracyclines are also stored in the dentine and enamel of unerupted teeth and are concentrated in the gingival crevicular fluid. The long-acting agents are concentrated to at least 4 times serum levels.

The various tetracyclines differ clinically in their duration of action, percent absorbed when taken orally, half-lives, and mechanism of elimination. Doxycycline is excreted in the feces, whereas tetracycline is eliminated essentially un-

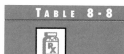

TABLE 8-8 Oral and Topical Tetracyclines

Drug Name	Serum Protein Binding (%)	Normal Serum T$_{1/2}$ (hr)	Usual Oral Adult Dosage	Lipid Solubility
Tetracycline* (Achromycin V)	20-65	6-10	250-500 mg q6h	Intermediate
Fibers (Actisite)†			12.7 mg/fiber	
Doxycycline caps (Vibramycin)‡	60-90	14-25	50 mg q12h or 100 mg q24h	High
Caps (Periostat)‡,§			20 mg bid	
Gels (Actridox)†				
Minocycline (Minocin)‡,‖	55-75	11-20	100 mg q12h	High

*Avoid concomitant administration with foot or divalent or trivalent cations.
†Used topically in sulcus.
‡May be taken with food or milk but not high concentration of divalent or trivalent cations.
§Systemic—very low doses; effect due to collagenase not antibacterial action.
‖Vestibular side effects, blue oral lesions.

changed by glomerular filtration and minocycline is metabolized in the liver and excreted in the urine. Both doxycycline and minocycline may be given safely to patients with renal dysfunction. All tetracyclines cross the placenta and enter the fetal circulation.

SPECTRUM

The tetracyclines are bacteriostatic and interfere with the synthesis of bacterial protein by binding at the 30S subunit of bacterial ribosomes. As broad-spectrum antibiotics, they are effective against a wide variety of gram-positive and gram-negative bacteria (both aerobes and anaerobes), *Rickettsia*, spirochetes *(Treponema pallidum)*, some protozoa *(Entamoeba histolytica)*, and *Chlamydia* and *Mycoplasma* organisms.

Bacterial resistance to the tetracyclines develops slowly in a stepwise fashion. Cross-resistance among tetracyclines is probably complete. This resistance is caused by a decreased uptake of the tetracycline by the organism. In the study of sensitivity of organisms isolated from dental infections, one fifth to three fifths of *S. viridans* and one fifth to two fifths of *S. aureus* were found to be resistant to tetracycline. The

advantage of penicillin over tetracycline in these aerobic gram-positive infections is clear.

ADVERSE REACTIONS

Although most adverse reactions to the tetracyclines occur infrequently, gastrointestinal distress is not uncommon.

Gastrointestinal effects. The gastrointestinal adverse effects include anorexia, nausea, vomiting, diarrhea, gastroenteritis, glossitis, stomatitis, xerostomia, and superinfection (moniliasis). The side effects are largely related to local irritation from alteration of the oral, gastric, and enteric flora.

If diarrhea occurs in a patient receiving tetracycline, the possibility of infectious enteritis such as staphylococcal enterocolitis, intestinal **candidiasis,** and pseudomembranous colitis (secondary to *Clostridium difficile* overgrowth) must be ruled out. Some patients taking tetracyclines have developed a yellowish-brown discoloration of the tongue. This can occur with either topical or systemic administration. Patients with ill-fitting dentures are likely to have candidiasis (moniliasis) caused by superinfection associated with the areas of the oral mucosa tissue where breakdown has occurred.

Effects on teeth and bones. Tetracyclines are incorporated into calcifying structures. If they are used during the period of enamel calcification, they can produce permanent discoloration of the teeth and enamel hypoplasia. Consequently, they should not be used during the last half of pregnancy or in children less than 9 years of age. Tetracycline will affect the primary teeth if given to the mother during the last half of pregnancy or to the infant during the first 4 to 6 months of life. If tetracycline is administered between 2 months and 7 or 8 years of age, the permanent teeth will be affected. The mechanism involves the deposition of tetracycline in the enamel of the forming teeth. These stains are permanent and darken with age and exposure to light. They begin as a yellow fluorescence and progress with time to brown. This process is accelerated by exposure to light. The permanent discoloration ranges from light gray to yellow to tan. With large doses of tetracyclines, a decrease in the growth rate of bones has been demonstrated in the fetus and infants.

The treatment of tetracycline-stained teeth is now done almost exclusively with veneers. In the past, heat plus 30% hydrogen peroxide (Superoxol) was applied to the affected teeth to bleach the stain. This process was often not as satisfactory because the stain sometimes returned and the bleaching process did not completely remove the existing stain

Minocycline can cause black **pigmentation** of mandibular and maxillary alveolar bone and the hard **palate.** When viewed through the mucosa, the pigment appears bluish. Other cases of oral pigmentation have been said to involve the crowns of the permanent teeth (half of incisal surface) and the gingival mucosa. The incidence of this oral pigmentation in adults is 10% after 1 year and 20% after 4 years of therapy. With discontinuation of minocycline, the pigmentation becomes less intense but is usually not completely reversible.

Hepatotoxicity. The incidence of liver damage increases with the intravenous use of tetracyclines. Deaths have occurred, especially in pregnant women. Renal impairment leads to accumulation of tetracycline and may increase the likelihood of hepatic damage.

Nephrotoxicity. Toxic renal effects with characteristic disorders of renal tubular function, producing Fanconi's syndrome, have been reported after the use of old (degraded) tetracycline. Old or outdated tetracycline should be discarded to prevent future use. Because the nephrotoxic effect of the tetracyclines is additive with that of other drugs, tetracyclines should not be used concomitantly with other nephrotoxic drugs.

Hematologic effects. Although uncommon, the hematologic changes hemolytic anemia, leukocytosis, and thrombocytopenic purpura have been reported after tetracycline therapy.

Superinfection. With superinfection, resistant organisms multiply and may cause disease. One common situation, especially prevalent in the compromised host, is an overgrowth of *C. albicans.* Oral or vaginal candidiasis can result from the administration of oral tetracycline.

Photosensitivity. Patients taking tetracyclines who are exposed to the sunlight sometimes react with an exaggerated sunburn. Although the incidence seems to vary with the different tetracyclines, patients receiving a prescription for a tetracycline should be told to use a sunscreen before exposure to the sun.

Other effects. Minocycline [min-oh-SYE-kleen] has been associated with CNS side effects, including lightheadedness, dizziness, and vertigo. Patients who will be driving a car should be warned about this reaction.

Allergy. Anaphylactic and various dermatologic reactions to the tetracyclines have occasionally occurred, but the overall allergenicity of these drugs is low. Glossitis and cheilosis have also been attributed to a hypersensitive reaction to tetracycline. A patient who is allergic to one tetracycline is almost certain to be allergic to all tetracyclines.

DRUG INTERACTIONS

Cations. Divalent (Ca^{++}, Mg^{++}, Fe^{++}, Zn^{++}) and trivalent (Al^{+++}) cations reduce the intestinal absorption of tetracyclines by forming nonabsorbable chelates of tetracycline with, for example, calcium. Dairy products containing calcium, antacids (Ca^{++}, Mg^{++}, Al^{+++}), and mineral supplements (**iron,** calcium, zinc, fortified foods) should not be taken within 2 hours of ingesting tetracycline. Reasonable quantities of dairy products can be taken with doxycycline and minocycline because there is less interference with absorption, but concomitant administration with antacids or mineral supplements should be avoided.

Enhanced effect of other drugs. Tetracycline enhances the effect of the oral sulfonylureas, which has the potential to result in hypoglycemia. The effects of digoxin, lithium, and theophylline may also be enhanced, which leads to toxicity from these agents with narrow therapeutic indices. Furosemide's toxicity may also be increased by tetracycline.

Reduced doxycycline effect. The barbiturates and phenytoin can reduce the action of doxycycline. The mechanism is stimulation of hepatic microsomal enzymes so that doxycycline is metabolized more rapidly.

General antibiotic interactions. Like all the antibiotics, tetracyclines may reduce the effectiveness of oral contraceptives or increase the effectiveness of oral anticoagulants. Also, in most instances, mixing tetracyclines with another antibiotic results in antagonism, especially if the other antibiotic is bactericidal.

USES

Tetracyclines, including both tetracycline and doxycycline, have extensive medical and dental use.

Medical. Although active against a wide variety of microorganisms, tetracyclines are rarely the drug of choice for a specific infection. Occasionally they are alternative drugs to treat chlamydial and rickettsial infections. They are used to treat acne (topically and systemically), pulmonary infections in patients with **chronic obstructive pulmonary disease (COPD),** and traveler's diarrhea. Tetracyclines should not be used for prophylaxis against infective endocarditis except in one unusual situation in dentistry as discussed next.

Dental. Tetracyclines are not indicated as the drug of choice or the alternative drug of choice for dental infections unrelated to periodontal disease. They are frequently used for certain periodontal conditions. Conventional treatment with local measures should have failed before tetracycline therapy is initiated. A potential advantage of the tetracyclines in treatment of certain periodontal situations relates to their ability to concentrate in the gingival crevicular fluid. Because long-acting tetracyclines are concentrated to a greater extent in the gingival fluid and they require once-daily dosing, they may have some advantage over tetracycline itself. The ideal tetracycline therapy would be delivered directly to the gingival crevice, thereby greatly reducing the systemic dose. A variety of plastic strips, hollow fibers, or collars to deliver the tetracycline directly to the sulcus are being used but continue to be evaluated. Table 8-9 lists the tetracyclines available to use for periodontal organisms.

Although tetracycline is not a drug of choice for prophylaxis of infective endocarditis before dental appointments, it has a role in one situation. Penicillin-resistant *Actinobacillus actinomycetemcomitans* organisms have been shown to produce endocarditis. It is also present in about one half of adult and almost all juvenile patients

TABLE 8-9   Periodontal Microbes and Their In Vitro Susceptibility to the Tetracyclines

Organisms	Tetracycline	Doxycycline
Actinobacillus actinomycetemcomitans	2–8	6
Porphyromonas gingivalis (Bacteroides gingivalis)	2	1
Prevotella intermedia (Bacteroides intermedius)	6	3
Eikenella corrodens	3–32	6
Fusobacterium spp.	2	2
Campylobacter rectus (Wolinella recta)	2	1

Modified from Slots J, Rams TE: Antibiotics in periodontal therapy: advantages and disadvantages, *J Clin Periodontol* 17:479-493, 1990.

with periodontitis. Therefore, to prevent endocarditis infection from *A. actinomycetemcomitans* after dental treatment in patients at risk, a full course (3 weeks) of tetracycline should be administered several weeks before dental treatment is begun. Amoxicillin (or clindamycin) should be administered according to the American Heart Association's guidelines.

A mixture of equal parts of tetracycline syrup and viscous lidocaine has been used for the management of recurrent aphthous stomatitis. Currently, it is thought that using lidocaine or diphenhydramine alone produces equivalent or even better results than the tetracycline mixture. Although local measures are preferred, acute necrotizing ulcerative **gingivitis** may also be treated with tetracycline.

CLINDAMYCIN

Clindamycin [klin-da-MYE-sin] (Cleocin) is a bacteriostatic antibiotic effective primarily against gram-positive organisms and anaerobic *Bacteroides* species. Clindamycin is produced by adding a −Cl group to lincomycin, which is elaborated by *Streptomyces lincolnensis*, found in a soil sample taken near Lincoln, Nebraska. Clindamycin is structurally unrelated to any other antimicrobial agent other than lincomycin, which is not used.

PHARMACOKINETICS

Clindamycin may be administered orally, topically, intramuscularly, or intravenously. Oral clindamycin is well absorbed, and food does not interfere with its absorption. It reaches its peak concentration in 45 minutes, with a half-life of about 2.5 hours. Clindamycin is distributed throughout most body tissues, including bone, but not to the cerebrospinal fluid. Concentration in the bone can approximate that in the plasma. It crosses the placental barrier, and it is more than 90% bound to plasma proteins. Only about 10% of the active drug is eliminated in the urine. The majority of clindamycin is excreted as inactive metabolites in the urine and feces (via the bile).

SPECTRUM

The antibacterial spectrum of clindamycin includes many gram-positive organisms and some gram-negative organisms. The antibacterial action results from interference with bacterial protein synthesis. Clindamycin is bacteriostatic in most cases, although occasionally it can be bactericidal at higher blood levels.

Similar to erythromycin, clindamycin's activity includes *S. pyogenes* and *S. viridans*, pneumococci, and *S. aureus*. In contrast to erythromycin, clindamycin is very active against several anaerobes, including *B. fragilis* and *Bacteroides melaninogenicus*, *Fusobacterium* species, *Peptostreptococcus* (anaerobic streptococci) and *Peptococcus* species, and *Actinomyces israelii*.

Bacterial resistance to clindamycin develops in a slow, stepwise manner. It occurs by mutations in the bacterial ribosomes that result in a decrease in affinity and binding capacity of these drugs. Cross-resistance between clindamycin and erythromycin is frequently noted. An antagonistic relationship has been observed between clindamycin and erythromycin because of competition for the same binding site (50S subunit) on the bacteria.

ADVERSE REACTIONS

Gastrointestinal effects. The most commonly observed side effects of clindamycin are gastrointestinal, including diarrhea, nausea, vomiting, enterocolitis, and abdominal cramps. Glossitis and stomatitis have also been reported with these agents. The incidence of diarrhea with clindamycin is approximately 10%.

PMC (AAC) possible but uncommon.

The development of pseudomembranous colitis, also known as *antibiotic associated colitis* has been a more serious consequence associated with clindamycin. It is characterized by severe, persistent diarrhea and the passage of blood and mucus. This colitis, which can be fatal, is caused by a toxin produced by the bacterium *Clostridium difficile*. It is associated not only with clindamycin but also with other antibiotics such as tetracycline, ampicillin, and the cephalosporins. Treatment of colitis includes discontinuation of the drug, vancomycin or cholestyramine administered orally, and fluid and electrolyte replacement. Systemically administered corticosteroids have sometimes proved helpful. Opioid-like agents such as diphenoxylate and atropine (Lomotil) may exacerbate the condition and should not be used. Pseudomembranous colitis may occur during treatment, several weeks after cessation of antibiotic therapy, or without any antibiotic use.

Superinfection. As with other antibiotics, superinfection by *C. albicans* is sometimes associated with the use of clindamycin.

Other effects. Adverse reactions affecting the formed elements in the blood include **neutropenia,** thrombocytopenia, and agranulocytosis.

Abnormal liver function tests and renal dysfunction have been noted.

Allergy. Morbilliform skin rashes occasionally occur in patients given clindamycin. Oral allergic manifestations include glossitis and stomatitis. More severe allergic reactions include urticaria, angioneurotic edema, erythema multiforme, serum sickness, and anaphylaxis.

USES

Although clindamycin is effective against many gram-positive organisms, other agents are available that are at least as effective as clindamycin and do not usually cause pseudomembranous colitis. The indications for treatment with clindamycin are limited to a number of infections caused by anaerobic organisms, especially *Bacteroides* species and some staphylococcal infections, when the patient is allergic to penicillin.

Many oral infections have been shown to contain a predominance of anaerobic organisms. Many of these anaerobes, such as *Bacteroides oralis*, *Peptostreptococcus*, *Fusobacterium*, and *Veillonella* species, as well as clostridia, are sensitive to oral penicillin V. Clindamycin is the drug of choice for some bacteroides species and other anaerobes, endocarditis prophylaxis with penicillin allergy, and some pelvic infections.

When one compares the list of microorganisms responsible for periodontal infections with the spectrum of action of clindamycin, its potential for use in a variety of anaerobic infections is evident (Table 8-10). As the importance of the anaerobes in both oral infections and a wide variety of periodontal conditions becomes documented in the literature, the use of clindamycin will increase. Mixed gram-positive and gram-negative anaerobic infections may be treated with clindamycin. The use of clindamycin when anaerobic osteomyelitis is suspected is indicated if the organism is susceptible. It is important to emphasize that clindamycin should be used only when specifically indicated, not indiscriminately,

TABLE 8-10   Periodontal Microbes and Their In Vitro Susceptibility to Clindamycin, Metronidazole, and Ciprofloxacin

ORGANISMS	CLINDAMYCIN	METRONIDAZOLE	CIPROFLOXACIN
Actinobacillus actinomycetemcomitans	Resistant	32	<1
Porphyromonas gingivalis (Bacteroides gingivalis)	<1	4	<1–2
Prevotella intermedia (Bacteroides intermedius)	<1	2	<1
Eikenella corrodens	R	R	<1
Fusobacterium spp.	<1	1	3
Campylobacter rectus (Wolinella recta)	1	2	Resistant

Modified from Slots J, Rams TE: Antibiotics in periodontal therapy: advantages and disadvantages, *J Clin Periodontol* 17:479-493, 1990.

and the patient should be warned of the potential for pseudomembranous colitis and informed about its symptoms (bloody diarrhea mixed with mucus). The dose of clindamycin is 150 to 300 mg q6h (qid).

METRONIDAZOLE

Metronidazole [me-troe-NI-da-zole] (Flagyl) is an antiinfective that is a synthetic nitroimidazole with trichomonacidal *(Trichomonas vaginalis)*, amebicidal (*Entamoeba histolytica* species), and bactericidal action. It has exceptional action against most obligate anaerobes such as *Bacteroides* species. As with all antibiotics, resistance to this agent is increasing. It freely enters cells and is reduced into unknown polar compounds that do not contain the nitro group. This short-lived product is cytotoxic, but it causes DNA to lose its cyclic structure and inhibits nucleic acid synthesis, leading to death of the organisms. It affects cells whether or not they are dividing.

In addition to its antiinfective effects, metronidazole also has antiinflammatory effects. It affects neutrophil motility, lymphocyte action, and cell-mediated immunity. What therapeutic purpose these actions might serve is yet to be identified.

PHARMACOKINETICS

Taken orally, metronidazole is well absorbed, with a peak level occurring between 1 and 2 hours after administration. Between 60% and 80% of a dose is excreted in the urine. Metabolites account for about 20% of the dose. Its half-life averages 8 hours, but with alcoholic liver disease it averages 18 hours. It is less than 20% protein bound. Metronidazole is somewhat concentrated in the gingival crevicular fluid, producing concentrations that are bacteriocidal to pathogenic periodontal organisms. Metronidazole is distributed into the cerebrospinal fluid, saliva, and breast milk in levels approximating that of the serum.

SPECTRUM

Metronidazole is bactericidal and penetrates all bacterial cells. The spectrum of action of metronidazole includes the protozoa *T. vaginalis* and *E. histolytica*. Metronidazole is active against obligate anaerobic bacteria such as *Bacteroides, Fusobacterium, Veillonella, Treponema, Clostridium, Peptococcus, Campylobacter,* and *Peptostreptococcus* organisms. The increased use of antibiotics is resulting in a continuing rise in the incidence of resistance. Compare the spectrum of action of metronidazole with the bacteria responsible for periodontal conditions and the concentration effective against those bacteria (see Table 8-10).

ADVERSE REACTIONS

Stomach distress common

Gastrointestinal tract effects. Metronidazole's most common adverse reactions involve the gastrointestinal tract. This side effect occurs in 12% of patients taking metronidazole. It includes nausea, anorexia, diarrhea, and vomiting. Epigastric distress and abdominal cramping have also been reported.

Central nervous system effects. Headache, dizziness, vertigo, and ataxia have been reported. Confusion, **depression,** weakness, insomnia, and serious convulsive seizures are rarely associated with metronidazole use.

Renal toxicity. Cystitis, **polyuria, dysuria,** and **incontinence** can occur with metronidazole. Rarely, darkening of the urine as a result of a metabolite has been reported.

Xerostomia, unpleasant metallic taste—yuk!

Oral effects. Another effect that has been reported is a dry mouth. Frequently, an unpleasant or sharp metallic taste has been reported. Altered taste of alcohol has been noted. Glossitis, stomatitis, and a black-furred tongue are side effects the dental health care worker might observe. These side effects may be related to monilial overgrowth. Appendix H discusses xerostomia in more detail.

Other effects. Transient neutropenia in humans and carcinogenicity, mutagenicity, and tumorigenicity in lower life-forms have been reported. Metronidazole is in Food and Drug Administration (FDA) pregnancy category B because administration to pregnant mice caused fetal toxicity. Administration of metronidazole for dental infections during pregnancy is contraindicated. Nursing mothers should not be given metronidazole unless milk is expressed and discarded beginning when the metronidazole is taken and continuing for 48 hours after discontinuing the drug.

DRUG INTERACTIONS

When alcohol is ingested with metronidazole, a reaction can occur that is a mild form of the reaction that occurs when a recovering alcoholic drinks alcohol while taking disulfiram (Antabuse), which reduces the chance that the alcoholic will drink alcohol (see Chapter 26). Symptoms include nausea, abdominal cramps, flushing, vomiting, or headache. Alcohol should be avoided during metronidazole administration and for 1 day after therapy has ceased. Products such as mouthwashes or elixirs that contain alcohol should not be used during this period. Metronidazole can potentiate the effect of warfarin. The combination of metronidazole and disulfiram has led to confusion and should be avoided. Drugs that stimulate liver microsomal enzymes, such as phenobarbital and phenytoin, can reduce the plasma levels of metronidazole. Before metronidazole is administered to patients the possibility of a drug interaction should be checked.

No alcohol with metronidazole

USES

Metronidazole is used for the treatment of infections caused by susceptible organisms in both medical and dental conditions. It has special usefulness because of its anaerobic spectrum.

Medical. The medical uses of metronidazole include treatment of trichomoniasis, giardiasis, amebiasis, and susceptible anaerobic bacterial infections. It is effective against serious anaerobic infections of the abdomen, skeleton, and female genital tract. Endocarditis and lower respiratory tract infections caused by *Bacteroides* species are treated with metronidazole. It is available as oral tablets, vaginal cream for vaginal infections, and topical cream for the treatment of rosacea.

Dental. Because of its anaerobic efficacy, metronidazole is useful in the treatment of many periodontal infections. Table 8-10 lists metronidazole's effect against peridontal organisms. One notable exception is that it has no action against *A. actinomycetemcomitans.* The combination of metronidazole with amoxicillin, sometimes called "poor man's Augmentin," can be useful in the treatment of some patients with juvenile or refractory periodontitis. One advantage of metronidazole is that when prescribed generically it is inexpensive (see Figure 8-3).

CEPHALOSPORINS

The cephalosporin [sef-a-loe-SPOR-in] group of antibiotics is structurally related to the penicillins. Cephalosporins

> "Kissing cousins" to the penicillins.

are active against a wide variety of both gram-positive and gram-negative organisms. The oral cephalosporins products, listed in Table 8-11, are divided into first-, second-, third-, and fourth-generation agents. Most third-generation cephalosporins are available for parenteral use. The orally active cephalosporins are discussed.

The source of the original cephalosporins was *Cephalosporium acremonium*, isolated from a sewer outlet near Sardinia, in Italy. Because cephalosporins are true antibiotics, they were originally produced by organisms. Those available for oral

TABLE 8-11 Cephalosporins, Oral

Drug Name	Protein Bound %	Bioavailability %	Peak (hr)	$T_{1/2}$ (hr)	$T_{1/2}$ (min)	$T_{1/2}$ Decrease Renal	Daily Dose* (gm)	Interval (hrs)
First generation								
Cephalexin (Keflex)	10	95	1	0.9-1.2	50-80	5-30	1-4	6
Cephradine (Velosef, Anspor)	8-17	95	1	0.8-1.3	50-180	8-15	1-4	6-12
Cefadroxil (Duricef, Ultracef)	20	95	1.5-2	1.2-1.5	80-95	20-25	1-2	12-24
Second generation								
Cefaclor (Ceclor)	25	95	0.5-1	0.6-0.9	35-54	2.3-2.8	0.75-1	8-12
Cefuroxime (Ceftin, Kefurox, Zinacef)	33-50	52ct† 37s	2.7-3.6	1.2-1.9	80	6	1 0.25-1	12
Cefprozil (Cefzil)	36	95	1.5	1.3	80	to 5.2	0.5-1.0	12-24
Third generation								
Cefixime (Suprax)	65	40-50	2.6	3-4	180-240	6.4-11.5	0.4	12-24
Cefpodoxime proxetil (Vantin)	25	50†	2-3	2.1-2.8	120-180	3.5-9.8	0.2-0.8	12
Cefdinir (Omnicef)			2-4	1.7			0.6	12-24
Carbacephams—relative								
Loracarbef (Lorabid)	25				60		0.4-0.8	12-24

*Dose varies with impaired renal function and type of infection.
†Absorption increases with food.

use are relatively acid stable and highly resistant to penicillinase, but they are destroyed by cephalosporinase, an enzyme elaborated by some microorganisms.

PHARMACOKINETICS

The cephalosporins can be administered orally, intramuscularly, or intravenously. The agents that cannot be used orally are too poorly absorbed to provide adequate blood levels. The cephalosporins used orally are well absorbed. They are bound 10% and 65% to the plasma proteins (see Table 8-11). After absorption, they are widely distributed throughout the tissues. Like penicillin, the cephalosporins are excreted by glomerular filtration and tubular secretion into the urine. Their half-lives vary between 50 and 240 minutes.

SPECTRUM

The cephalosporins, which are bactericidal, are active against most gram-positive cocci, penicillinase-producing staphylococci, and some gram-negative bacteria. They inhibit most *Salmonella* and *Klebsiella* organisms, some paracolon strains, and *E. coli. Serratia* and *Enterobacter* species, *H. influenzae*, indole-positive *Proteus*, methicillin-resistant staphylococci, and most *Pseudomonas* strains are unaffected. The generation of the cephalosporin (first, second, or third) designates the width of antimicrobial action, with the first generation being narrower (gram-positive, few gram-negative) than the second generation (gram-positive, more gram-negative and anaerobes), and the third generation (gram-positive weaker, many gram-negative and anaerobes) possessing the broadest spectrum of action. Figure 8-1 provides a visual representation of the spectrum of action of dentally useful antiinfective agents against the most common organisms associated with dental infections—gram-positive aerobes, gram-positive anaerobes, and gram-negative anaerobes.

MECHANISM OF ACTION

The mechanism of action of the cephalosporins is like that of the penicillins—inhibition of cell wall synthesis. They bind to enzymes in the cell membrane involved in cell wall synthesis. The cephalosporin acts as an analog of acyl-D-alanyl-D-alanine to produce a deficiency in the cell walls, leading to lysis. They are more effective against rapidly growing organisms (explains the potential drug interaction between bacteriostatic and bactericidal antibiotics).

ADVERSE REACTIONS

In general, the cephalosporins have a low incidence of adverse reactions (excluding allergic reactions) and are well tolerated. They have more adverse reactions than penicillin VK. The following adverse reactions may occur.

Gastrointestinal effects. The most common adverse reaction associated with the cephalosporins is gastrointestinal, including diarrhea, nausea, vomiting, abdominal pain, anorexia, dyspepsia, and stomatitis.

Nephrotoxicity. Evidence suggests that the cephalosporins may produce nephrotoxic effects under certain conditions. Although some have suggested that this is a toxic reaction, it may be an allergic reaction.

Superinfection. As with all antibiotics, especially those with a broader spectrum of action, superinfection has been reported. Resistant gram-negative organisms are often the culprits.

Local reaction. As with penicillin, the irritating nature of the cephalosporins can produce localized pain, induration, and swelling when given intramuscularly and abscess and thrombophlebitis when given intravenously.

Hemostasis and disulfiram-like reaction. Certain parenteral cephalosporins can impair hemostasis or produce a disulfiram-like reaction. The *N*-methylthiotetrazole side chain appears responsible. Dental health care workers do not use parenteral cephalosporins, and therefore this side effect is of no concern to dentistry.

Allergy. Various types of hypersensitivity reactions have been reported in approximately 5% of patients receiving cephalosporins. These reactions include fever, eosinophilia, serum sickness, rashes, and anaphylaxis. Large doses frequently produce a direct positive Coombs' reaction. This can lead to a significant degree of hemolysis.

The cephalosporins and penicillin have similar structures; some cross-hypersensitivity can occur. Clinically, the incidence of hypersensitivity reactions to the cephalosporins is higher in patients with a history of penicillin allergy. The degree of cross-hypersensitivity reported is about 10%. Cephalosporins are frequently given to patients with a history of penicillin allergy, especially if the reaction was mild and in the distant past.

Uses

The cephalosporins are indicated for infections that are sensitive to these agents but resistant to penicillin. They are especially useful in certain infections caused by gram-negative organisms such as *Klebsiella*. Their dental use includes prophylaxis for patients with "at-risk" joints who are undergoing dental procedures likely to produce bleeding. They are also used to treat infections with sensitive organisms when other agents are ineffective or cannot be used. Their doses are listed in Table 8-11. They are not a substitute for penicillin VK, if this agent is effective.

RATIONAL USE OF ANTIINFECTIVE AGENTS IN DENTISTRY

Figure 8-5 shows the progression of most dental infections. The early phase, stage 1, is primarily gram-positive organisms; the mixed stage, stage 2, has both aerobes and anaerobes; and the last stage, stage 3, is exclusively anaerobes. If incision and drainage is possible, most dental infections in patients with normal immunity, whether the infection is in stage 1, 2, or 3, do not need antiinfective agents.

Stage 1. Acute abscess and **cellulitis** are primarily gram-positive. The drug of choice in patients without a penicillin allergy is penicillin VK, 500 mg q6h for 5 to 7 days (actually the patient needs to take the antibiotic every day as long as symp-

FIGURE 8-5 *Odontogenic infections in the oral cavity (early to late).*

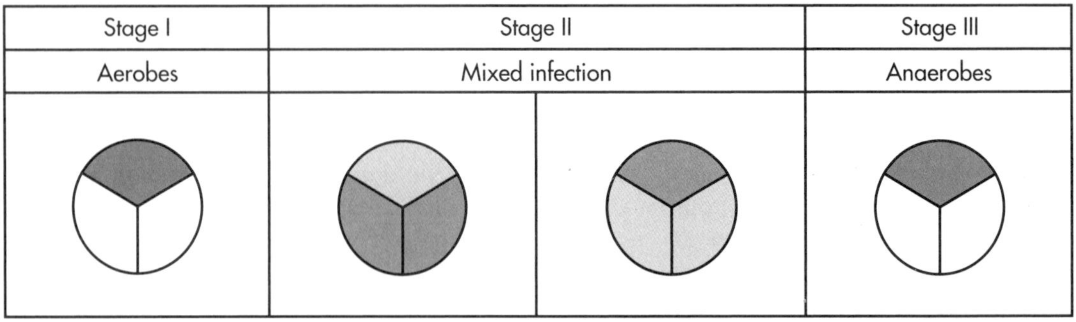

Stage I	Stage II	Stage III
Aerobes	Mixed infection	Anaerobes

toms persist plus 2 or 3 days). For those with an allergy to penicillin, erythromycin ethylsuccinate or clindamycin may be used (see Appendix G for a flowchart). Sample prescriptions for the antiinfective agents discussed are included in Appendix C.

Stage 2. During stage 2, the infection is mixed. This can be handled by attacking either the gram-positive organisms or the anaerobes. The gram-positive organisms can be managed with the same drugs as in stage 1. To attack the anaerobes an antiinfective with good anaerobic coverage is needed. The two antibiotics with the most anaerobic coverage are clindamycin and metronidazole. Penicillin VK also has anaerobic coverage. If drainage can be established, antiinfective agents are not indicated in the immunocompetent patient.

Stage 3. In stage 3, the organisms have coalesced into one area and are almost solely anaerobic. Most often incision and drainage is sufficient. In fact, this sometimes happens spontaneously and the patient is "cured" (in their mind because they do not have pain). If chronic infection persists or if the patient is immune-compromised, use of an antibiotic with anaerobic coverage is warranted.

When a prescribed antiinfective is not effective, there may be several reasons for this outcome. If an antibiotic failure occurs, the patient must be reevaluated taking into account the following reasons why an antibiotic may be ineffective:

- **Patient compliance.** The patient may not be taking the antibiotic.
  - ◆ *Did not get the prescription filled.* Was the patient informed about the benefit that the medicine would have? Was the patient informed about the risk of not taking the medicine? Consequences?
  - ◆ *Tried to get the prescription filled.* There was a long wait at the pharmacy. The children have to be picked up from

school. The checkbook was forgotten. When the patient was told the price of the prescription, he or she was not able to pay for it. The patient was told that antibiotics can interfere with the effectiveness of birth control pills and she did not want to get pregnant.
  - ◆ *Got prescription filled but. . . .* The patient noticed that the tablets "smelled bad" or were "hard to swallow" or "I decided to take an herbal product."
  - ◆ *Did not complete prescription.* Patients state that they "began to feel better," "forgot to take some pills," "took a few but then quit," "saved them for the next time I have a toothache," and so on.
- **Wrong antibiotic.** The antibiotic chosen may not be effective against the organism producing the infection. If antibiotics do not spawn a response after 2 or 3 days, consideration should be given to changing the antibiotic (check compliance first).
- **Poor debridement.** Dead tissue, purulent exudate, or foreign bodies were not completely removed from the site of infection.
- **Resistant organism.** The antibiotic may not be effective because the organism is resistant to the antibiotic chosen. Knowledge about the resistance patterns in your area is important to consider before prescribing an antibiotic.
- **Concentration did not reach the site of the infection.** There are several mechanisms by which an adequate concentration of the antibiotic does not reach the site of the infection. Lack of penetration may occur because of decreased vascularity, an isolated location or "walled off" area, or a drug interaction inactivating the antibiotic before absorption. Microvascular disease, often seen in diabetics, further reduces the blood flow and the amount of antibiotic sent to the area.
- **Host defenses inadequate.** The ability of the host's immune system to fight the infection

is very important in ridding the body of the infection.

ANTIMICROBIAL AGENTS FOR NONDENTAL USE

VANCOMYCIN

Used IV for systemic effect; PO for local effect.

Vancomycin [van-koe-MYE-sin] (Vancocin) is an antibiotic elaborated by *Streptomyces orientalis*, an actinomycete found in soil samples from India and Indonesia. It is unrelated to any other antibiotic currently marketed. Because it has very poor gastrointestinal absorption and it causes irritation when used intramuscularly, it is usually administered only intravenously, for a systemic effect. When used by mouth, it is being used to eradicate organisms within the gastrointestinal tract (see discussion of pseudomembranous colitis, p. 175).

Spectrum. Vancomycin is bactericidal and has a narrow spectrum of activity against many gram-positive cocci, including both staphylococci and streptococci. It acts by inhibition of bacterial cell wall synthesis. In the past, resistance did not develop readily, but recently vancomycin-resistant organisms have appeared. When resistance was uncommon, vancomycin was rarely used. After resistance to other organisms increased, the use of vancomycin increased. This led, predictably, to an increase in resistance to vancomycin. Cross-resistance with other antibiotics is not believed to occur, because it has a different structure from other antibiotics.

Adverse reactions. Except when vancomycin is given in large doses, significant toxic reactions are infrequent. With oral use, nausea, vomiting and a bitter taste may be experienced. With intravenous use, an erythematous rash on the face

and upper body has been reported (red man syndrome). Hypotension accompanied by flushing, chills, and drug fever are also associated with vancomycin.

AMINOGLYCOSIDES

As the name implies, the aminoglycoside [a-mee-noe-GLYE-koe-side] antibiotics are made up of amino sugars in glycosidic linkage. In 1943, a strain of *Streptomyces griseus* was isolated that elaborated streptomycin. Further strains of *Streptomyces* species furnished neomycin, kanamycin, tobramycin, and amikacin, and *Micromonospora* organisms produced gentamicin and netilmicin. They are bacteriocidal and appear to inhibit protein synthesis and to act directly on the 30S subunit of the ribosome. The aminoglycosides are as follows:

Neomycin (Mycifradin)
Streptomycin
Kanamycin (Kantrex)
Gentamicin (Garamycin)
Tobramycin (Nebcin)
Amikacin (Amikin)
Netilmicin (Netromycin)

Pharmacokinetics. Because these agents are poorly absorbed after oral administration, they must be administered intramuscularly or intravenously for a systemic effect. Aminoglycosides are used orally for their local effect within the intestines. Before gastrointestinal surgery, aminoglycosides reduce the intestinal bacterial flora.

Spectrum. The aminoglycosides are bactericidal and have a broad antibacterial spectrum. Their use is primarily in the treatment of aerobic gram-negative infections when other agents are ineffective. They have little action against gram-positive anaerobic or facultative bacteria.

Adverse reactions. The adverse reactions of the aminoglycoside antibiotics seriously limit their use in clinical practice. Their major adverse effects include the following:

OTOTOXICITY The aminoglycosides are toxic to the eighth cranial nerve, which can lead to auditory and vestibular (in ear) disturbances. Patients may have difficulty maintaining equilibrium and can develop vertigo. Hearing impairment and deafness, which can be permanent, have resulted from the administration of these agents. This side effect is more common in patients with renal failure because the drug accumulates in the body. The elderly are also more susceptible.

NEPHROTOXICITY The aminoglycosides can cause kidney damage by concentrating in the renal cortex. The blood levels and total amount of drug given correlate with the incidence of nephrotoxicity.

Uses The aminoglycosides are indicated for the treatment of hospitalized patients with serious gram-negative infections. In past American Heart Association recommendations, these agents were used prophylactically in heart valve replacement. Now oral therapy (like all other indications) is recommended.

CHLORAMPHENICOL

Chloramphenicol [klor-am-FEN-i-kole] (Chloromycetin), a broad-spectrum, bacteriostatic antibiotic, inhibits bacterial protein synthesis by acting primarily on the 50S ribosomal unit. It is active against a large number of gram-positive and gram-negative organisms, rickettsiae, and some chlamydia. It is particularly active against *Salmonella typhi.*

Chloramphenicol has fallen into disuse primarily because of its serious adverse effects, which include fatal blood dyscrasias such as aplastic anemia, agranulocytosis, hypoplastic anemia, and thrombocytopenia. Chloramphenicol can produce bone marrow suppression with

pancytopenia. Although the incidence is low (1:40,000), this condition is often fatal. Chloramphenicol has no use in dentistry.

SULFONAMIDES

Strictly speaking, the sulfonamides [sul-FON-a-mides] cannot be classified as *antibiotics* because they are not produced by living organisms. They may be termed *antiinfectives* or *antimicrobials.*

The introduction of many newer antibiotics limited the use of the sulfonamides until the introduction of trimethoprim-sulfamethoxazole combination. This combination, the most common use of the sulfonamides, is discussed.

Mechanism of action. The structural similarity between the sulfonamide agents and *p*-aminobenzoic

> PABA analogue—inhibits synthesis of folic acid.

acid (PABA) is the basis for most of their antibacterial activity. Unlike humans, many bacteria are unable to use preformed **folic acid,** which is essential for their growth. They must synthesize folic acid from PABA. Because of their structural similarity to PABA, the sulfonamides competitively inhibit dihydropteroate synthetase, the bacterial enzyme that incorporates PABA into dihydrofolic acid, an immediate precursor of folic acid (Figure 8-6). Drugs that are metabolized to PABA (e.g., ester local anesthetics) could theoretically interfere with the action of the sulfonamides.

Spectrum. The sulfonamides are bacteriostatic against many gram-positive and some gram-negative bacteria. They are frequently used in medicine to treat acute otitis media in children *(H. influenzae)*, acute exacerbations of chronic bronchitis in adults *(S. pneumoniae)*, and urinary tract infections *(Klebsiella* and *Enterobacter* organisms and *E. coli)*. They are ineffective against *S. viridans* but are active against some *Chlamydia* organisms. Sulfonamides are also used for pro-

FIGURE 8-6 *Location of action of sulfonamides and trimethoprim. They inhibit the synthesis of folic acid at two different locations.*

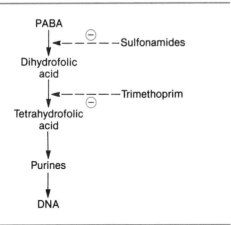

phylaxis of *Pneumocystis carinii* pneumonitis and for traveler's diarrhea caused by enterotoxigenic *E. coli* or *Cyclospora* organisms.

The readily absorbed sulfonamides are used for their systemic effects and are distributed throughout the body. Some poorly soluble sulfonamides, when given orally, act locally in the treatment of ulcerative colitis or before surgical procedures on the bowel.

Adverse reactions. The most common side effect of the sulfonamides is allergic skin reactions. Patients with an allergy to "sulfa" drugs may exhibit some cross-hypersensitivity with thiazide diuretics and the sulfonylureas (used orally to treat diabetes). There is no cross-hypersensitivity between sulfa drugs and either sulfites, sulfates, or sulfur.

The allergic reactions may manifest as rash, urticaria, **pruritus,** fever, a fatal exfoliative dermatitis, or periarteritis nodosa. Other cutaneous allergic reactions include erythema nodosum, erythema multiforme, Stevens-Johnson syndrome, and epidermal necrolysis.

Other relatively common side effects include nausea, vomiting, abdominal discomfort, head-

ache, and dizziness. Liver damage, depressed renal function, blood dyscrasias (agranulocytosis, thrombocytopenia, aplastic and hemolytic anemia), and precipitation of lupus erythematosus are seen less frequently.

Patients with **human immunodeficiency virus (HIV)** are much more likely to exhibit adverse effects (65%) such as rash, fever, or leukopenia and to discontinue therapy. In patients with HIV the sulfisoxazole-trimethoprim combination is used prophylactically to prevent *Pneumocystis carinii* **pneumonia.**

The possibility of renal crystallization (crystalluria) must always be kept in mind with the sulfonamides. The earlier sulfonamides had low solubility in the urine, and there was danger of crystallization in the kidney. The new sulfonamides are more soluble and therefore less likely to precipitate in the kidney. This is the reason patients taking sulfonamides are encouraged to drink plenty of water.

> Drink plenty of water.

Uses. These agents have no use in dentistry.

SULFAMETHOXAZOLE-TRIMETHOPRIM

Trimethoprim [trye-METH-oh-prim] (cotrimoxazole, SMX-TMP), an antibacterial and antimalarial agent, and sulfamethoxazole [sul-fa-meth-OX-a-zole], a sulfonamide, are commonly used in combination (co-trimoxazole, SMX-TMP, Bactrim, Septra). Because sulfamethoxazole inhibits the incorporation of PABA into folic acid and trimethoprim inhibits the reduction of dihydrofolate to tetrahydrofolate (see Figure 8-6), this combination inhibits two separate steps in the essential metabolic pathway of the bacteria, thus delaying resistance and leading to a synergistic effect.

SMX-TMP (Bactrim, Septra) is bacteriostatic against a wide variety of gram-positive bacteria and some gram-negative bacteria. Its adverse effects are similar to those of the sulfonamides. About 75% of the adverse reactions associated with this combination involve skin disorders.

SMX-TMP is indicated in the treatment of selected urinary tract infections and selected respiratory and gastrointestinal infections. It is used extensively to treat acute otitis media in children, which is often caused by *H. influenzae*. A combination of erythromycin and sulfisoxazole (Pediazole) is also used to treat otitis media in children. SMX-TMP is used prophylactically to prevent *Pneumocystis carinii* pneumonia in patients with AIDS, *Serratia* sepsis, and systemic *Salmonella* (ampicillin-resistant) and *Shigella* infections. SMX-TMP has no documented use in dentistry, but pediatric patients coming to the dental office may be taking it prophylactically for prevention of chronic ear infections.

NITROFURANTOIN

Nitrofurantoin [nye-troe-fyoor-AN-toyn] (Macrodantin) possesses a wide antibacterial spectrum including both gram-positive and gram-negative bacteria. It is bacteriostatic against many common urinary tract pathogens, including *E. coli*. Many strains of *Klebsiella* and *Enterobacter* and all strains of *P. aeruginosa* are resistant. The most common adverse reactions are nausea, vomiting, and diarrhea, but taking the drug with food decreases these effects. Many hypersensitivity reactions are associated with nitrofurantoin. Nitrofurantoin is used in the treatment or prophylaxis of certain urinary tract infections.

QUINOLONES (FLUOROQUINOLONES)

Orally effective and active versus *Pseudomonas* organisms.

A group of orally effective antibacterial agents, called the quinolones [KWIN-a-lones], are chemically related to nalidixic [nal-i-DIX-ik] acid (NegGram). The number of agents in this group of drugs has risen

BOX 8-4   FLUOROQUINOLONES

Ciprofloxacin (Cipro)
Enoxacin (Penetrex)
Grepafloxacin (Raxar)
Lomefloxacin (Maxaquin)
Norfloxacin (Noroxin)
Ofloxacin (Floxin)
Trovafloxacin (Trovan)

exponentially. This group may have potential use in dentistry because of their spectrum of action. Like other new antibiotics, their overuse produces resistance. They are bactericidal against most gram-negative organisms and many gram-positive organisms. They are the first orally active agents against certain *Pseudomonas* species. There is no cross-resistance with other antimicrobial agents.

The mechanism of action of the quinolones is unique and involves antagonism of the A subunit of DNA gyrase; the enzyme is involved in DNA synthesis. It also inhibits the relaxation of supercoiled DNA and promotes breakage of double-stranded DNA. Because interference with DNA gyrase results in cell death, resistance is not transferred from one resistant bacteria to an unexposed bacteria. Plasmid and chromosomal DNA are destroyed. DNA gyrase is found only in microorganisms, and therefore human cells are unaffected by the quinolones' action. The members of the fluoroquinolones are listed in Box 8-4. The discussion concentrates on ciprofloxacin [sip-roe-FLOKS-a-sin], a prototype of the quinolones.

Pharmacokinetics. Ciprofloxacin is well absorbed orally and is eliminated with a half-life of 4 hours. Both antacids and probenecid interfere with ciprofloxacin's absorption and serum concentration. Patients should be well hydrated to prevent any possibility of crystalluria (drink water while taking).

Spectrum. Ciprofloxacin is bactericidal against a wide range of gram-negative organisms including *Klebsiella* and *Enterobacter* species, *E. coli, P. aeruginosa,* and gram-positive organisms such as *S. aureus.* Its special spectrum is against *Pseudomonas* organisms. Unlike other antiinfective agents, an additive action may result when ciprofloxacin is combined with other antimicrobial agents. The emergence of organisms resistant to the fluoroquinolones and the cross-resistance among the fluoroquinolones is increasing. Use of fluoroquinolones in chickens may be partially responsible for increasing resistance.

Ofloxacin [o-FLOKS-a-sin] is the quinolone with activity against organisms present in dental infections. When the spectrums of ciprofloxacin and ofloxacin are compared, ofloxacin's spectrum of action most closely parallels the spectrum of microbes found in dental infections. After consulting many sources for information about the spectrum of action of the fluoroquinolones the conclusion reached is that intraspecies variation is at least as great as interspecies variation. In other words, spectrum of action is difficult to predict and depends on which sample of microorganisms is tested. Because of this action, ciprofloxacin or other quinolones may be used in dentistry in the future.

Adverse reactions

GASTROINTESTINAL TRACT Nausea, diarrhea, vomiting, painful oral mucosa, bad taste, and oral candidiasis have been reported. Pseudomembranous colitis has been seen in patients taking quinolones.

CENTRAL NERVOUS SYSTEM EFFECTS CNS adverse reactions include headache, restlessness, lightheadedness, and insomnia. CNS stimulation has been noted.

HYPERSENSITIVITY Rash, pruritus, urticaria, hyperpigmentation, and edema of the lips have been noted. Fluoroquinolones are associated with photosensitivity reactions when the patient

is exposed to the sun. The patient should be advised to use sunscreen or wear clothes that cover the whole body. A few anaphylactic reactions have been reported.

OTHER EFFECTS Disturbed vision, joint pain, renal problems, and palpitations have rarely been reported. An unusual reaction affecting the Achilles tendon has become fairly common in patients taking quinolones. These agents can produce tendonitis or tendon rupture in the Achilles tendon, so exercise should be limited. Hepatotoxicity has rarely been attributed to the quinolones.

PREGNANCY AND NURSING Ciprofloxacin is contraindicated in the pregnant or nursing woman.

Uses. Ciprofloxacin is indicated for lower respiratory tract, skin, bone and joint, and urinary tract infections caused by susceptible organisms. Because of the spectrum of the quinolones, future use may include dental periodontal disease. In summary, the new quinolones have an advantage over other antimicrobial agents because of their unique mechanism of action, making the development and transfer of resistance more difficult. Their gram-negative spectrum coupled with their oral efficacy and bactericidal action makes these agents a welcome addition to the antimicrobial armamentarium. Many more members of this group of agents currently have been released, and more wait in the wings. Overuse of these agents has already begun, and it is hoped that they do not become much less useful as a result of overprescribing.

ANTITUBERCULOSIS AGENTS

The treatment of tuberculosis (TB), a disease caused by the acid-fast bacterium *Mycobacterium tuberculosis,* is difficult for several reasons. First, patients with TB often have inadequate defense mechanisms (e.g., AIDS). Second, tubercle bacilli develop resistant strains easily and possess unusual metabolic characteristics, including long periods of inactivity (they become dormant) when they are resistant to treatment. Next, most of the drugs available are not bactericidal and because of their toxicity often cannot be used in sufficient doses. Lastly, people using antituberculosis agents often do not take them as prescribed. For these reasons, the development of multidrug-resistant TB (MDR TB) has continued to increase because of its spread in patients with HIV and homeless patients and spread in other countries. (On an airline flight a patient with active TB has been reported to have infected several other passengers. The latest report of the spread of TB infection occurred in a fast food line.) The newest development in the world-wide problem with TB is the practice of manufacturing and selling drugs used for treatment of TB containing only a fraction of the labeled amount (counterfeit tablets).

Treatment of TB relies almost entirely on chemotherapy (Table 8-12). Because of the problem of resistance, at least three drugs are administered concurrently in all active cases. Isoniazid, rifampin, and pyrazinamide are combined for the treatment of pulmonary tuberculosis. The isoniazid and rifampin are continued every day for 9 to 12 months. The pyrazinamide is continued for 2 months. With susceptible organisms, a patient, if compliant, usually becomes noninfective within 2 to 3 weeks. This compliance presents a problem because patients often stop taking their medication before the designated time.

The Centers for Disease Control and Prevention (CDC) recommends that the following pa-

TABLE 8-12 Antituberculosis Agents

Drug Name*	Dose	Side Effects	Comments
Isoniazid (INH, Laniazid)	300 mg/d; 900 mg 2 × wk	Hepatitis (acetaminophen, alcohol exacerbates); peripheral neuropathy, give pyridoxine (vitamin B_6); CNS toxicity, GI	Alone for conversion or prophylaxis; combined with other TB drugs for treatment
Rifampin (Rifadin, Rimactane) Rifapentine (Priftin)†	600 mg/d	GI (nausea, vomiting, anorexia, pseudomembranous colitis); rash; kidney (hematuria, pyuria, or proteinuria); hepatitis (alcohol exacerbates), CNS (mood changes fatigue); blood dyscrasias	Reddish-orange to reddish-brown discoloration of urine, feces, saliva, sputum, sweat, and tears (discolor contact lenses permanently); induces enzymes
Pyrazinamide (PZA)	50-70 mg/kg 2 × wk	Hepatotoxicity; nausea, vomiting; hyperuricemia (gouty attack)	Used with ciprofloxacin for MDR TB
RIFATER		ISONIAZID + RIFAMPIN + PYRAZINAMIDE	
Ethambutol (Myambutol)	15 mg/kg/d	Retrobulbar optic neuritis, (eye examination visual fields and acuity and red-green discrimination), peripheral neuritis; gouty arthritis; GI symptoms; CNS (confusion)	
Streptomycin	15 mg/kg/d; max 1 gm	Ototoxicity (vertigo), nephrotoxicity	Given by IM injection; dose adjusted per renal function

*Rifater, rifampin, isoniazid, pyrazinamide.
†Cyclopentyl rifamycin.
CNS, Central nervous system; *GI*, gastrointestinal; *IM*, intramuscular; *MDRTB*, multidrug-resistant tuberculosis; *TB*, tuberculosis.

tients receive isoniazid because they are at risk of developing TB: close contacts of recently diagnosed patients, patients with a positive skin test and radiographic findings consistent with patients with nonprogressive TB, patients whose skin test has become positive (converted), and immunosuppressed patients. If patients have been vaccinated against TB (with **Bacillus** Calumet Guérin [BCG]), skin tests (purified protein derivative [PPD]) will always be positive, and chest x-rays are required for screening.

ISONIAZID

Isoniazid [eye-soe-NYE-a-zid] (Laniazid, INH) is bactericidal only against actively growing tubercle bacilli. The mechanism of action may relate to inhibition of mycolic acid synthesis resulting in disruption of the bacterial cell wall. "Resting" bacilli exposed to the drug are able to resume normal growth when the drug is removed. Within a few weeks after beginning therapy, resistant strains develop.

Pharmacokinetics. INH is readily absorbed from the gastrointestinal tract and is distributed throughout the body. Its metabolism varies by race. Most Eskimos and Japanese are fast acetylators, whereas whites and blacks in the United States are split 50-50 between fast and slow acetylators. The ability to acetylate rapidly is inherited as an autosomal dominant trait. Whether this ability to metabolize INH rapidly is related to the chance of developing INH-induced hepatitis is unknown. The half-life for fast acetylators is 1.5 hours; for slow, 3 hours.

Adverse reactions. The incidence of all adverse reactions to INH is approximately 5%. The most common adverse reaction, occurring in about 20% of patients, involves the nervous system. Peripheral and **optic** neuritis, muscle twitching, toxic encephalopathy, insomnia, restlessness, sedation, incoordination, convulsions,

and even psychoses have been reported. These neurotoxic symptoms can be prevented by coadministration of pyridoxine (vitamin B_6).

The other major adverse effect associated with INH is hepatotoxicity. About 1% of patients taking INH exhibit clinical hepatitis, and up to 10% develop abnormal laboratory values. Some cases of hepatitis have been fatal. The risk for development of this adverse effect is age related; that is, it rarely occurs in patients less than 20 years old, whereas 2.5% of patients older than 50 develop hepatitis. This differential in incidence of hepatitis by age may modify the treatment plan for an individual patient. Other side effects include hematologic effects, gastrointestinal effects, dryness of the mouth, and a lupus-like reaction or rheumatic syndrome with arthralgia. Urinary retention and gynecomastia have been noted in males. Hypersensitivity reactions, including rashes, hepatitis, lymphadenopathy, and fever, are occasionally reported. The choice of whether to use INH or not depends on many factors such as patient age, presence of renal or hepatic deficiency, history of seizures, gastrointestinal disturbances, alcoholism, or history of neurotoxicity.

INH is both an inhibitor and an inducer of cytochrome P-450 2E isoenzymes. The benzodiazepines that are oxidized in the liver, such as diazepam and midazolam, may have an increased effect in patients taking INH. Foods (e.g., cheese and fish) and drugs that are contraindicated with MAO inhibitors may also react with INH.

Uses. INH is used alone for prophylaxis or for converters (change in TB test results). It is used in combination with other antituberculosis agents. The usual adult dose is 300 mg daily.

RIFAMPIN

Rifampin [RIF-am-pin] (Rifadin, Rimactane) is a semisynthetic derivative of rifamycin, an antibiotic produced by *Streptomyces mediterranei*. Its mechanism of action involves inhibition of DNA-dependent ribonucleic acid (RNA) polymerase, which then suppresses the initiation of chain formation. It is active against *Mycobacterium tuberculosis* and many gram-positive and some gram-negative bacteria. Rifampin's spectrum also includes *S. aureus, N. meningitidis, H. influenzae,* and *Legionella* species. In TB, resistance quickly develops to rifampin administered alone in a one-step process as a result of a change in the RNA polymerase. Administering rifampin with other antituberculosis agents reduces the development of resistance.

Pharmacokinetics. Rifampin is absorbed from the gastrointestinal tract and eliminated in the bile, where enterohepatic circulation occurs. Its half-life is 1.5 to 5 hours and is increased in hepatic disease but unaltered by renal disease. The half-life is reduced by INH coadministration because of enzyme induction. By blocking the hepatic uptake of rifampin, probenecid increases the concentration of rifampin in the serum.

Adverse reactions. The most common adverse reactions are gastrointestinal, including anorexia, stomach distress, nausea, vomiting, abdominal cramps, and diarrhea. Occasionally, rashes, thrombocytopenia, nephritis, and impairment of liver function are seen. A flulike reaction can occur with infrequent administration. Rifampin gives a red-orange color to body fluids, including tears (which affects contact lenses), urine, feces, saliva, and sweat.

Uses. Rifampin is used in combination with other agents for treatment of TB. The adult dose is 600 mg daily. It is used to treat meningococcal carriers prophylactically in and children exposed to *H. influenzae* meningitis.

PYRAZINAMIDE

Pyrazinamide [peer-a-ZIN-a-mide] (PZA), a relative of nicotinamide, is well absorbed and widely distributed throughout the body. It is hepatotoxic and can produce rash, hyperuricemia, and gastrointestinal disturbances. The Centers for Disease Control and Prevention currently recommends PZA for use during the first 2 months with INH and rifampin to treat TB. Pyrazinamide, which used to be a tertiary drug, now plays a much more important role than it has in the past.

Treatment. One regimen includes the use of isoniazid and rifampin every day for 9 to 12 months. The pyrazinamide is continued for 2 months (Figure 8-7).

If a patient is compliant and the organisms susceptible, the patient usually becomes noninfective within 2 to 3 weeks to 2 to 3 months. A negative sputum sample is required to ensure that the patient is noninfective.

ETHAMBUTOL

Ethambutol [e-THAM-byoo-tole] (Myambutol) is a synthetic tuberculostatic agent effective against *M. tuberculosis.* Resistance among tubercle bacilli develops very rapidly when this drug is used alone.

The most important side effect is optic neuritis, resulting in a decrease in visual acuity and loss of ability to perceive red and green. Periodic ophthalmologic examinations are recommended. Other side effects include rash, joint pain, gastrointestinal upset, malaise, headache, and dizziness. This drug is used when other antituberculosis agents cannot be used or resistance is encountered.

TOPICAL ANTIBIOTICS

In general, the use of topical antibiotics is discouraged. Systemic administration is superior in most cases. If an agent is used topically, it should be one that cannot be used systemically. One old and one newer product are mentioned briefly.

FIGURE 8-7   *Treatment and time course of tuberculosis—a minimum of three drugs used. Depending on the recommended regimen, treatment with rifampin and INH may last between 9 and 12 months.*

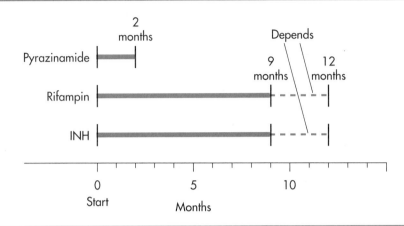

NEOMYCIN, POLYMYXIN, AND BACITRACIN

The combination of an aminoglycoside, neomycin [nee-oh-MYE-sin], and two polypeptide antibiotics, polymyxin [pol-i-MIX-in] and bacitracin [bass-i-TRAY-sin], is available in ointment form (Neosporin, triple antibiotic ointment).

Neomycin affects gram-negative organisms, and polymyxin and bacitracin affect gram-positive organisms. This combination product is used topically on scratches; if the wound is infected, systemic antibiotics are indicated.

MUPIROCIN

Mupirocin [myoo-PEER-oh-sin] (Bactroban) is a topical antibacterial produced by *Pseudomonas fluorescens*. Mupirocin inhibits protein synthesis by binding to bacterial isoleucyl transfer-RNA synthetase. It shows no cross-resistance with other antibiotics. It is active versus certain *Streptococcus* and *Staphylococcus* organisms, and is indicated for the topical treatment of **impetigo.** Local itching and stinging have been reported.

Mupirocin is as effective as the usual systemic treatments (penicillinase-resistant penicillins) and has fewer side effects.

In dentistry, mupirocin can be used to treat the bacterial infection with streptococci or staphylococci that are occasionally present with angular cheilitis. The secondary infection can be determined by its clinical presentation. Because angular cheilitis most commonly is a fungal infection, topical antifungal agents should be used first.

ANTIBIOTIC PROPHYLAXIS USED IN DENTISTRY

Infective endocarditis is caused by an infection of the heart valves or endocardium with an organism. The incidence of infective endocarditis is a fraction of 1%, with more cases occurring in males with a median age of 50. More cases are now caused by fungi and gram-negative organisms.

Infective endocarditis often begins with sterile vegetative cardiac lesions consisting of amalgamations of platelets, fibrin, and bacteria. When bacteria are introduced into the bloodstream, they may infect the damaged valves. Infective endocarditis can also occur in patients without predisposing cardiac factors. The difficult question, to which there is currently no proved answer, is this: "Which factors will be predictive in identifying patients in whom appropriate antibiotics will prevent infective endocarditis when specific dental procedures are performed?"

PREVENTION OF INFECTIVE ENDOCARDITIS

- Dental
- Cardiac
- Drug

Prophylaxis for infective endocarditis is based on the concept (which may not be true) that giving certain antibiotics to certain patients before certain procedures can prevent these patients from getting infective endocarditis. In 1997, the *Journal of the American Medical Association*[2] published the current American Heart Association's guidelines for antibiotic prophylaxis before dental procedures to prevent infective endocarditis. The trend is toward the use of fewer but higher doses of an antibiotic. For every situation in which it may be appropriate to use prophylactic antibiotics, the following three factors should be considered:

1. The specific dental procedure being performed (examine the mouth, obtain consult)
2. The cardiac and medical condition of the patient (check the drugs being taken)
3. The drug and the dose that may be needed (consider allergy history)

The following are reasons for the failure of antibiotic prophylaxis for infective endocarditis:
- A portion of the patients who get infective endocarditis are not in any identifiable risk group, so they would not be medicated.
- The endocarditis can be caused by organisms that are not covered by the antibiotic given (many of these organisms do not originate in the mouth).
- Historically, the incidence of infective endocarditis today is the same as it was before the discovery of antibiotics.
- Because historically antibiotics have been used in certain cardiac conditions, providers are hesitant to omit an antibiotic (even though it has not been shown to be helpful. In fact bacterial endocarditis is just as common today as before antibiotics were available). The risk of a lawsuit is also a consideration in provider's minds.

Even though the effectiveness of this practice is in question, it is continued because no other method is known to be effective. As long as there are official recommendations, dental health care workers should follow the current practice of infective endocarditis prophylaxis. The dental health care worker must consider the legal ramifications of both *prescribing* (commission) and *withholding* (omission) prophylactic antibiotics (evaluate the risk-to-benefit ratio) and should routinely check the literature for the newest regimen. The number of doses and the situations for use of antibiotics has been reduced with each update of the recommendations.

Even with antibiotic coverage, infective endocarditis may occur. Other than antibiotic prophylaxis, the incidence of infective endocarditis can best be minimized by patients maintaining exemplary oral hygiene. Additional practices that reduce bacterial counts in the oral cavity include having the patient rinse mouth with chlorhexidine or water before each dental procedure.

Dental procedures. When dental treatment is rendered (including periodontal probing), organisms are more likely to enter the blood supply, producing bacteremia. Bacteremia is also produced when eating potato chips, brushing teeth, or chewing wax. The organisms can then produce infective endocarditis.

To determine whether prophylactic antibiotic coverage is needed before a dental procedure see the infective endocarditis decision tree in Appendix C. Note the following:

1. Does the cardiac/medical condition warrant prophylaxis?
2. Will the dental procedure to be performed produce significant bleeding?

Only if *both* of these questions are answered in the affirmative would prophylaxis be indicated. Some providers are hesitant to use this currently recommended practice.

Depending on the dental procedure being performed, patients may or may not need prophylactic antibiotic coverage. Box 8-5 divides dental procedures into those likely to produce significant bleeding (and therefore produce bacteremia and therefore *may* require prophylactic antibiotic coverage for susceptible patients) and those that produce little bleeding and for which prophylaxis is not indicated. The amount of bleeding can also be influenced by the oral health of the patient. Clinical judgment will determine the need either for or against antibiotic coverage for each patient.

Cardiac conditions. Antibiotic prophylaxis before dental procedures, patients with cardiac conditions can be divided into groups based on the cardiac condition (Box 8-6). The first group contains patients at risk for developing infective

---

Box 8-5 INFECTIVE ENDOCARDITIS PROPHYLAXIS RECOMMENDATIONS— DENTAL PROCEDURES*

Prophylaxis recommended

* Producing significant gingival/mucosal bleeding
* Oral prophylaxis
* Scaling and root planing
* Intraligamentary injections

No prophylaxis

* Not producing much bleeding
* Block or infiltration injection
* Oral radiographs
* Impressions
* Sublingual placement of antibiotic fibers/strips
* Sealant placement
* Fluoride treatments

*Box lists selective cases and is not all-inclusive.

Box 8-6 INFECTIVE ENDOCARDITIS PROPHYLAXIS RECOMMENDATIONS— CARDIAC CONDITIONS*

Prophylaxis recommended

* Prosthetic heart valve
* History of infective endocarditis
* Congenital heart conditions, unrepaired
* Rheumatic heart disease
* Hypertrophic cardiomyopathy
* Mitral valve prolapse *with* regurgitation
* Pathologic murmur
* Systemic lupus erythematosus

No prophylaxis

* >6 mo after surgical repair of septal defects/patent ductus arteriosus
* Coronary artery bypass surgery
* Mitral valve prolapse *without* regurgitation
* Functional murmur
* History of rheumatic fever without valve dysfunction
* Cardiac pacemaker/defibrillator

*Box lists selective cases and is not all-inclusive.

endocarditis (e.g., prosthetic heart valve, a history of bacterial endocarditis, or rheumatic heart disease). Oral antibiotic prophylaxis is required for these patients if the dental procedure warrants it. The second cardiac group includes those conditions that most clinicians believe do not require prophylactic antibiotic coverage (e.g., coronary bypass surgery after 6 months).

Several cardiac conditions are "depending on" situations (see Box 8-6). With **mitral valve prolapse** the presence or absence of insufficiency or regurgitation determines whether prophylaxis is indicated. Without complete information, prophylaxis is recommended until clarification is received. Two other "depends" situations include rheumatic fever (may or may not have rheumatic heart disease) and murmur (pathologic or physiologic). Typical physiologic murmurs include murmurs of childhood or pregnancy that have resolved. Without clarification, prophylactic antibiotics are indicated

Antibiotic regimens for dental procedures. Table 8-13 lists the antibiotic regimens for prophylaxis of endocarditis before dental procedures. These situations include no allergies, allergy to penicillin, and other alternatives.

When a patient's physician is contacted concerning the patient, the current medical condition of the patient should be explored. Based on the patient's medical status and the current rec-

ommendations, the dental health care worker determines whether antibiotics are indicated. Explain to the medical provider that the choice of therapy will be determined based on the patient's medical condition and the dental treatment being rendered. An agreement between the dentist and medical provider should be reached, but the dentist should not agree to practice outside the recommendation. This will minimize suggestions of inappropriate antibiotics or regimens. When no recommendations exist and the literature is contradictory, the choice should be based on a consensus between the dental health care worker and the patient's physician.

When the patient's medical condition and dental procedure indicate prophylaxis, the use of the current recommendations is appropriate. To use another regimen, overwhelming justification for the change would need to be available. For example, prophylaxis uses 1 dose of the antibiotic 1 hour before the dental appointment. Recommendations of long-term therapy do not fit with current thinking. When a medical consult is indicated, ask the provider about the status of the patient's medical condition. Inform them that the current recommendations for that condition will be used. If the condition has no recommendation, come to agreement with the patient's provider. Do not ask, "What do you want to give this patient for (insert dental procedure here)?" Explain how much bleeding you ex-

TABLE 8-13 Prophylactic Oral Antibiotic Drug Regimens

Use: 1 dose 1 hour before dental procedures likely to produce bleeding

Situation	Drug	Oral Dose Adult (mg)	Oral Dose Child (mg/kg)	Parenteral dose <30 min before appointment Adult (mg)	Parenteral dose <30 min before appointment Child (mg/kg)
No allergy	Amoxicillin (Amoxil)	2000	50	Ampicillin 2000 IM/IV	Ampicillin 50 IM/IV
Allergy to penicillins	Clindamycin (Cleocin)	600	20	600 mg IV	20 mg IV
	Azithromycin (Zithromax)	500	15		
	Clarithromycin (Biaxin)	500	15		
	Cephalexin (Keflex)*	2000	50	Cefazolin 1000 IM/IV	Cefazolin 25 IM/IV
	Cefadroxil (Duricef)	2000	50		

Modified from Dajani, AS et al: Prevention of bacterial endocarditis: recommendations by the American Heart Association, *JAMA* 277(22):1794-1801, 1997.
*Only if penicillin allergy is distant and minor.

pect and what the guidelines are for similar conditions.

Tetracycline is never indicated for infective endocarditis prophylaxis just before dental procedures likely to produce bacteremia. (It is sometimes used a few weeks early in treatment to clear organism in localized juvenile periodontitis.) If risk factors for infective endocarditis are present, the usual regimens should be administered before providing dental treatment.

PROSTHETIC JOINT PROPHYLAXIS

> Most prosthetic joint prostheses do not need prophylactic antibiotic coverage.

The *Journal of the American Dental Association*[3] has published an article providing guidelines for antibiotic prophylaxis for prosthetic joints. Like other preprocedure prophylaxis situations, the joint condition, the dental procedures, and the appropriate drugs must be considered.

See Appendix G for a flowchart to determine when prophylaxis is needed in a patient with a joint prosthesis.

Most patients with prosthetic joints do not need prophylactic antibiotic coverage before dental procedures. Only in patients with an at-risk joint and a dental procedure likely to cause significant bleeding might prophylactic antibiotics be indicated (Box 8-7).

Whether the use of antibiotics is indicated should be determined by those involved most closely with the patient's condition. For example, when a patient with a prosthetic hip replacement is seeking dental treatment, the dental health care provider should contact the patient's orthopedic surgeon. The provider should be questioned about whether the joint is an at-risk joint. Examples should be provided, such as multiple replacements, on steroids, or diabetic. See Appendix G for a decision tree on total joint replacement.

Documentation should be placed in the chart, and a letter summarizing the conversation should be sent to the provider and a copy retained.

NONCARDIAC MEDICAL CONDITIONS

Patients with noncardiac medical conditions may also require prophylactic antibiotic cover-

---

BOX 8-7 INCREASED RISK FACTORS IN PATIENTS WITH TOTAL JOINT REPLACEMENT

Most patients with total joint replacements do not need antibiotic prophylaxis, but prophylaxis may be needed in the following situations:

- Less than 2 years after implantation of prosthesis
- Previous prosthetic joint infections, multiple replacements, unstable (wobbly joints)
- Immunocompromised patients *may* be at higher risk for hematogenous infections
- Drugs that suppress immunity—corticosteroids (e.g., prednisone), cyclo-

sporin (Sandimmune), antineoplastic/antimetabolic agents used for autoimmune disorders such as azathioprine (Imuran), cyclophosphamide (Cytoxan), methotrexate (Rheumatrex); used to treat inflammatory diseases such as systemic lupus erythematosus, psoriasis, rheumatoid arthritis
- Diseases—Type 1 diabetes mellitus, rheumatoid arthritis (not osteoarthritis), systemic lupus erythematosis, malnourishment, and hemophilia
- Radiation treatments

age before dental procedures, but lack of agreement among practitioners for these situations causes confusion.

For some conditions in this group there is consensus that antibiotics are indicated or that antibiotics are not indicated For other conditions there is poor consensus.

Conditions with almost complete agreement for using prophylaxis include patients with renal dialysis shunts or ventriculoatrial hydrocephalic shunts. Conditions in which prophylactic antibiotics are not indicated include ventriculoperitoneal hydrocephalic shunt (drains into **peritoneal** cavity), splenectomy (more than 2 years from surgery), and lens and breast **implants.**

A condition without consensus is penile implant. Some recommend prophylaxis for 6 months to 2 years after the procedures. No prophylaxis is recommended thereafter (consensus poor). The practitioner must exercise clinical judgment when situations exist that do not fall within these guidelines. Also, patients at-risk may not be identified by a health history.

References

1. Hersh EV: Adverse drug interactions in dental practice: interactions involving antibiotics, *JADA* 130(2):236-251, 1999.
2. Dajani, AS et al: Prevention of bacterial endocarditis: recommendations by the American Heart Association, *JAMA* 277(22):1794-1801, 1997.
3. Fitzgerald RH et al: Antibiotic prophylaxis for dental patients with total joint replacements, *JADA* 128(7):1004-1007, 1997.

REVIEW QUESTIONS

1. Explain the rationale for the use of agents effective mainly against gram-positive organisms in the treatment of most dental infections.
2. Describe the proper use of prophylactic antibiotics in dentistry (other than for infective endocarditis).
3. Define the following terms:
   a. spectrum
   b. bacteriostatic
   c. bactericidal
   d. blood level
   e. synergism
   f. antagonism
   g. resistance
4. List the three groups of penicillins and explain the differences among these groups.
5. State the most serious adverse reaction associated with the penicillins.
6. Describe how the dentist should determine whether a patient has a "true" allergy to penicillin. State one procedure that would be extremely inadvisable.
7. List the two most commonly used penicillins in dental practice.
8. Explain the use of erythromycin in dentistry.
9. Name the major adverse reaction associated with the macrolides, and state the one adverse reaction associated primarily with erythromycin estolate ester.
10. Explain the major adverse reaction associated with clindamycin. Can it also occur with other antibiotics?
11. Describe two major therapeutic uses for the clindamycin antibiotics. Explain its special interest (renewed) to dentistry.
12. Name one oral cephalosporin used in the dental patient. State for which prophylaxis and its regimen (dose and time).
13. State two similarities and one difference between the cephalosporins and penicillins.
14. List one aminoglycoside, and state two major adverse reactions associated with use of aminoglycosides.
15. State one major adverse reaction associated with the tetracyclines that is seen in the dental office.
16. What two special instructions should be

given to a patient being prescribed tetracycline?

17. Name two differences between tetracycline and doxycycline.
18. Name two unusual side effects (one dental) associated only with minocycline.
19. Describe metronidazole's special spectrum of interest in dentistry. Name an action to avoid while ingesting it.
20. Describe one situation in which cephalosporins are used in dental practice.
21. Explain why the quinolones may have dental use in the future.
22. State the major spectrum of action of the aminoglycosides and list two routes of their administration.
23. Explain the advantage of SMX-TMP over a sulfonamide drug alone.
24. State the mechanism of action and the spectrum of action of the quinolones.
25. State three agents commonly used together in the treatment of active tuberculosis.
26. Describe the drug regimen for the prophylaxis of infective endocarditis in patients with a history of rheumatic heart disease, both with no allergy to penicillin and with an allergy to penicillin.

27. State the dental procedures for which antibiotic prophylaxis may be indicated.
28. Name three cardiac conditions listed under "it depends." State what conditions must be present before prophylaxis may be needed.
29. State what drug, if any, should be given to a patient with a prosthetic joint before dental procedures, such as oral prophylaxis or an amalgam restoration. State an alternative to use if the patient has a history of allergies. Describe the factors, if any, that would influence the decision.
30. Describe what additional information is needed about the patient to make a decision about antibiotic prophylaxis.
31. For each of the following patient conditions state whether prophylactic antibiotics would be required before periodontal surgery: heart transplant, penile implant, hydrocephalic shunts, renal dialysis shunts, metal plates in head, breast implant, and patients taking cyclosporin, probenecid, prednisone, amitriptyline, methotrexate, or azathioprine.

Antifungal and Antiviral Agents

The antibiotics and antiinfectives discussed in Chapter 8 are effective against a certain spectrum of organisms—bacteria, protozoa, rickettsia, trichomonads, amoebas, and spirochetes. These agents are not effective against either fungal or viral infections. This chapter discusses treatment and management of fungal and viral infections commonly encountered in the dental office: the fungus *Candida albicans* (candidiasis or thrush) and the herpes simplex virus. The viral infection acquired immunodeficiency syndrome (AIDS) and the different types of **hepatitis (A, B, C, D, Ex)** are discussed with reference to factors that might affect dental treatment. Other fungal and viral infections that are common in the population are briefly mentioned.

ANTIFUNGAL AGENTS

Although fungal infections are not frequently encountered

Candida albicans—most common oral fungus

in dental practice, when they are present, they are often difficult to treat. Unlike bacterial infections, fungal infections are more insidious. Fungal infections are more likely to occur in patients who are immunocompromised, and these infections can become chronic. Fungal infections can be divided into those that affect primarily the skin or mucosa (mucocutaneous) and those that affect the whole body (systemic). The dental health care worker usually is treating skin or mucosal lesions, most commonly within the mouth. These mucosal lesions may be treated with a topical or systemic antifungal agent.

Although there are different groups of fungi, two common groups are the candida-like and tinea. Dental health care workers manage mucocutaneous candidal infections, primarily caused by *C. albicans*, with nystatin, clotrima- zole, ketoconazole, or fluconazole (Table 9-1). Infections with tinea affect the skin and produce athlete's foot, **"jock itch,"** and ringworm. Both over-the-counter (OTC) and prescription products are used to manage these conditions (Table 9-2) topically.

Mucocutaneous candidal infections com-

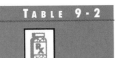

TABLE 9-1   Dentally Useful Antifungal Agents for Oral Candidiasis

Drug Name	Dentally Useful Dosage Forms	Comments	Dose	Sugar Dose (gm)
Nystatin (Mycostatin, Nilstat, others)	Aqueous suspension, vaginal tablets, cream, ointment, pastilles	Side effects uncommon	Suspension: 5 ml qid Vaginal tab: 1 qid Pastilles: 1 4–5 ×/day	2.5* (50%) — 1.2†
Clotrimazole (Mycelex)	Troches (lozenges)	Nausea	Troches: Dissolve 1 5 ×/d	0.9‡ (90%)
Ketoconazole (Nizoral)	Oral tablets (200 mg), cream	Hepatoxicity anaphylaxis, teratogenic, drug interactions	Tablet: 1 or 2 daily Cream: apply	N/A N/A
Fluconazole (Diflucan)	Oral tablets (50, 100, 200 mg)		200 mg first day; then 100 mg daily	N/A

*Sucrose
†0.4 sucrose + 0.8 glucose.
‡Glucose

TABLE 9-2   Topical Antifungal Agents

Drug Name	Route	Spectrum
OTC		
Undecylenic acid (Desenex, Cruex)	Powder, ointment, cream, liquid, foam, soap	Tinea
Tolnaftate (Tinactin, Aftate)	Cream, powder, liquid, solution, aerosol, gel	Tinea
Miconazole (Micatin, Monistat-Derm)	Cream, powder, spray	Candida
Clotrimazole (Lotrimin, Mycelex)	Cream, lotion, solution	Candida
Butoconazole (Femstat)	Cream	Candida
Sulconazole (Exelderm)	Cream, solution	
Triacetin (Enzactin, Fungoid)	Cream, ointment	
Haloprogin (Halotex)	Cream, solution	Tricophyton, tinea
Rx		
Terbinafine (Lamisil)	Cream, ointment	Candida, tricophyton
Butenafine (Mentax)	Cream	Tinea
Naftifine (Naftin)	Cream, gel	Tinea
Ciclopirox (Loprox)	Lotion	Candida, tinea
Econazole (Spectazole)	Cream	Candida, tinea
Ketoconazole (Nizoral)	Cream, shampoo	Candida, tinea

monly occur in the vaginal canal. If the patient can recognize the symptoms (by having had a previous infection), an antifungal OTC product can be purchased and used.

Systemic mycoses produced by fungi include aspergillosis, blastomycosis, coccidioidomycosis, cryptococcosis, histoplasmosis, mucormycosis, and paracoccidioidomycosis. Chromomycosis, mycetoma, and sporotrichosis may progress to deep mycotic infections. These serious infections are medical management situations beyond the scope of this chapter. Amphotericin B and miconazole are used to treat these serious infections. Figure 9-1 divides the antifungal agents into related groups, and Figure 9-2 provides comparative acquisition.

F I G U R E   9 - 1   *Related groups of antifungal agents.*

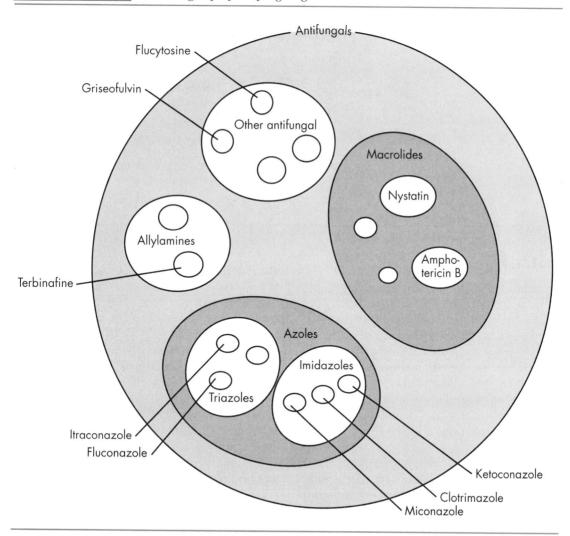

FIGURE **9 - 2**   *Relative cost of antifungal prescriptions.*

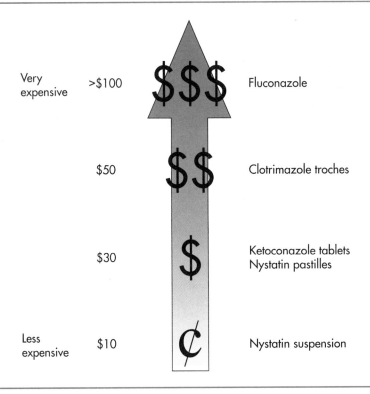

Very expensive	>$100	Fluconazole
	$50	Clotrimazole troches
	$30	Ketoconazole tablets / Nystatin pastilles
Less expensive	$10	Nystatin suspension

NYSTATIN

Nystatin [nye-STAT-in] (Mycostatin, Nilstat), which is a prescription antifungal agent, is a polyene macrolide antibiotic that is produced by *Streptomyces noursei*. Its mechanism of action involves binding to sterols in the fungal cell membrane. This produces an increase in membrane permeability and allows leakage of potassium and other essential cellular constituents. Because bacteria do not contain sterols in their cell membranes, nystatin is not active against these organisms.

Nystatin is not absorbed from the mucous membranes or through intact skin; taken orally, it is poorly absorbed from the gastrointestinal tract. In usual therapeutic doses, blood levels are not detectable. When administered orally, it is not absorbed but is excreted unchanged in the feces. Nystatin is fungicidal and fungistatic against a variety of yeasts and fungi. In vitro, nystatin inhibits *C. albicans* and some other species of *Candida*.

The adverse reactions associated with nystatin are minor and infrequent. Applied topically or taken orally (through the gastrointestinal tract), there is little if any absorption. When higher doses have been used, nausea, vomiting, and diarrhea have occasionally occurred. Rarely, hypersensitivity reactions have been reported.

Nystatin is used for both the treatment and prevention of oral candidiasis in susceptible cases. Although *C. albicans* is a frequent inhabitant of the oral cavity, only under unusual conditions does it produce disease. Frequently, patients affected are immunocompromised (see Box 8-1).

For the treatment of oral candidiasis, nystatin is available (see Table 9-1) in the form of an aqueous suspension (100,000 U/ml) containing 50% sucrose. The directions to the patient are to swish, swirl, and spit (swallow) 5 ml (1 tsp.) 4 times daily. The suspension should remain in the mouth 2 minutes for the best effect. For infants and small children with thrush, half of a dropperful (2.5 ml) is placed in each side of the mouth and rubbed into the recesses of the mouth and on the lesions. If swallowed, diabetics using this suspension must take the sugar content into account (2.5 gm sucrose per tsp.) when planning their meals and insulin use.

Nystatin pastilles are licorice-flavored, rubbery, and also contain sugar. Informal feedback has indicated that patients with xerostomia might not find this dosage form acceptable. The advantage of this preparation is that it takes 15 minutes for the lozenge to dissolve in the mouth, thus bathing lesions in the antifungal agent for a longer period. It is allowed to dissolve in the mouth 4 times daily. The dental health care worker must discuss patients' oral health habits, especially when patients are chronically ingesting these cariogenic agents.

Nystatin is available in vaginal tablets for use in vaginal infections. These vaginal tablets can be used orally. They are dissolved in the mouth 4 times daily. The advantages of the vaginal tablet used as a lozenge are that the drug remains in contact with the infected oral mucosa longer than it does when in the suspension form and it contains no sugar. The disadvantage is that it is not flavored for oral use.

Patients should be instructed to use the nystatin product for between 10 to 14 days, depending on the severity of the infection, or for 48 hours after the symptoms have subsided and cultures have returned negative. Cultures are typically not performed. Some patients, especially if immunocompromised, may require long-term

prophylactic antifungal agents to control candidiasis.

IMIDAZOLES

Several imidazoles useful in dentistry include clotrimazole, miconazole, and ketoconazole.

Clotrimazole. Clotrimazole [kloe-TRIM-a-zole] (Mycelex) is a synthetic antifungal agent available in the form of a slowly dissolving, sugar-containing, lozenge for oral use. It is also available as an OTC cream for topical application to the skin or vaginal canal.

Clotrimazole's mechanism of action involves alteration of cell membrane permeability. It binds with the phospholipids in the cell membrane of the fungus. As a result of the alteration in permeability, the cell membrane loses its function, and the cellular constituents are lost.

Clotrimazole oral lozenges dissolve in approximately 15 to 30 minutes. Patients with xerostomia may have difficulty dissolving this product. Saliva concentrations that are sufficient to inhibit most *Candida* species are maintained in the mouth for about 3 hours. The drug is bound to the oral mucosa, from which it is slowly released. The amount of clotrimazole absorbed systemically by this route is unknown, but some absorption occurs. Each lozenge also contains 0.9 gm of glucose. The spectrum of action of clotrimazole is primarily against the *Candida* species.

The most common adverse reactions associated with clotrimazole involve the gastrointestinal tract, including abdominal pain, diarrhea, and nausea. Clotrimazole has been reported to produce elevated liver enzyme (aspartate aminotransferase) levels in approximately 15% of patients.

Systemic clotrimazole has been assigned to Food and Drug Administration (FDA) pregnancy category C. Very high doses have been embryotoxic in rats and mice. High doses have caused impairment of mating and a decrease in both the number and survival of the young. No teratogenic effects have been found in several other species tested. No carcinogenicity has been demonstrated in rats.

> Clotrimazole troches: 1 box = 70 lozenges

Clotrimazole is indicated for the local treatment of oropharyngeal candidiasis. Patients should be instructed to dissolve the lozenge in the mouth slowly, like a cough drop, to minimize gastrointestinal discomfort. They should also be told to take all of the medication prescribed to minimize relapse. The usual adult dosage is 1 lozenge (10 mg) 5 times daily for 10 to 14 days (or longer for immunosuppressed patients) or for 48 hours after the symptoms have cleared. Some clinicians advocate dissolving 1 100-mg clotrimazole (Mycelex) vaginal tablet 4 times daily in the oral cavity, like a lozenge or troche. The advantages of the vaginal tablet used as a lozenge are that the drug remains in contact with the infected oral mucosa longer than it does when in the suspension form and it contains no sugar. The disadvantage is that it is not flavored for oral use.

Ketoconazole. Ketoconazole [kee-toe-KON-a-zole] (Nizoral), another imidazole used in dentistry, alters cellular membranes and interferes with intracellular enzymes. By interfering with the synthesis of ergosterol, a cellular component of fungi, membrane permeability is altered and purine transport inhibited. The imidazoles inhibit the C-14 demethylation of lanosterol, an ergosterol precursor. It also inhibits sex steroid biosynthesis, including testosterone, perhaps by blocking several P-450 enzyme steps.

> Systemic imidazole— ketoconazole

PHARMACOKINETICS For the adequate systemic absorption of ketoconazole, an acidic environment is required. Patients with achlorhydria should take ketoconazole with hydrochloride acid (use straw to minimize damage to teeth). Medications that interfere with the normal production of stomach acid, such as H_2-blockers or H_2-receptor antagonists (H_2-RA), and proton pump inhibitors, reduce the absorption of ketoconazole. If ketoconazole must be taken with drugs that reduce the stomach acid, the ketoconazole should be taken as long a time as possible before or after the acid-reducing drug. All imidazole antifungal agents require an acidic environment for optimal absorption. With the exception of the cerebrospinal fluid (CSF), it is well distributed in humans. It crosses the placenta and is excreted in breast milk. The peak serum concentration occurs between 1 and 4 hours after administration. Ketoconazole is metabolized in the liver, and approximately 13% is excreted by the kidney, with a half-life between 2 and 8 hours. Because of the small contribution of the kidney to the excretion of ketoconazole, patients with renal impairment do not generally require a reduction in their dose. Because the primary route of excretion for ketoconazole is biliary, patients with hepatic impairment may require a lower dose.

SPECTRUM Ketoconazole is effective against a wide variety of fungal infections. It is indicated in many systemic fungal infections, including blastomycosis, candidiasis, coccidioidomycosis, and histoplasmosis. Although effective against organisms causing tinea, it is not the drug of choice unless traditional agents have failed.

ADVERSE REACTIONS

Gastrointestinal The most frequent adverse reactions (3% to 10%) associated with ketoconazole are nausea and vomiting, which can be minimized by taking ketoconazole with food.

Hepatotoxicity The most serious adverse reaction associated with ketoconazole is hepatotoxicity. Its incidence is at least 1:10,000. It is usually reversible on discontinuation of the drug, but occasionally it has been fatal. It is thought to be an idiosyncratic reaction that can happen at any time. With extended use the patient should have periodic liver function tests. Patients taking other hepatotoxic agents, those with liver disease (e.g., alcoholic hepatitis), or those on prolonged therapy should be watched closely because they may be more susceptible to this hepatotoxicity.

Ketoconazole, in higher doses, inhibits the secretion of the corticosteroids and lowers the serum levels of testosterone. This effect can, in men, produce gynecomastia and impotence. This adverse effect is specific to ketoconazole.

Other effects Other adverse reactions reported include headache, dizziness, drowsiness, photophobia, skin rash or pruritus, and insomnia. Fever, chills, dyspnea, tinnitus, arthralgias, and thrombocytopenia have occurred in a few patients. When ketoconazole is applied topically, irritation, pruritus, and stinging are the most commonly reported side effects.

Pregnancy and nursing Animal studies have shown that ketoconazole can produce **syndactyly, oligodactyly,** dystocia, and **embryotoxicity.** The FDA pregnancy category for ketoconazole is C. Because ketoconazole is excreted in breast milk, the risk-to-benefit ratio must be considered before it is used in the nursing mother.

DRUG INTERACTIONS Ketoconazole has many drug interactions that have been reported in the literature. Because an acidic environment is required for dissolution and absorption of ketoconazole, agents that alter the amount of stomach acid could theoretically reduce the absorption of ketoconazole (H_2-RA, H^+-pump inhibitors, anticholinergic agents, and antacids). At least 2 hours should elapse between the ingestion of these agents and ketoconazole's administration.

Ketoconazole inhibits the CYP P-450 3A4 hepatic microsomal isoenzyme, which can produce drug interactions with many other drugs also metabolized by this isoenzyme. Ketoconazole can increase the blood levels of cyclosporine, warfarin, corticosteroids, phenytoin, digoxin, lovastatin, and simvastatin, to name a few.

Isoniazid, phenytoin, and theophylline can decrease ketoconazole serum levels. Ketoconazole should not be used with rifampin, because rifampin renders its blood level undetectable. Ketoconazole may decrease the effect of oral contraceptives; an alternative method of birth control should be suggested. Ketoconazole may produce a disulfiram-like reaction or enhance hepatotoxicity with alcohol.

USES

Dental Ketoconazole is indicated in the treatment and management of mucocutaneous and oropharyngeal candidiasis (oral thrush). It can be used prophylactically in chronic mucocutaneous candidiasis. Because of its adverse reaction profile, ketoconazole should be used only after topical antifungal agents have been ineffective or there is reason to believe that they will be ineffective.

Medical Ketoconazole is indicated in the treatment of candidiasis, histoplasmosis, and paracoccidioidomycosis. It is also used to treat certain recalcitrant cutaneous dermatophytoses such as tinea corporis, tinea cruris, tinea versicolor, and seborrheic dermatitis.

DOSE The usual adult dose of ketoconazole for the treatment of *Candida* species is 200 to 400 mg PO qd. It should be used for at least 2 weeks, and 6 to 12 months may be required for chronic mucocutaneous candidiasis. Maintenance therapy may be necessary for certain patients. Ketoconazole is available for topical administration in a 2% aqueous vehicle (cream) for tinea or candidal infections. It is applied once or twice daily for at least 2 weeks. Ketoconazole (Nizoral) shampoo is used twice weekly to treat dandruff, a condition caused by the fungus.

Others. Other imidazoles, such as fluconazole [floo-KON-a-zole] (Diflucan), an oral triazole antifungal agent, are used to treat certain fungal infections. Fluconazole prevents the synthesis of ergosterol in the fungal cell membranes by inhibiting fungal cytochrome P-450 enzymes. Phospholipids and unsaturated fatty acids accumulate in the fungal cells.

Fluconazole is indicated for treatment of oropharyngeal and esophageal candidiasis, and serious systemic candidal infections. One tablet of fluconazole is now indicated to treat vaginal candidiasis. Fluconazole is used prophylactically against candidiasis in immunocompromised patients or for the treatment of candidal infections that do not respond to other agents.

Itraconazole [it-ra-KON-a-zole] (Sporanox), another systemic imidazole, is used for blastomycosis, histoplasmosis, and aspergillosis. It is the first antifungal agent to be effective in the treatment of onychomycosis of the toenail or fingernail (pulse therapy is used; i.e., on–off–on–off).

OTHER ANTIFUNGAL AGENTS

Amphotericin B. An important agent in the treatment of many serious systemic fungal infections is amphotericin B [am-foe-TER-i-sin] (Fungizone). Because of its side effects, it has earned the nickname "amphoterrible." It must be administered parenterally because it is poorly absorbed from the intestinal tract.

For serious fungal infections— systemic

Amphotericin is an amphoteric polyene macrolide antibiotic produced by *Streptomyces nodosus*. It binds to the sterols in the fungus cell membrane, altering membrane permeability and allowing the loss of potassium and small molecules from the cells. Because renal cells and erythrocytes contain sterols, the adverse reactions of amphotericin often affect these cells.

The spectrum of amphotericin includes many fungi, such as certain strains of *Aspergillus, Paracoccidioides, Coccidioides, Cryptococcus, Histoplasma, Mucor,* and *Candida* organisms. It is also effective against the protozoa *Leishmania.*

The adverse reactions associated with amphotericin are wide ranging and potentially serious, but it is often the only effective treatment for certain serious systemic fungal infections. Most patients experience hypokalemia, headache, chills (50%), fever, malaise, muscle and joint pain, gastric complaints, and nephrotoxicity (80%). Amphotericin has many potentially serious drug interactions.

Topical amphotericin has produced burning, itching, and in rare cases an allergic contact dermatitis. It is available as a 3% cream or ointment. The parenteral forms of amphotericin include liposomal and cholesteryl forms.

Griseofulvin. Griseofulvin [gri-see-oh-FUL-vin] (Fulvicin P/G, Grisactin Ultra, Gris-PEG) is an antibiotic produced by *Penicillium griseofulvum.* Its antifungal action is produced by disrupting the cell's mitotic spindle structure and arresting cell division in metaphase. Unlike many drugs, griseofulvin's absorption is enhanced by taking it with a fatty meal. It is tightly bound and preferentially deposited in diseased keratin precursors (hair, nails, skin). Its spectrum includes tineas (e.g., ringworm), *Trichophyton, Microsporum,* and *Epidermophyton* species but does not include *Candida* organisms.

The adverse reactions of griseofulvin include headache, gastrointestinal complaints, and overgrowth of *Candida* organisms in the oral cavity (thrush).

Commonly used for tinea capitis (ringworm of scalp).

Hypersensitivity reactions include urticaria, photosensitivity, and lupuslike reactions. The possibility of some cross-sensitivity with penicillins should be considered because the organism that makes griseofulvin is in a family related to

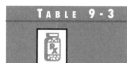

TABLE 9-3 Antiviral Agents, Excluding HIV Drugs

Drug Name	Route(s)*	Indication(s)	Comments
Acyclovir (Zovirax)	Oral, topical, IV	Primary and recurrent herpes in immunocompromised patients*	Local: burning Oral: nausea, CNS effects
Vidarabine (Ara-A, Vira-A)	IV, ophthalmic ointment	Herpes encephalitis, keratoconjunctivitis, recurrent epithelial keratitis	
Idoxuridine (IDU, Herplex, Stoxil)	Ophthalmic ointment, solution	Herpes simplex keratitis	Irritaion, pruritus, edema, inflammation
Gancyclovir (Cytovene)	IV, IM, SC	CMV retinitis (AIDS): CMV disease prevention (transplant)	Granulocytopenia
Ribavirin (Virazole)	Aerosol	Infants with severe respiratory syncytial virus	Very costly, difficult to administer, requires special machine
Amantadine (Symmetrel)	Oral	Prophylaxis of influenza A virus	Also used to treat parkinsonism
Interferon (Intron A, Roferon-A, Betaseron)	IM, SC IM	Hairy cell leukemia, chronic Hepatitis, multiple sclerosis	Many investigations currently under way

*AIDS, Autoimmune deficiency syndrome; *CNS*, central nervous system; *CMV*, cytomegalovirus; HIV, human immunodeficiency virus; *IV*, intravenous; *IM*, intramuscular; *SC*, subcutaneous.

that which produces penicillin. Depression of hematopoietic functions and carcinogenicity in animals have been demonstrated. It can also produce a disulfiram-like reaction.

Griseofulvin is indicated in the treatment of susceptible infections of the skin, hair, and nails. Because the drug is deposited only in the growing tissues, the duration of treatment depends on the time it takes for the affected area to completely grow out, which may be from 2 weeks to 8 months. Although there is no known use in dentistry, the side effects of griseofulvin—hematopoietic suppression and oral candida infection—must be considered when a dental patient is taking this drug.

ANTIVIRAL AGENTS

The search for drugs useful in the treatment of viral infections has posed the greatest problem of all infectious organisms. This is because viruses are obligate intracellular organisms that require cooperation from their host's cells. Therefore, to kill the virus, often the host's cell must also be harmed. The herpes virus, because of the location of the lesions around the oral cavity or, in some cases, on the dentist's or hygienist's finger (herpetic whitlow), has been of the most interest to the dental health care worker. Now, with the symptoms of AIDS being seen clinically in the mouth, the treatment of this virus takes on more importance. Table 9-3 lists some antiviral agents along with their routes of administration and indications. Figure 9-3 separates the antivirals into related groups.

HERPES SIMPLEX

Herpes viruses are associated with "cold sores," and dental practitioners are asked for "something to help." Most antiviral agents are either purine or pyrimidine analogues that inhibit DNA synthesis.

FIGURE   9 - 3   *Related groups of antiviral agents.*

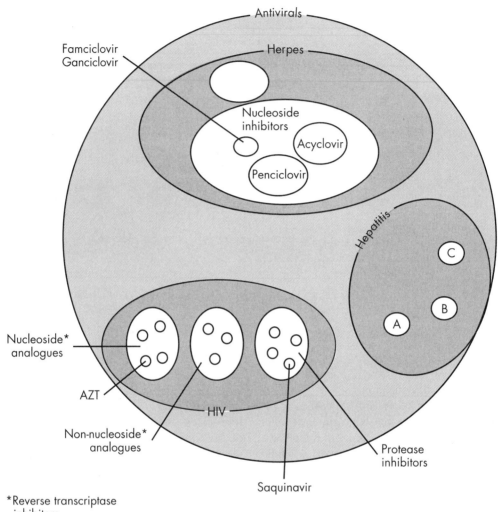

Famciclovir
Ganciclovir

Antivirals

Herpes

Nucleoside
inhibitors

Acyclovir

Penciclovir

Hepatitis

C

B

A

Nucleoside*
analogues

AZT

HIV

Non-nucleoside*
analogues

Saquinavir

Protease
inhibitors

*Reverse transcriptase
inhibitors

| Acyclovir—activated by herpes enzymes |

Acyclovir. Acyclovir [ay-SYE-kloe-veer] (Zovirax), a purine nucleoside, is first converted to acyclovir monophosphate by thymidine kinase, an enzyme present in the herpes simplex virus. Cellular enzymes convert the monophosphate to the diphosphate and then to the triphosphate. The triphosphate exerts its antiviral action on herpesviruses by interfering with DNA polymerase and inhibiting DNA replication. It is much less toxic to normal uninfected cells because it is preferentially taken up by infected cells. In the host's cells, acyclovir is only minimally phosphorylated. This explains its excellent adverse reaction profile.

PHARMACOKINETICS When acyclovir is taken orally, between 15% and 30% is absorbed. Peak concentrations occur within about 2 hours. Food does not affect the drug's absorption. Acyclovir is distributed widely throughout the body. In animals, acyclovir crosses the placenta but its presence in human placenta or milk is unknown. The half-life of acyclovir in the initial phase is 0.3 hour and in the terminal phase is 2.1 to 3.5 hours. As the patient's creatinine clearance rises, the half-life of the drug is prolonged. Approximately 10% of a dose of acyclovir is metabolized in the liver. It is excreted primarily unchanged in the urine by glomerular filtration and tubular secretion.

SPECTRUM The antiviral action of acyclovir includes various herpesviruses, including herpes simplex types 1 and 2 (HSV-1 and HSV-2), varicella-zoster, Epstein-Barr, *Herpesvirus simiae* (B virus), and cytomegalovirus. Several mechanisms of resistance to acyclovir have been found.

ADVERSE REACTIONS The type and extent of the adverse reactions experienced depend on the route of administration of acyclovir.

Topical When administered topically, acyclovir produces burning, stinging, or mild pain in about one third of patients. Itching and skin rash have also been reported.

Oral One of the most common adverse effects associated with oral acyclovir is headache (13%). Other central nervous system (CNS) effects include vertigo, dizziness, fatigue, insomnia, irritability, and mental depression. Oral acyclovir also commonly produces gastrointestinal adverse reactions, including nausea, vomiting, and diarrhea. Anorexia and a funny taste in the mouth have also been reported rarely. Other side effects associated with oral acyclovir include acne, accelerated hair loss, arthralgia, fever, menstrual abnormalities, sore throat, lymphadenopathy, thrombophlebitis, edema, muscle cramps, leg pain, and palpitation.

Parenteral With parenteral administration, local reactions at the injection site are the most common side effects reported; these include irritation, erythema, pain, and phlebitis. Because acyclovir can precipitate in the renal tubules, it can occasionally affect the blood urea nitrogen or serum creatine levels. Symptoms of encephalopathy, including lethargy, obtundation, tremors, confusion, hallucination, agitation, seizures, and coma, have been reported in about 1% of patients given parenteral acyclovir.

USES

Topical The indications for topical acyclovir include initial herpes genitalis and limited non–life-threatening initial and recurrent mucocutaneous herpes simplex (HSV-1 and HSV-2) in immunocompromised patients. Topical acyclovir has not been effective in the treatment of recurrent herpes genitalis or herpes labialis infections in nonimmunocompromised patients. It does produce a limited shortening in the duration of viral shedding in males by a few hours. It does not prevent the transmission of infection, nor does it prevent recurrence. The available literature does not support the use of topical acyclovir for management of herpes labialis in dentistry. But guess what—it is used extensively. No acyclovir products are approved for the treatment of recurrent herpes labialis in the immunocompetent patient.

Oral The oral form of acyclovir is indicated in the treatment of initial herpes genitalis and management of recurrent herpes genitalis infections in both immunocompromised and nonimmunocompromised patients. It is effective in the prophylaxis of recurrent herpes genitalis infections in both patient groups. It is not indicated for the suppression of recurrent herpes genitalis in patients with mild infections. In the treatment of herpes labialis, oral acyclovir has shown unimpressive results. Even with hundreds of patients in some studies, only a small difference in a few measured parameters are seen. Higher doses may prove to be effective.

Injectable The parenteral form of acyclovir is used for severe initial herpes genitalis infections in the nonimmunocompromised patient. It is also indicated for the treatment of initial and recurrent mucocutaneous herpes simplex infections in the immunocompromised patient. Other uses include herpes zoster and varicella-zoster treatment.

DOSE The usual oral adult dosage of acyclovir for the treatment of initial **genital herpes** is 200 mg q4h while the patient is awake 5 times daily for 10 days. Treatment should be started as soon as the prodromal stage is noticed. The prophylactic dosage for recurrent episodes is 400 mg bid not to exceed 12 months. Some patients may need up to 200 mg 5 times daily. For intermittent therapy of recurrent episodes the dose is 200 mg q4h 5 times a day for 5 days. This is the common dose that has been studied in herpes labialis. Acyclovir has not been shown to effectively treat herpes labialis in topical, tablet, or capsule forms. The slight decrease in crusting or pain does not warrant its use. A larger dose is used in the treatment of herpes zoster (shingles) or chickenpox. It does not prevent the postherpetic **neuralgia** produced by shingles.

Penciclovir. Penciclovir [pen-CY-klo-veer] (Denavir), available topically, has been shown to reduce both the duration of the lesion and the pain of the lesions on the lips and face associated with both primary and recurrent herpes simplex. The advantages of penciclovir over acyclovir are that it can achieve a higher concentration within the cell and that the drug remains in the cells longer.

Famciclovir [fam-CY-klo-veer] and valacyclovir [val-a-Cy-klo-veer] are prodrugs converted to penciclovir and acyclovir, respectively, as they pass through the intestinal wall. They are indicated in the treatment of recurrent episodes of genital herpes. They have not been studied for use in herpes labialis. Organisms that have resistance to acyclovir often have cross-resistance with these other agents. Famciclovir and valacyclovir are indicated for acute localized varicella-zoster infections. Intravenous ganciclovir is indicated for serious cytomegalovirus retinitis in immunocompromised patients.

ACQUIRED IMMUNODEFICIENCY SYNDROME

Acquired immunodeficiency syndrome (AIDS) is the disease produced by infection with the retrovirus human immunodeficiency virus (HIV).

Antiretroviral agents are used in combinations called "cocktails" to manage AIDS. Nucleoside reverse transcriptase inhibitors, nonnucleoside reverse transcriptase inhibitors, and protease inhibitors are the groups discussed in this chapter. Table 9-4 lists current drugs used in the management of AIDS. The usual combination includes one choice from each of the

TABLE 9-4	HIV Drugs
DRUG NAME	DRUG NAME
Nucleoside analogs	Didanosine (ddI) (Videx)
	Lamivudine (3TC) (Epivir)
	Stavudine (d4T) (Zerit)
	Zalcitabine (ddC) (Hivid)
	Zidovudine (AZT, ZVD) (Retrovir)
Nonnucleoside analogs	Delavirdine (Rescriptor)
	Nevirapine (NVP) (Viramune)
Protease inhibitors	Indinavir (Crixivan)
	Nelfinavir (Viracept)
	Ritonavir (Norvir)
	Saquinavir (Invirase, Fortavase)

three groups, combined by selecting one from each column (Table 9-5). **Opportunistic infections** often occur in patients with AIDS, so they may be taking various antiinfective agents to prevent diseases such as tuberculosis, *Pneumocystis carinii* pneumonia, herpes infections, and candidiasis (Table 9-6).

Nucleoside reverse transcriptase inhibitors [NRTIs].
Zidovudine [zye-DOE-vue-deen] (AZT, Retrovir), a thymidine analogue, is converted into zidovudine triphosphate by cellular enzymes. This AZT derivative is then incorporated into DNA polymerase (reverse transcriptase) so that synthesis of viral DNA is terminated. The re-

verse transcriptase of HIV is 100 times more susceptible to inhibition than are normal human cells. The nucleoside antiretroviral agents block viral replication and conversion into a form that can get into an uninfected host cell. It has no effect on cells already containing HIV. AZT is well absorbed orally, metabolized by the liver, and excreted by the kidneys with a half-life of about 1 hour. It is distributed to most body tissue, including the cerebrospinal fluid. AZT inhibits HIV synthesis and reduces the **morbidity** and mortality from AIDS and AIDS-related complex. Opportunistic infections are reduced in both number and frequency.

The toxicity of AZT is related to bone marrow depression, which can lead to anemia, granulocytopenia, and thrombocytopenia. Transfusions are often required. CNS effects include headache, agitation, and insomnia. Nausea occurs in almost half the patients. A causal relationship to AZT has not been established, but oral manifestations reported include taste perversion, edema of the tongue, bleeding gums, and mouth ulcers. Adverse reactions sometimes limit treatment with AZT.

Acetaminophen, indomethacin, and aspirin can inhibit AZT's glucuronidation and potentiate the toxicity of both drugs. Other nonsteroidal antiinflammatory agents have not been implicated, but current literature should be consulted. A higher incidence of granulocytope-

TABLE 9-5 Antiretroviral Combinations to Treat HIV Infections

Column A	Column B
Indinavir	ZDV + ddI
Nelfinavir	d4T + ddI
Ritonavir	ZDV + ddC
Ritonavir	ZDV + 3TC
Saquinavir	d4T + 3TC

3TC, Lamivudine; *d4T*, stavudine; *ddC*, zalcitabine; *ddI*, didanosine; *ZDV*, zidovudine.

TABLE 9-6 Opportunistic Infections of HIV Patients and Their Drugs of Choice

Organism	Effect	Treatment
Cryptococcus neoformans	Meningitis	Amphotericin B
Candida	Esophagitis	Clotrimazole, ketoconazole
Pneumocystis carinii	Pneumonia	Trimethoprim-sulfamethoxazole, pentamidine
Cytomegalovirus	Lungs Pneumonitis	Gancyclovir
Mycobacterium tuberculosis	Lungs	INH + rifampin + pyrazinamide
Toxoplasma gondii	Encephalitis	Pyrimethamine-sulfadiazine

nia was reported when acetaminophen was used with AZT.

Nonnucleoside reverse transcriptase inhibitors [NNRTIs].

Nevirapine [ne-VYE-ra-peen] (VP, Viramune), a nonnucleoside reverse transcriptase inhibitor, is specific for HIV-1. These agents inhibit the same enzymes as the nucleoside analogues, but they do not require bioactivation. Adverse reactions include CNS effects (headache, drowsiness), rash, gastrointestinal effects (diarrhea, nausea), and elevated liver function tests (LFTs). When these agents are used alone, resistance to them develops quickly. This group is combined with the nucleoside analogues and the protease inhibitors.

Protease inhibitors.

Saquinavir (sa-KWIN-a-veer), a protease inhibitor, prevents the cleavage of viral protein precursors needed to generate functional structural proteins in and modulation of reverse transcriptase activity, preventing the maturation of HIV-infected cells. The difference between the protease inhibitors and the other two groups is that the protease inhibitors can interfere with the action of the HIV-infected cells. Its adverse reactions include rash, hyperglycemia, and paresthesias. Gastrointestinal adverse reactions include pain, diarrhea, and vomiting. Oral adverse reactions involve buccal mucosal ulceration. Ketoconazole significantly increases the levels of saquinavir. Patients taking saquinavir should take it 2 hours after a full meal and avoid sunlight. Although adverse reactions can occur, they are generally less serious than with the older agents. The discovery of the protease inhibitors has made a substantial difference in both the mortality and morbidity of AIDS patients.

Combinations.

In the management of HIV and AIDS, drugs are combined to produce an improved effect. The combinations of drugs, called "cocktails," used to manage HIV or AIDS are changing constantly. Table 9-5 has two columns, and cocktails are made by combining one choice from each column. Rapid changes in retroviral drug therapy makes predicting what specific agents will be used in a few years impossible. Within each group, the agents chosen are often the newest agents, which have quickly been brought to the market. Because the drugs patients with AIDS will be taking will be the newest agents, it is important to obtain information about these drugs before planning dental treatment. Normally patients with HIV will be taking three drugs—a nucleoside, a nonnucleoside reverse transcriptase inhibitor, and a protease inhibitor. An example of this combination is lamivudine, nevirapine, and saquinavir.

Other antiviral agents

AMANTADINE Amantadine [a-MAN-ta-deen] (Symmetrel) inhibits the penetration of the adsorbed virus into the host's cells or inhibits the uncoating of the influenza A viruses. Its common side effects include nausea, dizziness, lightheadedness, and insomnia. It can be used prophylactically for prevention of an influenza A viral infection or for treatment to reduce the symptoms of the infection. It is used in institutional patients (e.g., nursing homes) to prevent the spread of infection during outbreaks. It also has antiparkinsonian action. A new relative of amentadine with similar action is rimantadine (Flumadine).

INTERFERONS The **interferons** [in-ter-FEER-ons] are a large group of endogenous proteins that have antiviral, cytotoxic, and immunomodulating action. Recombinant DNA technology now produces interferons. The FDA has approved several interferons currently classified as alfa* (α), beta (β), and gamma (γ) for certain indications but they are used for other, unapproved indications. Many more are available that have not been marketed; for example, there are 16 known subtypes of alfa interferons. The types

---

*Spanish spelling is used for global consistency.

TABLE 9-7 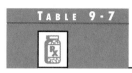		Interferons
INTERFERON TYPE	TRADE NAME	INDICATIONS, SELECTED
Alfa-2a	Roferon-A	Hairy cell leukemia, chronic hepatitis C
Alfa-2b	Intron-A	Hairy cell leukemia, chronic nonA, non B/C hepatitis AIDS-related **Kaposi's sarcoma**
Alfa-n3	Alferon N	Condyloma acuminatum
Beta-1a	Avonex	Multiple sclerosis, relapsing
Beta-1b	Betaseron	Multiple sclerosis, relapsing

of interferons available and their indications are listed in Table 9-7. All currently available interferons are parenteral. The most common uses of the interferons are for hepatitis C and for **multiple sclerosis.**

Interferons are used parenterally, and injection site reactions such as necrosis can occur. The interferons interact with cells through cell surface receptors. Activation of these receptors produces the following effects: induction of gene transcription, inhibition of cellular growth, alteration of the state of cellular differentiation, and interference with oncogene expression. Other effects include alteration of cell surface antigen expression, increasing phagocytic activity of macrophages, and augmenting the cytotoxicity of lymphocytes. With so many actions, it is no wonder that these agents are being explored for other indications.

Adverse reactions vary depending on the interferon, but some can be serious and even require discontinuation of the drug. A flulike syndrome, consisting of myalgias, fatigue, headache, and arthralgia, occurs in many patients. Other side effects include CNS effects (fatigue, fever, headache, depression, and chills), gastrointestinal tract effects (nausea, vomiting, diarrhea), and rash. Oral effects include taste changes, reactivation of herpes labialis, and excessive salivation.

REVIEW QUESTIONS

1. Name the least toxic antifungal agent useful in the treatment of oral candidiasis. State three dosage forms useful in dentistry and describe their pros and cons.
2. State two agents (other than those from question 1) useful for oral candidiasis. State one problem with each agent. Explain when administration of each is appropriate.
3. Describe the reason for the difficulty associated with the treatment of herpes labialis with antiviral agents. Describe any useful clinically proved effect of either the topical or systemic use in dentistry.
4. Explain the significance of a patient taking AZT, ddI, ddC, d4T, NVP, and ritonavir.
5. Describe the serious adverse reactions associated with AZT.
6. Describe how drug combinations are used to manage HIV.
7. List the therapeutic use of two different interferons.

Local anesthetics—frequently used drugs in dentistry

No drugs are employed more often in the dental office than the local anesthetic agents. Because their use can become routine, it is easy to forget that these agents have a potential for systemic effects in addition to the desired local effects. Dentists and, in some states, dental hygienists are responsible for the administration of local anesthetic agents in certain situations. With this duty comes the need for an in-depth knowledge of the local anesthetic agents.

HISTORY

First local anesthetic—cocaine

"Painless" dentistry, through the use of a local anesthetic, is a relatively recent development. It began with the observation that the indigenous people of the South American Andes chewed certain leaves that made them feel better. The active ingredient of the leaves was cocaine, isolated by Niemann in 1860. He noted that tasting this substance produced the loss not only of taste but also the sensation of pain. In 1884, Koller noted that cocaine instilled in the eye produced complete anesthesia. Its use in eye surgery was immediately adopted. During this time Sigmund Freud was also experimenting with cocaine and its effects on the central nervous system (CNS). CNS stimulation, toxicity, and the potential for abuse were quickly recognized as major problems with the widespread use of cocaine as a local anesthetic.

The search for a more acceptable local anesthetic for dentistry continued. Einhorn synthesized procaine in 1905, but it was not until many years later that its use in dentistry became common. In 1952, the amide lidocaine (Xylocaine) was released, and mepivacaine (Carbocaine) was released in 1960. More recently, bupivacaine (Marcaine) has been made available for dental use. The search for the perfect local anesthetic agent continues.

IDEAL LOCAL ANESTHETIC

Although local anesthesia can be produced by several different agents, many are not clinically acceptable. The ideal local anesthetic should possess the following properties:
- Potent local anesthesia
- Reversible local anesthesia
- Absence of local reactions
- Absence of systemic reactions
- Absence of allergic reactions
- Rapid onset
- Satisfactory duration
- Adequate tissue penetration
- Low cost
- Stability in solution (long shelf life)
- Sterilization by autoclave
- Ease of metabolism and excretion

No local anesthetic agent in use today meets all of these requirements, although many acceptable agents are available.

CHEMISTRY

Local anesthetic agents are divided chemically into two major groups—the esters and the amides (Table 10-1). A few agents fall outside these two groups and are called *other*. The clinical importance of this division is associated with potential allergic reactions. A patient who has an allergy to one group is more likely to exhibit a hypersensitivity reaction to other agents within the same group. Cross-hypersensitivity between the amides and the esters is unlikely. The structure of local anesthetics is composed of the following three parts:

1. Aromatic nucleus (R)
2. Linkage (either an ester or an amide, followed by an aliphatic chain, R)

3. Amino group

The aromatic nucleus (R) is lipophilic (lipid soluble), and the amino group is hydrophilic (water soluble). The esters are largely metabolized in the plasma and the amides in the liver.

MECHANISM OF ACTION

ACTION ON NERVE FIBERS

A resting nerve fiber has a large number of positive ions (cations) on the outside (electropositive) and a large number of

> Interfere with function of the neurons

negative ions (anions) on the inside (electronegative). The nerve action potential results in the opening of the sodium channels and an inward flux of sodium, resulting in a change from the -90-mV-potential to a $+40$-mV potential (Figure 10-1; Box 10-1). The outward flow of potassium ions repolarizes the membrane and closes the sodium channels. Local anesthetics attach themselves to specific receptors in the nerve membrane. After combining with the receptor, the local anesthetics block conduction of nerve impulses by decreasing the permeability of the nerve cell membrane to sodium ions. This then decreases the rate of depolarization of the nerve membrane, increases the threshold for excitability, and prevents the propagation of the action potential. Local anesthetics may reduce permeability by competing with **calcium** for the membrane

TABLE 10-1 Local Anesthetic Agents Grouped by Chemical Structure

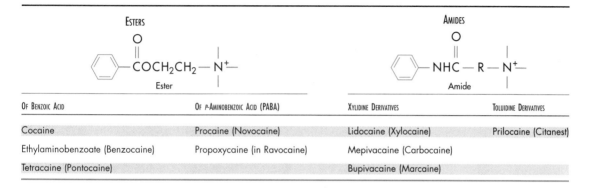

OF BENZOIC ACID	OF p-AMINOBENZOIC ACID (PABA)	XYLIDINE DERIVATIVES	TOLUIDINE DERIVATIVES
Cocaine	Procaine (Novocaine)	Lidocaine (Xylocaine)	Prilocaine (Citanest)
Ethylaminobenzoate (Benzocaine)	Propoxycaine (in Ravocaine)	Mepivacaine (Carbocaine)	
Tetracaine (Pontocaine)		Bupivacaine (Marcaine)	

FIGURE 10-1   *A, Nerve action potential resulting in the opening of the sodium channels and an inward flux of sodium, which causes a change from the −90-mV potential to a +40-mV potential. B, An action potential involves opening both Na+ and K+ channels.*

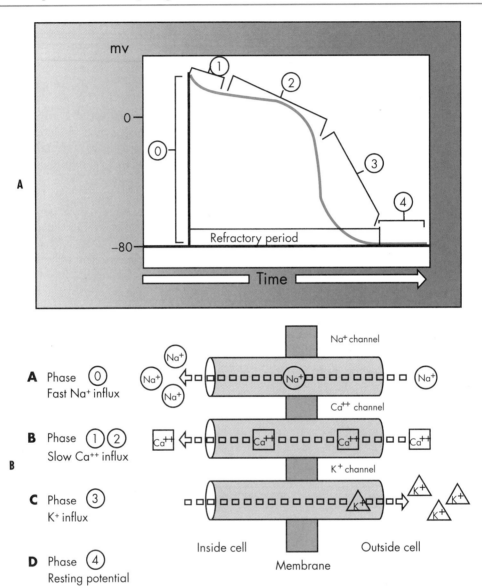

binding sites and by preventing the onset of nerve conduction.

IONIZATION FACTORS

> Ionization equilibrium depends on pH and pK_a.

The local anesthetic agents are weak bases occurring equilibrated between their two forms, which are the fat-soluble (lipophilic) free base and the water-soluble (hydrophilic) hydrochloride salt (Figure 10-2). The proportion of drug in each form is determined by the pK_a* of the local anesthetic and the pH of the environment. In the acidic pH of the dental cartridge (4.5), the proportion of the drug in the ionized

_____

*pH at which half is in each form (salt and base equal).

> **Box 10-1   MECHANISM OF ACTION = BLOCKADE OF VOLTAGE-GATED SODIUM CHANNELS**
>
> 1. Membrane potential = -90 to -60 mV
> 2. Excitatory impulse
> 3. Na channels open
> 4. Na flows in (depolarizes membrane [$+40$ mV])
> 5. Na channels close
> 6. K channels open
> 7. K flows out
> 8. K^+ channels close
> 9. Na^+/K^+ exchange
> 10. Repolarizes membrane (-95 mV)

FIGURE 10-2   *Properties of base and salt forms of local anesthetics.*

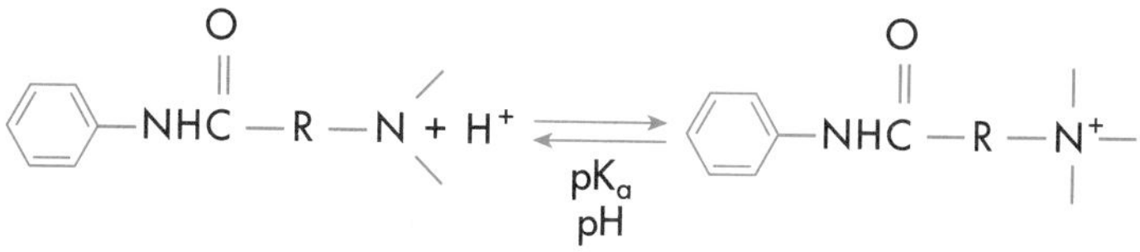

or written simply as

$$RN + H^+ \rightleftharpoons RNH^+$$

Free base	Salt
• Viscid liquids or amorphous solids	• Crystalline solids
• Fat soluble (lipophilic)	• Water soluble (hydrophilic)
• Unstable	• Stable
• Alkaline	• Acidic
• Uncharged, nonionized	• Charged, cation (ionized)
• Penetrates nerve tissue	• Active form at site of action
• Form present in tissue (pH 7.4)	• Form present in dental cartridge (pH 4.5–6.0)

form increases, thereby increasing solubility. Once injected into the tissues (pH 7.4), the amount of local anesthetic in the free-base form increases. This provides for greater tissue (lipid) penetration (Figure 10-3). In the presence of an acidic environment such as infection or inflammation (pH lower), the amount of free base is reduced (more in ionized form). This is one reason dental anesthesia with a local anesthetic is more difficult when infection is present. Other reasons include dilution by fluid, inflammation, and vasodilation in the area. Although the free base form is needed to penetrate the nerve membrane, it is the cationic form that exerts blocking action by binding to the specific receptor site.

PHARMACOKINETICS

ABSORPTION

The absorption of a local anesthetic depends on its route. When it is injected into the tissues the rate of absorption

> Systemic absorption greater, especially with inflammation.

depends on the vascularity of the tissues. This is a function of the degree of inflammation present, the vasodilating properties of the local anesthetic agent, the presence of heat, or the use of massage. It is important to reduce the systemic absorption of a local anesthetic when it is used in dentistry.

FIGURE   10-3   *Distribution of base and salt forms of local anesthetics in normal (pH 7.4) and infected (pH 6.5) tissue. If 1000 U of the local anesthetic were injected into the body, it would distribute according to the numbers in this figure. At the normal pH (left), 1000 U, with proportional distribution, would produce 180 U at the site of action. In contrast, 1000 U in the presence of infection would produce only 8 U at the site of action.*

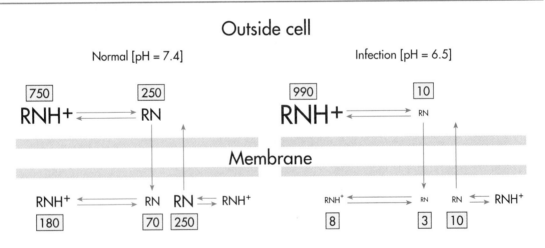

With reduced systemic absorption, the chance of systemic toxicity is reduced. To reduce absorption, a vasoconstrictor is added to the local anesthetic. The vasoconstrictor reduces the blood supply to the area, limits systemic absorption, and reduces systemic toxicity.

With topical application, especially on the mucous membranes or if the surface is denuded, absorption can approximate that produced by intravenous injection. Absorption is also determined by the proportion of the agent present in the free-base form (nonionized).

DISTRIBUTION

After absorption, local anesthetics are distributed throughout the body. Highly vascular organs have higher concentrations of anesthetics. Local anesthetics cross the placenta and blood-brain barrier. The lipid solubility of a particular anesthetic affects the potency of the agent. For example, bupivacaine, used as a 0.5% solution, is about 10 times more lipid soluble than lidocaine used as a 2% solution.

METABOLISM

> Metabolism Esters: plasma
> Amides: liver

The local anesthetic agents are metabolized differently, depending on whether they are amides or esters. Esters are hydrolyzed by plasma pseudocholinesterases and liver esterases. Procaine is hydrolyzed to *p*-aminobenzoic acid (PABA), a metabolite that may be responsible for its allergic reactions. Some patients who have an atypical form of pseudocholinesterase that does not allow them to hydrolyze these esters may exhibit an increase in systemic toxicity if an ester is administered.

Amide local anesthetics are metabolized primarily by the liver. In severe liver disease or with alcoholism, amides may accumulate and produce systemic toxicity. A small amount of prilocaine is metabolized to orthotoluidine, which can produce methemoglobinemia if given in very large doses. By reducing hepatic blood flow, cimetidine can interfere with the metabolism of the amides. (This is usually unimportant in dentistry because only one dose is given. No accumulation can result if repeated doses are not administered.)

EXCRETION

The metabolites and some unchanged drug of both esters and amides are excreted by the kidneys. With end-stage renal disease, both parent drug and metabolites can accumulate.

PHARMACOLOGIC EFFECTS

PERIPHERAL NERVE CONDUCTION (BLOCKER)

The main clinical effect of the local anesthetics is reversible blockage of peripheral nerve conduction. These agents inhibit the movement of the nerve impulse along the fibers, at sensory endings, at myoneural junctions, and at synapses. Therefore they may have wide-reaching effects on many kinds of nerves. Because they do not penetrate the myelin sheath, they affect the myelinated fibers only at the nodes of Ranvier. The local anesthetics affect the small, unmyelinated fibers first and the large, heavily myelinated fibers last. This is probably related to the ability of these agents to penetrate to their site of action. The losses of nerve function are in the following order:

1. Autonomic
2. Cold
3. Warmth
4. Pain
5. Touch
6. Pressure

7. Vibration
8. Proprioception
9. Motor

Although this is generally the order in which the senses are lost, some individual variation occurs among patients. In some patients the pain sensation is lost before the cold sensation. The functions of the individual nerves return in reverse order.

ANTIARRHYTHMIC

Local anesthetics have a direct effect on the cardiac muscle by blocking cardiac sodium channels and depressing abnormal cardiac pacemaker activity, excitability, and conduction. They also depress the strength of cardiac contraction and produce arteriolar dilation, leading to hypotension. These properties make them useful intravenously in the treatment of arrhythmias.

ADVERSE REACTIONS

The adverse reactions and toxicity of the local anesthetics are directly related to the plasma level of drug.

Considering the widespread use of these agents, their potential for danger must be minimal. Deaths from local anesthetics are difficult to document, but dental-related mortality is even rarer. Table 10-2 lists the maximum safe doses for common local anesthetics. Factors that influence toxicity include the following:

- *Drug:* Both the inherent toxicity of the particular local anesthetic and the amount of vasodilation it produces can contribute to toxicity.
- *Concentration:* The higher the concentration injected, the more drug that enters the systemic circulation.
- *Route of administration:* Inadvertent intravenous injection can produce extremely high blood levels. Even topical administration can produce high blood levels and lead to toxicity.
- *Rate of injection:* The faster the injection is made, the lower the chance that the local area can accept the volume injected. The operator, who has control over this variable, may find that counting the seconds is helpful.
- *Vascularity:* The presence of inflammation, infection, or vasodilation produced by the agent will increase the vascularity and therefore the systemic toxicity.
- *Patient's weight:* The same dose administered to a child and an adult will produce different blood levels because of their differences in weight.

TABLE 10-2 Maximum Safe Dose* (MSD) of Local Anesthetics

			Absolute Maximum	
Local Anesthetic (Concentration)	Epinephrine	Dose (mg/lb)	(mg)	# Cart
Lidocaine 2%	1:50,000	2 (3.5)*	200 (500)*	5.5
	1:100,000	2 (3)*	300 (500)*	8.5
Mepivacaine 3%	None (plain)	2 (3)*	300 (400)*	5.5
Mepivacaine 2%	1:20,000†	2 (3)*	300 (400)*	11
Prilocaine 4%	None (plain) and 1:200,000	2.7	400	5.5
Bupivacaine 0.5%	1:200,000	0.6	90	10

*Manufacturer's recommendations.
†Vasoconstrictor-levonordefrin.

- *Rate of metabolism and excretion:* Amides may accumulate with liver disease; both amides and their metabolites and ester metabolites may accumulate in renal disease.

Children, elderly individuals, and debilitated persons are more susceptible to the adverse reactions of the local anesthetic agents. The symptoms of an overdose of the local anesthetic agents are directly proportional to the blood level attained.

Toxicity. The two main systems affected by local anesthetic toxicity are the CNS and the cardiovascular system.

Central nervous system effects. CNS stimulation may occur before CNS depression. CNS stimulation caused by depression of the inhibitory fibers results in restlessness, tremors, and convulsions. CNS depression resulting from depression of both the inhibitory and facilitative fibers, respiratory and cardiovascular depression, and coma follow.

Cardiovascular effects. The local anesthetic agents can produce myocardial depression and cardiac arrest with peripheral vasodilation. The usual concentrations that are achieved with administration of dental anesthesia would not be expected to result in any of these adverse reactions, although deaths have been reported with the use of lower doses of anesthetic. It is postulated that the effect of these agents on heart conduction may have produced a fatal arrhythmia.

Local effects. Local effects can occur with the administration of local anesthetic agents. This is most commonly due to physical injury caused by the injection technique or the administration of an excessive volume too quickly to be accepted by the tissues. Occasionally a hematoma may be produced.

Malignant hyperthermia. Malignant hyperthermia is an inherited disease that is transmitted as an

Malignant hyperthermia—not related to amides

autosomal dominant gene with reduced penetration and variable expression. Its symptoms include an acute rise in calcium, which produces muscular rigidity, metabolic acidosis, and extremely high fever. Its mortality rate is about 50%. Treatment of malignant hyperthermia includes supportive measures and the administration of dantrolene (Dantrium). In the past it was thought that the amide local anesthetics might precipitate malignant hyperthermia, but currently they are no longer implicated. Patients with a family history of malignant hyperthermia can be given amide local anesthetic agents. Halothane, the inhalation anesthetic, and succinylcholine, the neuromuscular blocking agent, are the most common agents precipitating malignant hyperthermia.

Pregnancy and nursing. Elective dental treatment should be rendered before a patient becomes pregnant. If dental treatment is needed, however, most sources suggest that lidocaine may be administered to a pregnant woman. Fetal bradycardia has been reported when larger doses are administered to the mother near term. Both lidocaine and prilocaine are in Food and Drug Administration (FDA) pregnancy category B, whereas mepivacaine and bupivacaine are category C drugs. If a local anesthetic is needed, lidocaine in the smallest effective dose should be used. Usual doses of local anesthetics given to nursing mothers will not affect the health of the normal nursing infant.

Allergy. Allergic reactions that result from local anesthetics have been reported, and they range from rash to anaphylactic shock. An

Probably no allergies to amides

allergy history should be elicited from each patient before a local anesthetic agent is chosen. Esters have a much greater allergic potential; in fact, there is some question about whether amides can produce allergic reactions at all. Cross-allergenicity exists between the esters, but does not seem to occur between the amides in the xylidine and toluidine groups.

Patients giving a history of allergies to all local anesthetic agents may be "tested" by giving them an amide by injection. Of course, before contemplating administering this test, trained emergency personnel, equipment, and drugs should be assembled. Use of skin testing to determine local anesthetic allergies is unreliable because it can give both false-positive and false-negative results.

Another approach to treating a patient with a history of allergies to all the local anesthetic agents is to use the antihistamine diphenhydramine (Benadryl) as a local anesthetic. Antihistamines, because of their similarity in structure to local anesthetics, have some local anesthetic action. Diphenhydramine (Benadryl) in a concentration of 1% plus 1:100,000 epinephrine is recommended to be given by injection to produce a block. There is no prepared product available, so this combination must be prepared from its constituents. Past histories of allergic reactions to local anesthetics may have been the result of the preservative methylparaben. It is no longer present in any local anesthetic dental cartridges.

Local anesthetics with vasoconstrictors also contain a sulfite that serves as an antioxidant. In sulfite-sensitive patients, the sulfites may produce a hypersensitivity reaction that exhibits itself as an acute asthmatic attack. This reaction is the same as the "salad bar" syndrome—a hypersensitivity reaction to sulfites. In the past, certain restaurant foods offered at salad bars, such as lettuce, contained sulfites to prevent browning. Sulfites were used to help the lettuce and other greens retain their green color. Some restaurant menus still describe salad bars as "sulfite free." Deaths from hypersensitive asthmatics who ate

in restaurants have been reported. The nature of the reaction involves bronchoconstriction and anaphylactic reactions. A patient with an allergy to "sulfa" drugs does not exhibit cross hypersensitivity with sulfites. Appendix G discusses the implications of a sulfite hypersensitivity in more detail.

COMPOSITION OF LOCAL ANESTHETIC SOLUTIONS

In addition to the local anesthetic agent, local anesthetic solutions usually contain several other ingredients such as the following:

- *Vasoconstrictor:* A vasoconstrictor such as epinephrine is added to local anesthetic solutions to retard absorption, reduce systemic toxicity, and prolong its duration of action.

- *Antioxidant:* An antioxidant (sodium metabisulfite, sodium bisulfite, or acetone sodium bisulfite) is included in local anesthetic solutions to retard oxidation of the epinephrine. The antioxidants such as sodium bisulfite or metabisulfite prolong shelf life. Asthmatic dental patients who are given local anesthetic agents with a vasoconstrictor, which also contains a sulfite agent, should be watched for symptoms of wheezing or chest tightness.

> Sulfites—asthmatic hypersensitivity reaction

- *Sodium hydroxide:* Sodium hydroxide alkalinizes, or adjusts, the pH of the solution to between 6 and 7.

- *Sodium chloride:* Sodium chloride makes the injectable solution isotonic.

- *Methylparaben and propylparaben:* Methylparaben and propylparaben are preservatives added to multiple-dose parenteral solutions to prevent bacterial growth. Unlike multiple-dose vials, dental cartridges are single-use containers and do not contain methylparaben. In the past, this preservative was added to dental cartridges. [A question you might ask is, "Why was methylparaben added to a dental cartridge?" Perhaps the manufacturer had a big vat of solution prepared for the multidose vials, which need a preservative, and used the same solution to fill the dental cartridges. The parabens may be responsible for some allergic reactions attributable to local anesthetic agents reported in the past. No dental cartridge currently contains methylparaben.

LOCAL ANESTHETIC AGENTS

Many local anesthetic agents are available with similar pharmacologic and clinical effects and systemic toxicity. Commonly used local anesthetics are discussed next. Table 10-3 lists the local anesthetics available in dental cartridges. For clinical applications, lidocaine with epinephrine 1:100,000 is the usual choice. The question to be answered is, "Under what conditions would a local anesthetic other than lidocaine with epinephrine 1:100,000 be indicated?"

AMIDES

The amide local anesthetic agents are the only class of anesthetics used parenterally. Esters are occasionally used topically. The relative lack of allergenicity of the amides is probably responsible for this usage.

Lidocaine. An amide derivative of xylidine introduced in 1948, lidocaine [LYE-doe-kane] (Xylocaine, Octocaine) quickly

> Lidocaine with epinephrine is good for almost all dentistry.

became an anesthetic standard to which other local anesthetics were compared. It has a rapid onset, which is related to its tendency to spread well through the tissues. Lidocaine 2% with vasoconstrictor provides profound anesthesia of medium duration. It is the most commonly used local anesthetic solution in dental offices.

No cross-allergenicity between the amide lidocaine, or other available amides, or esters has been documented. Some patients appear to experience some sedation with lidocaine, and in toxic reactions one is likely to observe CNS depression initially rather than the CNS stimulation characteristic of other local anesthetics (Figure 10-4).

Adverse reactions include hypotension, positional headache, and shivering. Lidocaine is used for topical, infiltration, block, spinal, epidural, and caudal anesthesia. It is also used intrave-

TABLE 10-3 **Local Anesthetic Combinations Available in Dental Cartridges**

LOCAL ANESTHETIC	PERCENT (%)	VASOCONSTRICTOR	CONCENTRATION
Lidocaine (Xylocaine, Octocaine)	2	Epinephrine	1:50,000
	2	Epinephrine	1:100,000
Mepivacaine (Carbocaine, Isocaine)	3	Plain	—
	2	Levonordefrin	1:20,000
Prilocaine (Citanest)	4	Plain	—
(Citanest Forte)	4	Epinephrine	1:200,000
Bupivacaine (Marcaine)	0.5	Epinephrine	1:200,000

FIGURE **1 0 - 4**   *Relationship between levels of local anesthesia in serum and the pharmacologic and adverse effects.*

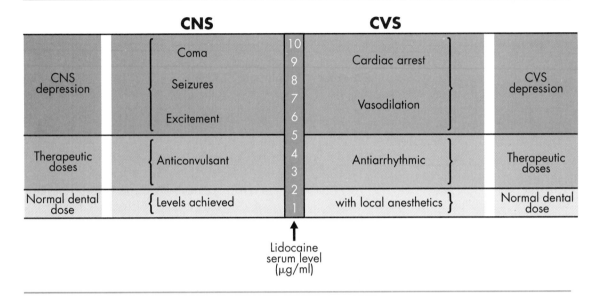

nously to treat cardiac arrhythmias during surgery.

In dentistry, lidocaine 2% with 1:100,000 epinephrine is used for infiltration and block anesthesia. Lidocaine is used for topical anesthesia as a 5% ointment, a 10% spray, and a 2% viscous solution. When used topically, its onset is rapid (2 to 3 minutes). Lidocaine with epinephrine 1:100,000 provides a 1- to 1.5-hour duration of pulpal anesthesia. Soft tissue anesthesia is maintained for 3 to 4 hours. Lidocaine with epinephrine 1:50,000 is used for hemostasis during surgical procedures. Rebound vasodilation (β effect) can be expected after the α effect (vasoconstriction) has occurred. A new dosage form of lidocaine is a patch that is applied to the mucosal membranes for local anesthesia. It provides good anesthesia, but its maximum effect occurs after about 10 minutes, which is probably too long to wait.

Mepivacaine. Another amide derivative of xylidine is mepivacaine [me-PIV-a-kane] (Carbo-caine, Polocaine, Isocaine). Introduced in 1960, its rate of onset, duration, potency, and toxicity are similar to those of lidocaine. No cross-allergenicity between the amide mepivacaine, other currently available amides, or the esters has been documented.

Mepivacaine is not effective topically; however, it is used for infiltration, block, spinal, epidural, and caudal anesthesia. The usual dosage form in dentistry is a 2% solution with the additon of 1:20,000 levonordefrin (Neo-Cobefrin) as the vasoconstrictor. Because mepivacaine produces less vasodilation than lidocaine, it can be used as a 3% solution without a vasoconstrictor (called *plain*). It can be used for short procedures when a vasoconstrictor is contraindicated (not often). Caution should be exercised when using the increased concentrations of the local anesthetic without a vasoconstrictor because systemic tox-

> To avoid vasoconstrictor, use mepivacaine plain.

icity is more likely. Except in unusual cases, the benefit of a shorter duration does not warrant eliminating the vasoconstrictor, especially when the concentration of the drug is increased.

Prilocaine. Prilocaine [PRILL-loh-kane] (Citanest, Citanest Forte) is related chemically and pharmacologically to both lidocaine and mepivacaine. Chemically, lidocaine and mepivacaine are xylidine derivatives, whereas prilocaine is a toluidine derivative. Prilocaine appears to be less potent and less toxic than lidocaine and has a slightly longer duration of action. It has been shown to produce satisfactory local anesthesia with low concentrations of epinephrine and without epinephrine.

Although toxicity of prilocaine is 60% of that occurring with lidocaine, several cases of **methemoglobinemia** have

Orthotoluidine— methemoglobinemia.

been reported after its use. Prilocaine is metabolized to *ortho*-toluidine and, in large doses, can induce some methemoglobinemia. A very large dose (greater than the maximum safe dose) would be required to produce clinical symptoms—cyanosis of the lips and mucous membranes and occasionally respiratory or circulatory distress. Although the small doses required in dental practice are not likely to present a problem in healthy, nonpregnant adults, prilocaine should not be administered to patients with any condition in which problems of oxygenation may be especially critical. Drugs that affect the hemoglobin, such as acetaminophen, may exacerbate the adverse reaction. Methemoglobinemia can be reversed by intravenous methylene blue.

Prilocaine is used for infiltration, block, epidural, and caudal anesthesia. It is available in dental cartridges as a 4% concentration both with and without 1:200,000 epinephrine.

Prilocaine's niche in dentistry involves situations in which the desired duration of action is somewhat longer than that obtained with mepivacaine (without and with). Prilocaine plain has

a duration of action slightly longer than mepivacaine plain, and prilocaine with epinephrine has a duration of action slightly longer than with epinephrine. The other potential advantage of prilocaine is that the concentration of epinephrine (1:200,000) is lower than in other local anesthetic amide combinations. Therefore, if prilocaine with epinephrine were to be used, the patient would be exposed to half of the amount of epinephrine as with lidocaine with epinephrine 1:100,000.

Bupivacaine. Bupivacaine [byoo-PIV-a-kane] (Marcaine) is an amide type of local anesthetic related to lidocaine

Bupivacaine—prolonged duration.

and mepivacaine. It is more potent but less toxic than the other amides. The major advantage of bupivacaine is its greatly prolonged duration of action. It is indicated in lengthy dental procedures when pulpal anesthesia of greater than 1.5 hours is needed or when postoperative pain is expected (e.g., endodontics, periodontics, and oral surgery). After the sensation begins to return, a period of reduced or altered sensation (analgesia) may last several hours. Compared with lidocaine with epinephrine, the onset of bupivacaine with epinephrine is slightly longer, but its duration is at least twice that of lidocaine. It is available in dental cartridges as a 0.5% solution with 1:200,000 epinephrine. It should not be used in patients prone to self-mutilation (mental patients or children under 12 years old). During its early use in anesthesiology and obstetrics, fatal unresuscitable cardiac arrests occurred. The doses used for obstetrics were much higher that those used in dentistry. After the maximum doses for obstetrics were lowered, these cardiac arrests essentially disappeared. Because much lower maximum doses are recommended for dental procedures, these adverse reactions are very unlikely to occur in dental practice. Bupivacaine has been used for infiltration, block, and peridural anesthesia.

Ropivacaine. Ropivacaine (Naropin) is a relatively new amide local anesthetic that has been used primarily for epidural blocks. Other routes of administration include major **nerve block** or infiltration anesthesia. It has not been used in dentistry.

ESTERS

There are currently no esters available in a dental cartridge. Esters, such as benzocaine, are commonly used topically.

Procaine. Procaine [PROE-kane] (Novocain) is a PABA ester. It is one of the safest local anesthetics known, and other local anesthetics are measured against it.

Procaine is used as an antiarrhythmic agent (procainamide) and is combined with penicillin to form procaine penicillin G. Procaine is not used in dentistry today.

Propoxycaine. Propoxycaine [proe-POX-i-kane] (Ravocaine), another ester of PABA, is not available in a dental cartridge.

Tetracaine. Tetracaine [TET-ra-kane] (Pontocaine), an ester of PABA, has a slow onset and long duration and is generally estimated to have at least 10 times the potency and toxicity of procaine. In view of this drug's high toxicity and the rapidity with which it is absorbed from mucosal surfaces, great care must be exercised if it is used for topical anesthesia. Dermatologic reactions include contact dermatitis, burning, stinging, and angioedema. A maximum dose of 20 mg is recommended for topical administration. Tetracaine is available in various sprays, solutions, and ointments for topical application. The concentration of tetracaine in most topical preparations is 2%.

OTHER LOCAL ANESTHETICS

Dyclonine [DYE-kloe-neen] (Dyclone) is a topical local anesthetic that is neither an ester nor an amide. Its side effects involving the cardiovascular system and CNS are similar to those of the other local anesthetics. Dyclonine may produce slight irritation and stinging when applied. Patients can exhibit allergic reactions to dyclonine, but, because of its unique structure, cross-allergenicity with other local anesthetics would not be expected. The onset of local anesthesia is 2 to 10 minutes, and its duration is 30 to 60 minutes. The solution and topical product are available as 0.5% and 1% concentrations.

Benzonatate. Benzonatate [ben-ZOE-na-tate] (Tessalon Perles) is a tetracaine congener (a near relative) indicated in the management of nonproductive cough. It is a topical anesthetic that acts on the respiratory stretch receptors, which produces its antitussive properties. Because the drug's local anesthetic activity can reduce the patient's gag reflex, care should be taken when working within the mouth to prevent foreign particles from entering the throat. Side effects include sedation, headache, dizziness, rash, gastrointestinal upset, and nasal congestion. It is used to treat cough.

VASOCONSTRICTORS

The **vasoconstricting** agents are included in local anesthetic solutions for the following reasons:

> Vasoconstriction keeps anesthetic in area injected.

1. Prolong the duration of action
2. Increase the depth of anesthesia
3. Delay systemic absorption
4. Reduce the toxic effect in the systemic circulation
5. Reduce the bleeding in the area of injection—visibility at surgical site

The vasoconstrictors are members of the autonomic nervous system drugs called the *adrenergic agonists* or *sympathomimetics* (see Chapter 5).

Whenever a local anesthetic solution does

not contain a vasoconstrictor, the anesthetic drug is more quickly removed from the injection site and distributed into systemic circulation than if the solution contained a vasoconstrictor. Plain (without vasoconstrictor) will exhibit a shorter duration of action and result in a more rapid buildup of a systemic blood level. Therefore any anesthetic given with a vasoconstrictor is more likely to be toxic than those given without a vasoconstrictor. Any advantage gained by eliminating the vasoconstrictor (shorter duration and increased possible systemic effect of the vasoconstrictor) must be

weighed against the potential for adverse effects from the epinephrine.

The decision about whether epinephrine should be used in a patient is made by weighing the risks and the benefits. Figure 10-5 shows the amount of epinephrine at rest and during mild to severe stress. Figure 10-6 compares the dose for anaphylaxis and dental use.

A sufficient concentration must be used to keep the local anesthetic localized at its sight of action and provide adequate depth, duration, and low systemic toxicity of the anesthetic. It has been shown that 1:100,000 and 1:200,000 pro-

F IGURE 1 0 - 5   *Blood levels of endogenous epinephrine during rest; with minor, moderate, or severe injury; myocardial infarction (before arrest); and cardiac arrest.*

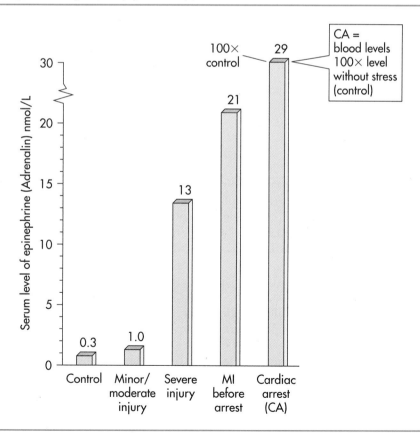

1:200,000 epinephrine would be "ducky." (It's a good thing.)

duce about the same amount of vasoconstriction and the same distribution of the local anesthetics. No justification exists for the use of epinephrine in a concentration greater than 1:200,000, except in cases in which local hemostasis is needed (1:50,000 is used). Lidocaine is available with 1:100,000 epinephrine, even though the weaker concentration has been shown to produce similar results.

In the 1940s, the literature stated that dental local anesthetics containing vasoconstrictors should not be used in patients with cardiovascular disease. This recommendation stemmed from the fear that the vasoconstrictor would elevate the blood pressure too much. It is now known that a patient can produce endogenous epinephrine far in excess of that administered in dentistry in the presence of inadequate anesthesia, which sometimes occurs when vasoconstrictors are avoided. Returned medical consults often recommend that epinephrine be avoided because physicians are familiar with the doses used in medicine (0.5 to 1.0 mg) rather than the dental dose (0.018 mg/cartridge [1.8 ml] of 1:100,000) of epinephrine (see Figure 10-6).

Patients with *uncontrolled* high blood pressure, hyperthyroidism, angina pectoris, or cardiac arrhythmias, as well as those who have had a myocardial infarction or cerebrovascular accident in the past 6 months, should make an appointment for elective dental treatment after their medical condition is under control. For a myocardial infarction or cerebrovascular accident, that would be after 6 months. Those undergoing general anesthesia with a halogenated hydrocarbon inhalation anesthetic should be monitored for arrhythmias if epinephrine is used for its hemostatic effect (used commonly with halothane). If arrhythmias occur, antiarrhythmic agents are administered.

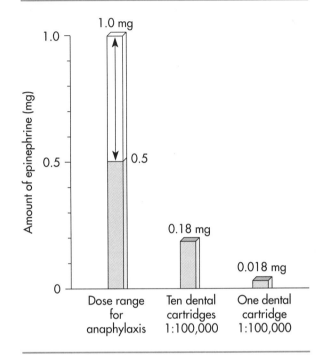

FIGURE **1 0 - 6**   *Histogram showing the dose range of epinephrine for anaphylaxis and the doses provided in dental cartridges.*

The patients with cardiovascular disease who are able to withstand elective dental treatment should receive administration of epinephrine-containing local anesthetic agents. The anesthetic should be administered in the lowest possible dose by means of the best technique, including aspiration and a very slow injection rate to minimize systemic absorption. Maximum cardiac doses should not be exceeded in patients with severe cardiovascular disease. Table 10-4 lists the maximum safe dose of epinephrine for the healthy patient (0.2 mg) and the cardiac patient (0.04 mg); the number of cartridges each of these doses represents is in-

Epinephrine cardiac dose = 0.04 mg.

TABLE 10-4 Vasoconstrictors, Maximum Safe Dose—Normal and Cardiac

| | | | MAXIMUM SAFE DOSE | | | | |
| | | | NORMAL ADULT | | CARDIAC PATIENT | | |
DRUG	CONCENTRATION	RELATIVE PRESSOR POTENCY	MG	NO. OF CARTRIDGES	MG	NO. OF CARTRIDGES	APPROXIMATE % OF (α/β) ACTIVITY
Epinephrine (Adrenalin)	1:50,000	1	0.2	5	0.04	1	50/50
	1:100,000	1	0.2	11	0.04	2	50/50
	1:200,000	1	0.2	22	0.04	4	50/50
Levonordefrin (Neo-Cobefrin)	1:20,000	1/5	1.0	11	0.2 or 1.0*	2 or 11*	75/25

*Data from Malamed SF: *Handbook of local anesthesia,* ed 4, St Louis, 1997, Mosby.

TABLE 10-5 Drug Interactions of Epinephrine (EPI)

MEDICAL DRUG GROUP	EXAMPLES	POTENTIAL OUTCOMES
Tricyclic antidepressants	Amitriptyline (Elavil) Imipramine (Tofranil)	Pressor response to IV EPI markedly enhanced
β-Blockers, nonselective	Pindolol (Visken) Propranolol (Inderal) Timolol (Blocadren)	Hypertension and reflex bradycardia
Antidiabetics	Tolbutamide (Orinase) Chlorpropamide (Diabinese)	Blood glucose increased
INTERACTIONS *NOT* SIGNIFICANT IN DENTISTRY		
Phenothiazines	Chloropromazine (Thorazine)	Reverse pressor response of EPI; avoid using EPI to raise BP
MAOI	Phenelzine Tranylcypromine	EPI not inactivated by MAO

NOTE: More details available in Table 26-6.
BP, Blood pressure; *EPI,* epinephrine; *IV,* intravenous; *MAO,* monoamine oxidase; *MAOI,* monoamine oxidase inhibitor.

cluded. For example, the cardiac patient could be given two cartridges of 1:100,000 epinephrine without exceeding the cardiac dose.

DRUG INTERACTIONS

Selected drug interactions of epinephrine are listed in Table 10-5. Of the most important drug interactions with epinephrine, two are clinically significant and two are not. The two epinephrine drug interactions that are most likely to be clinically significant are those with tricyclic antidepressants and nonselective β-blockers. With tricyclic anti-

> Significant drug interactions with epinephrine—tricyclic antidepressants and nonselective β-blockers.

depressants, administration of epinephrine may produce an exaggerated increase in pressor response (increased blood pressure). With the nonselective β-blockers, hypertension and reflex bradycardia may be exhibited. These are not absolute contraindications to the use of epinephrine, but patients taking these agents should be monitored for symptoms of alterations in their blood pressure. The two drug interactions that are commonly mentioned but are not usually clinically significant are with monoamine oxidase (MAO) inhibitors and phenothiazines. Epinephrine can be given to patients taking MAO inhibitors (MAOI) because epinephrine is eliminated primarily by reuptake and secondarily by catechol *O*-methyltransferase (COMT) rather than by MAO. If any small interaction exists, it would be due to "denervation hypersensitivity." In contrast to epinephrine, the indirect-acting sympathomimetic agents (e.g., pseudoephedrine) should be avoided in patients taking MAO inhibitors because they are inactivitated in significant amounts by MAO. The drug interaction between epinephrine and phenothiazines occurs because the phenothiazines are α-blockers, and when an α and β agonist (epinephrine) is given the β effects (vasodilation) predominate. Therefore if epinephrine is used for its vasopressor effect (to raise the blood pressure) the blood pressure is likely to decrease. When epinephrine is used in a local anesthetic solution, it is not being given for its vasopressor effect, so this interaction is not clinically significant.

CHOICE OF LOCAL ANESTHETIC

Practitioners should choose a few local anesthetic solutions to use, depending on the duration of local anesthesia desired

> Pick two local anesthetics solutions.

and the side effects that must be avoided. Table 10-6 lists the local anesthetics by their durations of action, including both pulpal and soft tissue anesthesia. Figures 10-7 and 10-8 illustrate the

TABLE 10-6   Categories of Duration of Action of Local Anesthetic Agents (Plain and Without)

GENERAL CATEGORIES		
SHORT DURATION (PULPAL = 30 MIN)	INTERMEDIATE DURATION (PULPAL 30-60 MIN)	LONG DURATION (PULPAL > 90 MIN)
Lidocaine plain (without)	Mepivacaine with	Bupivacaine with
Mepivacaine plain (without)	Prilocaine plain (block) (without)	
Prilocaine plain (infiltration)	Prilocaine with (60-90 min)	

PULPAL AND SOFT TISSUE			
LOCAL ANESTHETICS		PULPAL (MIN)	SOFT TISSUE (HRS)
Lidocaine	with	60	3-5
Mepivacaine	without (plain)	40 (20)*	2-3
	with	60-90	3-5
Prilocaine	without (plain)	60 (10)*	2-4 (1.5-2)*
	with	60-90 (45-60)*	3-8 (2-4)†
Bupivacaine	with	90-180	4-9 (12)

*With infiltration.
†With 1:200,000 epinephrine.

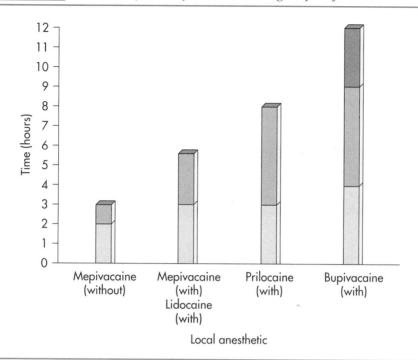

FIGURE **1 0 - 7** *Duration of action of local anesthetic agents for soft tissue.*

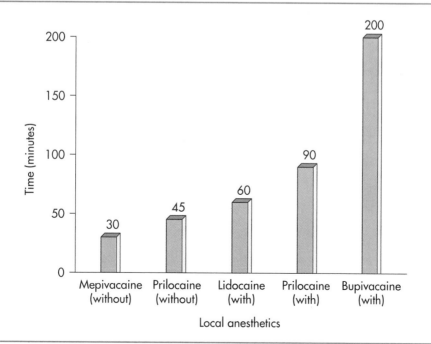

FIGURE **1 0 - 8** *Duration of action of local anesthetic agents for pulpal anesthetics.*

durations of action of local anesthetic agents for soft tissue and pulpal anesthetics, respectively. Several properties of local anesthetic agents determine their differences in pharmacokinetics. Table 10-7 lists these physical properties for some local anesthetics. For example, the pK_a is related to the onset of action. With a lower pK_a, the local anesthetic is distributed more in the base form and so is better absorbed. The duration of action of the local anesthetics is primarily related to its protein binding capacity. Its lipid solubility may also play some part. The duration is unrelated to

the local anesthetic's half-life, because its action is terminated when the drug is removed from the receptor. The lipid solubility determines the potency of a local anesthetic agent. The vasodilating property of a local anesthetic can affect both the potency and duration of action. Note that the vasodilating effect of lidocaine (1) is more than that of mepivacaine (0.8) and prilocaine (0.5). Because mepivacaine and prilocaine have less vasodilating effect, they can be used without vasoconstrictor. In contrast, lidocaine (1) and bupivacaine (2.5) produce too much vasodilation to be used without a vaso-

TABLE 10-7   Physical Properties of Local Anesthetics

Local Anesthetic	pK_a[a]	Vasodilating[b]	$T_{1/2}$[c]	Lipid Solubility[d]	Protein Binding[e] [%]
Lidocaine	7.9	1	90	2.9	65
Mepivacaine	7.6	0.8	90[f]	0.8	75
Prilocaine	7.9	0.5	80	0.9	55
Bupivacaine	8.1	2.5	76	27.5	95

[a]pK_a, Dissociation constant; rate of onset; [b]Vasodilating—lidocaine given value of 1; [c]Half-life (min); [d]Lipid solubility—oil/water solubility; **intrinsic** potency, increased penetrability; [e]Protein binding—duration of action; [f]Estimated.

TABLE 10-8   Contraindications to the Use of Local Anesthetic Combinations

Categories	Situation	Preferred Anesthetic
History of allergy	To amides (very unlikely)	Amides, with informed consent
	To esters	Amide
	Sulfa	Any
	Sulfite hypersensitivity (asthma)	Any without vasoconstrictor
Choice of local anesthetic agent	Pregnancy	Lidocaine
	Congenital cholinesterase deficiency	Amides
	Malignant hyperthermia	Any amide
	Methemoglobinemia	Any but prilocaine
	Severe renal disease	Any, but limit dose
	Severe liver disease	Any, but limit dose
Vasoconstrictor limits	Very severe cardiovascular disease	Limit to cardiac dose
	Untreated (or drug treated) hyperthyroidism	Limit to cardiac dose
	Tricyclic antidepressants	Limit to cardiac dose
	β-Blockers, nonselective	Limit to cardiac dose

constrictor. The dental practitioner should become familiar with a short-, an intermediate, and a long-acting agent. The duration of the procedure and any patient-specific information will determine the anesthetic of choice. Table 10-8 lists some common contraindications to the use of local anesthetic agents.

TOPICAL ANESTHETICS

Benzocaine, an ester, is the most commonly used topical anesthetic; lidocaine, an amide, is the second most commonly used. Some topical anesthetics are listed in Table 10-9. Comparison among the agents should take into account their onset, duration of action, and allergenic potential. The patient should be instructed to avoid eating for 1 hour after application to oral mucosa so that the gag reflex can become fully functional.

AMIDES

Lidocaine. Lidocaine (Xylocaine) is available as the base or hydrochloride salt. The base is pre-

ferred when large areas of the mucosal surfaces are ulcerated, abraded, denuded, or erythematous. Because it is poorly water soluble, its penetration and absorption are much less than the base. The hydrochloride salt is water soluble and penetrates the tissue better. Therefore its propensity for systemic absorption is greater than with the base. Lidocaine base is available as a jelly and an oral topical solution, and hydrochloride is available as an ointment, an oral topical, and an oral aerosol. Concentration of the creams ranges from 2% to 5%. Viscous lidocaine (2%) is available for oral rinse to manage aphthous lesions or reduce gagging.

Lidocaine and prilocaine. Lidocaine and prilocaine (EMLA), an amide local anesthetic combination, has an onset of action of about 1 hour and a peak effect in 2 to 3 hours. Its duration of action is 1 to 2 hours after the cream is removed. This product has no current use in outpatient dentistry because its onset of action is long, its duration is long, and it must be physically removed to terminate its action.

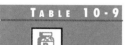

TABLE 10-9 **Selected Topical Local Anesthetics**

	Local Anesthetic Agent	Dosage Forms	Concentration (%)	Maximum Dose (mg)	Peak (min)	Duration (min)	Chemical Group
LIDOCAINE	Xylocaine	Spray, ointment, solution, viscous, jelly	2-10	750	2-5	15-45	Amide
BENZOCAINE	Hurricaine Orajel Mouth-Aid Maximum Strength Anbesol Americaine Anesthetic lubricant	Liquid, gel, spray, ointment	7.5-20	5000	1	15-45	Esters
	Tetracaine (Pontocaine, in Cetacaine)	Solution	0.5-2	50	3-8	30-60	
	Cocaine	Has no dental use, highly abused					
	Dyclonine (Dyclone)	Solution	0.5-1	100	<10	<60	Other

ESTERS

Benzocaine. Benzocaine [BEN-zoe-kane] (Hurricaine, Anbesol, Benzodent, Orabase-B), an ester of PABA, cannot be converted to a water-soluble form for injection. Because it is poorly soluble, it is poorly absorbed and lacks significant systemic toxicity. Local reactions reported include burning and stinging. Dermatologic reactions have included angioedema and contact dermatitis, which can occur if the operator does not wear gloves (an unacceptable practice today). Benzocaine is available in dental products and in many over-the-counter (OTC) products for teething, sunburn, hemorrhoids, or insect bites (up to 20% for many, but not all). Benzocaine is used in many dental offices, even though a hypersensitivity reaction is possible.

Cocaine. Cocaine [koe-KANE] is a naturally occurring ester of benzoic acid that is potent and extremely toxic. Its onset of action is less than 1 minute and its peak is within 5 minutes. Its duration of action is about 30 minutes. Although cocaine has ideal pharmacokinetics, the systemic absorption and subsequent CNS stimulation makes the use of cocaine as a local anesthetic untenable. Its CNS effects are discussed in Chapter 26. It has no dental application.

PRECAUTIONS IN TOPICAL ANESTHESIA

Some local anesthetics are absorbed rapidly when applied topically to mucous membranes. To avoid toxic reactions from surface anesthesia, the dental health care provider should consider the following:

- Know the relative *toxicity* of the drug being used.
- Know the *concentration* of the drug being used.
- Use the *smallest volume*
- Use the *lowest concentration*
- Use the *least toxic* drug to satisfy clinical requirements.
- Limit the *area of application* (avoid sprays).

DOSAGES OF LOCAL ANESTHETIC AND VASOCONSTRICTOR

The amounts of local anesthetic and vasoconstrictor contained in a certain volume of solution can be calculated from the concentration of that solution. The local anesthetic percent, for example, 2%, may be expressed as follows:

$$2\% = \frac{2\ gm}{100\ ml} \times \frac{2000\ mg}{gm} = \frac{2000\ mg}{100\ ml} =$$

$$\frac{20\ mg}{1\ ml} = 20\ mg/ml$$

amount in 1 cartridge =

$$\frac{20\ mg}{1\ ml} \times \frac{1.8\ ml}{cartridge} = \frac{36\ mg}{cartridge}$$

For the amount of epinephrine is calculated as follows:

$$1:100{,}000 = \frac{1gm}{100{,}000\ ml} \times \frac{1000\ mg}{1\ gm} =$$

$$\frac{1000\ mg}{100{,}000\ ml} = \frac{1mg}{100\ ml} \times \frac{1000\ \mu g}{1\ mg} =$$

$$\frac{1000\ mg}{100\ ml} = \frac{10\ \mu g}{ml}$$

[concentration of epinephrine in 1:100,000]

amount in 1 cartridge =

$$\frac{10\ \mu g}{ml} \times \frac{1.8\ ml}{cartridge} = \frac{18\ \mu g}{cartridge} = \frac{.018\ mg}{cartridge}$$

The dental health care provider should be able to determine the number of milligrams of both local anesthetic and vasoconstrictor given in any clinical situation. The maximum safe dose for each component should not be exceeded.

Each dose should be recorded in the patient's chart as soon as possible after the injection. The information placed in the chart should include the strength of both ingredients and the volume of solution used or the number of milligrams of each given. For example, if a patient were given one cartridge of lidocaine 2% with 1:100,000 epinephrine, the chart would read: lidocaine 2% with epinephrine 1:100,000—1.8 ml, or lidocaine 36 mg with epinephrine 0.018 mg.

One reason for including this information in the chart is to minimize questions that might arise later if the patient or future practitioner has concerns about the treatment. Because of the increasing incidence of lawsuits against dentists and hygienists, maintaining a complete chart to prevent any ambiguity is extremely important.

REVIEW QUESTIONS

1. Name the properties of the ideal local anesthetic.
2. Differentiate between the two major chemical groups of local anesthetic agents.
3. Contrast the allergenicity and metabolism of the ester and amide local anesthetics.
4. List the systemic adverse reactions to the local anesthetics.
5. List five injectable local anesthetic agents and give their composition.
6. Explain the presence in a dental cartridge of agents other than the local anesthetic.
7. State the rationale for the inclusion of vasoconstricting agents in local anesthetic solution.
8. Give the maximum recommended dose of three common local anesthetics.
9. State the maximum safe dose of the two vasoconstrictors used in dentistry for both the normal patient and the cardiac patient.
10. Explain how to determine the amounts of vasoconstrictor and local anesthetic agent present in a given solution. State the reason for recording this information in the chart.
11. Name an agent that could be used as a local anesthetic if a patient is allergic to both esters and amides.
12. If a patient has an allergy to sulfites, what types of local anesthetic products should be avoided?
13. Describe a new dosage form for lidocaine.

Antianxiety Agents

CHAPTER OUTLINE

> Dental professionals often do not recognize or relate to a patient's stress level while dental treatment is being provided.

Both the dentist and the dental hygienist recognize the value of having a relaxed patient. Often patient anxiety is sufficiently reduced by a calm, patient, confident, and understanding attitude on the part of the dental health care workers. However, individual responses to dental treatment vary widely, ranging from total relaxation and even sleeping to severe apprehension and inability to approach the dental office, much less the dental chair. Each dental patient should be provided with the most pleasant experience possible within the limits of safety. When the patient is relaxed, appointments can be more productive, and the dentist, hygienist, and patient all benefit.

Dental professionals, because of their familiarity with all of dentistry's components and ramifications, often do not understand the basis of anxiety in the dental patient. Frequently, dental health care workers lack empathy and even commonly blame or fault the patient for his or her discomfort. Members of the dental team often become defensive because they do not feel comfortable and do not know how to manage these intense feelings. By acting perturbed, the dental team reinforces the patient's negative feelings about the dental appointment. A dental practitioner who decides that anxiety control is only necessary for the first third of a dental appointment does not have an understanding of patient anxiety and its treatment.

Many patients who require dental care never go to the dental office because of fear and apprehension. A common misconception is that dental patients who express anxiety are just "looking for drugs." The average dental patient who is being treated for dental anxiety during the appointment does not get the opportunity to abuse antianxiety agents. The appropriate use of antianxiety agents might encourage more patients to seek needed dental treatment. If, in order to treat many nervous dental patients, an occasional patient who was "seeking" antianxiety agents obtains them, that is an appropriate balance in the use of antianxiety agents. It would be unlikely for a person in search of drugs to sit for an hour in the dental chair, have dental treatment performed, and then pay for the treatment all to obtain 1 tablet of an antianxiety drug that was taken in the dental office. However, prescribing 20 tablets of an antianxiety drug for a patient nervous about getting dentures would be inappropriate.

It is necessary to objectively assess the patient's anxiety on both the first and subsequent visits. A patient who is clutching the dental chair arms and has white knuckles is not in a relaxed state (Figure 11-1). By questioning and observing the patient, a determination can be made about the need for antianxiety agents. Thus the patient can feel comfortable and relaxed during subsequent dental appointments. Remember that whatever procedure you are performing, you have performed it many times. However, for many patients this may be their first experience with the procedure, and their reactions may be altered by their interpretation of what is happening. [That sharp, pointy thing is going to hurt! What are those gunlike weapons?]

Of the agents discussed in this chapter, the dental team will most commonly use orally administered drugs to provide relaxation for the anxious patient. Intravenous administration is used infrequently because it requires more training and experience than most general dentists possess. Most states require a separate certificate to administer intravenous agents or to provide conscious sedation. The malpractice insurance is much more expensive. Even though orally administered sedatives provide inconsistent or poorly predictable results, practitioners should become familiar with one or two drugs and use them repeatedly. In the long run this practice will produce greater benefits than changing from drug to drug.

> Appropriate dose to use is difficult to determine (in fact, it's a "shot in the dark").

The dose of a particular antianxiety agent effective for a particular patient is vastly variable, involving both intrapatient and interpatient variation. Predicting the correct dose is a guess at best. The amount needed is poorly related to the degree of the patient's anxiety or the dental procedure to be performed. The normal sedative dose (calms normal patient without dental appointment) is not expected to produce calmness in a dental patient, but the hypnotic dose (that which induces sleep in the normal patient) can often produce the desired degree of sedation before dental treatment.

This chapter discusses some of the agents that can be used to allay anxiety—primarily the benzodiazepines. Nitrous oxide, which is used in dentistry as an antianxiety agent, is discussed in Chapter 12 because it is classified as a general anesthetic. It is very useful in decreasing apprehension during the dental appointment and is underutilized in many dental practices. Some drugs with properties of both the antihistamines and phenothiazines, such as hydroxyzine and

FIGURE 11-1 *White-knuckle syndrome. (From Clark MS, Brunick A:* Handbook of nitrous oxide and oxygen sedation, *St Louis, 1999, Mosby, Inc.)*

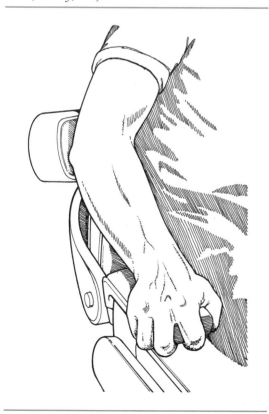

promethazine, have weak antianxiety properties and are discussed in Chapter 18.

DEFINITIONS

The sedative-hypnotic agents can produce varying degrees of central nervous system (CNS) depression depending on the dose administered. A small dose will produce mild CNS depression described as *sedation* (reduction of activity and simple anxiety). This level of CNS depression has some anxiolytic effects. A larger dose of the same drug, the *hypnotic* dose (inducing sleep), will produce greater CNS depression. Thus the

FIGURE 11-2 *Sedative-hypnotics. Range of effects with increasing doses.*

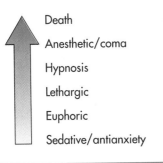

Death
Anesthetic/coma
Hypnosis
Lethargic
Euphoric
Sedative/antianxiety

same drug may be either a sedative or a hypnotic depending on the dose administered. In even larger doses, sedative-hypnotics may produce anesthesia and finally death (Figure 11-2).

The term *tranquilizer* refers to two quite different groups of agents—the *minor tranquilizers*, whose action is like that of the sedative-hypnotics, and the *major tranquilizers*, which have antipsychotic activity. Table 11-1 lists differences between the minor and major tranquilizers. The minor tranquilizers are used in the treatment of anxiety, and the major tranquilizers are used to treat psychoses. The minor tranquilizers produce sedation similar to that produced by alcohol. With larger and larger doses, these agents can produce coma and finally death. Even with large doses, the patient taking major tranquilizers can be easily aroused from the sedation. The minor tranquilizers relax voluntary muscles (usually in conjunction with CNS depression), whereas the major tranquilizers produce extrapyramidal effects, including involuntary muscle movement and rigidity. Minor tranquilizers have a potential for addiction, whereas the sedation produced by major tranquilizers is not reinforcing. In fact, patient compliance with the major tranquilizers is a problem. Major tranquilizers have a strong anticholinergic effect that commonly produces xerostomia. (Minor tranquilizers have very weak anticholinergic effects.) The

TABLE 11-1   Tranquilizers—Major Versus Minor

PHARMACOLOGIC GROUP	SEDATIVE-HYPNOTIC AGENTS	ANTIPSYCHOTIC AGENTS
TRANQUILIZER	MINOR	MAJOR
EXAMPLES:	DIAZEPAM (VALIUM)	CHLORPROMAZINE (THORAZINE), THIORIDAZINE (MELLARIL)
Therapeutic use	Anxiety relief	Controls psychotic behavior
Side effects (CNS)	Ataxia, disinhibition, drunkenness	Easy arousal
Lethality	Anesthesia, depression, and death	Cardiac toxicity
Seizures	Anticonvulsant	Convulsions
Muscle relaxation	Voluntary	Extrapyramidal; parkinsonism
Addiction	Physical dependence, habituation	Not addicting
Other side effects		Autonomic—anticholinergic

major tranquilizers are discussed in detail in Chapter 11.

This chapter discusses both the minor tranquilizers (the benzodiazepines and meprobamate) and the classic sedative-hypnotic agents (the barbiturates, chloral hydrate, and zolpidem). The benzodiazepines are discussed first because they are used most frequently.

BENZODIAZEPINES

The benzodiazepines [ben-zoe-dye-AZ-e-peens] currently account for 10 slots in the list of the top 200 most commonly prescribed drugs (see Appendix A). For years diazepam was in the top 10, but last year the highest-ranked benzodiazepine, alprazolam, was listed as 57. Alprazolam was listed 4 times (under different brands), lorazepam twice, clonazepam twice, and diazepam and temazepam once. The members of this group differ mainly in their onset and duration of action, dose, and dosage forms available. They are sometimes referred to as *minor tranquilizers.*

CHEMISTRY

The benzodiazepines are so called because of their structure—a 1,4-benzodiazepine nucleus. Chlordiazepoxide [klor-dye-az-e-POX-ide] (Librium), the first derivative, was synthesized in 1955. After its success, thousands of other benzodiazepine derivatives were screened for psychopharmacologic activity. As a result of this search, diazepam (Valium) was synthesized in 1959 and marketed in 1963. Many benzodiazepines are now available (Table 11-2).

When an additional ring was added to the original nucleus, another high-potency benzodiazepine, triazolam, was synthesized. Next, two imidazobenzodiazepines, midazolam and flumazenil, were synthesized. Midazolam is a potent water-soluble benzodiazepine, whereas flumazenil is a benzodiazepine antagonist without any pharmacologic action of its own.

PHARMACOKINETICS

The benzodiazepines are well absorbed when administered by the oral route. The rapidity of the onset of action of the benzodiazepines is related to their lipid solubility. Diazepam, which is highly lipid soluble, has a quick onset and is concentrated in the adipose tissue. Storage in adipose tissue prolongs the action of lipid soluble benzodiazepines. The benzodiazepines are available in the following dosage forms: tablets, capsules, oral solution, rectal gel, and injectable forms. The intramuscular route, for benzodiazepines other than midazolam, gives slow, erratic, and unpredictable results. In contrast, the intravenous route, for those available in parenteral form, produces a rapid, predictable response that makes them ideal for conscious sedation. Once a benzodiazepine is absorbed, the rate at which it crosses into the cerebrospinal fluid (CSF) through the blood-brain barrier is dependent on protein binding, lipid solubility, and the ionization constant of the compound. Most benzodiazepines are highly protein bound and are present in the un-ionized, lipid-soluble form. They easily cross the blood-brain and placental barriers to produce an effect in the CNS and on the fetus (Food and Drug Administration [FDA] categories D or X), where they can accumulate with repeated doses.

After absorption, the benzodiazepines are metabolized by phase II metabolism alone or by phase I metabolism, which is followed by phase

> Phase I metabolism = HARD—reduced by some drugs and by age.

II metabolism (Figure 11-3). Phase I metabolism involves oxidation, reduction, hydrolysis, dealkylation, and hydroxylation. Phase I metabolism is *hard* (difficult) metabolism. Phase I metabolism is decreased in the elderly, in patients taking certain drugs that inhibit hepatic metabolism, and in the presence of hepatic disease. Certain drugs, such as cimetidine and erythromycin, inhibit the metabolism of benzodiazepines that

TABLE 11-2 Benzodiazepines and Miscellaneous Sedative-Hypnotic Agents

Drug Name Generic (Trade)	Hypnotic Dose (mg)	Onset of Action (General)	(min)	Peak (hr)	Half-Life (hr)	Metabolism	Half-Life (hr) of Major Metabolism	FDA
Alprazolam (Xanax)	0.25-0.5	I[o]	45-60	1-2	6-27	IM[b], O[c], G	—	D[d]
Chlordiazepoxide (Librium)	5-20	I	15-45	0.5-4	5-30	AM, O	30-200	D
Clonazepam (Klonopin)[e]	1.5	I[f]	20-60	1-2	18-50	IM[g], R[h]	—	C
Clorazepate (Tranxene)	7.5	F[i]	30-60	1-2	40-50	AM, S[i]	30-200	C
Diazepam (Valium)[k,l]	5-10	V[m]	15-45	0.5-2	20-80	AM, O	30-200	D
Estazolam (ProSom)	1-2			0.5-2	10-19	IM, O	—	X
Flunitrazepam[n]	0.5-1	F	15-45	1-2	16-35	AM		
Flurazepam (Dalmane)	15-30	I	15-45	0.5-1	47-100 (metab)	O	47-100	D
Halazepam (Paxipam)	20-40	S[o]	25-60	1-3	14	AM, O	30-200	D
Lorazepam (Ativan)[a,p]	2-4	I	15-30	1-6	10-20	G[q]	—	D
Midazolam (Versed)[a,s]	— / Titrate	F / F	PO 30 / IV 1-5	PO 0.5-1 / IV 3-5 min	11 / 11	AM, OH[t] + G	1-1.3	D
Oxazepam (Serax)	15-30	S	45-90	2-4 (1-2)	5-20	G	—	C
Quazepam (Doral)	7.5-15			1-2	39	O, G	40-75	X
Temazepam (Restoril)	15-30	S	25-60	2-3	8-38	G	—	X
Triazolam (Halcion)[l]	0.125-0.5	F	15-30	2, 0.5-2	1.5-5	IM, F[c], G	—	X

NONBENZODIAZEPINE, NONBARBITURATE SEDATIVE-HYPNOTICS

Drug Name Generic (Trade)	Hypnotic Dose (mg)	Onset of Action (General)	(min)	Peak (hr)	Half-Life (hr)	Metabolism	Half-Life (hr) of Major Metabolism	FDA
Zolpidem (Ambien)[x]	10	F		0.5-2	1.5-4.5	IM,		C
Chloral hydrate (Noctec)	500-1000[y]		30			AM, L and E[z]	7-10[aa]	C

[a]I, Intermediate; [b]AM, active metabolite; [c]O, metabolized by oxidation; [d]pregnancy category determined by the FDA; [e]used as adjunct to treat certain kind of seizures; (unlabeled uses are bipolar affective disorder, tics, adjunct for schizophrenia, leg movements in sleep); [f]I, intermediate; [g]IM, inactive metabolite; [h]R, nitroreduction; [i]F, fast; [j]metabolized in stomach; [k]injectable contains propylene glycol—can produce thrombophlebitis; [l]amnesia can occur with parenteral administration; [m]VF, very fast; [n]used in association with date rape, amnesia with oral use, not available in United States; [o]S, slow; [p]available parenterally; [q]G, metabolized by glucuronidation; [r]available parenterally; [s]midazolam administered intravenously in United States; intravenous form can be given orally; [t]OH, metabolized by hydroxylation (?); [u]therapeutic index may be less than others; [v]amnesia with oral use; [w]first-pass hepatic extraction; [x]not a benzodiazepine; [y]child's dose 50 mg/kg up to 1000 mg; [z]liver and erythrocytes; [aa]of metabolite trichloroethanol.

FIGURE 11-3 *Benzodiazepine metabolism. Some (diazepam and chlordiazepoxide) are metabolized to active metabolites (phase I), whereas others (oxazepam and lorazepam) are glucuronidated to inactive metabolites (phase II metabolism).*

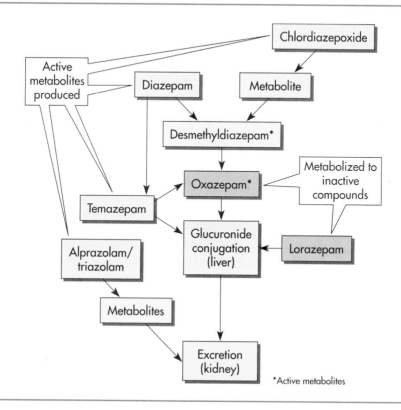

*Active metabolites

undergo phase I metabolism. This drug interaction prolongs the duration of action and increases the half-lives of the benzodiazepines that undergo phase I metabolism, such as diazepam and chlordiazepoxide. Phase I metabolism results in active metabolites that, with repeated administration, can accumulate. The half-lives of these drugs and their metabolites range from 2 to 200 hours (see Table 11-2).

Phase II metabolism involves glucuronidation and is *easy* (unaffected by external factors). Benzodiazepines that undergo only phase II metabolism, such as lorazepam and oxazepam, are much less affected by drugs or hepatic disease. One type of phase II metabolism, glucuronidation, involves the drug itself or its metabolite (from phase I) being conjugated with glucuronic acid. This process requires glucuronyl transferase, an enzyme present in many tissues. Therefore this process is not as sensitive to the presence of liver disease, age, or drug interactions. For the elderly patient or patient taking drugs that inhibit metabolism of benzodiazepines, use of a benzodiazepine that is metabolized solely by the process of glucuronidation (Phase II) is preferred. An example of a benzodiazepine that un-

Phase II metabolism = EASY—not affected by drugs or age.

dergoes both phase I and II metabolism is diazepam (see Figure 11-3). Diazepam undergoes phase I metabolism, resulting in desmethyldiazepam, an active metabolite of diazepam. The half-life of diazepam itself (phase I metabolism) is 20 to 50 hours. Desmethyldiazepam, the active metabolite, is then glucuronidated (phase II metabolism), with a half-life of 50 to 100 hours. With benzodiazepines that undergo both phase I and phase II metabolism, phase I (hard) precedes phase II (easy) metabolism. Because the glucuronide metabolite is eliminated mainly in the urine, kidney disease causes accumulation of the glucuronide metabolites, but these have no pharmacologic effect.

MECHANISM OF ACTION

Benzodiazepines facilitate GABA-mediated transmission.

Benzodiazepines enhance or facilitate the action of the neurotransmitter by exerting their effects in the CNS mediated by γ-aminobutyric acid (GABA), a major inhibitory transmitter in the CNS. It acts in the limbic, thalamic, cortical, and hypothalamic levels of the CNS. Benzodiazepines act as agonists at the benzodiazepine receptor, forming a BZ-GABA-receptor-chloride-ionophore-complex. The benzodiazepines bind to the omega 1, 2, and 3 $GABA_A$ receptors (BZ_1, BZ_2, and BZ_3). The combination of GABA and the benzodiazepines increases the frequency of the chloride channel opening. With hyperpolarization, the excitation transmission and subsequent depolarization is decreased so that the inhibitor effect of GABA is enhanced. There are thought to be at least three benzodiazepine receptor subtypes called BZ_1, BZ_2, and BZ_3 ($omega_1$, $omega_2$, $omega_3$), with more likely to be identified. Some other actions of the benzodiazepines are GABA-receptor independent.

The benzodiazepine receptor ligands in the brain are currently thought to be of three types: agonists such as the useful benzodiazepines, antagonists such as flumazenil that block the action of the benzodiazepines, and anxiogenic benzodiazepines. Administered alone, this last group may produce anxiety and convulsions, which may explain why they are not used clinically.

PHARMACOLOGIC EFFECTS

The pharmacologic effects of the benzodiazepines have qualitatively similar actions but vary in potency.

Behavioral effects. The effects of benzodiazepines on behavior have been determined mainly through animal studies and may differ greatly from the actual effects in humans. In animals these agents are able to suppress behavior motivated by punishment, restore behavior suppressed by lack of regard, and alter behavior accompanying stress and frustration. They also have the ability to reduce aggression and hostility in animals. These effects in animals allow the screening of many derivatives for anxiolytic action in animals.

The clinical effects of these agents in humans are anxiety reduction at low doses and production of drowsiness and even sleep at higher doses. Repeated doses of benzodiazepines reduce rapid eye movement (REM) sleep. Usual doses produce a marked reduction in stages 3 and 4 sleep (deep sleep) (Figure 11-4).

Anticonvulsant effects. The benzodiazepines, such as diazepam, have anticonvulsant activity (i.e., they increase the seizure threshold). Diazepam, used parenterally, has been shown to be an effective anticonvulsant for the prevention of seizures associated with local anesthetic toxicity and for the treatment of status epilepticus. Some oral benzodiazepines are used in combination with other anticonvulsants to manage epilepsy. The benzodiazepines prevent the spread of seizures in tissues surrounding the anatomic seizure focus (when such a focus exists) but have little effect on the discharges at the focus itself.

FIGURE 11-4 *Sleep cycle. Lines point to REM and NREM sleep. Stages of sleep range from 1 to 4. In REM sleep, blood pressure, heart rate, and respiratory rate increase. This is the stage where dreams and erections occur. In NREM sleep, blood pressure, heart rate, respiratory rate, and muscle tone decrease. Dreams also occur in this stage.*

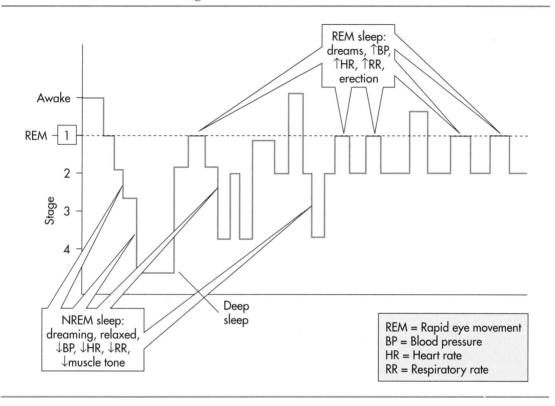

Muscle relaxation. Like all CNS depressants, benzodiazepines can produce relaxation of skeletal muscles. Some studies show benzodiazepines to be superior to other skeletal muscle relaxants for relief of musculoskeletal pain; other studies show pain relief effect be no better than aspirin or placebo. Benzodiazepines are effective for muscle spasticity secondary to pathologic states, such as cerebral palsy or paraplegia.

ADVERSE REACTIONS

In general, benzodiazepines, used alone, have a wide margin of safety. They all have similar adverse effects, but differ in their frequency.

Agents with long-elimination half-lives tend to accumulate and produce more side effects.

Central nervous system effects. The most common side effect attributed to benzodiazepines is CNS depression manifested as fatigue, drowsiness, muscle weakness, and ataxia. These side effects are more likely to occur in elderly persons and less likely to occur in heavy cigarette smokers. The patient may also experience lightheadedness and dizziness. Tolerance to this effect occurs over time. Paradoxical CNS stimulation that produces talkativeness, anxiety, nightmares, tremulousness, hyperactivity, and increased muscle spasticity can occur. This reaction is more common in psychiatric patients, and benzodiazepines should be discontinued if this reaction occurs.

When benzodiazepines are used in dentistry to produce conscious sedation, this side effect of CNS depression is used as the primary effect. The use of parenteral benzodiazepines such as diazepam, midazolam, or lorazepam during a dental appointment reduces the patient's anxiety and alters his or her perception of time.

The amount of the benzodiazepine used to provide conscious sedation is titrated to the patient's response. The appearance of ptosis is used as an initial endpoint for the dose administered. These agents have a rapid onset of action and an initial effect of 45 minutes to 1 hour.

Diazepam was the most common benzodiazepine used parenterally until newer benzodiazepines were developed. Diazepam's long half-life and its metabolism to an active metabolite prolonged its duration of action. Its effect lasted past the dental appointment time, and even into the next day.

Midazolam, a water-soluble benzodiazepine, is metabolized primarily to inactive metabolites. This produces an advantage for its intravenous use over diazepam in conscious sedation. Because these benzodiazepines are inactivated either by metabolism or by metabolism of their active metabolites, the duration and depth of sedation can be magnified by administration of drugs that inhibit the hepatic microsomal enzymes. Agents that inhibit these enzymes include cimetidine and erythromycin.

> "Roofies" are used before date rape; amnesia makes prosecution difficult.

A potent benzodiazepine named flunitrazepam (flew-nye-TRAY-ze-pam) (Rohypnol) is a benzodiazepine available in Europe but not the United States, is being used inappropriately in this country. Acquired illegally from Europe or Mexico, this benzodiazepine, nicknamed "roofies," has been secretly administered to women who were then "date raped." The amnesia and muscle flaccidity produced by this agent makes it difficult for the victim to testify or resist. Increasing the penalty for possession of this agent is being considered.

Anterograde amnesia. It can be easily demonstrated that parenteral benzodiazepines such as diazepam and midazolam produce amnesia beginning when the drug is taken. This effect is used to therapeutic advantage in patients scheduled for an unpleasant dental procedure. Clinical use has produced episodes of amnesia that can sometimes last several hours and can occur with several benzodiazepines. Oral triazolam seems to have a greater likelihood to produce amnesia than other oral benzodiazepines. Patients should be warned not to sign important papers or make important decisions after benzodiazepines are administered. The mechanism of amnesia results from an impairment of consolidation processes that store the information in the brain.

Respiratory effects. Usual doses of benzodiazepines have no adverse effect on respiration. However, doses of diazepam administered for outpatient dental procedures have been occasionally reported to produce respiratory depression. An isolated case of **apnea** after intravenous diazepam has also been observed. These respiratory effects are more common in elderly patients. The minimal respiratory depression can be exacerbated by opioids or alcohol.

Cardiovascular effects. Therapeutic doses of benzodiazepines have no adverse effect on circulation. The relief of anxiety may result in a fall in blood pressure and pulse rate. The pulse rate has also been reported to rise (tachycardia) and then return to normal after a few minutes.

Visual effects. Benzodiazepines are contraindicated in angle-closure (narrow angle) glaucoma and can produce other visual changes such as diplopia, **nystagmus,** and blurred vision. They may be used in treatment of wide-angle glaucoma (the most common kind of glaucoma).

Dental effects. The benzodiazepines have been reported to produce xerostomia, increased salivation (recognize these are opposite), swollen tongue, and a bitter or metallic taste.

Thrombophlebitis. Parenteral diazepam can produce thrombophlebitis. Because diazepam is poorly soluble in water, the vehicle propylene glycol is used to solubilize it. The vehicle is responsible for the thrombophlebitis. The incidence is lower when the intravenous **infusion** is given in the antecubital space rather than the dorsum of the hand (more blood and faster blood flow). Because midazolam is soluble in water and propylene glycol is not used to solubilize it, it is much less likely to produce this effect. With parenteral use, apnea, hypotension, bradycardia, and cardiac arrest have been reported. These are more frequent with rapid administration. Equipment for respiratory and cardiovascular assistance must be available if these agents are to be used parenterally (e.g., conscious sedation in the dental office). Special training of the dental team administering benzodiazepines is required.

Other effects. Benzodiazepines can affect the gastrointestinal tract, producing cramps or pain, and the genitourinary tract, producing difficulty in urination. They can also produce allergic reactions, including skin rash or itching.

Pregnancy and lactation. An increased risk of congenital malformation in infants of mothers taking benzodiazepines in the first trimester has been reported. **Cleft lip and palate,** microencephaly, and gastrointestinal and cardiovascular abnormalities were greater in the group taking benzodiazepines. Most of these agents are classified as FDA pregnancy category D drugs; triazolam and temazepam are in FDA pregnancy category X (see Chapter 24).

Near-term administration of benzodiazepines to the mother has resulted in floppy infant syndrome. This syndrome includes hypoactivity, hypotonia, hypothermia, apnea, and feeding problems. Because these agents are seldom absolutely needed (except for epilepsy), they should be avoided in women who are or may become pregnant and in nursing mothers. Before administering a benzodiazepine, the pregnancy status of the female patient should be determined. The first trimester, often before the patient knows that she is pregnant, is the time benzodiazepines are more likely to be teratogenic, or cause problems in the fetus.

ABUSE AND TOLERANCE

Benzodiazepines can be abused, and physical dependence and tolerance have been documented. Physiologic addiction can occur if large doses are taken over an extended period. However, their abuse and addiction potential is less than that of the other sedative-hypnotic agents such as the barbiturates.

Prolonged intake of large doses of benzodiazepines can result in a degree of CNS tolerance. Cross-tolerance also exists between the benzodiazepines and other CNS depressants. This may explain why benzodiazepines can be substituted for ethyl alcohol to relieve the symptoms of delirium tremens precipitated by acute alcohol withdrawal.

One of the advantage of benzodiazepines over barbiturates is their wider therapeutic index | Very wide therapeutic index. | (their range of safe dosage). Overdose poisoning with these drugs has been rare and appears to be difficult to achieve when used alone, although apnea has rarely been reported. In most instances, excessively large doses must be ingested to produce respiratory or central vasomotor depression. Combining benzodiazepines with other CNS depressants can reduce the safety so that the combination can be lethal. The addition of alcohol can result in coma, respiratory depression, hypotension, or hypothermia.

Treatment of overdose. Rarely does the ingestion of a benzodiazepine alone result in severe symptoms. Supportive therapy should be undertaken if symptoms result. With recent ingestion, emesis may be induced. Activated charcoal and a saline cathartic may be administered. The patient's respiration and blood pressure should be monitored.

> Chronic use in insomnia is not recommended.

To reverse some of the effects of a benzodiazepine flumazenil, [floo-MAZ-ee-nill] (Romazicon), a benzodiazepine antagonist available for intravenous administration, may be used. It has been shown to reverse the sedating and psychomotor effects, but reversing the respiratory depression produced by the benzodiazepines is incomplete. The amnesia is not consistently reversed. It has an initial half-life of about 10 minutes and a terminal half-life of about 60 minutes. Side effects include pain at the injection site, agitation, and anxiety. An increase in inadequate analgesia did not occur. Some patients became resedated before the end of 3 hours when high doses of long-acting benzodiazepines were ingested (the antagonist wore off before the agonist had been metabolized and excreted). Administering flumazenil to benzodiazepine-dependent individuals could precipitate withdrawal symptoms (similar to naloxone to opioids).

DRUG INTERACTIONS

Like other antianxiety agents, benzodiazepines interact in an additive fashion with other CNS depressants, notably alcohol, barbiturates, anticonvulsants, and phenothiazines. Because diazepam and desmethyldiazepam are cytochrome P-450 2C enzyme substrates, enzyme inducers may increase their metabolism and enzyme stimulators may decrease their metabolism.

Smoking reduces the effectiveness of the benzodiazepines. The tars produced by smoking cigarettes stimulate the hepatic microsomal enzymes in the liver. The increased number of liver enzymes increases the rate of metabolism of the benzodiazepines, so a higher dose of a benzodiazepine is required to produce the same effect.

Drugs that inhibit oxidative metabolism (phase I metabolism), such as cimetidine (ranitidine is less of a problem), disulfiram, isoniazid, cisapride, and omeprazole, may increase the effect of benzodiazepines that undergo phase I metabolism (hard). Benzodiazepines that only undergo phase II metabolism (easy) are not affected (see Table 11-2).

Valproic acid may displace diazepam from binding sites, which may result in an increase in sedative effects. Selective serotonin reuptake inhibitors (e.g., fluoxetine, sertraline, paroxetine) have greatly increased diazepam levels by altering its clearance. Benzodiazepines may reduce the effectiveness of levodopa, and parkinsonism has been exacerbated in these patients. Benzodiazepines may increase the effect of digoxin, phenytoin, and probenecid (Table 11-3).

USES

Medical. Benzodiazepines are useful in short-term treatment of anxiety, insomnia, and alcohol withdrawal. They are used for the acute treatment of seizures. Some neuromuscular diseases can be treated with the benzodiazepines. They

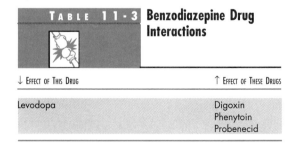

TABLE 11-3	Benzodiazepine Drug Interactions
↓ EFFECT OF THIS DRUG	↑ EFFECT OF THESE DRUGS
Levodopa	Digoxin
	Phenytoin
	Probenecid

are used in conscious sedation, general anesthesia, or during surgery.

ANXIETY CONTROL Generalized anxiety disorder and **panic disorder** are common indications for use of benzodiazepines in general medicine. Anxiety produces a physiologic response resembling fear, with manifestations including restlessness, tension, tachycardia, and dyspnea. Most well-controlled clinical trials have shown that the antianxiety effect of benzodiazepines is better than those of placebo, barbiturates, and meprobamate. Benzodiazepines also produce less sedation than the classic sedative-hypnotic agents.

| For dental anxiety |

INSOMNIA MANAGEMENT If insomnia is a manifestation of anxiety, sleep will usually improve when a benzodiazepine is administered at bedtime as an antianxiety drug. The benzodiazepines are preferable to the barbiturates as hypnotics because the risk of physical addiction or serious poisoning is much less. The efficacy of the benzodiazepines in the treatment of chronic insomnia has not been demonstrated past 1 month.

The occasional use of the benzodiazepines within controlled limits can be useful. For example, limiting the number of tablets to 10 per month for insomnia will limit tolerance, dependence, and withdrawal. Underlying causes of insomnia, such as depression or alcoholism, should be identified and treated. Nonaddicting agents such as trazodone may be useful in the treatment of insomnia, and, unlike the benzodiazepines, no tolerance or dependence is produced even with chronic use. Nonpharmacologic management of sleep disorders should be instituted before any benzodiazepine is prescribed. Several patients with new prescriptions for "sleeping pills" have discussed the pot of coffee they drink after dinner. [What's wrong with this picture?] (Box 11-1).

TREATMENT OF EPILEPSY (SEIZURES) Diazepam or lorazepam is the drug of choice for treatment of repetitive, intractable seizures (status epilepticus) that require intravenous therapy. They are also used for treatment of seizures caused by local anesthetic toxicity. Orally administered diazepam is of little value, even as a maintenance anticonvulsant. Oral clonazepam is used as an adjunct to other anticonvulsants for some difficult-to-control types of seizures. It is also used in the management of mood disorders.

TREATMENT OF ALCOHOLISM The benzodiazepines are used in the treatment of the alcohol withdrawal syndrome. Administration of an adequate amount of a benzodiazepine can prevent the emergence of the signs and symptoms of acute alcohol withdrawal, such as agitation and tremor. It has not been shown that they prevent hallucinations or delirium tremens.

CONTROL OF MUSCLE SPASMS Benzodiazepines are used to control the muscle spasticity that accompanies various diseases such as multiple sclerosis and cerebral palsy. They are used for the relief of pain and spasm of back strain. Studies have suggested that the benzodiazepines are more effective than other muscle relaxants such as methocarbamol, carisoprodol, and chlorzoxazone.

MANAGEMENT OF THE DENTAL PATIENT TAKING BENZODIAZEPINES

The dental implications of the benzodiazepines are described in Box 11-2.

Dental procedures. Orally administered diazepam has been shown to be more effective than placebo in allaying apprehension in patients undergoing restorative procedures. It is used in combination with other agents such as opioids and anticholinergic agents. If diazepam is used for the initial treatment of patients with dental anxiety, it is hoped that future appointments may

Box 11-1 Nonpharmacologic Management of Sleep Disorders

Before patients are given agents to treat insomnia, they should be questioned about their sleep hygiene habits. Insomnia can be due to many organic, psychologic, or situational causes. The following is a list of several habits that should be followed to minimize insomnia:

- Regular bedtime—regardless of whether slept
- Remain in bed no more than 20 minutes without sleeping
- Get up if not sleeping and perform a quiet activity
- Regular awakening—awake at 6 AM even if sleep only began at 5 AM
- Limit sleeping to fewer hours—go to bed later, get up earlier
- Exercise during the day (not within 3 hours of bedtime)
- Light snack (warm milk) at bedtime
- No naps during the day regardless of sleep problems
- Avoid caffeine within 8 hours of bedtime (cola, sodas [check label for caffeine], coffee, tea).
- No smoking within 8 hours of bedtime

- Get ready for bed by engaging in quiet activities such as reading or listening to music. Use "noise" to disguise noise—listen to white noise.

Repeated use of a sedative-hypnotic leads to tolerance and a need for an increased dose to produce the same effect. Most agents become increasingly less effective with regular use. These agents can also alter sleep architecture (REM sleep).

The normal sleep cycle is illustrated in Figure 11-4. *Latency* is the time it takes to get to sleep. Sleeping is distributed between rapid eye movement (REM) sleep (30%) and non-rapid eye movement (NREM) sleep. NREM sleep has four stages.

Benzodiazepines reduce the latency, REM sleep, and NREM sleep stages 3 and 4, while increasing stage 2. When benzodiazepines have been used chronically and are discontinued, rebound REM sleep frequently occurs, resulting in an increase in vivid dreams. Some patients continue to take benzodiazepines because they do not want to experience these scary dreams.

be completed successfully without benzodiazepines increases. For preoperative dental anxiety, a benzodiazepine should be chosen that has a fast onset of action and a relatively short half-life. This reduces the patient's waiting time and allows resumption of normal functions as soon as possible. The dose used should be in the range of the usual hypnotic dose (see Table 11-2). Examples of agents used for dental anxiety might include triazolam [trye-AY-zoe-lam] (fast onset and short half-life) and diazepam (very fast onset, but long half-life). Lorazepam [lor-A-ze-pam] or alprazolam [al-PRAY-zoe-lam] (inter-

mediate onset, but relatively short half-lives) could also be used, especially in the elderly. Midazolam [MID-ay-zoe-lam], is available for parenteral (Versed injection) and oral (Versed syrup) use in the United States and is used to sedate children. The parenteral midazolam product can be administered orally to sedate children. Patients given either oral or parenteral benzodiazepines should not be allowed to oper-

> Ensure that the patient has a responsible driver before releasing.

BOX 11-2 MANAGEMENT OF THE DENTAL PATIENT TAKING BENZODIAZEPINES

- Additive CNS depression with other CNS depressants (including alcohol).
- Avoid in addicts or women who could be pregnant (women age 11-63).
- Keep track of exact number prescribed and usage rate in patient's chart.
- Use glucuronidated type in elderly and in patients on cimetidine.
- Warn about sedation and amnesia.
- Match onset and duration with dental procedure requirements.
- Make sure patient has arranged for transportation to and from dental appointment.

ate a motor vehicle, and the dental staff should ensure that a driver is present before dismissing the patient.

Premedication. The benzodiazepines have been used before surgical procedures to allay anxiety. They may be used orally or parenterally. The amnesia that occurs with parenteral administration is especially useful during stressful dental procedures. Diazepam is used as a premedication before general anesthesia, endoscopy, cardioversion, gastroscopy, sigmoidoscopy, and cystoscopy.

Conscious sedation. Conscious sedation using the benzodiazepines is usually accomplished by intravenous administration. Diazepam, lorazepam, or midazolam, given intravenously, provides muscle relaxation and anterograde (amnesia occurs to events after the injection) amnesia during dental procedures. Although amnesia quickly follows the intravenous injection of diazepam and midazolam, it depends on several variables. Amnesia may be expected to persist for up to 45 minutes; therefore postoperative instructions

should be provided in writing. Benzodiazepines available for parenteral administration (diazepam, midazolam, lorazepam) are used for conscious sedation. The patient maintains reflexes, but time perception is lost and amnesia reduces the patient's memory. Because parenteral benzodiazepines have been associated with respiratory depression and arrest when used for conscious sedation, they require continuous monitoring of respiratory and cardiac function. Emergency drugs, equipment, and personnel must be available. Because some states and insurance companies are placing controls on the use of intravenous sedation in dentistry, those dentists without additional training cannot use conscious sedation. Additional training is now a requirement before dentists can administer parenteral benzodiazepines.

BARBITURATES

Barbiturates [bar-BI-tyoo-rates], the original sedative-hypnotic agents, are chemically related to each other and have similar pharmacologic effects. The barbiturates differ from each other mainly in their onset and duration of action. Because these agents have been used for years, the problems with their use have been well documented. Although nonbarbiturate sedative-hypnotics have been developed in an attempt to overcome the problems of the barbiturates, these agents seem to possess little if any clinical advantage over the barbiturates. Benzodiazepines have almost completely replaced barbiturates in clinical use, except for the barbiturates' use as anticonvulsants and to induce general anesthesia.

CHEMISTRY

The clinically useful barbiturates are formed by substitution of R groups (organic groups) on the barbiturate nucleus—sites A and B. Another modification of the barbiturate nucleus involves replacing the oxygen atom with a sulfur atom—

site C. Compounds with the S-substitution are effective as intravenous agents such as thiopental.

PHARMACOKINETICS

Barbiturates are well absorbed orally and rectally. Because the injectable solutions are highly irritating, the intramuscular route is avoided and the drugs are used intravenously. The intravenous agents are inactivated mainly by redistribution from their site of action in the CNS to the muscles and finally to adipose tissue. The short- and intermediate-acting barbiturates are rapidly and almost completely metabolized by the liver. Long-acting barbiturates are largely excreted through the kidneys as the free drug. Patients with liver damage may have an exaggerated response to short- and intermediate-acting agents, and patients with renal impairment may have an accumulation of the long-acting agents.

MECHANISM OF ACTION

Barbiturates produce their effect by enhancing GABA receptor binding. They prolong the opening of the chloride channels. In higher doses they may also act directly on the chloride channels without GABA presence. This mechanism is less specific than that of the benzodiazepines, which may account for their ability to induce surgical anesthesia and produce pronounced generalized CNS depressant effects.

PHARMACOLOGIC EFFECTS

Central nervous system depression. The principal effects of the barbiturates are on the CNS. When normal doses of these agents are administered, relaxation occurs and the EEG speeds up. With larger doses, the inhibitory fibers of the CNS are depressed, resulting in disinhibition and euphoria. If excitation occurs at this point, it is due to depression of the inhibitory pathways.

Anxiety relief cannot be separated from the sedative effects. When higher doses are administered, hypnosis can be produced. The administration of even higher doses can result in anesthesia, with respiratory and cardiovascular depression and finally arrest. This progressive CNS depression parallels that caused by most CNS depressants, including general anesthetics (see Chapter 11).

The CNS depression produced by the barbiturates is additive with other agents that produce this effect. For example, a patient who takes an alcoholic beverage or is given an opioid analgesic will show additive CNS depression.

Analgesia. Barbiturates have no significant analgesic effects. Even doses that produce general anesthesia do not block the reflex response to pain. Patients in pain may become agitated and even delirious if barbiturates are administered without analgesic agents.

Anticonvulsant effect. The barbiturates possess anticonvulsant action. The long-acting agents such as phenobarbital are used in the treatment of epilepsy (see Chapter 16).

ADVERSE REACTIONS

Sedative or hypnotic doses. In the usual therapeutic doses, barbiturates are relatively safe. However, one should be aware that CNS depression may be exaggerated in elderly and debilitated patients or those with liver or kidney impairment. In some patients, especially the elderly, barbiturates can have an idiosyncratic effect, causing stimulation instead of sedation. Barbiturates can cause fetal harm if administered to a pregnant woman.

Anesthetic doses. With higher doses, barbiturate concentrations attained in the blood can be lethal. High concentrations are used for **intubation** or very short procedures. Coughing and laryngospasm have been reported with intravenous use of barbiturates. High doses may reversibly depress liver and kidney function, reduce gastrointestinal motility, and lower body temperature.

Acute poisoning. When barbiturates are prescribed, the possibility that acute poisoning can occur must be considered. Although a lethal dose can only be approximated, severe poisoning will follow the ingestion of 10 times the hypnotic dose, and life is seriously threatened when more than 15 times the hypnotic dose is consumed. The cause of death when an overdose occurs is respiratory failure. The treatment includes conservative management and treatment of specific symptoms.

CHRONIC LONG-TERM USE

Chronic use of barbiturates can lead to physical and psychologic dependence. Long-term use produces a state similar to alcohol intoxication. The barbiturate addict becomes progressively depressed and is unable to function. Tolerance develops to most effects of barbiturates but not to the lethal dose. Therefore a larger and larger dose must be used to produce an effect and this dose can approximate the lethal dose. Cross-tolerance occurs among barbiturates and between the barbiturates and nonbarbiturate sedative-hypnotic agents. Chapter 26 discusses the abuse of the barbiturates.

CONTRAINDICATIONS

The use of barbiturates is absolutely contraindicated in patients with intermittent porphyria or a positive family history of porphyria. This is because barbiturates can stimulate and increase the synthesis of porphyrins, which are already at an excessive level in this metabolic disease. In fact, the barbiturates have been reported to precipitate an acute attack of porphyria.

DRUG INTERACTIONS

Because barbiturates are potent stimulators of liver microsomal enzyme production, they are involved in many drug interactions. These enzymes are responsible for the metabolism of many drugs, so that an increase in these enzymes could increase the rate of drug destruction and decrease the duration of action. For example, an epileptic patient who is currently receiving phenytoin (Dilantin) is subsequently given phenobarbital. The phenobarbital stimulates the liver microsomal enzymes that destroy the phenytoin, as well as the phenobarbital, more rapidly, which could cause convulsions. This drug interaction requires repeated doses and is not significant with a single dose. Some barbiturate drug interactions are listed in Box 11-3.

USES

The therapeutic uses of barbiturates are determined by their duration of action (Table 11-4).

Box 11-3 BARBITURATE DRUG INTERACTIONS	
Barbiturates Reduce These Drugs' Effects	**Barbiturate's Effect Enhanced by These Drugs**
Acetaminophen β-Blocker Birth control pills Chlorpromazine Doxycycline Estrogens Griseofulvin Phenytoin Quinidine Steroids Tricyclic antidepressants Warfarin	Disulfram Monoamine oxidase inhibitors Propoxyphene **Enhanced or Additive CNS Depressant Effect** Alcohol CNS depressants Opioid analgesics

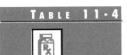

TABLE 11-4 Barbiturates

Barbiturate Groups	Route of Administration*	Onset†	Duration‡ of Action (hr)
Ultrashort acting			
Methohexital (Brevital)	IV	Immediate	Minutes
Thiamylal sodium (Surital)	IV	Immediate	Minutes
Thiopental sodium (Pentothal)	IV	Immediate	Minutes
Short acting			
Pentobarbital (Nembutal)	PO, IM, IV, rectal	10-15 min	3-4
Secobarbital (Seconal)	PO, IM, IV, rectal	10-15 min	3-4
Immediate acting			
Amobarbital (Amytal)	PO, IM, IV, rectal	40-60 min	6-8
Butabarbital (Butisol)	PO	40-60 min	6-8
Long acting			
Phenobarbital (Luminal)	PO, IM, IV	30>60 min	10-16
Mephobarbital (Mebaral)	PO	30>60 min	10-16

*IV, Intravenously; PO, orally; IM, intramuscularly.
†Onset = time until the drug's action begins.
‡Duration = length of drug's action.

The ultrashort-acting agents such as thiopental [thye-oh-PEN-tal] are used intravenously for the induction of general anesthesia. For very brief procedures they may be used alone. For more extensive procedures they are used to induce stage III surgical anesthesia (see Chapter 12).

The short- and intermediate-acting agents have little medical use. Benzodiazepines have replaced them for insomnia and anxiety relief. The short-acting agents were popular agents of abuse because of their fast onset of action.

The long-acting barbiturates, such as phenobarbital [fee-noe-BAR-bi-tal], are used for the treatment of epilepsy.

NONBARBITURATE SEDATIVE-HYPNOTICS

During the last half of the nineteenth century the bromides and chloral hydrate began to replace opium, alcohol, and belladonna as drugs for the production of sedation. The barbiturates were introduced in 1904 and, until the benzodiazepines, remained the principal sedative-hypnotic drugs used in dental and medical practice. Benzodiazepines are now used almost exclusively over barbiturates.

Nonbarbiturate sedative-hypnotics offer few advantages over barbiturates. Preoperative sedation in dental practice can usually be obtained with a properly selected dose of a benzodiazepine. Because of tradition, chloral hydrate has been used for sedation of children in dentistry.

ZOLPIDEM (AMBIEN)

Zolpidem [zole-PI-dem] (Ambien) is a sedative-hypnotic agent that was recently developed and is indicated for the short-term management of insomnia. Its structure is unlike the benzodiazepines. In contrast to some sedative-hypnotic agents that act at all BZ receptors, zolpidem interacts with the $GABA_A$

> Zolpidem is a newer sedative-hypnotic used for insomnia.

receptor at the BZ_1 receptor. Although zolpidem retains its hypnotic and anxiolytic effects, its receptor specificity gives zolpidem less muscle relaxant and anticonvulsant effects. It may be less likely to produce depression of sleep stages 3 and 4. Side effects include headache, drowsiness, dizziness, and diarrhea. Myalgia, arthralgia, sinusitis, and **pharyngitis** have been reported. Amnesia may also occur. Withdrawal can occur if abruptly stopped after 1 to 2 weeks of use. Rebound insomnia may be experienced. Its quicker onset of action makes it useful to initiate sleep. Because of its fast onset of action, it should be taken immediately before bedtime. It is claimed that zolpidem is less addicting and that less tolerance develops to this agent. [Time will tell!]

Zolpidem is likely to be useful in dentistry when an oral anxiolytic agent is desired for relaxing an anxious dental patient. Like all anxiolytic agents used orally, use of this agent requires another person to transport the patient to and from the dental appointment. Its quick onset of action may allow the patient to come to the office to receive medication.

CHLORAL HYDRATE

Chloral hydrate [KLOR-al HYE-drate] (Noctec) is an inexpensive, orally effective sedative-hypnotic drug with a rapid onset (20 to 30 minutes) and fairly short duration of action (about 4 hours). Therapeutic doses do not produce pronounced respiratory or cardiovascular depression. An exaggerated effect occurs in patients with advanced liver or kidney disease. Large doses or long-term use may produce peripheral vasodilation and hypotension with some degree of myocardial depression. Gastric irritation can be minimized by taking chloral hydrate in diluted solutions with milk or food. The highly irritating effect of chloral hydrate on the mucosa can produce aspiration, especially in struggling children. Its disagreeable odor and taste can be partially masked in a flavored syrup. As with all sedative-hypnotic agents, psychologic or physical dependence may follow prolonged use of this drug.

Chloral hydrate has been used in dentistry for the preoperative sedation of children. The child's hypnotic dose of chloral hydrate, when used alone, is 50 mg/kg, up to a maximum of 1 gm. Benzodiazepines are a safer choice for sedation of children.

MEPROBAMATE

Meprobamate [me-proe-BA-mate] (Equanil, Miltown) was developed to enhance the central muscle-relaxing action of mephenesin. Its assumed potential to relieve anxiety furthered its rapid acceptance, but abuse of this agent quickly followed.

Although meprobamate's action is difficult to differentiate from that of barbiturates, it is classed by some

> Used extensively in earlier years.

sources as a minor tranquilizer. It has sedative properties and anticonvulsant action. With increasing dosage, the relief of anxiety is accompanied by a slower reaction time and a definite slowing of learning. Meprobamate has some muscle-relaxing properties.

In the usual therapeutic doses meprobamate has few side effects. With an acute overdose, meprobamate produces excessive CNS depression manifested as unconsciousness, cardiovascular collapse, respiratory depression, and death. As with barbiturates, the treatment of an overdose is supportive and symptomatic.

Chronic long-term administration of meprobamate can lead to CNS tolerance, compulsive use, and physical dependence. When the drug is abruptly stopped, the withdrawal syndrome can occur.

The use of meprobamate with other CNS depressants will produce an additive effect. With chronic use, cross-tolerance develops between meprobamate and other sedative-hypnotics, including alcohol.

Minor tranquilizers such as meprobamate have been associated with an increased risk of congenital malformations during the first trimester of pregnancy. Their use in pregnant women should be avoided. Meprobamate crosses the placenta and is present in the fetal circulation and in breast milk.

Meprobamate is occasionally used for the treatment of anxiety and as a daytime sedative or nighttime hypnotic. It is used in products that are a combination of agents (e.g., Equagesic [meprobamate plus aspirin]) and has been employed in dentistry as an antianxiety agent and muscle relaxant. No current clinical trials are available.

Centrally Acting Muscle Relaxants

Drugs classified as centrally acting muscle relaxants exert their effects on the CNS to produce skeletal muscle relaxation.

Pharmacologic Effects

Some degree of sedative effect is exhibited by all the CNS muscle relaxants because their action is on the CNS. Xerostomia is common with these agents.

Clinical tests have shown that the sedative effects dominate over the "selective" [NOT!] muscle relaxant activity. When administered intravenously in humans, these agents have been shown to be useful in treating muscle spasm and producing muscle relaxation for certain orthopedic procedures. When these agents are given orally, they do not produce the flaccidity obtainable with intravenous administration. Thus, until better studies are produced, the beneficial effects of these drugs can be logically ascribed to their sedative action. They are used for back and neck pain and in patients with muscle spasms related to a car accident.

Individual Centrally Acting Muscle Relaxants

Centrally-acting skeletal muscle relaxants exert their muscle relaxing properties indirectly by producing CNS depression. They act in the CNS and have no direct effect on striated muscle, the motor endplate, or nerve fibers. They do not directly relax tense skeletal muscles.

They share many common side effects, including gastrointestinal upset, sedation, and dizziness (results of CNS depression). All of the muscle relaxants have the potential to produce allergic reactions. Most of these agents can produce xerostomia, and the dental health care worker should question the patient about self-treatment for this adverse effect.

Structurally related to the tricyclic antidepressants, cyclobenzaprine [sye-kloe-BEN-za-preen] (Flexeril) is considered to be the strongest muscle relaxant. Because sedation occurs in about 40% of the patients taking cyclobenzaprine, it is the most sedating muscle relaxant. It also is most likely to produce xerostomia with an incidence of 30%. (This demonstrates typical effects and adverse reactions of drugs—the more pharmacologic effect [wanted], the more adverse reactions [unwanted].)

A relative of meprobamate is carisoprodol [kar-eye-soe-PROE-dole] (Soma). Chlorzoxazone [klor-ZOX-a-zone] (Paraflex) may discolor the urine purple-red. The patient should be warned about this harmless property. Other muscle relaxants include methocarbamol [meth-oh-KAR-ba-mole] (Robaxin) and orphenadrine [or-FEN-a-dreen] (Norflex). Diazepam (Valium), a benzodiazepine, also possesses muscle relaxant properties and is used for spastic muscles such as occurs in multiple sclerosis. Table 11-5 lists the muscle relaxants that function via the brain and their selected side effects and usual doses.

Use. The muscle relaxants are all indicated as an adjunct to rest and physical therapy for relief of muscle spasm associated with acute painful musculoskeletal conditions. Questions about their

TABLE 11-5   Centrally Acting Skeletal Muscle Relaxants

Drug	Comments	Dose (mg)*
Carisoprodol (Soma)	Tachycardia, flushing	350 tid-qid
Chlorzoxazone (Parafon Forte DSC)	GI distress, hypersensitivity, CNS depression	250 tid-qid
Methocarbamol (Robaxin)	CNS depression, GI distress, rash	1000-1500 qid
Orphenadrine (Norflex)	Xerostomia, GIT, vision changes	100 bid
Cyclobenzaprine (Flexeril)	Sedation (40%), zerostomia (30%)	10 tid
Diazepam (Valium)	Benzodiazepine	5-10 bid-tid

*bid, Twice per day; tid, 3 times per day; qid, 4 times per day; ONS, central nervous system; GI, gastrointestinal; GIT, gastrointestinal tract.

efficacy still linger in the literature. They are also used in the treatment of temporal mandibular disorder (TMD) because relaxation of the muscles is helpful to the symptoms. The success of muscle relaxants in the management of TMD has not been documented.

MISCELLANEOUS AGENTS

BACLOFEN

Baclofen [BAK-loe-fen] (Lioresal) inhibits both monosynaptic and polysynaptic reflexes at the spinal level. It also inhibits GABA, but whether this is related to its action is unknown. It is indicated for spasticity from multiple sclerosis or spinal cord injuries or diseases. Baclofen has been used to treat trigeminal neuralgia, although it is not FDA-approved for this purpose. Drowsiness, weakness, headache, and insomnia have been reported. Nausea, dry mouth, taste disorder, and urinary frequency have been seen. Lowering of the seizure threshold and an increase in ovarian cysts in rats have also occurred.

TIZANIDINE

Tizanidine [tye-ZAN-i-deen] (Zanaflex) is a short-acting muscle relaxant. It is a centrally act-ing α-adrenergic receptor agonist (like clonidine) that increases presynaptic inhibition of motor neurons. Like clonidine it can produce sedation, drowsiness, hypotension, and xerostomia.

DANTROLENE

Dantrolene [DAN-troe-leen] (Dantrium) affects the contractile response of the skeletal muscle by acting directly on the muscle itself. It dissociates the excitation-contraction coupling, probably by interfering with the release of calcium from the sarcoplasmic reticulum. It is indicated in the treatment of spasticity from upper motor neuron disorders such as spinal cord injury, cerebral palsy, or multiple sclerosis. It is also used orally to prevent and intravenously to treat malignant hyperthermia brought on by succinylcholine or inhalation of general anesthetics. The hepatotoxicity it produces is more common with higher doses and in older female patients taking concomitant medications. This agent may cause drowsiness or photosensitivity.

BUSPIRONE

Buspirone [byoo-SPYE-rone] (BuSpar) is unique in structure and action. It is the only member of this anxiolytic group. Its onset of action is about 1 week. It is discussed separately because of its unique structure and pharmacology. Its mechanism of action is unknown, but it is believed to be related to interactions with neurotransmitters in the CNS, including serotonin (5-HT_{1A}), dopamine, and cholinergic and α-adrenergic receptors. Buspirone undergoes first-pass metabolism and has a half-life of 2 to 4 hours.

The pharmacologic effect of buspirone is called *anxioselective* because of its selective anxiolytic action without hypnotic, anticonvulsant, or muscle relaxant properties. It produces much less CNS depression than other sedative-hypnotic agents and does not affect driving skills. Some patients experience nervousness or insomnia. Buspirone does not produce tolerance or dependence. It does not appear to be addicting and there is no withdrawal syndrome. Due to the mechanism by which buspirone produces its anxiolytic effect, most patients prefer the benzodiazepines [surprise?].

GENERAL COMMENTS ABOUT ANTIANXIETY AGENTS

ANALGESIC-SEDATIVE COMBINATIONS

The use of an analgesic and a sedative-hypnotic agent to provide concomitant sedation and analgesia is rational for the following reasons:
* Relief of both anxiety and pain is frequently required in one patient.
* Sedatives potentiate analgesic agents.
* Sedatives may induce excitation when given without an analgesic to patients with uncontrolled pain.
* Anxiety can lower the pain threshold.

Both sedation and analgesia can be obtained from the opioid analgesics alone. However, it is not desirable to prescribe an opioid to add sedation to analgesia unless the analgesic potency is required. In cases in which anxiety is an important component in pain relief either a nonopioid or opioid can be used concomitantly with a sedative. This combination may be prescribed separately, although a few fixed-dose products are available. A combination of a sedative with an analgesic is available in butalbital compound (Fiorinal) or butalbital/APAP (Fioricet). If the patient's pain is more severe, then an opioid and a sedative-hypnotic agent can be prescribed. The above-mentioned agents are available mixed with codeine (#3 contains 30 mg codeine), to make Fiorinal #3. In a dental patient in whom anxiety is magnifying the pain reaction, the prescribing of a combination agent might be useful.

SPECIAL CONSIDERATIONS

Certain generalizations should be kept in mind when discussing the use of the antianxiety agents. The dental practitioner plays an important role in helping the patient understand the possible effects of the drugs used to allay anxiety. The patient may raise questions about these agents, and their effects should be explained. Dental patients who are to use antianxiety agents should be driven to and from the dental appointment.

Drugs are not to be used as a substitute for patient management. The practitioner should not rely exclusively on drugs to provide a calm and cooperative patient. The dental team should exhibit a confident and relaxed manner. A pleasant, soothing office atmosphere is of great importance in relaxing an anxious patient. Appropriate use of music of the patient's choice can reduce anxiety. Drugs should not be substituted for patient education or for the proper psychologic approach to patient care.

> Psychologic management must accompany use of antianxiety agents.

When an agent for anxiety relief is required, the selection of the specific drug should be based on a knowledge of the advantages and disadvantages of the agents available and an understanding of the needs and contraindications related to the case at hand.

CAUTIONS

Regardless of the antianxiety agent selected, the following precautions pertain:

- Patients with impaired elimination may experience exaggerated effects of these medications. These persons include the young, the elderly, the debilitated, and those with liver or kidney disease.
- Depression caused by all sedative-hypnotics will add to depression caused by other CNS depressants that the patient may be taking. The patient should be made aware of this, particularly in regard to alcohol; over-the-counter sleep aids may also be a potential source of hazard.
- The patient should understand that the drug prescribed will make it unsafe to perform acts requiring full alertness and muscle coordination, such as driving a car. *The patient should be accompanied by a responsible adult who can drive the patient home.* The patient should be warned against signing any important papers or documents. These cautions are particularly important if the patient has not taken the drug previously and, consequently, his or her response is less predictable.
- Psychic and physical dependence has been observed with almost all drugs used to allay anxiety. The dentist should realize that these drugs have abuse potential and should limit their use accordingly. This is particularly important in regard to the treatment of chronic conditions or persons with a history of addiction or alcoholism.
- Suicide may be attempted by taking sedative-hypnotic drugs. Consequently, the amount of drug prescribed should be limited to the minimum required to accomplish the therapeutic objective. With benzodiazepines the therapeutic index is wide unless mixed with alcohol.

- These drugs should never be administered to pregnant women or those who may be pregnant unless the potential benefit to the mother outweighs the risk to the fetus.
- Sedatives do *not* provide analgesia. In fact, the use of a sedative without adequate pain control may cause the patient to become highly excited and act irrationally. However, sedatives may potentiate the effect of an analgesic taken concomitantly.

REVIEW QUESTIONS

1. Define the following terms:
   a. sedative
   b. hypnotic
   c. minor tranquilizer
   d. major tranquilizer
2. State four differences between the major and minor tranquilizers.
3. Name two major pharmacologic effects of barbiturates.
4. List the four groups of barbiturates, and state what differentiates these groups from one another.
5. Describe the major adverse reactions of barbiturates.
6. Name the one absolute contraindication to the use of barbiturates.
7. Describe the mechanism of the most important drug interaction of barbiturates. Explain its clinical implication with an example.
8. Explain the important differences between barbiturates and nonbarbiturate sedative-hypnotic agents.
9. Name four benzodiazepines, two that are short-acting and two that are long-acting.
10. State the major differences between benzodiazepines and barbiturates.
11. Explain why sedative-hypnotic agents are controlled substances and how their abuse determines on what schedule (II, III, or IV) they are listed.
12. Describe the adverse effect that can occur

with intravenous administration of diazepam but not with oral administration.

13. Describe the parenteral use of diazepam and midazolam in dentistry. State a benefit over oral use.
14. State three uses of benzodiazepines.
15. Review the following terms:
    a. tolerance
    b. withdrawal
16. Describe the specific treatment for a benzodiazepine overdose.
17. Describe the inappropriate use of "ruffies."
18. State the potential advantages of zolpidem.
19. Explain why chloral hydrate is still used by some dentists as premedication for children.

CHAPTER 12

General Anesthetics

> . . . reversible loss of consciousness and insensibility to painful stimuli . . .

The state of general anesthesia is produced by a heterogeneous group of potent central nervous system (CNS) depressants. They produce a reversible loss of consciousness and insensibility to painful stimuli. Contemporary general anesthetic techniques employ balanced anesthesia that uses a combination of drugs to minimize adverse reactions, taking into account the patient's physical status and preanesthetic and postanesthetic needs. Respiratory depression and loss of protective reflexes are associated with general anesthesia; thus the patient must be constantly monitored and evaluated. Because of the variety of anesthetic agents and techniques employed, special training and a complete working knowledge of the pharmacology of each anesthetic is essential.

The hospital operating room provides the optimum setting for procedures requiring general anesthesia because of the ready availability of monitors for vital signs, resuscitative equip-

> Hospital = General anesthesia

ment, and trained anesthesia personnel. However, oral and maxillofacial surgeons have used general anesthetic drugs in their offices for many years with an excellent safety record. Nitrous oxide, because it is not a complete anesthetic, is not useful alone as a general anesthetic. In the dental office, it is commonly employed to allay patient anxiety. Other general anesthetic drugs, in less than anesthetic doses, are now used to provide conscious sedation in the dental office. In today's practice the dental health team should have an understanding of the principles of general anesthesia because it is an indispensable tool for the needs of special patients, as well as for extensive oral and maxillofacial surgery.

> Dental office = Conscious sedation

HISTORY

The original method to produce general anesthesia involved either strangulation or cerebral concussion. Later, opium, belladonna, hemp, and alcohol were used to render patients unconscious. During this time the surgeries were "quick and dirty." About the middle of the 1800s, true general anesthetics were discovered in the United States.

Colton began giving public demonstrations of "laughing gas" (nitrous oxide) for 25¢ admission (similar to the "hits" of nitrous oxide placed in balloons that are sold in New Orleans). Wells, a dentist, attended one of Colton's lectures, at which a drug clerk volunteered to receive the gas. A fight commenced, and the clerk gashed his leg; under Wells questioning, the clerk said that he felt no pain. The next day Wells extracted one of his own teeth after having administered nitrous oxide and felt no pain. Nitrous oxide was produced

> Dentists—significant contributions to discovery

in 1776, and 20 years later Davy suggested that the administration of nitrous oxide might be useful in surgery.

Wells began using nitrous oxide in his own dental practice. Finally, he persuaded William T. G. Morton, a former dental partner who was studying medicine, to arrange a demonstration of nitrous oxide before the Harvard University medical faculty. During the demonstration the patient awoke too soon and began screaming. Nitrous oxide's low potency accounted for its failure (it is an incomplete anesthetic without anoxia).

> Dentists Wells and Morton recognized N_2O and ether's use.

Soon after, ether was manufactured and ether "jags" (sort of like parties) were held. Another dentist, William Morton, knew of both ether and nitrous oxide. He practiced administering these drugs to himself and the family dogs and cats. His demonstration of the use of ether began with the surgeon turning to Morton and stating, "Well, sir, your patient is ready." After using ether successfully to anesthetize the patient, Morton said to the surgeon, "Here's your patient!" The surgeon replied, "Gentlemen, this is no humbug."

In the following months, Morton attempted to patent ether and spent the remainder of his life futilely trying to collect claims for compensation from the U. S. government. Both Wells and Morton became insane and committed suicide because they did not get credit for their "finds." Even though the accomplishments of these dentists were not recognized during their lifetimes, the medical and dental professions today applaud their contribution to methods of alleviating pain.

MECHANISM OF ACTION

Many theories have been proposed to explain the mechanism of action of the various general anesthetic agents, but, unfortunately, none of them does so completely. It may seem relatively simple to say that these drugs are CNS depressants. However, the way in which they depress the normal functions of the CNS is a matter complicated by lack of knowledge of the physiologic and biochemical events of arousal and unconsciousness. Proposed mechanisms for the action of different general anesthetics involve an increase in the threshold for firing, facilitation of inhibitory γ-aminobutyric acid (GABA), and a decrease in duration of opening of nicotinic receptor–activated cation channel. The increase in the threshold or hyperpolarization is a result of the activation of the potassium channels.

STAGES AND PLANES OF ANESTHESIA

The degree of CNS depression produced by general anesthetics must be carefully titrated to avoid excessive cardiorespiratory depression. In 1920, Guedel described a system of stages and planes to describe the effects of anesthetics (Figure 12-1). Although

> Guedel described four stages and planes of anesthesia.

FIGURE 12-1 *Stages and planes of anesthesia. In, Inspiration. (Modified from Meyers FH, Jawetz E, Goldfien A:* Review of medical pharmacology, *ed 7, Los Altos, Calif, 1980, Lange Medical Publications.)*

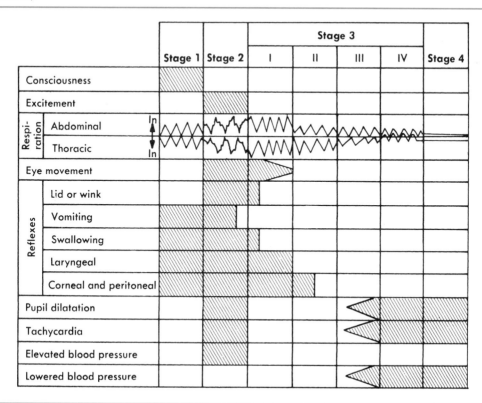

| | | Stage 1 | Stage 2 | Stage 3 | | | | Stage 4 |
				I	II	III	IV	
Consciousness								
Excitement								
Respiration	Abdominal							
	Thoracic							
Eye movement								
Reflexes	Lid or wink							
	Vomiting							
	Swallowing							
	Laryngeal							
	Corneal and peritoneal							
Pupil dilatation								
Tachycardia								
Elevated blood pressure								
Lowered blood pressure								

Guedel's classification applied to the effects produced by ether when using the open drop method of administration, modern anesthetic techniques seldom show these exact stages. However, the four stages are briefly described because Guedel's terminology is still used to describe the depth of anesthesia.

Induction is the term used to refer to the quick change in the patient's state of consciousness from stage I to stage III.

1. **Stage I—analgesia.** This stage is characterized by the development of analgesia or reduced sensation to pain. The patient is conscious and can still respond to command. Reflexes are present and respiration remains regular. Some amnesia may also be evident. Nitrous oxide, as used in the dental office, maintains the patient in stage I. The end of this stage is marked by the loss of consciousness.

2. **Stage II—delirium or excitement.** This stage begins with unconsciousness and is associated with involuntary movement and excitement. Respiration becomes irregular and muscle tone increases. Sympathetic stimulation produces tachycardia, mydriasis, and hypertension. This can be an uncomfortable time for the patient because emesis and incontinence can occur. As the depth of anesthesia increases, the patient begins to relax and proceeds to stage III.

   For the patient's comfort and safety it is important to have a smooth and rapid induction. The ultrashort-acting barbiturates accomplish this readily. When balanced anesthesia is used, the patient does not pass through each stage as listed. Adjunct drugs reduce the side effects of each of the drugs used during surgery.

3. **Stage III—surgical anesthesia.** This is the stage in which most major surgery is performed. This stage is further divided into four planes that are differentiated on the basis of eye movements, depth of respiration, and muscle relaxation. The onset of stage III (planes I and II) is typically charac-

terized by the return of regular respiratory movements, muscle relaxation, and normal heart and pulse rates. Reflexes associated with the eye disappear during planes I and II. Vomiting reflex stops during stage II, but swallowing reflex is maintained until stage III, plane I [good plan?]. Plane III is associated with decreased skeletal muscle tone, dilated pupils, tachycardia, and hypotension. Beginning in plane III and progressing to plane IV is characterized by intercostal muscle paralysis (diaphragmatic breathing remains), absence of all reflexes, and extreme muscle flaccidity. If the depth of anesthesia is allowed to increase, the patient will rapidly progress to the last stage with cessation of all respiration.

4. **Stage IV—respiratory or medullary paralysis.** Stage IV is characterized by complete cessation of all respiration (diaphragmatic respiration last to go) and subsequent circulatory failure. At this point pupils are maximally dilated and blood pressure falls rapidly. If this stage is not reversed immediately, the patient will die. Respiration must be artificially maintained.

Modern anesthetic techniques now employ more rapidly acting agents than those associated with the four stages of Guedel. Flagg's approach, used to describe the levels of anesthesia (Figure 12-2), includes the following categories:

1. **Induction.** The induction phase encompasses all the preparation and medication necessary for a patient up to the time the operation begins, including preoperative medications, adjunctive drugs to anesthesia, and anesthetics required for induction.

2. **Maintenance.** The maintenance phase begins with the patient at a depth of anesthesia sufficient to allow surgical manipulation and continues until completion of the procedure.

3. **Recovery.** The recovery phase begins with the termination of the surgical procedure and continues through the postoperative period until the patient is fully responsive to the environment.

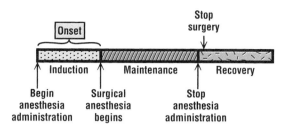

FIGURE 12-2 *Levels of anesthesia. Induction, maintenance, recovery.*

TABLE 12-1   Adverse Reactions to General Anesthetics

SYSTEM	EFFECT/COMMENT
Cardiovascular system	Cardiovascular collapse Cardiac arrest
Arrhythmias	Ventricular fibrillation Halogenated hydrocarbons
Blood pressure	Hypertension (stage II) Hypotension
Respiration	Depressed respiration (stage III) Respiratory arrest (stage IV) Laryngospasm—ultrashort-acting barbiturates "Boardlike" chest—neuroleptanalgesia
Explosions/flammability	Cyclopropane Ether
Teratogenicity (either male or female exposure)	Chronic exposure—fetal abnormalities Spontaneous abortions
Hepatotoxicity (repeated exposure)	Operating room personnel Halogenated hydrocarbons
Other	Headache, fatigue, irritability, addicting

ADVERSE REACTIONS

> Risk of general anesthesia must always be compared with the benefit of surgery.

The goals of surgical anesthesia are good patient control, adequate muscle relaxation, and pain relief. To produce anesthesia, potent CNS depressants are given in relatively high doses, and many combinations of drugs are employed in balanced anesthesia.

The hazards encountered with the administration of general anesthetics are summarized in Table 12-1. Current knowledge dictates that dental offices in which inhalation anesthetics are used should adopt methods to minimize exposure to the operator, including scavenging systems, adequate ventilation, good technique, and safe equipment.

GENERAL ANESTHETICS

CLASSIFICATION OF ANESTHETIC AGENTS

The general anesthetic agents can be classified according to their chemical structure or route of administration. Table 12-2 categorizes the agents according to their routes of administration.

Inhalation anesthetics. Inhalation agents can be divided into gases and volatile liquids. The liquids are vaporized and carried to the patient in the form of gas. The inhalation agents are often used in combination, using oxygen as a carrier gas.

The volatile general anesthetics are liquids that evaporate easily at room temperature because of their low boiling

> Volatile anesthetics—liquids that easily evaporate

points. They are classified chemically as halogenated hydrocarbons because they contain fluorine, chlorine, or bromine in their structure. These are potent agents with limited solubility in body tissues, and they have successfully replaced the use of ether in anesthesia. Both methoxyflurane and halothane are used infrequently; enflurane and isoflurane are the more popular volatile liquids in current use.

TABLE 1 2 - 2 **Classification of General Anesthetics by Route of Administration**

INHALATION AGENTS		INTRAVENOUS AGENTS
GASES	VOLATILE LIQUIDS	

Nitrous oxide
Cyclopropane*
	Halogenated hydrocarbons
	  Chloroform*
	  Trichoroethylene*
	  Halothane (Fluothane)
	Halogenated ethers
	  Methoxyflurane (Penthane)
	  Enflurane (Ethrane)
	  Isoflurane (Forane)
	Ethers
	  Diethyl ether (ether)*
		Barbiturates
		  Methohexital (Brevital)
		  Thiamylal (Surital)
		  Thiopental (Pentothal)
		Dissociative
		  Detamine (Ketalar)
		Opioids
		  Morphine
		  Fentanyl (Sublimaze)
		  Sufentanil (Sufenta)
		  Alfentanil (Alfenta)
		Neuroleptic
		  Fentanyl with droperidol (Innovar)
		Benzodiazepines
		  Diazepam (Valium)
		  Midazolam (Versed)
		Others
		  Etomidate (Amidate)
		  Propofol (Diprivan)

*Of historic interest only.

TABLE 1 2 - 3 **Physical Properties of Selected Inhalation General Anesthetics**

	BLOOD:GAS PARTITION COEFFICIENT*	BRAIN:BLOOD PARTITION COEFFICIENT	MAC† (%)	COMMENTS
Nitrous oxide	0.47; very low solubility in blood; quick onset	1.1	Need >100%	Incomplete anesthetic, rapid onset and recovery
Halothane	2.3	2.9	0.75	Intermediate onset and recovery
Methoxyflurane	12; high solubility in blood; slow onset	2	0.16; small % anesthetized	Slow onset and recovery

*Partition coefficient (relative distribution by area; blood, brain, gas).
†Minimal alveolar concentration (amount that anesthetizes 50% of people).

Physical factors. The concentration of anesthetic in the inspired mixture is proportionate to its partial pressure or tension. The depth of anesthesia produced is a function of the tension (partial pressure) of the anesthetic agent in the brain. The most important physical factors that influence brain anesthetic tension are the tension of the anesthetics in the inspired gases, the rate and volume of delivery of anesthetics to the lungs, and anesthetic's solubility in body tissues. Induction can be hastened with high initial anesthetic concentrations and hyperventilation. As anesthesia depth develops, both the concentration and rate of delivery are reduced to maintenance levels.

Table 12-3 gives the physical properties of some of the anesthetics. The solubility in blood is expressed by the blood/gas partition coefficient. The less soluble the anesthetic is in body tissues, the more rapid the onset and recovery. The low solubility of nitrous oxide (0.47) correlates well with its rapid onset and recovery. This physical factor allows the anesthesiologist to adjust quickly the desired level of anesthesia. In contrast, halothane, with its higher solubility (2.30), has a longer induction and recovery and changes in level of anesthesia occur more slowly.

The term *minimum alveolar concentration* (MAC) is used to compare the potency of general anesthetic inhalation agents. *MAC* is defined as the minimal alveolar concentration of an anesthetic at 1 atmosphere required to prevent 50% of patients from responding to a supramaximal surgical stimulus. The MAC of nitrous oxide is greater than 100, whereas halothane has a MAC of 0.75, isoflurane of 1.15, and enflurane of 1.68. The lower MAC values indicate the more potent anesthetics. The volatile anesthetics are given in combination with nitrous oxide to reduce the concentration of each while improving MAC values.

Intravenous anesthetics. The intravenously administered general anesthetics are a diverse group of CNS depressants that include the opioids, the ultrashort-acting barbiturates, and the benzodiazepines. Although most injectable general anesthetics are administered intravenously, one agent, ketamine, can also be given intramuscularly. These drugs find their greatest utility in induction of general anesthesia, but may occasionally be used as single agents for short procedures. Although they offer the advantage of convenience, the depth and duration of anesthesia are less easily controlled compared with the inhalation agents. Certain drugs of this group are used in less than anesthetic doses to produce conscious sedation (reflexes retained).

NITROUS OXIDE

Nitrous [NYE-trus] oxide (N_2O) is a colorless gas with little or no odor and is the least soluble in blood of all the inhalation anesthetics. Because of its low potency (MAC greater than 100), nitrous oxide used alone is unsatisfactory as a general anesthetic agent. However, if anesthesia is first induced with a rapidly acting intravenous agent and nitrous oxide–oxygen combination (N_2O-O_2) is administered in combination with a volatile anesthetic, excellent balanced anesthesia is produced. This synergistic combination permits the use of reduced doses of the more potent inhalation anesthetics. N_2O-O_2 is given throughout most surgical procedures that necessitate the use of general anesthesia because it reduces the concentration of other agents needed to obtain the desired depth of anesthesia.

Administration of nitrous oxide–oxygen (N_2O-O_2) has become a primary part of dental office anxiety reduction procedures. This use should not be confused with general anesthesia, because the intent is to provide for a lightly sedated and relaxed patient. When nitrous oxide is properly administered, the patient remains conscious with the protective reflexes intact. Nitrous oxide provides anxiety relief coupled with analgesia. Thus the N_2O-O_2 sedation technique may be adopted to offer increased patient cooperation and comfort in a wide range of dental office procedures. The dental practitioner should be thoroughly familiar with this use of nitrous oxide. The dentist (and in some states the hygienist) may legally administer nitrous oxide.

| Provides anxiety relief |

N_2O-O_2 sedation technique involves increasing the concentration of nitrous oxide to titrate the patient to a desired level of sedation. The gas mixture is delivered to the patient by flow meters that control both the volume flow and the ratio of nitrous oxide to oxygen. Starting with 100% oxygen for 2 to 3 minutes, nitrous oxide is gradually added in 5% to 10% increments until

| Onset rapid—a few minutes |

the patient response indicates that the desired level of sedation has been achieved. Once the nitrous oxide is added, onset occurs rapidly within 3 to 5 minutes. Table 12-4 shows the typical responses observed with increasing concentrations of nitrous oxide. The percent of nitrous oxide required for patient comfort is variable and may range from 10% to 50% (average 35%).

At the termination of a N_2O-O_2 sedation procedure, the patient should be placed on 100% oxygen for at least 5 minutes. Recovery occurs rapidly as nitrous oxide is quickly re-

moved from the tissues. If the mask is removed without the oxygen recovery period and the patient allowed to breathe room air, a phenomenon known as *diffusion* **hypoxia** may result. This occurs because of the rapid outward flow of nitrous oxide accompanied by oxygen and carbon dioxide. The loss of carbon dioxide, a stimulant to respiratory drive, could decrease ventilation with resultant hypoxia. Patients may complain of headache or other side effects if this occurs. Recovery with 100% oxygen avoids this problem.

As has been implied, the N_2O-O_2 technique has sufficient advantages to recommend its consideration in many dental procedures. Among its advantages are the following:

- **Rapid onset.** Because of the poor solubility of nitrous oxide in blood, it has a rapid onset of action (less than 5 minutes).
- **Easy administration.** No injection is required to obtain an effect. The patient merely breathes through his or her nose.
- **Close control.** The proper depth of sedation can be maintained by adjusting the percentage of nitrous oxide administered.
- **Rapid recovery.** Recovery is obtained rapidly with a full return to presedative psychomotor capacity. Thus the need for the patient to be accompanied to the dental appointment can often be eliminated.
- **Acceptability for children.** Nitrous oxide is a valuable adjunct in managing some apprehensive children. However, it cannot be used when a child's behavior is openly defiant or hysterical, and it is not a substitute for good behavioral management techniques. The analogy of "going into space" can be effective.
- **Relaxed dental team.** The N_2O-O_2 technique will not only offer comfort to the patient and increase the acceptance of dental procedures but will also afford more relaxed treatment; that is, the dental team should be less tense and fatigued at the end of the office day.

TABLE 12-4   Signs and Symptoms in Response to Nitrous Oxide and Oxygen Conscious Sedation

CONCENTRATION N_2O	RESPONSE
10% to 20%	Body warmth Tingling of hands and feet
20% to 30%	Circumoral numbness Numbness of thighs
20% to 40%	Numbness of tongue Numbness of hands and feet Droning sounds present Hearing distinct but distant Dissociation begins and reaches peak Mild sleepiness Analgesia (maximum of 30%) Euphoria Feeling of heaviness or lightness of body
30% to 50%	Sweating Nausea Amnesia Increased sleepiness
40% to 60%	Dreaming, laughing, giddiness Further increased sleepiness, tending toward unconsciousness Increased nausea and vomiting
50% and over	Unconsciousness and light general anesthesia

From Bennett CR: *Conscious-sedation in dental practice*, St Louis, 1974, Mosby.

Pharmacologic effects.

CENTRAL NERVOUS SYSTEM SEDATION Sedation is the main pharmacologic effect of nitrous oxide on the CNS, resulting in analgesia and amnesia. Although there is sensory depression, auditory perception is not affected to the same degree. Therefore a tranquil, quiet environment is required for N_2O-O_2 analgesic procedures. The use of personal audio input may be useful.

CARDIOVASCULAR Peripheral vasodilation is produced by nitrous oxide administration. This property may facilitate venipuncture should an intravenous route be desired after starting the N_2O-O_2.

GASTROINTESTINAL Nausea and vomiting with N_2O-O_2 analgesia are uncommon, but can occur. The patient should eat a light meal before the appointment but should be warned to avoid a large meal within 3 hours of the appointment.

Changing the concentration of nitrous oxide slowly and monitoring the patient closely can minimize this response. When nitrous oxide is administered slowly, its effects may be evaluated according to Table 12-4 and are summarized as follows:

- The best indicator of the degree of sedation is the patient's response to questions. The patient may exhibit slurred speech or a slow response. Do not evaluate only as anesthesia is adjusted. Perform repeated evaluations throughout the dental procedure. Examples of evaluations are asking the patient to "open your mouth" or "move one finger" and noting the patient's response (can be slow, but should respond).
- The patient is relaxed and cooperative and reports a feeling of euphoria. Local anesthetic injections elicit little if any response at this time. Analgesia produced by nitrous oxide is variable but can be equivalent to morphine injection in patients.
- The patient is easily able to maintain an open-mouth position in the desired plane.
- The patient's eyes may be closed but can be opened easily.
- The respiration, pulse rate, and blood pressure are within normal limits.

In addition to the features already mentioned, the patient often indicates that the time frame the procedure occupied in his or her consciousness has been dramatically decreased. The operating time may appear to the patient to be one third or one half as long as it is in reality. This can be especially beneficial in long procedures, particularly in dental schools. Interesting audio input acts as a distractor for both hearing and feeling sensations.

Adverse reactions.

Invariably, complications that have occurred with the use of N_2O-O_2 techniques have been the

> Be smart, think, monitor patient.

result of misuse or faulty installation of equipment. Obviously, an installation that crossed oxygen and nitrous oxide lines could be disastrous if nitrous oxide were given under the assumption that it was oxygen! [This has occurred, and taking off the mask would have saved the patient's life!] Cases of dentists abusing N_2O, including use of solely N_2O, and taping the mask to the face have resulted in reported deaths.

All cylinders are now colored in a standardized manner. Nitrous oxide cylinders are blue, and oxygen cylin-

> O_2 = Green tank
> N_2O = Blue tank

ders are green. The cylinders are also "pin coded" to prevent inadvertent mixing of cylinders and lines.

Equipment with built-in safety features is now available. The inhalation administration equipment in every dentist's office should automatically limit the percentage of nitrous oxide that can be administered and have a fail-safe system that shuts down the nitrous oxide if the oxygen runs out.

The combination of nitrous oxide with other sedative regimens can increase the potential danger of causing a general anesthetic state. The limits of this sedation technique must be understood by every member of the dental health team. If inhalation sedation is combined with other modes of sedation, the entire dental staff must be trained and prepared for the possibility that general anesthesia might be produced.

Contraindications

RESPIRATORY OBSTRUCTION Because the nasal passages are used for gaseous exchange, upper respiratory obstruction or a stuffy nose is an absolute contraindication to this technique. Other respiratory diseases must also be carefully evaluated.

CHRONIC OBSTRUCTIVE PULMONARY DISEASE In the normal person, the drive for ventilation (breathing) is stimulated by an elevation in the partial pressure of carbon dioxide ($PaCO_2$). The partial pressure of oxygen (PaO_2) can vary widely without stimulating ventilation in the normal patient. Patients with chronic obstructive pulmonary disease (COPD), because their ventilation is compromised, experience a gradual rise in $PaCO_2$ over time. Because this mechanism becomes resistant to this stimuli, a new stimulant emerges—the partial pressure of $PaCO_2$. The patient's ventilation is then driven by a decrease in PaO_2. If a patient with COPD is given oxygen and the PaO_2 rises, the stimulant to breathing is removed and there is the possibility of inducing apnea. For patients with COPD ASA III and IV it is suggested that oxygen be limited to less than 3L/min. Another recommendation is that patients with severe COPD should be given oxygen by nasal cannula during a dental appointment, especially if pain or stress is expected (increased oxygen demand).

EMOTIONAL INSTABILITY Because patients may experience euphoria or an altered sensorium with nitrous oxide analgesia, a patient's emotional instability is a relative contraindication to its use. Patients taking psychotherapeutic medication must be carefully evaluated before nitrous oxide is used. These medications include phenothiazines, tricyclic antidepressants, and lithium. Fanciful dreams occurring during a procedure may be interpreted on recovery as having actually occurred; therefore a female staff member must be in attendance when a female patient is being treated by a male dentist or dental hygienist and nitrous oxide is used. Aberrant sensations may lead to unfounded accusations unless this requirement is strictly enforced. This is required to minimize legal liability (record in chart).

Pregnancy. Safety of the use of nitrous oxide in pregnant patients or administration by pregnant operators is in question. Although no direct correlation

> Pregnant dental practitioners should determine levels in dental operatory before exposure.

has yet been found, several epidemiologic studies cast doubt on the safety of exposure to nitrous oxide during pregnancy. The incidence of spontaneous abortion or miscarriages is higher in female operating personnel chronically exposed to anesthetic agents or in wives of male operators. Women exposed to high levels of nitrous oxide (greater than 5 hours per week) were significantly less fertile than unexposed women. This is especially important to female dentists and dental hygienists because dental operatories have been found to have higher concentrations of gases than even hospital operating rooms (poorer ventilation).

Dental health care workers should be aware of the concentration of nitrous oxide that is present in the dental operatories in which they practice. Machines are available that monitor the concentration of nitrous oxide. Scavenger systems can that retrieve much of the expired gas can be installed, and room air turnover of the room air can be increased. Checking of the nitrous oxide concentration in the dental operatory should be repeated, especially if the usage changes or personnel are pregnant.

Abuse. The dental team should be knowledgeable about the potential hazards associated with the abuse of nitrous oxide. Case histories describing the chronic abuse of nitrous oxide (self-administration) have reported examples of nitrous–induced **neuropathy**. Symptoms include numbness and paresthesia of the hands or legs that progresses to more severe neurologic symptoms with continued abuse. Nitrous oxide has been shown to reduce the activity of methionine synthetase, the enzyme involved with the function of vitamin B_{12}. Thus it appears that the chronic abuse of nitrous oxide and attendant neurologic symptoms may be related to its effect on the utilization of vitamin B_{12}. Liver and kidney problems have also been mentioned in association with nitrous oxide abuse. The profile of the average dentist who abuses nitrous oxide is male, white, and in his 40s. He has abused many drugs in the past (polydrug abuser) and has previously self-administered nitrous oxide "therapeutically." As his abuse progresses, he spends more time at the office alone. The number of missed appointments with patients increases, and his attention is focused on issues other than his patients (using the drug again).

Situations that determine that abuse has begun include self-using nitrous oxide, using nitrous oxide for anything other than dental anxiety, using nitrous oxide during lunch or after work, sneaking nitrous oxide use, begin missing appointments, not keeping promises, and problems with family or money.

HALOGENATED HYDROCARBONS

Halothane. Halothane [HA-loe-thane] (Fluothane) has a fruity, pleasant odor, and is nonflammable and nonexplosive. Both induction and recovery are relatively rapid. The MAC for halothane is 0.77, but is improved to 0.29 when combined with 70% nitrous oxide. Because halothane is nonirritating to bronchial mucous membranes, it is considered safe for use on asthmatics. As with the other volatile agents, the halothane dose must be carefully regulated to prevent overt respiratory depression. Muscle relaxation is incomplete, and peripheral neuromuscular blocking drugs such as *d*-tubocurarine are required. Halothane also depresses renal function and can cause uterine muscle relaxation.

Halothane's effects on the cardiovascular system are manifested by increased vagal activity producing bradycardia and peripheral vasodilation that lowers the blood pressure. It sensitizes the myocardium to the cardiac stimulatory effects of injected epinephrine and norepinephrine, leading to serious cardiac arrhythmias such as ventricular fibrillation (Figure 12-3). During surgery epinephrine is used (Box 12-1) with halothane and cardiac rhythm is monitored. If arrhythmias occur, antiarrhythmics are administered.

Evidence indicates a causal relationship between halothane use and postanesthetic hepatitis. Approximately 15% of halothane is metabolized in the liver, and these metabolites have been suggested as a cause of liver damage. Even though halothane has proved to be a reliable and effective general anesthetic for many years, the occurrence of this adverse effect has diminished its popularity. For this reason, halothane is contraindicated in patients in whom a previous exposure to halothane or other halogenated hydrocarbons has been followed by postanesthetic

FIGURE 12-3 *Hydrocarbon inhalation can produce fatal arrhythmias; don't imitate KISS.*

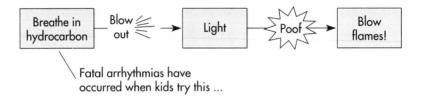

Don't imitate the rock group KISS...

Breathe in hydrocarbon → Blow out → Light → Poof → Blow flames!

Fatal arrhythmias have occurred when kids try this ...

liver toxicity. Patients with impaired liver function should be treated only with care.

Enflurane. Enflurane [EN-floo-rane] (Ethrane) is a halogenated ether anesthetic with a pleasant smell. Induction and recovery are rapid because of its low tissue solubility. The MAC is 0.57 when combined with nitrous oxide. Enflurane depresses respiration, but this effect is controlled with assisted ventilation. It provides good analgesia and muscle relaxation, but supplemental muscle relaxants are still required. The heart is depressed and blood pressure is reduced. Myocardial sensitization to injected epinephrine is less than that associated with halothane.

Adverse effects associated with enflurane use include alteration in electroencephalographic activity; thus excessive motor activity may occur during anesthesia. Careful regulation of anesthetic depth prevents such muscular activity. Enflurane is metabolized less than other volatile agents, which may account for the absence of hepatotoxicity. Enflurane also produces a transient depression of renal function.

Isoflurane. A drug chemically related to enflurane is isoflurane [eye-soe-FLURE-ane] (Forane). Its low tissue solubility allows for rapid induction and recovery. Isoflurane has a slightly pungent smell, limiting the induction concentration, which otherwise could provoke coughing.

When isoflurane is combined with 70% nitrous oxide, the MAC is 0.5. The pharmacologic effects of isoflurane are similar to those of the other halogenated ethers and include respiratory depression, reduced blood pressure, and muscle relaxation. Only a small amount of isoflurane undergoes metabolism, and liver toxicity does not seem to be a problem. Limited if any myocardial sensitization to injected epinephrine occurs. Nausea, vomiting, and shivering on recovery are comparable to responses to other anesthetic agents. The most undesirable side effect is respiratory acidosis associated with deeper levels of anesthesia. Isoflurane has proved to be a useful and popular drug for general anesthesia.

Desflurane and sevoflurane. The newest halogenated hydrocarbons include desflurane and sevoflurane. They have the

> Desflurane requires special vaporizer.

advantage of having low blood:gas partition coefficient so that they have a more rapid onset and a shorter duration of action than the other halogenated hydrocarbon anesthetics. Unfortunately they have other difficulties. Desflurane's low volatility requires a special vaporizer. Because it induces cough and laryngospasm, it cannot be used for induction. Its recovery, despite its physical properties, does not appear to be faster

Box 12-1 TYPICAL DRUGS ADMINISTERED DURING GENERAL ANESTHESIA

Here is a list of the drugs administered to a patient before and during a surgery for mandibular osteotomy together with a short explanation of their effects and the reasons they were given:

1. Valium 10 mg orally preoperative morning of surgery to relieve anxiety in the immediate preoperative period.
2. Xylocaine 1%—skin wheal to start IV provided localized numbness so the insertion of the IV needle can be accomplished without pain.
3. Fentanyl (Sublimaze) (0.05 mg/ml) 1 ml—a synthetic narcotic that is a strong *analgesic* and provides some degree of sedation. Given intravenously at the beginning of anesthesia administration.
4. Neo-Synephrine Nose Drops 1.0%—6 gtts in each side. Shrinks the nasal mucosa and allows passage via the nose of the plastic endotracheal tube.
5. Warmed normal saline (NS) to soften the endotracheal tube.
6. Xylocaine jelly 2%—to lubricate the endotracheal tube.
7. Xylocaine IV solution (20 mg/cc) 5 ml (100 mg)—IV about 2 minutes before insertion of the endotracheal tube to obtund reflex cough.
8. *d*-Tubocurarine (Curare)—pretreatment for succinylcholine (Anectine) given to prevent fasciculations and postoperative myalgia.
9. Na Pent (Sodium Pentothal)—an ultrashort-acting barbiturate given intravenously to induce sleep. The dose is 4 to 7 mg/kg and averages 210 to 280 mg for an average-size adult. It produces sleep pleasantly and quickly, allowing the other anesthetic agents to be added without discomfort to the patient.
10. Succinylcholine (Anectine) 100 mg—short-acting muscle relaxant that facilitates endotracheal intubation by relaxing the small muscles that operate the vocal cords.
11. Droperidol (Inapsine) 2.5 mg/ml 1.25 mg (0.5 ml)—for nausea control.
12. Nitrous oxide (N_2O)—inhalational agent that produces analgesia and anesthesia.
13. Oxygen—given in a proportion roughly 2 to 2.5 times that normally present in the atmosphere.
14. Isoflurane (Forane)—inhalation anesthetic which produces analgesia, anesthesia, and amnesia.
15. Lacrilube eye ointment—protects the corneas from drying out during the length of time that the anesthesia is administered.
16. Marcaine 0.5% with epinephrine 1:200,000—*injected* into the gums to add a greater degree of analgesia and to retard blood loss during the procedure.
17. Penicillin G Potassium 5 million units IV—given prophylactically to prevent infection with organisms that normally reside in the mouth.
18. Solu-Medrol 250 mg IV—given to retard postoperative soft tissue swelling.

These are some of the medications given after the surgery:

1. Dalmane—a benzodiazepine for sleep.
2. Emete-Con—for control of nausea.
3. Meperidine (Demerol)—an opioid analgesic, duration 2-4 hours, onset 10 to 15 minutes.
4. Phenergan—Phenothiazine, duration 4 to 6 hours, pronounced sedation, *antiemetic*.
5. Kenalog cream—topical corticosteroid (lip).
6. Afrin—topical nasal decongestant.

than that of older agents. Sevoflurane is chemically unstable when exposed to CO_2 absorbents, producing a potentially nephrotoxic compound. Because it releases fluoride (F^-) when metabolized, renal damage may occur.

OTHER GENERAL ANESTHETICS

Ultrashort-acting barbiturates. The ultrashort-acting barbiturates used include methohexital [meth-oh-HEX-i-tal] sodium (Brevital), thiopental [thye-oh-PEN-tal] sodium (Pentothal), and thiamylal [thye-AM-i-lal] sodium (Surital). Although the basic pharmacology of the barbiturates is discussed in Chapter 11, certain facts about these drugs are discussed here.

These ultrashort-acting agents have a rapid onset of action (about 30 to 40 seconds) when given intravenously. Figure 12-4 demonstrates the percent of the dose in each tissue over time. Note that the dose begins in the blood, rapidly goes to the brain (lipid soluble), redistributes to lean tissues (muscles with high vascularity), and finally moves to the fat (lipid soluble, but low perfusion). If repeated doses are given, as is often the case during anesthesia, the drug accumulates in body tissues, resulting in prolonged recovery.

If these drugs are employed as the sole anesthetic for short procedures, the patient will re-

spond to painful stimuli. Because no analgesia is observed with doses that allow the patient to breathe spontaneously, the intravenously administered barbiturates function more effectively when used with a local anesthetic agent as part of a balanced anesthetic technique.

A serious complication with the use of intravenous barbiturates occurs when the solution is accidentally injected extravascularly or intraarterially. Symptoms with extravascular infiltration can range from tissue tenderness to necrosis and sloughing. Intraarterial injection is extremely dangerous and can lead to arteriospasm associated with **ischemia** of the arm and fingers and severe pain.

Other complications with ultrashort-acting barbiturates include laryngospasm and bronchospasm. In some patients, hiccoughs, increased muscle activity, and delirium occur on recovery. Premedication with atropine or opioids has proved reasonably effective in reducing these recovery problems.

The absolute contraindications to the use of ultrashort-acting barbiturates include an absence of suitable veins for administration, status asthmaticus, porphyria, or known hypersensitivity. The dosage should be adjusted, and caution should be taken in patients with asthma or hepatic, renal, or cardiovascular impairment. These drugs can be used alone by trained and qualified practitioners for very short dental procedures or as part of a balanced anesthesia to induce surgical anesthesia (going from stage I to stage III). Because these drugs are potent anesthetics, they should be administered only by qualified individuals, with resuscitative equipment readily available.

Propofol. One of the genral anesthetics that is unrelated to any other general anesthetic is propofol [PROE-po-fole] (Diprivan). It is an intravenous anesthetic that produces an onset of anesthesia in 30 seconds (similar to the barbitu-

> Patient feels good; used for day surgery.

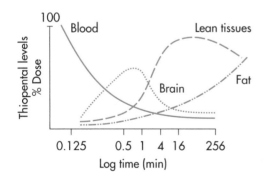

FIGURE 12-4 *Thiopental concentrations in various tissues: fat, muscle (lean tissues), blood, and brain.*

rates) and a duration of action of about 5 minutes. Patients "feel better" and begin ambulation sooner than with other agents. It produces little vomiting and may have antiemetic effects. Propofol can be used for induction and for maintenance of balanced anesthesia. It is very popular for outpatient surgery. Propofol is metabolized in the liver by conjugation to glucuronide and sulfate and excreted in the kidneys with a half-life of 30 to 60 minutes.

Propofol can produce a marked decrease in blood pressure during induction because it produces vasodilation. Apnea occurs in 50% to 80% of patients given propofol. Bradycardia and pain at the injection site can occur. Gastrointestinal adverse reactions have been reported. Hypersensitivity reactions involving hypotension, flushing, and bronchospasm occurred when propofol was dissolved in the original vehicle (polyoxyethylated caster oil) (Cremophor), but this reaction does not occur when it is dissolved in a fat emulsion (Intralipid) or soybean oil. Propofol is a relatively costly anesthetic.

Ketamine. The anesthetic ketamine [KEET-a-meen] (Ketalar) is related chemically to phencyclidine (PCP), a hallucinogen. The anesthetic state ketamine produces has been given the name *dissociative anesthesia* because ketamine appears to disrupt association pathways in the

> Chemically related to phencyclidine (PCP), produces *dissociative* anesthesia.

brain. Under ketamine, the patient appears to be catatonic and has amnesia; ketamine produces analgesia without actual loss of consciousness.

Ketamine may be given intravenously or intramuscularly, with a rapid (1 to 2 minutes) onset of action occurring with either route. It is distributed first to lipid tissues then to more vascular areas. Pharyngeal and laryngeal reflexes remain active, and there is little respiratory change. Ketamine increases cerebral blood flow and stimulates the heart to increase cardiac output. Because excessive salivation is a common finding with ketamine, atropine is a necessary premedication. Muscle tone may increase during its use.

The principal drawback to the use of ketamine is the occurrence of "emergence phenomena," including delirium and hallucinations during recovery. This happens most often in adults, older children, and drug abusers. Reactions of this type can be minimized if visual and auditory stimuli are reduced during recovery. Small doses of an ultrashort-acting intravenously administered barbiturate or benzodiazepine have been employed to control the recovery problem. Specific contraindications include a history of cerebrovascular disease, hypertension, and hypersensitivity to the drug. Psychiatric problems present a relative contraindication. Because protective reflexes of the **pharynx** and **larynx** are active, care should be taken not to stimulate the pharynx. This increase in reflexes in the throat may discourage use in dentistry.

Opioids. The opioids [OH-pee-oyds] have long been used as adjunctive drugs to general anesthesia in preanesthetic medication and to provide analgesia during and after a surgical procedure. Now opioids are used as anesthetic agents as well. The opioids used include morphine, fentanyl (Sublimaze), sufentanil (Sufenta), and alfentanil (Alfenta). These drugs do not significantly alter cardiovascular function or peripheral resistance. Prolonged respiratory depression is the major disadvantage and requires careful attention to ventilatory function throughout the anesthetic period. Reversal of this depression can be produced by the opioid antagonist naloxone.

Droperidol plus fentanyl. The term *neuroleptanalgesia* refers to the so-called wakeful anesthetic state produced by the combination of a neuroleptic drug, droperidol (Inapsine), and a potent opioid analgesic, fentanyl (Sublimaze). Droperidol produces marked sedation and a catatonic state. It is a close relative of haloperidol, an antipsychotic agent. The combination of drugs is marketed as Innovar and is usually given intravenously for a rapid onset. Adding nitrous oxide results in *neuroleptanesthesia*. Return to consciousness appears to be rapid, but the effects of droperidol are long-lasting and recovery is slow.

The adverse effects can be quite serious and include those that would normally be associated with the opioids and major tranquilizers. Respiratory depression and extrapyramidal tremors have occurred. This combination of drugs should be used with great care, especially in patients with pulmonary insufficiency and parkinsonism. A boardlike chest, associated with intercostal muscle paralysis and requiring ventilatory support, has occurred in some patients using IV opioids. Fentanyl is sometimes employed as a sole agent for sedation.

Benzodiazepines. The anxiolytic benzodiazepines have been an integral part of conscious sedation and preanesthetic medication for years. Diazepam (Valium) has been used intravenously for many years. Midazolam (Versed), which is water soluble, does not need a solvent for solution, so one of diazepam's major side effects, thrombophlebitis, can be avoided. Other advantages include that it has a shorter duration of action and produces more amnesia than diazepam. Parenteral lorazepam is also available for similar uses. The benzodiazepines find their greatest application as adjunctive drugs in the balanced anesthesia technique or for conscious sedation. They are discussed in detail in Chapter 11.

BALANCED GENERAL ANESTHESIA

The goals of surgical anesthesia are good patient control, adequate muscle relaxation, and pain relief. There are many agents that can produce general anesthesia. Each drug has its own adverse reaction profile. The many specific steps in Guedel's classification were developed for describing the effects obtained when ether was used alone. Box 12-1 lists all the drugs administered to a single patient who was undergoing retrognathic surgery. Note the use of many agents to keep the patient's consciousness and side effects smooth. When balanced anesthesia is used, the patient readily passes from stage I to stage III (surgical anesthesia), skipping over the signs of stage II. The ultrashort-acting intravenous barbiturates accomplish this readily. These barbiturates are combined with the gases nitrous oxide and oxygen (N_2O-O_2) in combination. These gases are then administered along with a volatile inhalation anesthetic (e.g., halogenated hydrocarbons). If local anesthetic blocks are administered before oral surgery procedures, the depth of general anesthesia can be lighter.

REVIEW QUESTIONS

1. Name and describe the four stages of anesthesia.
2. Differentiate between the three routes of administration of the general anesthetics.
3. State the pharmacologic effects of the general anesthetics.
4. Describe the effects observed with varying concentrations of nitrous oxide.
5. Explain the rationale for the use of several agents during general anesthesia.
6. List the contraindications to the use of nitrous oxide.
7. State the potential hazards associated with the general anesthetic agents.
8. Describe which general anesthetics would be useful in the following situations:
   a. a general dentist's office to allay anxiety without training
   b. a general dentist's office to allay anxiety with training
   c. a periodontist or oral surgeon doing surgery in his or her own office
   d. a periodontist or oral surgeon doing surgery with an anesthetist in his or her office

CHAPTER 13

Vitamins and Minerals

Vitamins—essential in small quantities for the maintenance of cell·structure and metabolism.

The vitamins [VYE-ta-mins], which are essential in small quantities for the maintenance of cell structure and metabolism, are a group of low-molecular-weight compounds. In normal quantities, a vitamin is used to replace that vitamin which is deficient. Vitamins are also employed to treat problems not associated with vitamin deficiency. When used as such they are regarded as drugs. However, few situations exist for which we have proof that vitamins are useful for the treatment of any condition except vitamin deficiency.

Vitamins are classified into two large groups: water soluble and fat soluble. The water-soluble vitamins include the B vitamins and vitamin C. The fat-soluble vitamins are vitamins A, D, E, and K. Vitamins act in three different ways: as coenzymes, antioxidants, or hormones. The water-soluble vitamins act as coenzymes, acting with a specific enzyme that catalyzes a specific reaction. Vitamins C and E act as antioxidants, and vitamin A and D act as hormones. Table 13-1 lists the common names of the vitamins and their deficiencies.

MEASUREMENTS OF VITAMIN NEEDS

RECOMMENDED DIETARY ALLOWANCE

Since the early 1940s, the Food and Nutrition Board of the National Academy of Sciences has been reviewing research to determine dietary recommendations. The original Recommended Daily Allowance (RDA) was designed with the goal of preventing the diseases produced by the deficiency of a certain nutrient. These values were meant to be used to make recommendations for populations (such as school lunches or nursing homes) rather than specific people. These RDAs are not synonymous with an individual's requirement. Individual requirements are influenced by many factors, including but not limited to physical characteristics, dietary habits, sex, pregnancy, lactation, and age. However, the RDAs are set high enough to allow for many variations in patient needs. During the subsequent years, because no other values were available, the RDAs began to be used (inappropriately) to address specific patient needs.

Since the discovery of vitamins, dietitians have been searching the literature for evidence for the vitamin needs of individuals and populations. After the release of the last published RDAs in 1989, a discussion of inappropriate use of the former RDAs was begun. Agreement was

TABLE 13-1   Vitamins and Their Deficiencies

	VITAMIN	NAME	DEFICIENCY	THERAPEUTIC USE
Water soluble	B_1	Thiamine	Beriberi, Wernicke's encephalopathy with alcoholism	Converted to NAD and NADP
	B_2	Riboflavin	Glossitis, chelitis	Converted into FMN and FAD
	B_3	Niacin (nicotinic acid)	Pellagra	Antihyperlipidemic; flushing
	B_6	Pyridoxine		
	B_{12}	Cyanocobalamin	Pernicious anemia	Watch with gout, needs intrinsic factor to be orally absorbed
	—	Folacin (folic acid)	Megaloblastic anemia	Treat deficiency
	C	Ascorbic acid	Scurvy	Antioxidant
Fat soluble	A	Retinoic acid, retinal, retinol (from plant carotene)	Night blindness	Topical/systemic for acne—analogues
	D	Cholecalciferol*, calcitriol (Rocaltrol), ergocalciferol† (Calciferol), dihyprotachysterol (Hytakerol)	Rickets, osteomalacia	Renal disease—preformed 1,25(OH)$_2$ cholecalciferol; osteoporosis in combination with calcium
	E	Tocopherol (α, β, γ)		Antioxidant (combined with selenium), for cardiovascular disease
	K	Phytonadione, menadione	Bleeding	Hepatic cirrhosis

*Called vitamin D_3.
†Form found in vitamin pills, vitamin D_2, product of sun on skin.
FAD, Flavin adenine dinucleotide; *FMN*, flavin mononucleotide; *NAD*, nicotinamide adenine dinucleotide; *NADP*, NAD phosphate.

reached that the use of this one number did not cover all the needs for nutrition information. In 1993, the Food and Nutrition Board initiated a review process, beginning with a symposium. This process of reviewing the literature to determine the appropriate recommendations reflecting the current research began and continues until today. The new RDAs are designed not only to prevent deficiency diseases but to minimize chronic diseases such as heart disease.

The original term, *RDAs* (old), that was used as reference for years has been divided into different more specific recommendations. The definitions of the five new terms appear in Box 13-1. The dietary reference intakes (DRIs) are used to develop diets for healthy people. The DRIs for individual vitamins and minerals began to be compiled and released. In 1997, vitamin D, magnesium, and fluoride were completed and in 1998, the B vitamins were addressed and recommendations released. In the next few years, the rest of the nutrients will be addressed. Currently,

the recommendations available are divided between the RDAs, and if that is unknown, the adequate intake (AIs). In general, the AI for a specific agent is less than the RDA because the RDA allows for some variation.

FALLACIOUS REASONING ABOUT VITAMINS

To determine whether certain vitamins might be useful as drugs, not as vitamin

> Use the scientific method

supplements, scientific principles must be followed. To prove an effect of a vitamin (as a drug, not a supplement) it has to be shown to repeatedly reverse or improve the condition being treated more than the placebo. Neither the person taking the medication nor the person giving the medication can be aware of who is receiving the active medication. These principles apply to the appropriate study of any drug. After the results of the study have been collected, statistical tests must be performed to determine if any statistically significant difference exists between the treatment and the placebo. Testimonies from a few people stating that they "felt better" taking the drug does not constitute a study. Only by use of double blind studies with a placebo control can correct conclusions be drawn.

In the realm of vitamins used for therapeutic effects the scientific thought process has historically been flawed. The fallacious thought process is as follows: If the lack of a certain vitamin produces a specific effect, for example gray hair with pantothenic acid deficiency, then giving that vitamin (pantothenic acid) should be effective in treating gray hair. This conclusion cannot be reached from the data given. This type of thinking is at the basis for many claims for uses of vitamins as drugs. With proper research certain vitamins may or may not be proved to act as drugs in higher doses. Proof is available in the case of niacin in the treatment of hyperlipidemias.

Box 13-1 TERMINOLOGY

Dietary reference intakes (DRIs)—The new standards for nutrition recommendations used to design diets for healthy people; it is a compilation of the four terms defined below.

Estimated average requirement (EAR)—Estimated to meet the requirements of half of the healthy population.

Recommended dietary allowance (RDA)—Related to the EAR, used for individual goals, meets nutrient needs for 97% to 98% of healthy people.

Adequate intake (AI)—Used when an RDA cannot be determined; best guess based on studies available.

Tolerable upper intake level (UL)—Highest amount that can be taken, on average, without any health risk to normal healthy population.

Another faulty thought process is as follows: If a condition improves after the patient takes a vitamin, then the vitamin produced the results. Changes cannot automatically be attributed to a preceding event. This is what spawns superstition.

WATER-SOLUBLE VITAMINS

ASCORBIC ACID (VITAMIN C)

Ascorbic [a-SKOR-bik] **acid,** or vitamin C, chemically is a sugar acid that readily undergoes oxidation to form dehydroascorbic acid. Because of this ability, ascorbic acid is an effective reducing agent. The active isomer is *l*-ascorbic acid.

Source. Good natural sources of ascorbic acid include citrus fruits, green peppers, tomatoes, strawberries, broccoli, raw cabbage, baked potatoes, and papaya. Some food products are fortified with vitamin C. Ascorbic acid is absorbed in the ileum by a Na^+-dependent carrier-mediated mechanism.

Because of its ability to be easily oxidized, ascorbic acid is readily destroyed through cooking, and as much as 50% of the ascorbic acid content of foods can be lost in this manner.

Recommended dietary allowance. The RDA of ascorbic acid for the normal adult is 60 mg. During pregnancy and lactation, stress, or tobacco smoking, the need for this vitamin increases.

Role. The metabolic role of ascorbic acid is probably related to the fact that ascorbic acid and dehydroascorbic acid form a readily reversible oxidation-reduction system. It is thought that this vitamin plays a role in biologic oxidations and reductions in cellular respirations. Ascorbic acid also plays a definite role in connective tissue metabolism, because it is required for the formation of collagen. The function of ascorbic acid can be dramatically demonstrated

in the wound healing process. Scorbutic wounds have a decrease in mature collagen fibrils associated with an accumulation of mucopolysaccharides or ground substance around a matrix of precollagenous fibers. The absence of mature collagen results in abnormal healing that reduces the tensile strength of the wound.

Deficiency. The deficiency of ascorbic acid produces a condition termed *scurvy*.

Scurvy

The manifestations of scurvy occur because of the inability of the connective tissue to produce and maintain intercellular substances such as collagen, bone matrix, dentin, cartilage, and vascular endothelium.

The functions of vitamin C include the following:
* Collagen formation
* Synthesis of epinephrine and norepinephrine
* Synthesis of carnitine, a protein that facilitates transport of fatty acids into mitochondria for β oxidation

The following are manifestations of defective connective tissue formation in vitamin C deficiency:
* Impaired wound healing resulting from a lack of collagen
* Inadequate response to infections
* Alterations in the integrity of capillary walls, manifested as hemorrhages in skin, mucous membranes, muscles, lungs, joints, and gingivae (spongy, edematous, inflamed)
* Lack of formation of bone matrix, resulting in disorganization of epiphyseal line, weakening of bones, pathologic fractures, and resorption of alveolar bone with loosening and loss of teeth

Because humans and other primates cannot synthesize vitamin C, they must obtain it daily from their diet. Diets completely deficient in vitamin C are unusual, and there are few cases of serious vitamin C deficiency (scurvy). After a prolonged period (4 to 5 months) without vitamin C, humans have symptoms of weakness, anorexia, suppressed growth, anemia, lower resistance to infection and fever, swollen and inflamed gums, loosened teeth, swollen wrists and ankle joints, petechial hemorrhages, fracture of ribs at costochondral junctions, and hemorrhaging resulting from capillary fragility in joints, muscle, and intestines. Sailors on ships that were on open seas for a prolonged period learned to carry limes to prevent scurvy.

Adverse reactions. Untoward effects have been reported with the use of megadoses of vitamin C. A daily intake of 1 gm of the vitamin may cause precipitation of oxalate stones in the urinary tract. For this reason, unwarranted use of large quantities of vitamin C is discouraged.

A rebound scurvy has been reported in adults and infants who received megadoses that were then stopped abruptly. Megadoses of ascorbic acid can destroy vitamin B, reduce copper absorption, and increase plasma cholesterol. The implications of these effects have not yet been elucidated.

Clinical considerations. As long ago as 1942, the suggestion was made that vitamin C could be therapeutically beneficial in preventing the common cold. Linus Pauling, reviewing available data, indicated that vitamin C has a substantial beneficial effect in preventing and treating the common cold. Other investigators, reviewing the data, concluded that little if any evidence existed to suggest the effectiveness of vitamin C in either preventing or treating the common cold. Based on current evidence, unrestricted use of ascorbic acid for these purposes cannot be advocated.

Another Pauling hypothesis suggested that large quantities of vitamin C may suppress neoplastic cellular proliferation. He indicated that vitamin C should be used in the management of all types of cancer. Other investigators have been unable to verify his claim. In conclusion, well-controlled, prospective clinical trials are needed to assess the value of ascorbic acid in the management of both the common cold and the cancer patient.

Because vitamin C enhances the absorption of iron, iron is either combined with vitamin C or taken with orange juice to treat **iron deficiency anemia.**

B-COMPLEX VITAMINS

The water-soluble vitamins, except for vitamin C, are known as the *B-complex vitamins.* On a functional basis these vitamins may be subdivided into the following three classes:
- Those that primarily release energy from carbohydrates and fats (thiamine, pyridoxine, niacin, riboflavin, pantothenic acid, biotin)
- Those that, among other functions, catalyze the formation of red cells (folic acid, vitamin B_{12})
- Those that have not been shown to be required in human nutrition (choline and inositol)

A close interrelationship among the B-complex vitamins exists. If a deficiency of one of them occurs, it will impair the utilization of others. Also, the signs and symptoms of a deficiency of individual B vitamins are similar. This is probably because a deficiency of a single member of the B complex seldom occurs. A diet deficient in one B vitamin is usually lacking in other B vitamins.

Thiamine (vitamin B_1). Thiamine [THYE-a-min] (vitamin B_1) is an essential water-soluble vitamin in humans. It is converted in the liver to its active coenzyme form, thiamine pyrophosphate (TPP).

SOURCE Thiamine is present in foods of both animal and vegetable origin. The best sources are pork, whole-grain and enriched breads, cereals and pastas, seeds of legumes such as peas, dried brewer's yeast, and wheat germ. The vitamin tends to be destroyed if heated to about 100° C; therefore significant amounts of this vitamin may be lost if foods are cooked too long above this temperature.

RECOMMENDED DIETARY ALLOWANCE The RDA for thiamine is 1.5 mg for adult (between 15 to 50 years old) males, 1.1 mg for adult females. Table 13-2 lists RDAs for other groups. Thiamine requirements parallel the caloric or carbohydrate content of the diet.

ROLE TPP plays a principal role in intermediary metabolism. It is a coenzyme required for the oxidative decarboxylation of α-keto acids. In this role TPP is sometimes referred to as *cocarboxylase.*

Beriberi

DEFICIENCY The severe deficiency of thiamine leads to a condition known as beriberi. Characteristics of beriberi are peripheral neuritis, muscle weakness, paralysis of the limbs, enlargement of the heart, tachycardia, and edema (typical of wet beriberi). Gastrointestinal tract effects include loss of appetite and intestinal atony, and constipation may also be present. The symptoms of mild thiamine deficiency are less characteristic. They include tiredness and apathy, loss of appetite, moodiness and irritability, pain and paresthesias in the extremities, slight edema, decreased blood pressure, and lowered body temperature.

Possible oral manifestations of thiamine deficiency are burning tongue, ageusia, and hyperesthesia of the oral mucosa.

The most common cause of thiamine deficiency in the United States is alcoholism. Both poor appetite and the effect of alcohol on the nerves may exacerbate this problem. Both Wernicke's encephalopathy and Korsakoff's psychosis can result if a severe deficiency exists.

ADVERSE REACTIONS Thiamine is usually nontoxic, even in large parenteral doses. However, in patients who are hypersensitive to thiamine, pruritus, sweating, nausea, respiratory distress with hypotension, vascular collapse, and death have occurred.

CLINICAL CONSIDERATIONS For treatment of a variety of manifestations

Wernicke's—alcoholism

of thiamine deficiencies, including beriberi and peripheral neuritis, which is associated with pellagra, thiamine is used. In acute Wernicke's encephalopathy, which occurs in some chronic alcoholics, thiamine is administered intravenously. It can temporarily correct certain genetic metabolic disorders (maple syrup urine disease and subacute necrotizing encephalomyelopathy). It has also been used as an insect repellent, but there is no evidence of its effectiveness.

Riboflavin (vitamin B₂). Riboflavin [RYE-boe-flay-vin] (vitamin B_2) is a water-soluble vitamin composed of flavin and D-ribitol.

SOURCE Riboflavin occurs abundantly in both plants and animals. However, dairy products and meat (especially organ meats such as liver) are the best sources of this vitamin. It is also present in green leafy vegetables and yeast. Riboflavin is relatively stable to heat, and cooking will not cause an appreciable loss. It is destroyed by ultraviolet radiation.

RECOMMENDED DIETARY ALLOWANCE The RDA for riboflavin ranges from 1.3 (adult females) to 1.8 mg (young adult men). See Table 13-2 for requirements for other groups. Requirements for riboflavin usually parallel caloric intake or metabolic body size.

ROLE Riboflavin functions in the body as a component of two flavoprotein coenzymes, ri-

TABLE 13-2 Food and Nutrition Board, National Academy of Sciences—National Research Council Recommended Dietary Allowances (RDAs),[a] Revised 1989 (Designed for the Maintenance of Good Nutrition of Practically All Healthy People in the United States)

Age (yr) and Sex Group	Weight[b] kg	Weight[b] lb	Height[b] cm	Height[b] inches	Protein (gm)	Fat-Soluble: Vit A (μg RE[c])	Vit D (μg[d])	Vit D AI (mg/day)	Vit E (mg α-TE[e])	Vit K (μg)	Water-Soluble: Vit C (mg)	Thiamin (mg)	Riboflavin (mg)	Niacin (mg NE[f])	Vit B6 (mg)	Folate (μg)	Vit B12 (μg)	Calcium RDA	Calcium AI (mg/day)	Phosphorus (mg)	Magnesium RDA (mg)	Magnesium AI (mg)	Iron (mg)	Zinc (mg)	Iodine (μg)	Selenium (μg)
INFANTS																										
0.0-0.5	6	13	60	24	13	375	7.5	5	3	5	30	0.3	0.4	5	0.3	25	0.3	400	210	300	40		6	5	40	10
0.5-1.0	9	20	71	28	14	375	10	5	4	10	35	0.4	0.5	6	0.6	35	0.5	600	270	500	60		10	5	50	15
CHILDREN																										
1-3	13	29	90	35	16	400	10	5	6	15	40	0.7	0.8	9	1.0	50	0.7	800	500	800	80		10	10	70	20
4-6	20	44	112	44	24	500	10	5	7	20	45	0.9	1.1	12	1.1	75	1.0	800	800	800	120		10	10	90	20
7-10	28	62	132	52	28	700	10	5	7	30	45	1.0	1.2	13	1.4	100	1.4	800	1000[g]	800	170		10	10	120	30
MALES																										
11-14	45	99	157	62	45	1000	10	5	10	45	50	1.3	1.5	17	1.7	150	2.0	1200	1300	1200	270		12	15	150	40
15-18	66	145	176	69	59	1000	10	5	10	65	60	1.5	1.8	20	2.0	200	2.0	1200	1300	1200	400		12	15	150	50
19-24	72	160	177	70	58	1000	10	5	10	70	60	1.5	1.7	19	2.0	200	2.0	1200	1000	1200	350	400	10	15	150	70
25-50	79	174	176	70	63	1000	5	5	10	80	60	1.5	1.7	19	2.0	200	2.0	800	1000	800	350	420	10	15	150	70
51+	77	170	173	68	63	1000	5	10	10	80	60	1.2	1.4	15	2.0	200	2.0	800	1200	800	350	420	10	15	150	70
FEMALES																										
11-14	46	101	157	62	46	800	10	5	8	45	50	1.1	1.3	15	1.4	150	2.0	1200	1300	1200	280	240	15	12	150	45
15-18	55	120	163	64	44	800	10	5	8	55	60	1.1	1.3	15	1.5	180	2.0	1200	1300	1200	300	360	15	12	150	50
19-24	58	128	164	65	46	800	10	5	8	60	60	1.1	1.3	15	1.6	180	2.0	1200	1000	1200	280	310	15	12	150	55
25-50	63	138	163	64	50	800	5	5	8	65	60	1.1	1.3	15	1.6	180	2.0	800	1000	800	280	320	15	12	150	55
51+	65	143	160	63	50	800	5	10	8	65	60	1.0	1.2	13	1.6	180	2.0	800	1200	800	280	320	10	12	150	55
PREGNANT					60	800	10	5	10	65	70	1.5	1.6	17	2.2	400	2.2	1200	1000-1300	1200	320	350-400	30	15	175	65
LACTATING																										
1st 6 months					65	1300	10	5	12	65	95	1.6	1.8	20	2.1	280	2.6	1200	1000-1300	1200	355	310-360	15	19	200	75
2nd 6 months					62	1200	10	5	11	65	90	1.6	1.7	20	2.1	260	2.6	1200	1000-1300	1200	340	310-360	15	16	200	75

[a] The allowances, expressed as average daily intakes over time, are intended to provide for individual variations among most normal persons as they live in the United States under usual environmental stresses. Diets should be based on a variety of common foods in order to provide other nutrients for which human requirements have been less well defined. See text for detailed discussion of allowances and of nutrients not tabulated.

[b] Weights and heights of reference adults are actual medians for the U. S. population of the designated age, as reported by National Health and Nutrition Examination Survey II. The median weights and heights of those under 19 years of age were taken from Hamill PVV, Drizd TA, Johnson CL, Reed RB, Roche AF, and Moore WM: Physical growth. National Center for Health Statistics Percentiles, Am J Clin Nutr 32:607, 1979. The use of these figures does not imply that the height-to-weight ratios are ideal.

[c] Retinol equivalents. 1 retinol equivalent = 1 μg retinol or 6 μg β-carotene. See text for calculation of vitamin A activity of diets as retinol equivalents.

[d] As cholecalciferol. 10 μg cholecalciferol = 400 IU of vitamin D.

[e] α-Tocopherol equivalents. 1 mg d-α tocopherol = 1 α-TE. See text for variation in allowances and calculation of vitamin E activity of the diet as α-tocopherol equivalents.

[f] 1 NE (niacin equivalent) is equal to 1 mg of niacin or 60 mg of dietary tryptophan.

[g] Approximated.

From National Research Council. Food and Nutrition Board Recommended Dietary Allowances, 10th ed., Washington, DC, National Academy Press, 1989.

boflavin phosphate (flavin mononucleotide [FMN]) and flavin adenine dinucleotide (FAD). Flavoprotein coenzymes in turn are proteins that act as electron acceptors and are involved in a variety of oxidation-reduction reactions. Riboflavin is also indirectly involved in maintaining the integrity of the erythrocytes.

DEFICIENCY Symptoms of riboflavin deficiency usually involve the lips, tongue, and skin. Sore throat and angular stomatitis (cheilosis) appearing as an ulceration with painful fissuring at the corners of the mouth are early and frequent findings. The lips may be either unusually red or whitish because of desquamation. Later, glossitis can occur, with the dorsum of the tongue becoming pebbly or granular. Contact with food or drink may produce pain or a burning sensation on the tongue. In some instances the tongue may become magenta or purplish-red. Excessive salivation and enlargement of the salivary glands may occur. Skin manifestations include a greasy, scaling inflammation around the nose, cheeks, and chin. Involvement of the scrotum and the vulva is frequent. Other manifestations of a severe riboflavin deficiency are normocytic, normochromic anemia, and neuropathy.

ADVERSE REACTIONS Riboflavin has not been associated with any toxicity.

CLINICAL CONSIDERATIONS Riboflavin deficiency is most likely to be seen in alcoholics, economically deprived individuals, or patients with severe gastrointestinal disease that causes loss of appetite, vomiting, and malabsorption syndromes. Oral contraceptives and probenecid may be associated with an increased need for riboflavin. The manifestations of riboflavin deficiency are difficult to distinguish from those of other B vitamin deficiencies because of the similarities in syndromes. The discovery of a deficiency of riboflavin warrants the use of a multivitamin because deficiency of several vitamins often coexists. The ease of measuring riboflavin

in the urine has prompted its use as a marker in drug studies to measure compliance.

Niacin or nicotinic acid (vitamin B$_3$). Niacin [NYE-a-sin], or nicotinic acid, is converted in the body to niacinamide or nicotinamide, its active form to serve as a vitamin. These water-soluble organic compounds have the ability to alleviate a deficiency syndrome known as *pellagra.*

SOURCE Good sources of niacin are lean meats, fish, liver, poultry, legumes, and whole grains. Pellagra was at one time a common disease of the southeastern United States among persons subsisting on a diet exclusively of corn products, because corn is extremely low in tryptophan, a precursor of this vitamin. Beans are often used in combination with corn to rectify this deficiency.

RECOMMENDED DIETARY ALLOWANCE Niacin requirement in the diet is somewhat dependent on both caloric and protein intake. Because tryptophan, an amino acid found in dietary protein, is metabolized to niacin in the body, intake of protein would reduce the amount of vitamin needed in the diet. The recommended dietary allowance for niacin is 15 to 20 mg niacin equivalents (NE) for adults (1 NE is equal to 1 mg of niacin or 60 mg of tryptophan). Oral doses of 15 to 20 mg of niacin daily are sufficient as a dietary supplement if patients have normal gastrointestinal absorption.

ROLE Nicotinic acid, like riboflavin, plays a key role in metabolism by participating in a variety of oxidation-reduction reactions (transfer of electrons). In the body it is converted into two active forms—the coenzymes nicotinamide adenine dinucleotide (NAD) and nicotinamide adenine dinucleotide phosphate (NADP). This vitamin serves as an essential coenzyme for dehydrogenases involved in the Krebs cycle. The Krebs cycle is responsible for anaerobic carbohydrate metabolism and lipid and protein metabolism.

3 Ds—dermatitis, diarrhea, and dementia

DEFICIENCY The clinical syndrome produced by niacin deficiency is pellagra, so named because the skin becomes rough (Latin: *pelle*, skin; *agra* rough), Early symptoms are an erythematous cutaneous eruption on the back of the hands, glossitis, and stomatitis. In advanced stages, pellagra can be diagnosed by the classic "three Ds": dermatitis, diarrhea, and dementia. The dermatitis consists of redness, thickening, and roughening of the skin followed by scaling desquamation and depigmentation. Diarrhea is caused by atrophy of the gastrointestinal tract mucosal epithelium, followed by inflammation of the mucosal lining of the esophagus, stomach, and colon. The dementia results from regressive changes in the ganglion cells of the brain and tracts of the spinal cord. Death may also result.

During the course of pellagra, symptoms are evident in the oral cavity. A burning sensation occurs throughout the oral mucosa. The lip and lateral margins of the tongue are initially reddened and swollen. In the later stages the entire dorsal surface of the tongue becomes red and swollen. In acute stages, vascular hyperemia, proliferation, hypertrophy, atrophy, and extinction occur successively in the papillae. Papillary loss may ultimately become complete, with the tongue surface becoming beefy red. Deep penetrating ulcers may appear on the tongue surface. In the gingiva, desquamative epithelial degeneration may occur, exposing the tissue to infection, inflammation, and fibrinous exudation. Gingivitis caused by pellagra is characterized by ulcers in the interdental papillae and marginal gingiva. Excessive salivary secretion with enlargement of the salivary glands also occurs.

Niacin deficiency occurs most frequently in poverty-stricken areas of the world because of inadequate intake. Deficiency may also arise from chronic alcoholism, gastrointestinal disturbances, pregnancy, hyperthyroidism, and infections.

ADVERSE EFFECTS Side effects that occur from ingestion of large doses of niacin include cutaneous flushing, pruritus, and gastrointestinal distress. These side effects can be reduced by administering an aspirin one-half hour before the niacin is ingested. Other adverse reactions include increased sebaceous gland action and increased gastrointestinal motility. With chronic use, dry skin, xerostomia, hyperuricemia, peptic ulcer, blurred vision, nervousness, panic, and hyperglycemia can occur. Abnormal liver function tests, prothrombin time, and hypoalbuminemia have been reported.

Aspirin prevents flushing and pruritus

CLINICAL CONSIDERATIONS Niacin or nicotinic acid and niacinamide are used as a vitamin in the treatment of pellagra. Only the niacin is useful in the treatment of hyperlipidemias. It reduces plasma **cholesterol**, triglycerides, very-low-density lipoproteins (VLDL), low-density lipoproteins (LDL), and chylomicrons. These effects are dose dependent. Niacin can also be used in combination with other **lipid-lowering agents,** so that a lower dose of each may be used.

Pyridoxine (vitamin B$_6$). Pyridoxine [peer-i-DOX-een] is one of three different pyridoxine derivatives known as vitamin B$_6$. The other two derivatives, pyridoxal and pyridoxamine, are chemically similar.

Source. Vitamin B$_6$ is present in most foods of both plant and animal origin. Good sources of this vitamin include whole-grain cereals, meat, legumes, eggs, and some vegetables. These similar foods are the sources of many of the B vitamins.

RECOMMENDED DIETARY ALLOWANCE The RDA for vitamin B$_6$ varies from 1.5 to 2 mg daily for adults (see Table 13-2).

ROLE To exert physiologic activity, all three forms of vitamin B_6 are converted to pyridoxal phosphate in the body. Pyridoxal phosphate is the active coenzyme form of vitamin B_6 and participates in all metabolic reactions that require the vitamin. Pyridoxal phosphate acts as a coenzyme in a variety of metabolic transformations of amino acids, including transamination and decarboxylation.

> B_6—cheilosis, stomatitis, glossitis

DEFICIENCY Vitamin B_6 deficiency is rare because of the widespread distribution of this vitamin in food. The characteristics of vitamin B_6 deficiency resemble those of riboflavin, niacin, and thiamine deficiencies. These include angular cheilosis, stomatitis, dermatitis, and erythema of the nasolabial folds. The dorsal mucosa of the tongue seems to be unusually sensitive to a single deficiency or mixed deficiencies of the B vitamins. Specifically, glossitis resulting from pyridoxine deficiency has been described in which the tongue's surface is smooth, slightly edematous, painful, and purplish.

ADVERSE REACTIONS Pyridoxine is usually nontoxic. When it is given parenterally in large doses, peripheral neuritis may be produced.

CLINICAL CONSIDERATIONS Vitamin B_6 can interact with other therapeutically useful drugs. For example, isoniazid (INH), a drug used to treat tuberculosis, inhibits the action of vitamin B_6 by blocking both the formation and the reaction involving pyridoxal phosphate, the active coenzyme. Isoniazid-induced vitamin B_6 deficiency can be prevented or treated by the administration of pyridoxine. For this reason, patients taking INH are usually also taking vitamin B_6. Long-term administration or high doses of steroids can require administration of folic acid. Because the anticonvulsants, such as carbamaze-pine and phenytoin, interfere with the absorption and storage of folic acid, patients taking these medications are given pyridoxine (see Table 13-4).

Vitamin B_6 administration can cancel the therapeutic and side effects of levodopa, a drug used to treat Parkinson's disease. If carbidopa, a peripheral decarboxylase inhibitor, is administered simultaneously with levodopa (the combination is Sinemet), pyridoxine may be administered concomitantly. In practice, Sinemet is currently used almost exclusively rather than levodopa alone.

Certain other drugs, such as cycloserine, hydralazine, and pyrazinamide, may produce a pyridoxine deficiency. Estrogenic steroids can produce vitamin B_6 deficiency in women. About 20% of women taking oral contraceptive agents can be shown to have a biochemical pyridoxine (B_6) deficiency. Usual RDAs seem to be enough to prevent this situation, and women taking birth control pills should routinely be encouraged to take supplemental pyridoxine.

The use of pyridoxine for many conditions has not been shown to be effective in well-controlled trials (premenstrual syndrome, acne, vertigo, tardive dyskinesia, asthma, alcohol intoxication).

Folic acid. Folic acid [FOE-lik] (pteroylglutamic acid, folacin, folate), although not usually referred to as a vitamin, meets the criteria of a vitamin. Normally it is grouped with the B vitamins.

Folic acid is made up of a pteridine heterocycle, *p*-aminobenzoic acid (PABA), and glutamic acid. After absorption, it is metabolized by dihydrofolate reductase to various folates, including tetrahydrofolic acid. Tetrahydrofolic acid is involved in 1-carbon transfer reactions. Folic acid acts as a cofactor in these transfers that are necessary for DNA synthesis. Reactions requiring folic acid include changing homocysteine to methionine and serine to glycine, the synthesis of purines and thymidylates, and the metabolism of histidine. Vitamin B_{12} is also involved in folate regeneration. Folic acid is sparingly soluble in water and is destroyed by heating in neutral or alkaline solution.

SOURCE Significant sources of folic acid include glandular meats such as liver, some fruits and vegetables, wheat germ, and yeasts. Because availability of folic acid from foods is highly variable, a wide margin of safety is allowed in the RDA. Synthetic folic acid is much better absorbed than that supplied from foods.

RECOMMENDED DIETARY ALLOWANCE The RDA for folic acid is 180 to 200 µg daily for adults.

ROLE The biologically active form of folic acid is the reduced derivative tetrahydrofolic acid, which is formed enzymatically in the body. Tetrahydrofolic acid functions primarily in the transfer and utilization of 1-carbon groups.

Certain microorganisms synthesize their own folic acid from PABA. The sulfonamides exert their bacteriostatic effect by antagonizing PABA and thereby interfering with the biosynthesis of folic acid in these organisms. This antagonism has no effect on humans because they require preformed folic acid and do not synthesize their own.

Megaloblastic anemia

DEFICIENCY Folic acid deficiency, the most common deficiency in the United States, produces megaloblastic anemia, which is indistinguishable from that caused by vitamin B_{12} deficiency. Other symptoms include weakness, weight loss, loss of skin pigmentation, and mental irritability. As with riboflavin deficiency, oral manifestations of folic acid deficiency include glossitis, angular cheilosis, and gingivitis. The glossitis begins with swelling and pallor of the tongue followed by desquamation of the papillae and accompanied by minute ulcers with fiery red borders.

Some causes of folic acid deficiency are inadequate diet, pregnancy, malabsorption syndrome, and chronic alcoholism. Pregnant women need supplemental synthetic folacin and should not rely solely on dietary sources. The absorption of folate decreases during pregnancy and in patients taking oral contraceptives.

Several drugs have been reported to produce folic acid deficiencies, including the anticonvulsants, oral contraceptives, and nitrofurantoin. Some drugs act as folic acid antagonists (e.g., pyrimethamine, trimethoprim) (see Table 13-4). The anticonvulsants produce a deficiency by interfering with the conversion of folate to a form of the vitamin that can penetrate the brain. Some cancer chemotherapy agents prevent the formation of tetrahydrofolic acid and interfere with DNA synthesis. Folic acid is not an antidote to an overdose from a folic acid antagonist (e.g., methotrexate); leucovorin calcium is used.

ADVERSE REACTIONS Folic acid is relatively nontoxic. Allergic reactions have been reported rarely and include rash, itching, and respiratory difficulty.

CLINICAL CONSIDERATIONS Although the administration of folic acid will cause remission of the hematologic effects of pernicious anemia, it will not prevent the neurologic effects caused by a deficiency of vitamin B_{12}. Therefore folic acid can mask a vitamin B_{12} deficiency. For this reason the Food and Drug Administration (FDA) has limited the dose of folic acid per tablet that can be purchased without a prescription to 0.4 mg in normal vitamin supplements and 0.8 mg for pregnant or lactating women (over-the-counter [OTC] prenatal vitamins). The use of folic acid several months before conception and early in pregnancy can help to prevent neural tube defects.

Vitamin B$_{12}$—cyanocobalamin

Cyanocobalamin (vitamin B$_{12}$). Cyanocobalamin [sye-an-oh-koe-BAL-a-min] (vitamin B$_{12}$) is a chemically complex substance that contains four extensively substituted pyrrole rings surrounding an atom of cobalt. A cyanide molecule is attached to the cobalt; hence the name *cyanocobalamin.* Vitamin B$_{12}$ is heat stable at a neutral pH but is readily destroyed by heat at an alkaline pH.

SOURCE The only sources of vitamin B$_{12}$ in nature are certain microorganisms that synthesize the vitamin. When vegetable produce is contaminated with these microorganisms it possesses the vitamin. Animals depend on synthesis within their own intestinal tracts. Human vitamin B$_{12}$, synthesized within the gastrointestinal tract, is not available for absorption.

Good sources of vitamin B$_{12}$ include foods of animal origin, such as liver, meat, milk, cheese, and eggs. Vegans (strict vegetarians who do not eat animal or dairy products) can become deficient because they do not eat these foods. In recent years some vegetable products such as soy milk have been fortified with vitamin B$_{12}$.

Vitamin B$_{12}$ is absorbed from the distal **ileum** by a receptor-mediated process. Without the presence of intrinsic factor, a protein-binding factor that aids in the absorption of vitamin B$_{12}$, it cannot be *well* absorbed. This system is saturated by about 3 mg of vitamin B$_{12}$. With very large doses of oral vitamin B$_{12}$ (1 mg) daily, the vitamin may be absorbed independent of intrinsic factor. Absorption of vitamin B$_{12}$ is decreased by damage to the stomach or ilium.

RECOMMENDED DIETARY ALLOWANCE The RDA of vitamin B$_{12}$ is 2 μg, with an additional 0.2 μg and 0.6 μg during pregnancy and lactation, respectively. Oral doses between 1 and 25 μg are adequate if the gastrointestinal absorption is normal. In pernicious anemia, a maintenance injection of vitamin B$_{12}$ is recommended once a month for life.

ROLE Vitamin B$_{12}$ serves as a coenzyme for the hydrogen transfer and isomerization process required in the conversion of methylmalonyl-CoA to succinyl-CoA. Thus vitamin B$_{12}$ is important in the metabolism of fats and carbohydrates.

DEFICIENCY The symptoms of vitamin B$_{12}$ deficiency include inadequate

Megaloblastic anemia

hematopoiesis, gastrointestinal tract disturbances, inadequate myelin synthesis, and generalized debility. The lack of this vitamin affects the cells that are most actively dividing, such as those in the bone marrow and gastrointestinal tract. The erythroblasts do not undergo proper division, resulting in **megaloblastic anemia.** Atrophic changes occur in the alimentary canal. The synthesis of abnormal fatty acids, which are then incorporated into cell membranes, may produce the neurologic manifestations of deficiency, including peripheral neuropathies and spinal cord and organic brain syndromes. The patient suffers from weakness, numbness, and difficulty in walking, symptoms that fluctuate with remission and relapses. The skin may have a distinctive lemon-yellow hue.

The most common cause of vitamin B$_{12}$ deficiency is **pernicious anemia,** an autoimmune disease that prevents the production of intrinsic factor. The secretory cells in the gastric mucosa do not produce intrinsic factor, and thus vitamin B$_{12}$ is very poorly absorbed. With a gastrectomy, usually for the treatment of peptic ulcer in the "old days," intrinsic factor secretion ceases. It then takes 3 to 6 years for a vitamin B$_{12}$ deficiency to develop. Other causes of vitamin B$_{12}$ deficiency include inadequate dietary intake and malabsorption syndromes.

Sore and red tongue, atrophy of papillae

Pernicious anemia results in several oral manifestations. Recurrent attacks of soreness and burning of the tongue occur followed by glossitis, at the peak of which the tongue is extremely painful and red. Atrophy of the filiform and fungiform papillae is a common occurrence. Involvement of the circumvallate papillae may cause diminution of taste. Painful, bright red lesions may occur in the buccal and pharyngeal mucosa and undersurface of the tongue.

ADVERSE REACTIONS Even large doses of vitamin B_{12} are usually nontoxic. Diarrhea, itching, urticaria, and swelling have occasionally been reported. If intrinsic factor is given with the vitamin B_{12}, an allergy to hog protein (a source of exogenous intrinsic factor) may be exhibited.

CLINICAL CONSIDERATIONS As mentioned previously, patients who are strict vegetarians (rarely) or who have had a gastrectomy can exhibit the symptoms of vitamin B_{12} deficiency. Ingestion of other agents can alter the absorption of vitamin B_{12}. For example, vitamin C may destroy the vitamin B_{12} levels in food. Pregnancy and use of the sweetener sorbitol increase vitamin B_{12} absorption. Absorption of vitamin B_{12} is decreased in persons with pyridoxine deficiency, iron deficiency, or hypothyroidism. Sustained-release potassium and anticonvulsants may decrease the absorption of vitamin B_{12}. Vitamin B_{12} has also been used, without any proof of efficacy, to treat trigeminal neuralgia, psychiatric disorders, and tiredness. Because intrinsic factor is not required for absorption from an intramuscular site, vitamin B_{12} can be administered intramuscularly (100 μg/month) in the absence of intrinsic factor. An oral dose of 1 mg daily is equivalent to the 100 μg/month intramuscularly. Because oral administration of vitamin B_{12} is unreliable, the intramuscular route is preferred.

Pantothenic acid. Pantothenic acid is another compound required to form acetyl-CoA. The active form of pantothenic acid is a component of the more complex compound, coenzyme A.

SOURCE Pantothenic acid is a part of all living material. Egg yolk, bran, yeast, and beef liver are excellent sources.

RECOMMENDED DIETARY ALLOWANCE It is suggested that a daily dietary intake of 5 to 10 mg is adequate for adults with normal gastrointestinal absorption. Table 13-3 lists the estimated safe and adequate daily dietary intake (ESADDI) for pantothenic acid.

ROLE The physiologically active form of pantothenic acid is coenzyme A, which serves as a coenzyme in various metabolic reactions, some of which involve the transfer of acetyl (2-carbon) groups. Pantothenic acid is required for gluconeogenesis and synthesis of fatty acids and sterols and steroid hormones. Both pantothenic acid and thiamine are required for the oxidative decarboxylation of pyruvate to produce acetyl-CoA. Pantothenic acid also functions as part of a glucose-carrier system to facilitate absorption through the intestinal mucosa. It is essential to normal epithelial function.

DEFICIENCY Because clinical deficiencies of pantothenic acid are extremely rare in humans, they are produced experimentally in humans only by using a pantothenic acid antagonist. Deficiency may develop in patients with liver disease or who drink excessive alcohol. The symptoms of pantothenic acid deficiency include fatigue, headache, malaise, nausea, abdominal pain, burning feeling of hands and feet, and cramping of leg muscles.

TABLE 13 - 3   **Estimated Safe and Adequate Daily Dietary Intake of Selected Vitamins and Minerals***

| | VITAMINS | | TRACE ELEMENTS† | | | | | |
AGE GROUP (YR)	BIOTIN (μg)	PANTOTHENIC ACID (mg)	COPPER (←―――――	MANGANESE ――――― mg	FLUORIDE ―――――→)	MAGNESIUM (←―――――	CHROMIUM ―――――― μg	MOLYBDENUM ――――――→)
INFANTS								
0-0.5	10	2	0.4-0.6	0.3-0.6	0.01	30‡	10-40	15-30
0.5-1	15	3	0.6-0.7	0.6-1.0	0.3	75‡	20-60	20-40
CHILDREN AND ADOLESCENTS								
1-3	20	3	0.7-1.0	1.0-1.5	0.7	80	20-80	25-50
4-6	25	3-4	1.0-1.5	1.5-2.0	1.1	130	30-120	30-75
7-10	30	4-5	1.0-2.0	2.0-3.0	2.0	240	50-200	50-150
11+	30-100	4-7	1.5-2.5	2.0-5.0	3.2	410	50-200	75-250
Adults	30-100	4-7	1.5-3.0	2.0-5.0	3.8	420§	50-200	75-250

From National Research Council. Food and Nutrition Board Recommended Dietary Allowances, 10th ed, Washington, DC, 1989 National Academy Press.
*Because there is less information on which to base allowances, these figures are not given in the main table of RDA and are provided here in the form of ranges of recommended intakes.
†Because the toxic levels for many trace elements may be only several times usual intakes, the upper levels for the trace elements given in this table should not be habitually exceeded.
‡Adequate intake.
§320 females.

CLINICAL CONSIDERATIONS Pantothenic acid has been used to treat gastrointestinal tract paralysis after surgery because it apparently promotes gastrointestinal motility. Even though a deficiency of pantothenic acid produces gray hair in black rats, there is absolutely no evidence that it reverses gray hair in humans.

Biotin. Biotin was initially demonstrated to be an essential growth factor for yeast, and it was later isolated from both yeast and egg yolk.

SOURCE Although biotin is present in almost all foods, good sources include liver, cow's milk, egg yolk, and yeast. It is also synthesized by the microflora in the intestinal tract, so that the amount of biotin excreted in the feces can actually exceed the intake.

RECOMMENDED DIETARY ALLOWANCE Although no minimum daily requirement of biotin has been established, the suggested adequate daily dietary intake for adults is 30 to 100 μg. Table 13-3 lists the ESADDI for biotin.

ROLE Biotin is a coenzyme required in metabolism in carbon dioxide fixation reactions, β-carboxylation, and deamination.

DEFICIENCY Biotin deficiency is extremely rare but can occur with long-term parenteral nutrition. A biotin deficiency can be induced by eating large quantities of raw egg white. Avidin, a component of egg white, combines with biotin in the gastrointestinal tract and prevents its absorption. If the egg white is cooked, the avidin is denatured and has no activity. When biotin deficiency is experimentally induced by concurrent administration of large amounts of raw egg white containing avidin, symptoms include loss of appetite, mental depression, hyperesthesia of the skin, nausea, malaise, and dry dermatitis.

CLINICAL CONSIDERATIONS Because the amount of biotin synthesized in the intestines is related to the number of microorganisms present, antiinfective agents such as the sulfonamides or tetracyclines can produce a biotin deficiency. Two types of infant dermatitis respond to biotin therapy.

Other B vitamins. Vitamin B_{15} and vitamin B_{17}, also known as *pangamic acid* and *amygdalin (Laetrile)*, respectively, have been shown to be neither vitamins nor important in human nutrition.

CHOLINE AND INOSITOL Neither choline [KOE-leen] nor inositol [EYE-nos-e-tal] has been demonstrated to be required in the human diet. They serve as lipotropic agents and prevent fatty infiltration of the liver. Choline serves as a precursor to acetylcholine. In humans, no deficiency for either choline or inositol has been demonstrated. Deficiencies of choline (in rats) and inositol (in mice) have been produced.

FAT-SOLUBLE VITAMINS

VITAMIN A

Vitamin A_1 and A_2 = retinoids

Vitamin A, which is an essential fat-soluble compound, is necessary for normal growth and for maintaining the health and integrity of certain epithelial tissues. The term *vitamin A* represents a group of retinoids (e.g., vitamin A_1 [retinol], vitamin A_2 [3-dehydroretinol]) and carotenoids. The retinoids include both naturally occurring and synthetic analogs of vitamin A. By cleavage of the carotene molecule, two molecules of vitamin A aldehyde (retinal) are formed.

Retinoids—in orange-colored fruit and vegetables (carrots)

Source. Vitamin A_1 occurs naturally in saltwater fish and animal tissues. Vitamin A_2 is found in freshwater fish. Preformed vitamin A is found in milk, liver, and some cheeses. Margarine can be fortified with vitamin A. However, carotenes provide the greatest source of vitamin A in most diets. Carotenes are found in various pigmented fruits such as apricots, peaches, tomatoes, and watermelon and in vegetables such as carrots, pumpkins, broccoli, spinach, and sweet potatoes. A dark green, yellow, or orange color indicates that a vegetable or fruit has carotene.

Recommended dietary allowance. The adult RDA for vitamin A is 800 to 1000 retinol equivalents (RE). One RE is equal to 1 μg of retinol or 6 μg of β-carotene.

Role. Vitamin A is essential for the maintenance of the photoreceptor mechanism of the retina; the integrity of the epithelia, such as the mucous membranes of the eye and the mucosa of the respiratory, gastrointestinal, and genitourinary tracts; and lysosome stability. Vitamin A plays a significant role in maintaining the integrity and controlling differentiation and possibly the normal permeability of the cell membrane and the membrane subcellular particles. Vitamin A prevents or reverses the transformation of premalignant cells to malignant cells. The importance of this finding is unknown. Vitamin A deficiency decreases the activity of osteoblasts and odontoblasts, thereby reducing the growth of bones and teeth. In contrast, excessive doses of vitamin A accelerate bone and cartilage resorption and new bone formation.

Deficiency. The human liver may store enough vitamin A to meet physiologic

Night blindness

demands for as long as a year, and therefore a deficiency of this vitamin is rare. Deficiencies, if they do occur, generally result from inadequate intake of the vitamin; a malabsorption syndrome, especially biliary tract disease; or severe liver disease. Deficiency of the vitamin leads to impaired vision in dim light called *night blindness (nyctalopia)*. It also results in keratinization of mucosa and cornea. Corneal keratinization leads to impairment of vision, called *xerophthalmia.* Irritation and inflammation may occur on the cornea, a condition called *keratomalacia.* Keratinization may also occur in the oral cavity and mucosa. The normal defense mechanisms of ciliary movement and mucous production are impaired, producing irritation and inflammation of these surfaces. Loss of the senses of taste and smell also occurs in vitamin A deficiency. Deficiency of vitamin A during pregnancy and infancy contributes to the development of enamel hypoplasia and caries in primary teeth.

Toxicity. Excessive intake of vitamin A results in a toxic condition called *hypervitaminosis A.* The characteristics of this toxic reaction include itching skin, desquamation, coarse or absent hair, painful subcutaneous swellings, gingivitis, hyperirritability, and limitation of motion. Hyperostosis in the bone is easily demonstrated on radiography. In infants, headache from increased intracranial pressure, gastrointestinal distress, jaundice, and hepatomegaly may occur. Because the margin of safety of vitamin A intake is large, a toxic reaction can occur only after long-term daily ingestion of more than 50,000 RE.

Acute poisoning has been reported in both infants and adults. When the Vikings landed in Iceland they ingested polar bear liver, a rich source of vitamin A, and died from acute poisoning. After ingestion of lesser amounts by infants, increased intracranial pressure with bulging fontanel and vomiting was reported.

Pregnancy. The use of or exposure to excess retinoids (vitamin A or its analogues) during pregnancy can have serious teratogenic effects. Excessive doses of both vitamin A and the analogues etretinate and isotretinoin are classified as FDA pregnancy category X drugs (see discussion of FDA category drugs in Chapter 24). Other retinoids such as adapalene (Differin) and tretinoin (Retin-A) are FDA category C drugs because the equivalent amount of vitamin A absorbed is substantially below the RDA.

Vitamin A analogues. Tretinoin [TRET-i-noyn] (Retin-A) is the acid form of vitamin A, a topical product that causes skin peeling and is used to treat acne. Another indication is in the treatment of wrinkles. Erythema, desquamation, and unusual sun sensitivity can occur.

Isotretinoin [eye-soe-TRET-i-noyn] (13-*cis*-retinoic acid, Accutane) is used orally for treatment of severe cystic acne. Side effects include corneal opacities, abnormal liver function tests, elevated plasma triglycerides, and, rarely, pseudotumor cerebri. It is highly teratogenic (FDA category X) and should not be used without adequate birth control measures. Remission of acne can remain after the drug has been withdrawn.

Etretinate [e-TRET-i-nate] (Tegison), another analogue of vitamin A, is used systemically to treat severe recalcitrant psoriasis. Like all vitamin A analogues, these agents are contraindicated in anyone who might become pregnant within the next few years, and they carry an FDA pregnancy category of X. Side effects are similar to those of hypervitaminosis A and relate to the mucocutaneous, musculoskeletal, hepatic, and CNS systems. Oral manifestations include gingival bleeding, inflammation, and xerostomia with its concomitant implications. A drug interaction with alcohol exists because they can both produce hypertriglyceridemia. Tetracyclines may increase the potential for a rare side effect, pseudotumor cerebri.

VITAMIN D

Source. *Vitamin D* is a collective term used to refer to both vitamin D_2 and vitamin D_3, two closely related sterols. Vitamin D_3 (cholecalciferol [koh-lee-kal-SIF-e-role] is produced in the skin of mammals by the action of sunlight (ultraviolet rays) on its precursor, 7-dehydrocholesterol. Cholecalciferol (vitamin D_3) is also present in some foods and is added as a supplement to dairy products. Ergocalciferol [er-goe-kal-SIF-e-role] (vitamin D_2), the form of vitamin D found in plants, is the form of vitamin D used in vitamin supplements. Vitamin D_2 is produced by the commercial irradiation (by ultraviolet light) of ergosterol.

Recommended dietary allowance. The RDA of cholecalciferol is 10 mg (400 IU of vitamin D) for a child, and 5 to 10 mg (200 to 400 IU of vitamin D) for adults. The AI for vitamin D is 200 IU.

Role. Vitamin D promotes normal mineralization of bone by stimulating intestinal absorption of calcium and decreasing the excretion from the kidney. Vitamin D_3 (cholecalciferol) is first hydroxylated in the liver to form 25-hydroxycholecalciferol (calcifediol [kal-si-fe-DYE-ole]) (see Figure 13-1), which is then transported to the kidney and converted to the physiologically active form, 1,25-dihydroxycholecalciferol (calcitriol [kal-si-TRYE-ole]). This active form, in conjunction with parathyroid hormone, stimulates intestinal absorption of calcium and mobilizes calcium from formed bones. These effects result in an elevation of serum calcium, which suppresses parathyroid hormone secretion and secondarily 1,25-dihydroxycholecalciferol synthesis. If the calcium level rises, the thyroid gland secretes calcitonin, which reduces the formation of 1,25-dihydroxycholecalciferol and increases the production of 24,25-dihydroxycholecalciferol. Low levels of phosphorus stimulate the production of 1,25-dihydroxycholecalciferol, whereas high phosphorus levels produce more 24,25-dihydroxycholecalciferol. Like vitamin D_3, exogenous ergocalciferol (vitamin D_2) is hydroxylated by the liver and then in the kidneys to 1,25 (OH)-D_2.

Rickets

Deficiency. The deficiency of vitamin D produces inadequate absorption of calcium and phosphate with a decrease in plasma calcium. Parathyroid hormone secretion is stimulated, which removes calcium from the bone to restore plasma levels. In children this deficiency results in rickets, a disease involving a decreased mineralization of newly formed bone and cartilage tissue. Children with rickets have bones that are unusually soft and easily bent, compressed, or fractured. Under the stress and strain of weight-bearing, the gross deformities of rickets, including spine curvature and bowing of the legs, become evident. Because of the excess formation of osteoids a squared appearance of the head occurs. Collapse of the ribs and protrusion of the sternum (pigeon breast syndrome) are also seen. Bone pain and muscle weakness may be present.

Vitamin D deficiency during pregnancy or in young children may result in enamel hypoplasia, but the teeth may remain caries free. In adults, vitamin D deficiency produces a disease state called **osteomalacia.** In general, there is decreased bone density because of inadequate mineralization, which results in an excess of osteoid matrix. Because of the weakness of the bones, pathologic fractures and deformities of weight-bearing bones occur. This happens most frequently during times of increased calcium usage such as pregnancy or lactation. Persons with malabsorption syndromes, alcoholics, those adhering to a low-fat diet, strict vegetarians, and those undergoing anticonvulsant therapy or using sedatives or tranquilizers are more prone to vitamin D deficiency.

Toxicity. The symptoms of hypervitaminosis D, which may result from either long-term or short-term ingestion of excessive quantities of vitamin D, are caused by abnormal calcium metabolism. The signs and symptoms of vitamin D toxicity include weakness, fatigue, headache, nausea, vomiting, and diarrhea. With prolonged hypercalcemia, calcification of the blood vessels, heart, lung, and kidney can occur. Continued ingestion of very large doses in a normal adult is likely to produce hypervitaminosis D.

Clinical considerations. Vitamin D is used to prevent and treat rickets. It is also used to treat chronic hypocalcemia, hypophosphatemia, osteodystrophy, and osteomalacia. Dihydroxycholecalciferol (calcitriol, 1,25 $[OH]_2D_3$) and dihydroxyergocalciferol ($[OH]_2$ D_2) do not require activation by the kidneys and are used for hypocalcemia in patients with chronic renal failure undergoing dialysis. Because of the need for a functioning kidney to activate vitamin D, the patient is given the preformed active vitamin D (Figure 13-1). Exogenous dihydrotachysterol (DHT), a close isomer of vitamin D, is hydroxylated in the liver to 25-hydroxy-DHT.

> Highest risk = Female, thin, white, and smoker

Osteoporosis. Normal bone is continuously being made and broken down in response to various stimuli. **Osteoporosis** occurs when the equilibrium between the resorption and formation of bone becomes negative. The loss of bone mass predisposes the patient to fractures. Patients who develop osteoporosis are much more likely to sustain fractures of their bones, including vertebra or hip, which often reduces their quality of life. The thin, white or Asian woman who smokes is most likely to develop osteoporosis. Patients taking chronic corticosteroids develop osteoporosis earlier. The most common occurrence of osteoporosis is in postmenopausal women because of inadequate sex hormones. Calcium intake of the equivalent of 1200 to 1500 mg of elemental calcium is recommended for postmenopausal women. Weight-bearing exercise may modulate osteoporosis. Estrogen replacement therapy (ERT) reduces the risk of osteoporosis and recent evidence has determined that the minimum dose of estrogen for this effect is 0.3 mg (0.625 mg was previously recommended). Some women fear the side effects of estrogens, including an increased risk of breast cancer (small increase in risk) and increased risk of uterine cancer (nullified by using progestin with the estrogen). Therefore they do not take supplemental estrogens and osteoporosis is not prevented. (They are also missing the benefit of supplemental estrogen on reducing cardiac disease.)

Calcium supplementation is encouraged to prevent osteoporosis in postmenopausal women. Osteoporosis is more effectively prevented when adequate intake of calcium begins in their 20s and 30s.

Three new drugs are indicated for the management of osteoporosis and have been recently released. The bisphosphonates include alendronate and etidronate.

Alendronate (Fosamax), a third generation bisphosphonate, has been shown to inhibit osteoclastic activity and reduce bone turnover. Under the influence of alendronate, bone formation is greater than bone resorption. It can produce an increase in bone density and reduces fractures for a 5-year period. It is taken on an empty

F IGURE 1 3 - 1 *Metabolism of vitamin D.*

Vitamin D_3
cholecalciferol

↓ + OH (in liver)

25-hydroxycholecalciferol

↓ + OH (in kidney)

1,25-dihydroxycholecalciferol

Must administer preformed 1,25-$(OH)_2$ in renal insufficiency stomach with plain water with instructions to refrain from lying down for 30 minutes thereafter. With higher doses, there is a potential for gastrointestinal adverse reactions. Salicylates can increase the gastrointestinal side effects.

Etidronate (Didronel) has been shown to increase bone mass and reduce the incidence of fractures for at least 2 years. It has been shown to increase the bone mass slightly.

Calcitonin (Miacalcin) is administered by intranasal inhalation. It has been shown to increase spinal bone mass in postmenopausal women with osteoporosis. Further study is needed to define the appropriate therapeutic use of these agents.

Although it is known that fluoride can stimulate bone formation, the use of sodium fluoride in the treatment of osteoporosis is controversial.

VITAMIN E

There are eight naturally occurring tocopherols possessing vitamin E activity. α-Tocopherol is the most active tocopherol. α-Tocopherol, from wheat, and γ-tocopherol, from corn and soybean oils, margarines, are about half as potent as the α form. The δ form, from sunflower oil, is almost inactive. Although the metabolic role of vitamin E is not understood, it is known that this vitamin functions as an antioxidant.

Source. The best sources of vitamin E are vegetable oils such as soybean, corn, and cottonseed oils. Other sources include fresh greens and vegetables.

Recommended dietary allowance. It has been estimated that a daily intake of 10 to 30 mg of vitamin E will keep the vitamin E serum level within a normal range. The Food and Nutrition Board of the National Research Council recommends between 8 and 10 α-tocopherol equivalents (TE) for adults per day (see Table 13-2).

Role. The action of vitamin E is probably exerted via its antioxidant effect. It prevents the oxidation of vitamins A and C, protects polyunsaturated fatty acids in membranes from attack by free radicals, and protects red blood cells against hemolysis. Vitamin E increases the absorption and utilization of vitamin A and protects against hypervitaminosis A.

Vitamin E is being intensely studied for its effect on clotting and on prevention of thromboses. It can be shown to interfere with clotting, but the exact mechanism is unknown (may be related to inhibition of prostaglandins). The evidence of vitamin E's role in cardiovascular disease is strengthened because studies have shown a decrease in both myocardial infarction and stroke.

Deficiency. Deficiency of vitamin E, produced in laboratory animals, can affect the reproductive, muscular, cardiovascular, and hematopoietic systems. Vitamin E deficiency in male rats has resulted in reproductive failure and sterility; in the pregnant female rat it has led to fetal death and resorption.

In humans, vitamin E has been used for the treatment of sterility and habitual abortion, but there is no conclusive evidence that this vitamin provides any beneficial effect in these conditions.

Although vitamin E has been used to treat several cardiovascular diseases, there is no scientific rationale for this use.

A deficiency of vitamin E can occur in malabsorption syndromes and in premature infants with impaired absorption ability. A deficiency of vitamin E has also been reported to cause anemia resulting from a decreased erythrocyte life span and abnormal hematopoiesis. Oxidizing agents can more easily hemolyze the erythrocytes from vitamin E–deficient animals.

Toxicity. Vitamin E is generally thought to have low toxicity. Levels of vitamin E greatly in excess of the normal dietary requirements have been administered to human subjects with no apparent adverse effect. Nausea, diarrhea, fatigue, weakness, and rash have occurred rarely.

Clinical considerations. Vitamin E therapy has been recommended for treatment of a wide variety of human diseases that are similar to conditions of vitamin E deficiency (see discussion of fallacious thinking on vitamins). Vitamin E has been used for many indications in which documentation is poor, such as intermittent claudication and protection against certain air pollutants. Other researchers have found that vitamin E supplementation had no effect on work performance, sexuality, or general well-being. At present, no therapeutic use of vitamin E has been proved by controlled scientific studies, with the exception of hemolytic anemia of the newborn.

Pharmacologic doses of vitamin E (used as a drug) have been employed as an antioxidant in premature infants exposed to high concentrations of oxygen to reduce the incidence and severity of retinopathy and bronchopulmonary dysplasia. Vitamin E has been used to treat both β-thalassemia and sickle cell anemia with questionable success. The usual dose of vitamin E for its protective cardiovascular effect is 400 IU.

VITAMIN K

Vitamin K was originally found to be a fat-soluble substance present in hog liver fat and alfalfa. Large quantities of the vitamin are also found in the feces of most species of animals. At least two distinct natural substances possess vitamin K activity: vitamin K_1 and vitamin K_2. Vitamin K_2 consists of several substances, with menaquinone-4 being the most active form. Vitamin K_1 (phytonadione [fye-toe-na-DYE-one], phytyl-menaquinone, phylloquinone) is found in plants. Vitamin K_2 (menaquinone, multi-prenyl-menaquinone) is synthesized by gram-positive bacteria present in the gastrointestinal tract. Both Vitamins K_1 and K_2 require bile salts for absorption from the intestines.

Source. Vitamin K occurs in green vegetables such as alfalfa, cabbage, and spinach and in egg yolk, soybean oil, and liver. Vitamin K is synthesized by gram-positive bacteria, and the microorganisms in the intestinal flora can provide humans with some vitamin K. Synthetic vitamin K is a form of vitamin K that has activity similar to that of naturally occurring vitamin K.

Recommended dietary allowance. The RDA for vitamin K is 40 to 80 μg for males and 45 to 65 μg for females. Generally the normal diet and intestinal bacteria provide all the necessary vitamin K.

Role. Vitamin K is essential for the hepatic synthesis of four of the clotting factors—II (prothrombin), VII, IX, and X. Without adequate clotting factors, normal blood clotting does not occur.

Deficiency. A vitamin K deficiency can produce hypoprothrombinemia. In the absence of this vitamin, bleeding will result. With a severe deficiency of vitamin K, the smallest trauma may produce hemorrhage. The most common sites of hemorrhage are operative wounds, skin (petechial bleeding), mucous membranes in the intestinal tract, and serosal surfaces. Ecchymoses, epistaxis, and **hematuria** are also common.

A vitamin K deficiency is usually caused by an inadequate intake or absorption (lack of bile salts) of the vitamin or by decreased normal bacterial flora resulting from prolonged antibiotic use. The newborn can have vitamin K deficiency because the intestinal organisms have not yet been established.

> Antibiotics can reduce vitamin K production

Toxicity. The naturally occurring vitamins K_1 and K_2 are essentially nontoxic in massive doses, and vitamin K (menadione) must be administered in large doses before toxicity can be demonstrated. It has been implicated in producing hemolytic anemia in newborns and hemolysis in persons suffering from glucose-6-phosphate dehydrogenase (G6PD) deficiency. Hypersensitivity reactions can occur.

Clinical considerations. Anticoagulant drugs such as warfarin competitively antagonize vitamin K and interfere with the production of prothrombin (II) and factors VII, IX, and X. Vitamin K, in the form of phytonadione, is used to treat excessive hypoprothrombinemia caused by warfarin toxicity. It is ineffective in reversing the hypoprothrombinemia caused by very severe liver disease.

In patients with severe hepatic disease, a deficiency of clotting factors can result in a prolonged prothrombin time without therapy. Vitamin K is administered to these patients and their prothrombin time measured before surgery. Other measures to help clotting include fresh frozen plasma or platelets.

SELECTED MINERALS

Table 13-3 lists the ESADDIs of selected minerals. Less information is available on minerals than on vitamins; selected minerals are discussed.

IRON

Fe = iron

Although **iron** (Fe) is widely distributed throughout the human body, it is principally found as hemoglobin. Approximately 80% of the iron in the body is functional or "essential" iron (e.g., in hemoglobin [70%] and myoglobin [10%]), whereas 10% to 20% remains as storage or "nonessential" iron (in ferritin and hemosiderin).

Source. Good sources of iron include organ meats such as liver and heart, wheat germ, brewer's yeast, egg yolks, oysters, red meats, and dried beans. Breads, flours, and cereals are commonly enriched with iron. Cooking utensils made of iron can raise the iron content of foods if the foods prepared in them are acidic. The percentage of iron absorbed from foods varies considerably, with absorption from meats being better. Numerous factors affect absorption, such as other foods eaten concomitantly, the bulk in the diet, the size of the dose of iron, the body's need, and the presence of achlorhydria. The H_2-receptor antagonists (H_2-RA) and proton pump inhibitors (PPI) can reduce the absorption of iron. If iron supplements are taken, they should be ingested as far away from the intake of these agents that increase pH.

Recommended dietary allowance. The body carefully conserves its iron and there is no mechanism for its excretion. Excess ingestion of iron over a long period may produce iron toxicity. The iron level is regulated by limiting its absorption from the intestinal tract. However, because iron is contained in each cell, when body cells are lost, iron is also lost. Women must replace the extra iron lost during menstruation. The RDA for iron is about 10 mg of iron per day for males and about 15 mg of iron daily for females to replace loss. Replacement of a donated pint of blood requires an additional 0.7 mg of absorbed iron daily for 1 year. Two percent to 10% of ingested iron is absorbed, and therefore men need about 1 mg of absorbed iron and women about 2 mg of absorbed iron each day. A pregnant woman's need for iron cannot be met by the usual American diet or the 18-mg supplement recommended for women. For this reason, 30 mg of iron is recommended for pregnant women. Of course, if they have iron deficiency anemia, the requirement is higher.

Role. The basic function of iron is to allow the movement of oxygen and carbon dioxide from one tissue to another. Iron accomplishes this task by being a part of both hemoglobin and myoglobin. Iron is also a component of enzymes involved in the uptake and release of oxygen and carbon dioxide, and therefore it is essential for protein metabolism.

Deficiency. Because the body is so efficient in conserving iron, a deficiency can occur only with growth, blood loss, or inadequate intake during pregnancy or lactation. The requirements of younger women cannot easily be reached without a supplement. Preschool children, adolescents, and elderly persons are also frequently found to be deficient in iron, probably because of inadequate intake.

Iron deficiency produces microcytic and hypochromic anemia. The symptoms are nonspecific, but include pallor, irritability, fatigue, decreased resistance to infection, and sore mouth. Anemia, a decrease in the quality or quantity of red blood cells, can be measured by laboratory tests.

Before treatment, patients with iron deficiency anemia should be checked for any sources of bleeding to rule out chronic problems such as colon cancer. After ruling out problems, iron deficiency is treated by the concurrent administration of adequate iron salt, usually in tablet form. Ascorbic acid, which increases the absorption of iron may be used concomitantly (e.g., take iron tablets with orange juice). When the hemoglobin becomes normal, which may require months, there is no reason to continue therapy if the diet has improved or the cause of the deficiency has been removed (e.g., by control of excessive bleeding).

Although iron has many salt forms, no product has been shown to be superior to another, but the dose of elemental iron must be calculated based on the specific salt. Because ferrous sulfate [FER-us SUL-fate] contains about 30% iron, 200-mg tablets contain about 60 mg of iron. If side effects occur, ferrous gluconate [FER-us GLOO-koe-nate] may be substituted, but the 300-mg (12% iron) tablets contain about 36 mg of iron. [Of course these will have fewer side effects because they have less iron.] Other preparations, including sustained-release products, have no advantage and in some cases may actually be less effective than ferrous sulfate. The actual amount of iron needed can be calculated based on the results of a laboratory test.

Toxicity. Complaints of gastrointestinal distress are common, even with therapeutic doses of iron. However, with an acute overdose, bleeding into the intestine can occur, resulting in shock or even death. Poisoning of children with iron has occurred and iron products, like all medications, should be placed out of the reach of children. Treatment of an acute overdose of iron involves removing the iron by gastric lavage and introducing phosphate into the stomach to decrease the iron's solubility. Chelating agents such as deferoxamine, which form a complex with iron, can be used if warranted.

With prolonged administration of iron, the intestinal mucosa, which normally regulates iron absorption, can be overcome. When an excess of iron accumulates, it produces hemochromatosis, a deposition of hemosiderin, in the organs. An iron overload can also occur with frequent blood transfusions. (Hemoglobin in blood is released and the iron is conserved within the body.) As with the treatment of acute overdose, chelating agents can be used to treat chronic toxic effects from iron. Removing a pint of blood from the patient weekly can also be used to remove iron from the body.

ZINC

Zinc has only recently been recognized as a mineral the body requires.

Source. The best sources of zinc are seafood and meat. Cereals and legumes also contain zinc, but it is more poorly absorbed from these foods because of the presence of phytic acid, which interferes with intestinal absorption.

Recommended dietary allowance. The RDA of zinc for adults is 15 mg.

Role. Zinc is required to transport carbon dioxide in the blood and eliminate it in the lungs. It is essential in the utilization of alcohol, and it rids the body of lactic acid formed during exercise. It is also a component of insulin.

At least 59 enzymes involved in digestion or metabolism contain zinc or need it to function. Zinc plays an integral part in some enzymatic reactions and is a catalyst for others.

Deficiency. Only in 1961 was zinc deficiency recognized in humans. A delay in sexual maturity, slow healing of wounds, and slowed growth are associated with this deficiency. In zinc-deficient rats, fetuses were either resorbed or born with congenital malformations. In humans, zinc-deficient mothers gave birth to low-birth-weight infants or infants with suggested malformations of the central nervous system. Both sexes have shown retarded gonadal development, and with severe deficiency, reproduction is impossible. In view of the drop in serum zinc produced by the oral contraceptives, speculation concerning subsequent pregnancies would be natural. A deficiency of zinc also stunts growth.

> Change in taste and smell

Hypogeusia, anorexia, and hyposmia have been reported in conjunction with zinc deficiency. Zinc seems to be essential to the growth and differentiation of the taste buds. It may also be a part of a "growth factor" for taste buds, appropriately named *gustin*. It may soon become routine to measure the zinc in saliva to correlate it with body zinc levels.

Toxicity. Long-term studies must be conducted to determine the effect of chronic zinc toxicity. Excessive intake of zinc has impaired the lymphocyte and polymorphonuclear leukocyte functions in healthy persons. Nausea, vomiting, fever, and diarrhea have been reported to follow acute ingestion.

Clinical considerations. Although it has long been known that zinc participates in wound healing, there is no known advantage to the administration of zinc in patients who have no zinc deficiency. The use of zinc supplements to promote wound healing is currently being studied for periodontal surgery. Zinc has also been used, without documented evidence, to treat acne, arthritis, and Wilson's disease. Zinc gluconate lozenges have been shown to reduce the duration of the common cold. Zinc lozenges are available over the counter.

CALCIUM

Calcium, the fifth most prevalent element in the body, is present in bones, teeth, and extracellular fluids. The level of calcium in the serum must be maintained within a very narrow concentration to prevent serious problems.

Source. Dairy products are the best source of calcium in the diet. These include milk, cheese, yogurt, and cottage cheese. Other good sources of calcium are sardines with bones, tofu, and shrimp.

Recommended dietary allowance. The RDA of elemental calcium is between 800 and 1500 mg for the adult. Pregnant and nursing women require 1500 mg daily. The recommended intake of calcium in postmenopausal women is 1500 mg per day. Postmenopausal women who add estrogen replacement therapy reduce their chance of exhibiting osteoporosis. Weight-bearing exercise also helps to prevent osteoporosis. Adequate vitamin D intake should be evaluated. Before a patient ingests exogenous calcium, the patient's diet should be evaluated to determine the baseline intake of calcium from food. Supplemental calcium should be taken to adjust the intake of calcium to 1500 mg. For example, if a diet analysis finds that the patient is taking 600 mg of calcium (two glasses of skim milk), then the calcium supplementation should be 900 mg for the post-menopausal woman.

Role. Calcium is essential for the function of the nervous, muscular, and skeletal systems and for cell membrane and capillary permeability. It is needed for skeletal muscle contraction, cardiac function, renal function, membrane integrity, and blood coagulation. The skeleton is a reservoir of calcium for the body. Parathyroid hormone, calcitonin, and vitamin D regulate calcium concentrations in the body.

Deficiency. A deficiency of calcium can occur when both calcium and vitamin D are withheld. Mobilization from the bone keeps tissue levels nearly normal. If levels in the blood fall, tetany, paresthesias, muscle cramps, and convulsions can result.

Adverse reactions. Oral calcium may be irritating to the gastrointestinal tract. It may cause constipation. Hypercalcemia may result if large doses of calcium are given to patients with chronic renal failure. Calcium can complex with tetracycline and the quinolones and inactivate them. Their oral administration should be separated by at least 2 hours.

Clinical considerations. Calcium is used to treat a deficiency of calcium, as well as tetany secondary to low calcium levels. When calculating the RDA of calcium the *amount of elemental calcium*, not the total weight of the calcium salt, must be used. For example, 1250 mg of calcium carbonate provides 500 mg of elemental calcium (40% Ca), whereas 500 mg of calcium gluconate provides 45 mg of elemental calcium (9%). So calcium gluconate has 90 mg of elemental calcium per gram, and calcium carbonate has 400 mg of elemental calcium per gram. Before choosing a calcium supplement, the labels of each product must be carefully compared. It is interesting that on the label of one bottle of calcium the weight of salt (1250 mg Ca $[CO_3]_2$) is printed in BIG letters and the weight of the elemental calcium (Ca) is in small letters.

Calcium may be used parenterally to elevate the serum calcium in an emergency. It is also used during **cardiopulmonary resuscitation,** in the treatment of hyperkalemia with secondary cardiac toxicity, and to treat hypermagnesemia.

DRUG-INDUCED VITAMIN DEFICIENCIES

Drugs from a large variety of drug groups have the ability to produce vitamin deficiency. Some actually produce a deficiency, whereas others tend to lower the levels of some vitamins. Table 13-4 lists drugs and the vitamin deficiency they produce.

Isoniazid (INH), a drug used for management of tuberculosis, can produce a neuropathy resulting from vitamin B_6 deficiency, so patients taking INH are given concomitant vitamin B_6. Patients taking the anticonvulsant phenytoin (Dilantin) may exhibit vitamin D deficiency because phenytoin stimulates the liver microsomal enzymes, resulting in an increase in vitamin D metabolism and a decrease in its blood levels. It may be necessary to give vitamin D to patients taking phenytoin. Folic acid levels may fall in patients taking phenytoin, but folic acid supplementation may lower the blood level of the anticonvulsant, requiring an increase in its dose.

Certain drugs such as oral contraceptives tend to induce a deficiency of vitamin B_1, B_2, and folic acid. The exact mechanism by which these vitamin deficiencies occur is not known, but an interference with absorption of the vitamin is a postulate. Drugs that produce a folic acid deficiency include methotrexate, sulfonamides, and triamterene. The anticonvulsants phenytoin,

▆ TABLE 13-4	Drug-Induced Vitamin Deficiencies
DRUG(S)	POTENTIAL DEFICIENCY
Methotrexate (MTX)	Folic acid
Isoniazid (INH)	Pyridoxine (B_6)
Sulfasalazine	Folic acid
Trimethoprim	Folic acid
Anticonvulsants	Vitamin D
Phenytoin	Folic acid
Birth control pills (oral contraceptives)	Vitamin A; B vitamins: thiamine (B_1), riboflavin (B_2), pyridoxine (B_6), folic acid and vitamin B_{12}; vitamins C and E
Levodopa	Avoid B_6 (antagonizes effect)
Smoking	Vitamin C
Colchicine	Vitamin B_{12}
Alcohol	Vitamin B_{12}

valproic acid, and phenobarbital are associated with folic acid deficiency.

REVIEW QUESTIONS

1. Name the water-soluble and fat-soluble vitamins.
2. For each of the vitamins, discuss the following, if applicable:
   a. source
   b. role
   c. recommended dietary allowance
   d. deficiency
   e. toxicity
   f. clinical considerations
3. For each of the vitamins, name the deficiency state and describe the major signs and symptoms.
4. Explain why certain vitamins have a greater likelihood for toxicity and name these vitamins.
5. Describe the conditions that are likely to produce iron deficiency anemia and explain its treatment.
6. Explain the potential use of zinc in dentistry.
7. List the vitamin deficiencies that may be induced by drug therapy with oral contraceptives and anticonvulsants.
8. Describe a use for niacin involving the patient with cardiovascular disease.
9. Describe a use for calcium in women and explain when its use should begin for this purpose. List two other groups of agents that may also be used.
10. List three drugs that can produce a vitamin deficiency.
11. List a benefit of vitamin E intake, unrelated to vitamin deficiency.

CHAPTER 14

Oral Conditions and Their Treatment

CHAPTER OUTLINE

The dental health care worker is the first professional that patients visit when they notice a lesion in the oral cavity. Patients often ask the dental care provider, "What is this? How do I get rid of it? How long will it take to go away? Why do I have it? Is it cancer?" Patients who have even visited several physicians may appear at the office with commonly seen oral lesions. The first step is the diagnosis. Obtaining an in-depth history of the problem (listening, open-ended questions) and examining the lesion can often result in a diagnosis or potential diagnoses. Depending on the diagnosis, the lesion may require only reassurance, palliative treatment, specific treatment, or even surgical intervention.

This chapter discusses a few of the more common oral lesions and medications used for the treatment of these conditions. Before discussing individual oral lesions, commonly used treatments for several types of lesions will be discussed.

INFECTIOUS LESIONS

ACUTE NECROTIZING ULCERATIVE GINGIVITIS

| ANUG = Vincent's infection |

Acute necrotizing ulcerative gingivitis (ANUG), which is also called *Vincent's infection* and *trench mouth*, has both bacteriologic (spirochetes) and environmental (stress, debilitation) factors.

ANUG is a spreading ulcer associated with a distinctive odor; the ulcerated area begins at the interdental papillae.

Good oral hygiene is the cornerstone of treatment, but other modalities have been recommended. Mouthwashes, such as hydrogen peroxide, or saline rinses assist by their flushing action. If pain or an elevated temperature accompanies ANUG, then aspirin or acetaminophen can be recommended. If eating is difficult, food supplements (Meritene, Sustacal, Sustagen) may be used instead of meals. Vitamin supplementation is useful only if the patient has a vitamin deficiency. The food supplements mentioned contain the required vitamins and minerals. Routine antibiotics should be condemned. Antibiotics should be considered only if the patient is immunosuppressed or there is evidence of systemic involvement (Table 8-1). Antibiotics useful for the immunosuppressed patient with ANUG include penicillin VK and metronidazole. Topical chlorhexidine gluconate, active against gram-positive and gram-negative organisms and *Candida* organisms, is used as a rinse for ANUG. The majority of ANUG cases respond dramatically to local treatment (oral prophylaxis with scaling).

HERPES INFECTIONS

Primary herpetic gingivostomatitis, or primary herpes, is the manifestation of the initial herpes infection. Occurring principally in infants

| *Herpes simplex, herpes labialis*—fever blister, cold sore |

and children, it is caused by the herpes simplex virus. Because it is frequently associated with or follows other infections it is also known as a *fever blister* or *cold sore*. The painful lesions may appear throughout the oral mucosa. Beginning as an erythematous area, numerous punctate ulcers with a circumscribed area of erythema appear. The ulcers can coalesce to form larger irregular ulcers with gray centers. Other signs of herpes include the formation of vesicles that become scabbed. Systemic symptoms that are more severe in infants can develop and, in some cases, can be life-threatening. Without treatment, herpes is self-limiting in the patient with normal immunity. Eighty percent to 90% of the adult population have been exposed to herpes simplex virus (HSV). HSV-1 is involved in most oral lesions and transmission is not sexual. HSV-2 is usually responsible for genital herpes and is transmitted venereally. Both HSV-1 and HSV-2 can spread to other parts of the body, for example, the eyes, genitals, and fingers (herpetic whitlow). When the lesions are in the vesicle stage, they are very contagious and the virus can survive for several hours on surfaces [think about possibilities in the dental office].

After the primary episode, the patient may experience recurrent herpes simplex (cold sores or fever blisters) outbreaks that occur at irregular and variable intervals. Events that may precipitate a herpetic outbreak include sunlight (ultraviolet light), hormonal changes such as menstruation, lip pulling, rubber dam, biting an anesthetized lip, emotional stress, or other infections (e.g., a viral respiratory infection). Repeatedly apply petroleum jelly to the lips, and be careful when manipulating the lips to minimize the trauma from a dental appointment. The effectiveness of the antiviral drugs varies depending on whether the outbreak is a primary episode or recurrence and whether the patient is immunocompromised or nonimmunocompromised.

Treatment. The treatment of herpes may include an antiviral agent, depending on the patient and the episode. Many instances of herpes simplex are not affected by antiviral therapy. Adequate clinical trials determine whether or not an antiviral agent should be prescribed.

Symptomatic treatment of lesions include swishing the mouth with topical diphenhydramine (Benadryl) elixir or viscous lidocaine and spitting it out.

Antiviral agents such as acyclovir and penciclovir are useful in certain *Herpes simplex* infections (Table 14-1).

ACYCLOVIR. Acyclovir is available as tablets, capsules, ointment, and parenteral injectable forms. This discussion is limited to the oral and topical products; parenteral products are not discussed in depth.

The approved indications for acyclovir include the treatment of primary and recurrent

TABLE 14-1	Dosing of Antiviral Agents in the Management of *Herpes Labialis*	
DRUG	INDICATION	DOSING
Acyclovir topical (Zovirax)	Primary and recurrent *Herpes labialis* in the immunocompromised patient. **Not** effective for recurrent herpes in immunocompetent patients	Apply q2h while awake
Acyclovir systemic (Zovirax)	Prophylaxis* for *Herpes labialis* in immunocompetent and immunocompromised patients. Treatment of only first episode of *Herpes labialis*	Acyclovir 400 mg bid
Penciclovir† topical (Denavir)	Recurrent *Herpes labialis* in immunocompetent patient	Apply q2h while awake

*If symptoms serious and more than six episodes per year.
†Only agent approved for use to treat recurrent herpes and immunocompetent patients.

Herpes simplex virus in the immunocompromised patient.

In the nonimmunocompromised patient, oral acyclovir is indicated for both treatment of the primary (first episode) outbreak and prophylaxis. Used prophylactically, it reduces the number and severity of recurrent outbreaks. Acyclovir should not be used prophylactically to prevent minor outbreaks because excessive use may lead to resistant strains of herpes.

> Oral acyclovir proven effective when taken prophylactically

Administration of oral acyclovir can be used before situations known to precipitate herpes lesions, such as a ski trip or wedding (stress) or a dental appointment that will produce trauma. The usual prophylactic dose of acyclovir is 400 mg bid. It has yet to be shown that oral acyclovir produces a significant clinical effect in the treatment of recurrent lesions in the immunocompetent patient. It may shorten the time to healing or the pain by a small amount of time.

Topical acyclovir ointment does not affect the course of recurrent herpes in the immunocompetent patient. This may be a result of poor penetration or delay in applying the ointment. Cell damage may be irreversible by the time symptoms are noticed.

Suggestions to add agents that increase penetration of the skin such as dimethyl sulfoxide (DMSO) to the acyclovir have not been studied thoroughly, but they may increase its effectiveness.

The incidence of resistance of the herpes organisms to acyclovir is increasing. If herpes lesions fail to respond to therapy, the virus should be tested for susceptibility to acyclovir. Resistant strains have been identified, especially in HIV-positive patients taking chronic acyclovir. This is the same principle that produces antibiotic resistance in the general population.

PENCICLOVIR Penciclovir (Denavir), which is available only topically, has been shown to reduce by one half day the duration and

> Penciclovir—reduces lesion duration and viral shedding by 0.7 days

pain of lesions on the lips and face associated with both primary and recurrent herpes simplex. The advantages of penciclovir over acyclovir are that penciclovir can achieve a higher concentration within the cell and it remains in the cells longer.

Table 14-1 summarizes the indications for the antiviral agents. Appendix C contains sample prescriptions for antiviral agents discussed here.

FAMCICLOVIR AND VALACYCLOVIR Both famciclovir and valacyclovir are prodrugs that are converted to active antiviral agents. They are indicated in the treatment of acute localized varicella-zoster infections and recurrent genital herpes in immunocompetent adults. Ganciclovir is indicated for serious cytomegalovirus retinitis in immunocompromised patients. It may be effective in some acyclovir-resistant organisms.

TREATMENT OF SYMPTOMS **Palliative treatment** involves treating the patient's symptoms.

> DPH or lidocaine topically

In a primary episode of herpes, fever may be managed by the administration of acetaminophen or by sponging the affected area with tepid water. The discomfort associated with herpes may be relieved by swishing diphenhydramine (DPH). This product is available under many trade names, for example, Diphen Cough, Diphenhist, Genahist, and Siladryl. All of these products are now alcohol-free liquids. Perhaps the most commonly available product is Benadryl. The strength of all the products is 12.5 mg of the active ingredient per 5 ml (1 teaspoonful). Other agents, such as viscous lidocaine (Xylocaine) or combinations of DPH with kaolin (Kaopectate), Maalox, or Mylanta are recommended for use in the oral cavity. Because antihistamines, such as diphenhydramine, have a structure (SAR) similar to local anesthetics, they have some local anesthetic action and can therefore reduce the pain.

Sodium carboxymethylcellulose paste (Orabase plain) or with benzocaine may reduce discomfort. Food supplements may be used if intake of food is impossible (because of oral discomfort). These remedies are the same as those used for patients receiving cancer chemotherapy agents. Corticosteroids are contraindicated because they suppress the cellular immunity that inhibits viral infections.

Candidiasis (Moniliasis)

Candidiasis, a fungal infection caused by *Candida albicans*, frequently affects the oral mucosa. Candidiasis occurs when the organisms multiply and predominate. Because candida is part of the normal oral flora, it is always present in small numbers. When other flora are suppressed, candida can predominate.

> Candidiasis often secondary to broad-spectrum antibiotics

When a patient presents with oral candidiasis, it is important that the dental health care worker search exhaustively for potential predisposing factors. A normal patient does not usually get oral candidiasis. Systemic antibiotic treatment, especially with broad-spectrum antibiotics such as tetracycline, can predispose a patient to candidiasis. A dental health care worker may be the first professional to diagnose HIV-positive patients or those with AIDS.

Although candidiasis can appear in several different forms, the lesions are typical and can usually be diagnosed by clinical appearance. They may be confirmed by culture. Topical products

available to treat oral candidiasis include nystatin products (aqueous suspension, vaginal tablets [used as lozenges], and lozenges [pastilles]) or clotrimazole troches (see Chapter 9).

With chronic candidiasis, ketoconazole tablets taken orally once daily can be used. Systemic alternatives include either fluconazole or itraconazole. All are effective, but they should be continued for at least 2 weeks and/or at least 2 to 3 days past the time when the symptoms have disappeared.

Angular Cheilitis/Cheilosis

Angular cheilitis appears as simple redness, fissures, erosion, ulcers, and crusting located at the angles of the

> Angular cheilitis—cracks in corners of mouth

mouth, which may or may not be painful. Most cases of cheilitis are associated with a mixed infection. Frequently, *C. albicans* infection is present, and not uncommonly both candida and gram-positive bacteria such as streptococci and/or staphylococci also invade the lesion.

Predisposing factors may include moisture from drooling (moist areas are more likely to be infected with fungus). In the past, a decrease in vertical dimension was thought to contribute to angular cheilitis, but recent evidence has not shown this to be true.

Depending on the presentation of the patient's lesion, therapy is addressed toward treating the secondary infection(s). If *Candida* organisms are present, treatment with an antifungal (Chapter 9) agent is indicated. Examples of topical antifungal agents include nystatin, clotrimazole, or miconazole. If inflammation is present, some practitioners prescribe a combination of an antifungal agent mixed with a topical steroid (e.g., Mycolog [miconazole {*Myco*statin}] plus triamcinolone acetonide {Kena*log*}). One concern, which may or may not be clinically significant, about using steroids with a fungal infection is that steroids inhibit the inflammatory reaction associated with cellular immunity (this is the reaction that normally fights fungal infections).

If a bacterial overgrowth is suspected, the organisms responsible are usually similar to those of impetigo—staphylococci and streptococci. To treat this bacterial infection, systemic penicillinase-resistant penicillins, such as dicloxacillin, are indicated (Chapter 8). A relatively new agent, mupirocin (Bactroban), is a topical antibacterial useful in the treatment of staphylococcal and streptococcal infections. Using mupirocin (Chapter 8) decreases the likelihood of adverse reactions, and mupirocin is as effective as systemic penicillinase-resistant penicillins. A topical antifungal agent and mupirocin can be used concomitantly if both are indicated.

Although rarely produced by a deficiency of vitamin B_6 (pyridoxine) or B_2 (riboflavin), cheilosis can result from deficiencies of these vitamins. Vitamin B supplements would be useful, but only if a vitamin deficiency exists.

ALVEOLAR OSTEITIS

> Dry socket increases with BCPs, smoking, and diabetes

Alveolar osteitis, or "dry socket," occurs in 2% to 3% of all tooth extractions, most commonly in the lower molar region, where the incidence is considerably higher than in other areas. Alveolar osteitis is thought to be caused by loss or necrosis of the blood clot that has formed in the extraction site, exposing the underlying bone. The exposed bone produces severe pain. Predisposing factors include oral contraceptive use and **menstrual cycle** phase. Smoking, especially after extraction, can increase the likelihood of dry socket. Inhaling on a cigarette produces a negative pressure in the oral cavity that may dislodge the clot.

Infection, swelling, elevated temperature, lymphadenopathy, and a foul odor may be present. Treatment consists of rinsing with saline water and debridement, placement of a pack, analgesics, and supportive therapy. Although there is some indication that local placement of antibiotics may reduce the incidence of dry socket, aseptic techniques, proper suturing techniques, and minimal trauma should be used as prophylactic measures. Most literature does not recommend the use of prophylactic antibiotics. If infection is present, antibiotics are indicated (treatment not prophylaxis). Antibiotics may be indicated in patients at high risk for infection.

IMMUNE REACTIONS

RECURRENT APHTHOUS STOMATITIS

Recurrent aphthous stomatitis, which is sometimes referred to as a **"canker sore,"** is a common

> RAS = canker sore

oral lesion occurring in about 20% of the population. It is seen after 20 years of age and has an unknown etiology, although an involvement of the immune system is suspected.

Recurrent aphthous stomatitis presents clinically as a few small to many large ulcers. These ulcers can even coalesce into giant ulcers. Although three distinct types have been clinically identified—minor, major, and herpetiforme; the most common form of aphthous ulcers is the minor type.

The etiology of aphthous stomatitis involves an immunologic component and may be associated with a focal immune dysfunction in which T lymphocytes play a significant role. There is a decreased ratio of T-helper (CD4+) cells to T-suppressor/cytotoxic (CD8+) cells. An increase in the CD8 cells is seen. The oral mucosa is destroyed by lymphocytes.

Many hypotheses have been considered concerning the etiology of recurrent aphthous stomatitis, including the following: an allergenic/hypersensitivity reaction (endogenous [autoimmune], exogenous [hyperimmune]), genetic, hematologic, hormones, infection, nutrition, and nonspecific events such as trauma and stress. Another hypothesis is that it is a hypersensitivity reaction to the sodium lauryl sulfate present in many over-the-counter (OTC) products, including most toothpastes (Table 14-2).

Corticosteroids. Steroids have been the mainstay of therapy for recurrent aphthous stomatitis for many years. Topical steroids, such as fluocinonide or betamethasone, are used to reduce the inflammation associated with the lesions. Topical corticosteroids are available in different strengths and potencies (Chapter 19). The amount of antiinflammatory action present depends on the strength of the steroid; however, the possibility for adverse reactions associated with the corticosteroids increases with increased strength of the steroid. Creams or gels are more easily applied than ointments (greasy base), but gels, because they contain alcohol, can cause burning. Examples of topical steroids are triamcinolone acetonide, clobetasol, and fluocinonide.

▮ **T**ABLE 14-2	**Toothpastes (Dentifrices) That Do Not Contain Sodium Lauryl Sulfate***

DENTIFRICE	AMERICAN DENTAL ASSOCIATION APPROVED
Arm and Hammer Dental Care Baking Soda tooth powder	No
Platinum Whitening Toothpaste with Fluoride	No
Pycopay Tooth Powder	No
Sensodyne Gel, Cool Mint	No
Sensodyne-SC Toothpaste	Yes

*Many products with almost identical names made by the same company do contain sodium lauryl sulfate. Mr. Toms contains sodium lauryl sulfate. The ingredients are listed on toothpaste tubes.

Another base, carboxymethylcellulose paste (Orabase), is a plasticized base that hardens into a plasticlike plaster. Steroids are incorporated into this paste, which is applied after drying the area. Patient opinions differ with respect to this base. Some like its plastic consistency and covering of the lesion, but others dislike the soft-shell-like inflexible lump of base. Orabase is available plain or mixed with either hydrocortisone or triamcinolone acetonide.

In severe cases of recurrent aphthous stomatitis, a short course of systemic steroids (40 mg/day) may be indicated.

Amelorex. Amelorex (Aphthasol) is a new drug used topically in treatment of aphthous ulcers. It is applied 4 times daily

> Amelorex reduces duration of aphthous (0.7 days)

and can produce a decrease in the duration of both healing and pain by 0.7 days.

Diphenhydramine. Diphenhydramine alone is now preferred because of its local anesthetic action. Tetracycline suspension mixed with nystatin and diphenhydramine has been advocated.

Immunosuppressives.
As a last resort, an immunosuppressive agent such as azathioprine (Imuran), methotrexate (Rheumatrex), and cyclosporin (Sandimmune) have

> Immunosuppressives—last resort

been used to treat severe aphthous. Other immunomodulating agents such as thalidomide and interferon also have been used. Whether thalidomide is effective in the treatment of aphthous and suppression of recurrences is controversial. Some studies found a positive effect, whereas others found none. Thalidomide was previously approved for use in Europe for insomnia in pregnant women. It was later found that as little as 1 tablet, taken on a certain day of gestation, could produce phocomelia (missing arm and or leg bones). It is currently used in certain South American countries to treat leprosy in men. Not unexpectedly, some thalidomide has been inappropriately transferred to women and teratogenic effects have been produced. The risk of teratogenic effects must be weighed against thalidomide's potential beneficial effects. The United States has approved thalidomide for use only with very limited distribution.

Tetracycline has been used in the past, but current thinking is that adding tetracycline suspension to mixtures does not add to the therapeutic effect. Chlorhexidine (Peridex) has been used to manage this condition.

LICHEN PLANUS

Lichen planus is a skin condition that frequently involves lesions on the oral mucous membranes. The oral lesions are present without the skin lesions in 65% of the cases. Lichen planus can present in three forms: striated, plaquelike, and erosive (contains the atrophic and bullous subtypes). The most characteristic type is hypertrophic lichen planus; this lesion has a white lacelike pattern that intersects to form a reticular pattern.

Symptoms of pain vary between no pain and extreme pain depending on the presence of ulceration. The etiology of lichen planus is unknown, but current hypotheses include a viral infection, an autoimmune disease, and a hypersensitivity reaction to an unknown agent.

MISCELLANEOUS ORAL CONDITIONS

GEOGRAPHIC TONGUE

With geographic tongue, the tongue may have lesions that typically appear to be a map of the world with the lesions appearing to be the continents. Usually, the lesions are ringed with erythema and their centers are white. There are changes in the patterns over time, and they may even disappear at times. The etiology of geographic tongue is unknown, but the condition may be related to hormonal changes, stress, infection, psoriasis, or autoimmune diseases. Often the burning becomes severe when eating spicy foods or drinking alcohol. Treatment includes reassurance and avoidance of irritating food and alcohol.

BURNING MOUTH OR TONGUE SYNDROME

Burning mouth or tongue syndrome has been called *glossodynia* and *glossopyrosis* (*pyro,* burn).

With this syndrome the oral cavity commonly appears normal, but the patient gives a history of experiencing a discomfort described as pain or a burning sensation that increases in severity through the day.

Glossodynia is a painful tongue and is divided into two types: with and without observable alterations on the tongue. It can be caused by many conditions, both local and systemic. Because the tongue is very sensitive, small inflammation of fungiform papillae or small trauma from a tooth can be extremely painful. Other visible changes in the tongue are atrophy of the filiform papillae and generalized redness. Burning, stinging, or itching may occur.

The nature of the psychologic component in this disease is unclear, but it is known that the presence of chronic disease can lead to depression and anxiety. Patients often are concerned that the cause of their problem may be related to malignancy. Scientific study must be done to determine its cause.

The etiology of burning tongue has not been elucidated, but numerous hypotheses have been proposed, including xerostomia, candidiasis, acid reflux, nutritional deficiency (B_{12}, folate, or iron), immunologic, hormonal changes, allergic reaction, inflammatory process, psychogenic, or an **idiopathic** reaction. (The variety of hypotheses indicates that the cause of burning tongue has not yet been determined.)

The treatment of burning tongue syndrome depends on the particular etiology the practitioner believes. Some clinicians treat the patient as they would if the patient had candidiasis. Others test for vitamin deficiencies. Palliative therapy involves using topical diphenhydramine (Benadryl) to relieve the symptoms. Tricyclic antidepressants, such as amitriptyline, can be used on a trial basis, beginning with a dose of 10 mg at bedtime and slowly increasing the amount until an effective dose is achieved. Amitriptyline is used for two effects. One is that it is thought that depression may play a role in this syndrome and the amitriptyline may treat the depression. However, this is unlikely because the dose used is not an antidepressant dose and the onset of action is much quicker than the antidepressant effect of amitriptyline. The second mechanism of amitriptyline's proposed effect is that amitriptyline is acting as an adjunct in the management of chronic pain. Amitriptyline has been shown to be effective in chronic pain. Additional studies are needed to determine whether any psychotropic agents might be effective in treating burning tongue.

INFLAMMATION

PERICORONITIS

Pericoronitis is inflammation of the tissue around the crown of the tooth. This term, most commonly applied to partially erupted third molars, refers to an inflammatory response that is produced when food and bacteria become trapped between the operculum and the tooth. Periodontal pockets can become painful and swell. If the condition is observed early in its course, debridement with saline irrigation and the use of warm saline rinses will rectify the situation. With severe pericoronitis, debridement is still the primary treatment. If the affected tooth is to be extracted, extraction can prevent further episodes of pericoronitis. With erupting third molars, repeated episodes may occur. Analgesics can be used for the discomfort. Infection, usually managed by local treatment, may rapidly spread in debilitated patients and should be aggressively treated with antibiotics.

POSTIRRADIATION CARIES

Changes in saliva after irradiation therapy and lack of proper plaque control can rapidly accelerate the rate of dental caries. Generalized cervical decay within the first year after radiation therapy can result. Meticulous oral hygiene, reinforced by the hygienist, short duration between subsequent recall appointments, artificial salivas, and self-application of sodium fluoride gel 4 times daily in a bite guard are recommended.

ROOT SENSITIVITY

Sensitivity of exposed root surfaces may be precipitated by heat, cold, and sweet or sour foods. Occlusal trauma may produce irritation to the exposed dentinal tubules; occlusal adjustment is the treatment. Roots exposed by periodontal surgery, extensive root planing, or accumulation of plaque and its by-products are more difficult to manage. Applications of glycerin with burnishing, sodium fluoride, stannous fluoride, and adrenal steroids have been used in the dental office in an attempt to reduce root sensitivity. Adequate clinical trials for these products are lacking. The patient may use home brushing with concentrated sodium chloride and 0.4% stannous fluoride. Sodium fluoride gel may also be self-applied in a bite guard. Desensitizing toothpastes have helped some patients, but controlled clinical trials with sufficient patient populations are lacking.

ACTINIC LIP CHANGES

Long-term exposure of the lip to the sun can cause irreversible tissue changes known as *actinic cheilitis*. These sun-related changes occur near the vermilion border of the lips and can progress to malignancy. Sunscreen preparations with higher (greater than 15) sun protective factors should be applied before sun exposure and reapplied as needed. If keratotic changes have occurred, treatment is topical 5-fluorouracil (5-FU), an antineoplastic agent that promotes sloughing of the skin (bad layers of cells are sloughed off). A topical steroid (see Chapter 19) may be used to relieve the irritation produced by 5-FU.

DRUG-INDUCED ORAL SIDE EFFECTS

Drug-induced oral side effects can be produced by a wide variety of drugs. Different kinds of lesions can be produced with the same drug, and the same kind of lesion can be produced by different agents. Some drugs that can cause changes in the oral cavity are listed in Box 14-1. Common oral side effects include xerostomia, drug-induced lichenoid-like reaction, and hypersensitivity reactions.

The most commonly listed oral side effect of drugs is xerostomia. Many drugs have been stated to produce xerostomia, but the effect is variable depending on the patient and the dose of the drug. An extensive list of xerostomia-producing drugs is available in Appendix H.

XEROSTOMIA

Xerostomia may result from a drug (e.g., atropine), a disease (e.g., Sjögren's syndrome), aging (may be caused by drugs rather than age), or radiation. Radiation therapy to the head and neck affects the salivary glands so that the consistency of saliva is altered and its volume is reduced substantially.

Many different groups of drugs produce xerostomia (Appendix H). For example, the anti-

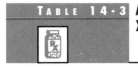

TABLE 14-3	Agents That Produce Xerostomia (Dry Mouth)	
DRUG GROUP	EXAMPLES
Anticholinergics*	Bentyl, Donnatal, Artane
Antihypertensives*	Aldomet, clonidine (Catapres), Minipress
Antipsychotics,* phenothiazines	Haldol, Navane, Mellaril
Tricyclic antidepressants*	Elavil, Norpramin
Antihistamines	Benadryl, Chlor-Trimeton, hydroxyzine
Adrenergic agents	Phenylpropanolamine, Sudafed
Diuretics	Dyazide, hydrochlorothiazide
Benzodiazepines	Xanax, Valium, Halcion

*Most likely to produce xerostomia.

cholinergics and other drugs with anticholinergic side effects are likely to produce xerostomia. With xerostomia, the patient has a dry mouth. Saliva washes the teeth; xerostomia, or dryness of the mouth, produces an increase in the incidence of caries, especially Class V lesions.

Treatment of xerostomia. Treatment of xerostomia consists of the following:
- *Caries prevention:* The use of fluoride trays and gels, as well as other topical agents, to counteract the formation of caries should be recommended and demonstrated.
- *Artificial saliva:* Artificial saliva may be suggested for use in these patients. Table 14-3 lists selected drug groups and examples most likely to produce dry mouth.
- *Home care:* The use of fluoride rinses or trays containing fluoride to deliver fluoride should be recommended before extensive caries occur. Using water or sugarless gum should be encouraged in place of gum and candies containing sugar.
- *Change medication or reduce dose:* With some drug groups, such as antidepressants,

BOX 14-1 ORAL SIDE EFFECTS OF DRUGS

Discoloration

Intrinsic

Tetracycline/doxycycline
Minocycline
Excessive fluoride (fluorosis)

Extrinsic

Stannous fluoride (extrinsic)
Chlorhexidine (extrinsic)
Liquid iron (extrinsic)

Sialorrhea (ptyalism)

Cholinergics
  Pilocarpine
Cholinesterase inhibitors
  Neostigmine
Ethionamide
Iodides
Ketamine
Lithium
Aldosterone
Apomorphine
Mercurials
Niridazole
Nitrazepam

Sialosis

Propylthiouracil (PTU)
Methimazole
Iodides
Isoprenaline
Methyldopa
Oxyphenbutazone
Sulfonamides

Gingival bleeding

Warfarin (Coumadin)
Ticlopidine (Ticlid)
Quinidine
Aspirin

Taste changes—(more listed in Appendix H)

Metronidazole
ACE inhibitors
Penicillamine
Griseofulvin
Gold salts

Gingival enlargement

Anticonvulsants
  Phenytoin
  Sodium valproate
  Phenobarbital
Cyclosporin
Calcium channel blockers
  Nifedipine
  Diltiazem
  Verapamil

Systemic lupus erythematosus

Antiarrhythmics
  Procainamide
  Quinidine
Hydralazine
Isoniazid
Anticonvulsants
  Hydantoins
  Ethosuximide
Lithium
Thiouracil

Parotitis

Cardiovascular drugs
  Methyldopa
  Guanethidine
  Clonidine
  Bretylium

Stomatitis

Antineoplastic agents
  Nitrogen mustard
  Methotrexate
  5-Fluorouracil
  6-Mercaptopurine
  Chlorambucil
  Doxorubicin
  Daunorubicin
  Bleomycin
Antiarthritic
  Penicillamine
  Gold salts
Local application
  Aspirin
  Valproic acid (inside capsule)
  Gentian violet

Pigmentation

Amalgam (e.g., tattoo)
Antineoplastics
  Cisplatin
  Doxorubicin
Oral contraceptives
Minocycline
Antimalarials

Candidiasis

Broad-spectrum antibiotics
Corticosteroids

Sialoadenitis

Phenylbutazone
Oxyphenbutazone
Nitrofurantoin
Isoproterenol
Iodine (iodides)
α-Methyldopa

Continued

Box 14-1 ORAL SIDE EFFECTS OF DRUGS—cont'd

Xerostomia—(more listed in Appendix H)

Antihypertensives
  Clonidine—centrally acting
  Diuretics
Psychotropic
  Antipsychotics
  Antidepressants
Antihistamines
Anticholinergics
Anticonvulsants
Laxatives
Muscle relaxants
  Cyclobenzaprine

Carisoprodol
Methocarbamol
Orphenadrine
Opioids
Sedative-hypnotics

Erythema multiforme

Antiinfectives
  Penicillins
  Tetracyclines
  Sulfonamides
  Clindamycin
Anticonvulsants

Caries

Xerostomia-producing agents
Sugar-containing medications

Muscle-related

Dystonic reactions
  Antipsychotic agents
  Metoclopramide
  Cisapride
Bruxism
  Amphetamines

---

there are drugs that produce significant xerostomia and others that produce much less xerostomia. For example, the antidepressant amitriptyline produces a significant amount of xerostomia while a different antidepressant, sertraline, produces much less. Any medication change must be coordinated with the patient's physician and would depend on many factors.

- *Pilocarpine:* Cholinergic agents (P+) such as pilocarpine can stimulate an increase in saliva in patients with functioning parotid glands. Chapter 5 discusses its dose and adverse effects.

SIALORRHEA

Certain drugs may produce an increase in saliva—termed *sialosis, sialism,* and *sialorrhea.* One example is the cholinergic agent pilocarpine. Mercurials and iodides also can cause sialosis.

HYPERSENSITIVITY-TYPE REACTIONS

Hypersensitivity reactions may be hyperimmune responses triggered by an antigenic component

on the drug or its metabolite. Contact stomatitis is more localized when gum and candy are responsible and is more diffuse with toothpaste use. The buccal mucosa and the lateral borders of the tongue are often involved. Even cinnamon-flavored products have been implicated in hypersensitivity reactions. The potential for a hypersensitivity reaction is determined by the particular drug, the frequency of administration, the route of administration (antibiotics administered topically are more likely to produce hypersensitivity reactions than those given parenterally), and the patient's immune system (IgE).

ORAL LESIONS THAT RESEMBLE AUTOIMMUNE-TYPE REACTIONS

Lichenoid-like eruptions. Many drugs are associated with eruptions that resemble lichen planus. Box 14-2 lists some drugs that have been associated with this type of reaction. The most common drug implicated is hydrochlorothiazide (HCTZ). Others include γ-blockers and antimalarials. Appendix H gives a more complete list.

BOX 14-2 DRUGS ASSOCIATED WITH LICHENOID ERUPTIONS

Heavy metals
Arsenic
Bismuth
Gold salts
Mercury (in amalgam)
Palladium
Antihypertensives
Methyldopa
β-Blockers
Labetalol
Oxprenolol
Practolol
Propranolol
Diuretics
Thiazides
Furosemide
Spironolatone
Antiarrhythmics
Quinidine
Procainamide

**Angiotensin-converting
enzyme inhibitors**
Captopril
Enalapril
Calcium channel blockers
Nifedipine
Ulcerative colitis agents
Sulfasalazine
Mesalazine
Antimalarials
Chloroquine
Hydroxychloroquine
Quinacrine (Atabrine)
Quinine
Levamisole
Antitubercular agents
Dapsone
Streptomycin
Pyrimethamine
p-Aminosalicylic acid
(PAS)
Ethambutol
Isoniazid

Antiinfectives
Tetracycline
Demeclocycline
Ketoconazole
Antineoplastic agents
Hydroxyurea
5-Fluorouracil
Sulfonylureas
Chlorpropamide
Tolbutamide
Tolazamide
Psychotropics
Phenothiazines
Chlorpromazine
Lithium
Others
Nonsteroidal antiin-
flammatory agents
Carbamazepine
Allopurinol
Triprolidine
Penicillamine

Lupus-like reactions. Oral manifestations can occur with systemic lupus erythematosus. These lesions may also be produced by a variety of drugs including antiarrhythmic agents and anticonvulsants.

Erythema multiforme-like. Some drugs, for example the anticonvulsants, can produce lesions that resemble those of erythema multiforme.

STAINS

Staining of teeth may occur either as the teeth are formed, or in a few cases in adult teeth. The tetracyclines are incorporated into forming teeth and thereby stain the teeth. Today, this adverse reaction is well known and pregnant women or very small children are not given tetracycline. With adults both intrinsic and extrinsic stains may occur. Minocycline is thought to produce a blue-gray coloration to the bone in adult teeth. Chlorhexidine rinse as well as liquid iron preparations can also cause extrinsic staining.

GINGIVAL ENLARGEMENT

Gingival **hyperplasia,** now known as *gingival enlargement*, has been renamed because hyperplasia is not the sole process that occurs in the gums. Gingival enlargement can occur in relation to several drug groups; the most common three are the following:
* ***Phenytoin (Dilantin):*** Chapter 16 discusses phenytoin and gingival enlargement. The

rate of occurrence varies with the patient population, but almost half of the patients exhibit this reaction. Occurrence of gingival enlargement in patients taking phenytoin may be dose related. Oral hygiene practices affect its incidence and severity.

- *Cyclosporin:* Cyclosporin is the antirejection drug used for every patient who has had a kidney transplant and for patients receiving many other transplants. Cyclosporin is associated with gingival enlargement.
- *Calcium channel blockers (CCB):* CCBs are used for hypertension and congestive heart failure. They have been associated with GE.
- *Others:* Other implicated drugs include some anticonvulsants such as carbamazepine (Tegretol) and valproic acid (Depakene).

COMMON AGENTS USED TO TREAT ORAL LESIONS

CORTICOSTEROIDS

For many oral lesions, especially those with a component of inflammation or immune response, corticosteroids are used. Depending on the severity of the lesions, the topical corticosteroids would be selected based on their potency. Weak, intermediate, and potent corticosteroids are used in turn until an agent is effective. The proper strength of steroid is the least potent that will ameliorate the lesion. (See the steroid topical chart in Chapter 19.) Hydrocortisone cream 1% is a low-potency topical steroid available over the counter. The 2.5% hydrocortisone cream is available on prescription. Triamcinolone acetonide (TAC) is more potent than hydrocortisone and is in the middle range of potency of the steroids. It is available as 0.025%, 0.1%, and 0.5 %; the first two strengths are classified as moderate, and 0.5% is stronger. Fluocinonide (Lidex) is more potent than TAC and is available as a 0.05% cream or solution. Clobetasol (Temovate), 0.05% cream or solution, is in

the most potent group. The later would be used only if the other agents were ineffective. Sample prescriptions are provided in Appendix C.

If topical corticosteroid therapy is ineffective or if the condition is severe, then systemic corticosteroids may be indicated. When systemic steroids are used, prednisone is the most commonly used. There is little reason to use other agents because all corticosteroids have virtually the same effect. When dosing systemic steroids, the dose begins high (usually between 40 and 60 mg of prednisone per day) and is then tapered (see Appendix C, sample prescriptions), depending on the progress of the lesions. In some cases, chronic systemic corticosteroids are required to control the oral lesion. When systemic steroids are used chronically, their adverse reactions must be managed (i.e., osteoporosis, fluid retention, diabetes, hypertension and the manifestations of moon face, buffalo hump, and abdominal striae).

PALLIATIVE TREATMENT

Palliative treatment is treatment designed to make the patient more comfortable. Agents that reduce the pain of the oral cavity can be topical and systemic. Topical agents are applied by swishing the liquid around in the mouth. These agents include a local anesthetic agent (viscous lidocaine) (Chapter 10) and an antihistamine with local anesthetic properties, diphenhydramine elixir (Chapter 19). Many combination products have been prescribed, but their benefit over plain diphenhydramine elixir is controversial. Mixtures of diphenhydramine, lidocaine, and magnesium-aluminum hydroxide have been advocated. Systemic analgesics can often provide relief from a painful oral lesion. Topical and systemic agents may be used together for an additive effect. One concern with the use of topical local anesthetics is that reduction in the sensations from the throat could lead to choking. This can be minimized by avoiding eating directly after application. If isolated lesions are present, the anesthetic can be painted on the lesion using a cotton-tipped swab.

REVIEW QUESTIONS

1. State the best way to prevent actinic lip changes.
2. Describe the treatment of a patient with acute necrotizing ulcerative gingivitis.
3. Describe the appropriate treatment for herpes labialis. State what has been proved to be effective in the treatment of recurrent *Herpes labialis* in nonimmunocompromised patients. Write a prescription for two anti-herpes agents.
4. Describe two appropriate treatments for recurrent aphthous stomatitis. Write a prescription for one agent.
5. State three drugs used for oral candidiasis and discuss when each agent would be appropriate.
6. Name two ways to reduce alveolar osteitis. Write a prescription for two agents, one topical and one systemic, used to treat oral candidiasis.
7. Describe three causes of xerostomia and state several drugs that can produce this effect.
8. Explain the management of xerostomia. Include preventive measures to be included.

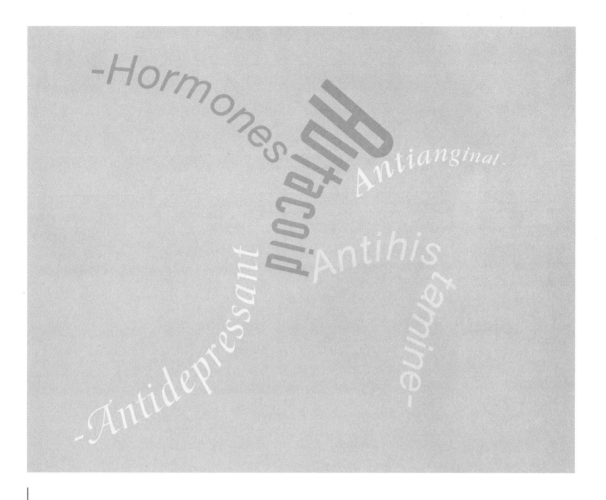

SECTION THREE

Drugs That May Alter Dental Treatment

Cardiovascular Drugs

> Cardiovascular disease affects many dental patients.

The term *cardiovascular disease* refers to a variety of diseases of the heart and blood vessels. Examples of these diseases include **hypertension,** angina pectoris, cerebrovascular accident, and congestive heart failure (CHF). Although cardiovascular disease is the leading cause of death in the United States, patients with it are now living longer, more productive lives because of cardiac care units, comprehensive drug therapy, and intensive screening procedures. This explains why cardiovascular disease affects such a large proportion of the dental patient population.

The dental health care worker first identifies the patient with cardiovascular disease while taking the medical or drug history. It is common for these patients to have several cardiovascular conditions, such as CHF, hypertension, and **hypercholesterolemia.** For each disease, a patient may take one or more medications. The importance of this group of drugs is demonstrated by the fact that about 25% of

> 1/4 of Top 200 are CV drugs

the top 200 drugs (Appendix A) are from this group.

Because cardiovascular medications are frequently given for the patient's lifetime, a knowledge of the actions, problems, and effects of these drugs on dental treatment is essential. Both the disease and the drugs used in their treatment can affect the management of a patient's dental care.

Before each group of drugs is discussed, the disease for which the drugs are used is briefly described, beginning with general considerations concerning the dental treatment of patients with cardiovascular disease.

DENTAL IMPLICATIONS OF CARDIOVASCULAR DISEASE

CONTRAINDICATIONS TO TREATMENT

Although most patients with cardiovascular disease can be safely treated in the dental office, circumstances may arise in which dental treatment should be delayed until the patient's disease is under better control.

Certain medical situations listed in Box 15-1 are absolute contraindications to dental treat-

Box 15-1 Cardiovascular Contraindications to Dental Treatment

- Acute or recent myocardial infarction (within the preceding 3 to 6 months)
- Unstable or the recent onset of angina pectoris
- Uncontrolled congestive heart failure
- Uncontrolled arrhythmias
- Significant, uncontrolled hypertension

ment until a consultation with the patient's provider has determined any special treatment alterations that might be warranted. These absolute contraindications apply only to uncontrolled or severe cardiovascular diseases. Examples of absolute contraindications to elective dental treatment include very high blood pressure and the period after the patient has experienced a **myocardial infarction.** Most patients with cardiovascular disease can be treated in the dental office. The type of procedure anticipated, the stress of the procedure, and the fact that many procedures are elective must be considered. By obtaining a thorough health history, a determination can be made about whether the patient's provider should be consulted before beginning dental treatment. When the health care provider is contacted, it is important to explain the procedure(s) that is indicated for the patient.

Vasoconstrictor Limit

Cardiovascular patients should receive epinephrine.

When a local anesthetic containing a vasoconstrictor is used in the treatment of patients with cardiovascular disease, the severity of the patient's disease must be considered. The majority of cardiovascular patients should benefit from the use of epineph-

rine in the local anesthetic agent. The amount and effect of the epinephrine administered must be weighed against the fact that poor pain management can produce the release of endogenous epinephrine. Limiting the dose of epinephrine to the cardiac dose (0.04 mg) may be warranted in a few severely affected patients (see Chapter 10 for a detailed discussion of vasoconstrictor limits).

Using a slow rate of injection and appropriate aspiration techniques to avoid intravascular injection reduces the chance of vasoconstrictor adverse reactions. A "fight or flight" reaction related to the patient's anxiety also results in the release of endogenous epinephrine—indistinguishable in effect from that of the exogenous epinephrine. [So, being *really scared* feels exactly like epinephrine—of course, you are making your own epinephrine!]

Infective Endocarditis

When a medical history is taken and the presence of rheumatic heart disease or other valvular or degenerative disease is discovered, the risk of producing infective endocarditis must be considered. In these cases, if warranted by the dental procedure being performed, antibiotics should be given prophylactically. Chapter 8 discusses the appropriate use of antibiotic prophylaxis in the prevention of infective endocarditis.

Cardiac Pacemakers

A cardiac pacemaker is an electrical device implanted in a patient's chest to regulate the heart rhythm. If not appropriately shielded,

Patients with pacemakers do not require antibiotic premedication.

some electrical devices commonly used in dentistry may interfere with proper pacemaker activity. Consultation with the patient's provider may be appropriate before treating a patient with a pacemaker. These patients do not require antibiotic prophylaxis.

PERIODONTAL DISEASE AND CARDIOVASCULAR DISEASE

Research has discovered a relationship between periodontal disease and both cardiovascular disease and stroke. An inherited phenotype, MO, is under both genetic and environmental influences, placing the patient at increased risk for severe periodontal disease, insulin-dependent diabetes mellitus, atherosclerosis, and emboli production. The monocytes in these patients secrete abnormally high levels of cytokines, including PGE_2, IL-1β, and TNF-α, all associated with both periodontal and cardiovascular disease. An increase in dietary intake of fat leads to an increase in low-density lipoproteins (LDL, bad cholesterol), which are known to upregulate the destructive monocyte response. Studies correlate the patient's periodontal condition to cardiovascular disease over time. In general the studies found that the presence of periodontal disease predicts an increase in morbidity and mortality resulting from cardiovascular disease.

CARDIAC GLYCOSIDES

CONGESTIVE HEART FAILURE (CHF)

> CHF—heart can't meet needs

The heart functions as a pump ensuring adequate circulation of the blood to meet the oxygen needs of all the body's tissues. When oxygen needs are increased, as in exercise, the normal heart adjusts its output to meet the increased oxygen needs. If the heart is unable to keep up with the body's needs, it becomes a "failing" heart and the pumping mechanism becomes inefficient. This occurs because the heart muscle has suffered an injury and cannot keep up its work. Some en-

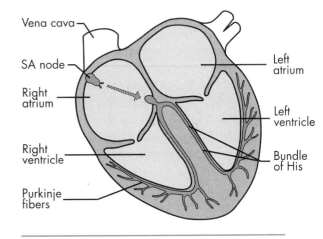

FIGURE 15-1   *Cross section of heart with conduction tissues.*

largement of the heart produces a more efficient heartbeat and cardiac output (Starling's law). However, over time, additional cardiac enlargement occurs (cardiac muscle stretched past its maximum effectiveness by the presence of excess blood that it cannot pump out), and the patient becomes tachycardiac. This inefficient pumping mechanism results in an inadequate cardiac output and unsatisfactory circulation. Various forms of injury to the heart, such as myocardial infarction (heart attack), arrhythmias, and valvular abnormalities from rheumatic heart disease, can contribute to a failing heart.

The heart has two-parts: the right and left sides (Figure 15-1). In congestive heart failure (CHF), the heart does not provide adequate cardiac output to provide for the oxygen needs of the body. Over time, the blood accumulates in the failing ventricle(s). The ventricle(s) enlarges, and finally becomes ineffective as a pump.

One or both sides of the heart can fail. Usually the left side fails first. If the left side of the heart fails, the blood backs up into the pulmonary circulation (lungs). Pulmonary edema results, producing **dyspnea** and **orthopnea.** Dental patients with left failure may need to have dental treatment performed with the patient in the semireclined position. If the right side of the heart fails, then the right ventricle is unable to remove all the blood from that side of the heart. Right-sided heart failure causes systemic congestion. Symptoms include peripheral edema with fluid accumulation evidenced by pitting edema (**pedal** edema). Over time, many patients experience failure of both sides of the heart, which causes symptoms from failure of both sides.

DIGITALIS GLYCOSIDES

The most common type of drug used in the treatment of CHF was first described by William Withering in 1785. At first he thought that these drugs affected the kidneys because they produced diuresis. Later these substances were referred to as *cardiac* or *digitalis glycosides, cardiac* because they affect the heart and glycoside because of their chemical structure. Although digitalis glycosides are not considered first-line therapy, they are discussed first. Several cardiac glycosides are available for clinical use, but digoxin [di-JOX-in] (Lanoxin), the most commonly used product, is used as the prototype.

> Positive inotropic effect

Pharmacologic effects. The major effect of digoxin on the failing heart is to increase the force and strength of contraction of the myocardium (positive inotropic effect). It allows the heart to do more work without increasing its oxygen usage. When the contractile force of the heart is improved, the heart becomes a more efficient pump and the cardiac output increases. After the patient takes digoxin, the heart is reduced to a more efficient size and can function more effectively.

Digoxin affects the heart rate in several ways. It has little effect on the heart rate of normal patients, but in CHF the heart rate is first increased. This occurs because of increased sympathetic action resulting from decreased cardiac output. As digoxin increases the cardiac output, the sympathetic tone is decreased, with a decrease in heart rate (bradycardia) as the end result.

Digoxin also reduces the edema that occurs with CHF. As a result of the improved pumping action, more blood circulates through the kidneys (increase in glomerular filtration rate), which mobilizes the edema from the tissues, producing diuresis. The diuresis is not due to an effect on the kidneys; it is due to its indirect effect produced by the improving heart's function. The size of the heart is reduced as the excess blood volume that has collected there is removed via the kidneys.

Digoxin can affect automaticity, conduction velocity, and refractory periods of different parts of the heart in different ways. It slows atrioventricular (AV) conduction, prolongs the refractory period of the AV node, and decreases the rate of the sinoatrial (SA) node. By prolonging the refractory period of the AV node, fewer impulses will be transmitted to the ventricle and the heart rate will fall. These effects are useful in the treatment of certain arrhythmias.

Uses. The most common use of digoxin is in the treatment of CHF. It is also used for atrial arrhythmias, including atrial **fibrillation** (AF) and paroxysmal atrial tachycardia (PAT). Patients with CHF and normal sinus rhythm may not experience long-term benefit in reducing mortality from the use of digoxin. A recent large trial comparing the mortality of patients taking digoxin with placebo determined that digoxin did not reduce mortality. For this reason, the use of digoxin is decreasing and other drugs such as calcium channel blockers are used more frequently.

Adverse reactions. Because of digoxin's narrow therapeutic index (see Chapter 3), toxic effects are not uncommon. Even slight changes in dosage, absorption, or metabolism can trigger toxic symptoms. In the elderly, toxicity is more likely to occur.

GASTROINTESTINAL Early signs of digoxin toxicity include **anorexia,** nausea and vomiting, and copious salivation. A reduction in the dosage of digoxin usually alleviates these adverse reactions.

ARRHYTHMIAS If a sufficient overdose is given, severe cardiac irregularities can develop. These arrhythmias can progress to ventricular fibrillation and death. Diuretics, often used in the treatment of CHF, can produce hypokalemia, which can predispose a patient to serious arrhythmias. Note that digitalis is used to treat arrhythmias and its toxicity can produce arrhythmias.

NEUROLOGIC The neurologic signs of toxicity include headache, drowsiness, and visual disturbances (green and yellow vision, halo around lights). A pain in the lower face resembling that of trigeminal neuralgia has been reported as a neurologic symptom of digitalis toxicity. Weakness, faintness, and mental confusion have also been reported.

ORAL Increased salivation is associated with digoxin toxicity. Increase in gagging reflex has been produced, which may interfere with taking an impression.

DENTAL DRUG INTERACTIONS With either increased or decreased blood levels, serious problems can occur when digoxin interacts with other drugs. One drug interaction between digoxin and the sympathomimetics may result in an increase in the chance of arrhythmias. Because both drugs can produce ectopic pacemaker activity, their concomitant administration can increase the chance of arrhythmias. For this reason, the vasoconstrictors added to local anesthetics, which are sympathomimetics, should be used with caution. In patients with severe cardiac disease, the epinephrine dose may be limited to the cardiac dose (0.04 mg). Erythromycin and tetracycline can increase the toxicity of digoxin in some patients.

Management of the dental patient taking digoxin. Box 15-2 summarizes the management of the dental patient taking digoxin.

GASTROINTESTINAL EFFECTS If a patient complains of nausea or vomiting, special care must be taken to prevent emesis. These symptoms may be associated with digitalis toxicity, and the patient's physician should be consulted if the nausea and vomiting have been protracted.

EPINEPHRINE ADMINISTRATION Because digoxin toxicity can sensitize the myocardium to arrhythmias, epinephrine should be used cautiously or limited to the cardiac dose in patients taking digitalis. Patients taking digitalis should be questioned about toxic symptoms before epinephrine is administered. Hypokalemia from diuretics can exacerbate this arrhythmogenic potential.

PULSE MONITORING Because digitalis can cause bradycardia or arrhythmias, the patient's pulse should be checked before each dental ap-

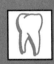

BOX 15-2 MANAGEMENT OF THE DENTAL PATIENT TAKING DIGOXIN

- Watch for overdose side effects such as nausea, vision changes, and copious salivation.
- Use epinephrine with caution to minimize arrhythmias.
- Monitor pulse to check for bradycardia.
- Tetracycline and erythromycin can increase digoxin levels (in ~10% of patients)

pointment for a normal rate and a regular rhythm. An abnormally slow rate or an irregular rhythm should be reported to the patient's provider for evaluation.

Other drugs

HYDRALAZINE AND NITRATE COMBINATION

Combining hydralazine and isosorbide dinitrate has been shown to decrease mortality of patients with CHF. Each of the components produces a different, but useful and additive, pharmacologic effect. Hydralazine, an arterial vasodilator, reduces the peripheral resistance by arterial vasodilation. With a reduction in the afterload, the work of the heart is reduced. Nitroglycerin, a venous dilator, reduces the preload, which reduces the work of the heart. With this combination, the heart is pumping against less resistance and is getting less blood returned to it (some blood remains in the venous circulation). The heart's workload is reduced and symptoms of CHF subside.

ANGIOTENSIN II RECEPTOR ANTAGONISTS

Angiotensin II receptor antagonists such as losartan have also been shown to reduce mortality and symptoms. They are now considered first-line therapy for CHF alone or combined with diuretics. In certain kinds of failure the α and β blockers, such as carvedilol, are effective in the treatment of CHF.

ANTIARRHYTHMIC AGENTS

The terms **arrhythmia** (*ar*, insensibility; *rhythmos*, rhythm) and **dysrhythmia** (*dys*, bad; *rhythmos*, rhythm) are used interchangeably to mean "abnormal rhythm." Arrhythmias may result from abnormal impulse generation or abnormal impulse conduction. Cardiac diseases such as myocardial anoxia, **arteriosclerosis,** and **heart block** can produce arrhythmias. The antiarrhythmic agents are drugs that are used to prevent arrhythmias.

AUTOMATICITY

The cells of the cardiac muscles, unlike those of skeletal muscles, have an intrinsic rhythm called *automaticity.* "Pacemaker" cells undergo slow spontaneous depolarization during diastole (as they rest, they leak ions). When the threshold is reached, a spontaneous action potential is generated. Any cardiac muscle cell left undisturbed, isolated from the rest of the heart cells, and supplied with appropriate nutrients and oxygen will beat spontaneously at its own rate. Each type of cardiac cell differs in its automaticity depending on the function of the particular cell. The cells that specialize in conduction functions have a faster rate of automaticity than other cardiac cells. "Pacemaker" cells spontaneously produce action potentials as they undergo slow spontaneous depolarization during diastole (as they rest, they leak ions). If any heart muscle cell is left undisturbed and isolated from the rest of the heart with appropriate nutrients and oxygen, each cell will beat spontaneously at its own rate. Each type of cardiac cell differs in its automaticity depending on the function of the particular cell. The cells that specialize in conduction functions have a faster rate of automaticity than other cardiac cells. This design ensures that the heart will beat in a coordinated manner.

The SA node has the fastest rate of depolarization and therefore directs all the other cells in the heart. It normally fires impulses about 80 times/min. The SA node is innervated by both the parasympathetic nervous system (PNS) and the sympathetic nervous system (SNS). If the SA node is called the "President of Cardiac, Inc." (Figure 15-2), then the President will "give the order." The President has a phone line (over the atrial muscles) to the Vice President, which is the AV node. When the impulse arrives at the

> Cardiac tissue has inherent automaticity (each part has different rate).

FIGURE **15-2**   *Organization of Cardiac, Inc.*

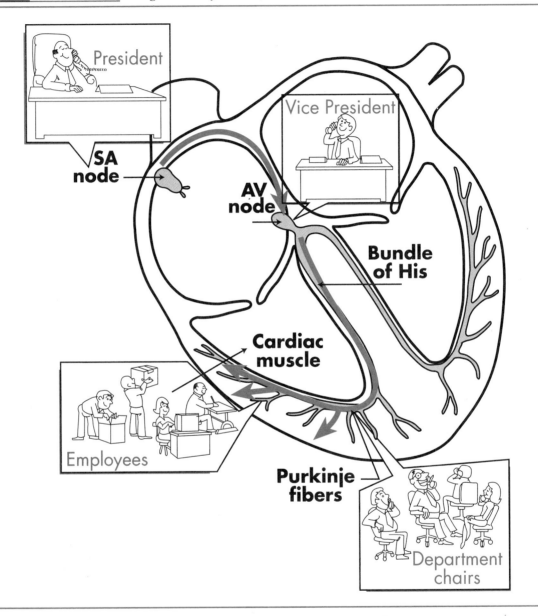

AV node (the Vice President) there is a slight delay because the phone lines beyond the Vice President are thinner. The Vice President sends the message via a major phone system (the bundle of His). The bundle of His then sends messages to the Department Chairs (Purkinje fibers). Many e-mail messages emanate from these Chairs to all the staff (cardiac muscle cells, to the apex of the ventricles), directing them all to contract as they get the message. This system is repeated with each heartbeat. [Naturally, these cells must act much faster than the response of the usual corporate structure.]

In the normal patient, this system functions seamlessly. In the patient with cardiac arrhythmias, diseased parts of the heart can produce abnormal conduction pathways, which may result in arrhythmias.

ACTION POTENTIAL

All action potentials have similar properties, but minor differences exist. During rest, the resting membrane potential varies, but is -75 mV for some cardiac tissues. Electrical excitation from the nerve produces movement of ions across the membrane, generating an action potential (Figure 15-3, *A*). Table 15-1 lists the four phases of ion movement. The electrical activity of the heart muscle as seen in the electrocardiogram **(EKG)** is shown below the action potential. There is a relationship between the action potential and the EKG tracing. During each of these phases there is a change in the ion flow that results in certain effects. These changes are seen in Figure 15-3, *B*.

ARRHYTHMIAS

There are many types of arrhythmias that produce various abnormalities of the heartbeat. These arrhythmias are usually divided into supraventricular (atrial) and ventricular types, depending on the location of the genesis of the arrhythmia. Abnormal arrhythmias may result in

TABLE 15-1 Different Phases of Ion Movement During an Action Potential

PHASE	IONIC EVENT	ION MOVEMENT
1	Fast influx of Na^+	Rapid depolarization
2	Slow influx of Ca^{++}	Maintains depolarization
3	Efflux of K^+	Repolarization
4	Influx of K^+??	Resting potential

tachycardia or bradycardia of the supraventricular (atrial) or ventricular parts of the heart or from ectopic foci. The ectopic foci are "emergent leaders" that preempt the SA or AV nodal rate. The electrical impulses begin at the SA node and travel to the AV node. At the conduction level, different patterns of conduction include the normal pattern, bifurcation (conduction splits and goes two ways), reentry, unidirectional block (action potential is blocked from being stimulated from one side of the tissue but not from the other), and prolonged refractory period.

Several recent deaths of fit adolescents during athletic events have been linked to congenital presence of a prolonged QT interval (Torsades de pointes; previously undiagnosed). Table 15-2 lists typical arrhythmias.

ANTIARRHYTHMIC AGENTS

The antiarrhythmic agents are placed in groups designated by Roman numerals I to IV. Subsets of these Roman numerals use capital letters (A, B, C). The specific actions of the antiarrhythmics are very complicated. The antiarrhythmic agents work by depressing parts of the heart that are beating abnormally. For example, if the Speaker of the House (an ectopic foci) attempts to take over the office of President (SA node) and send additional messages to the other officers, then the antiarrhythmic agents can "quiet" these foci.

FIGURE **15 - 3**   *Electrical excitation from the nerve produces movement of ions across the membrane, generating an action potential.*

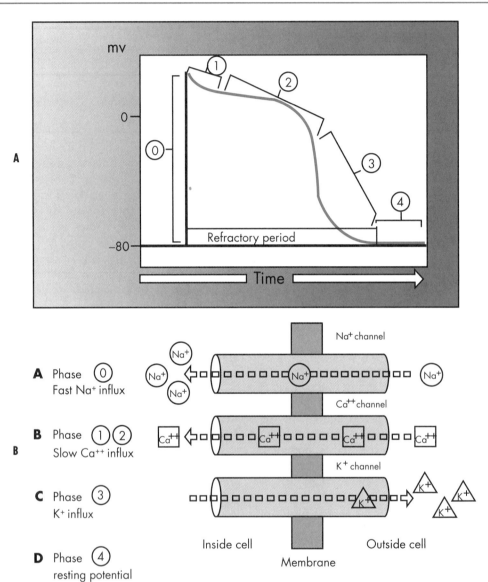

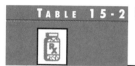

TABLE 15-2 Selected Arrhythmias and Antiarrhythmics Indicated*

Part of Heart	Abnormality	Antiarrhythmic Class				Other Agents Used
		I	II	III	IV	
Atrial	Premature beats		✔			
	Flutter (>300 beats/min)	✔	✔	✔	✔	DOC = **digoxin**
	Fibrillation	✔	✔	✔	✔	DOC = **digoxin;** warfarin
Supraventricular	Tachycardia (SVT)	✔A	✔		✔	**Adenosine** [α_1-agonist]
	AV nodal reentry		✔		✔	Digoxin
Ventricular	Tachycardia	✔**B**, C		✔		
	PVT		✔			
	Fibrillation	✔**B**				Epinephrine
	Torsades de pointes (prolonged QT interval)					**Mg^{++}**, β-agonist
	Arrest					Epinephrine
Digitalis-induced arrhythmias		✔**B**				

Bold, Drugs of choice; others are alternatives.
DOC, Drug of choice; *PVT*, paroxysmal ventricular tachycardia; *SVT*, supraventricular tachycardia.

Antiarrhythmics may change the slope of depolarization, raise the threshold for depolarization, and alter the conduction velocity in different parts of the heart. For example, by decreasing the slope of depolarization there would be a decrease in the frequency of discharge and the rate would slow. By raising the threshold for producing an action potential, extra beats may be suppressed. Examples of specific actions of these drugs include decrease in the velocity of depolarization, decrease in impulse propagation, and inhibition of aberrant impulse propagation. Tables 15-3 and 15-4 describe the classification and mechanism of action of the antiarrhythmics, the dental-related adverse reactions, and the dental implications of the antiarrhythmics.

> Long-term effects of drugs must be studied.

Conclusions that are drawn from data must be carefully analyzed to arrive at appropriate conclusions that can be applied clinically. One study demonstrated that IC antiarrhythmics can prevent postmyocardial infarction arrhythmias. [Good for the patient, right?] Although it would seem that this action would be beneficial, with additional data it was determined that although these drugs prevented arrhythmias, patient mortality doubled or tripled. [Not good for the patient.] Before this study was completed, these deaths were thought to be due to fatal arrhythmias unrelated to the drug. It pays to look at future outcomes (such as death) to determine whether a drug is "beneficial."

Digoxin. Although digoxin is not included in the other groups of antiarrhythmics, it is used to treat some arrhythmias. It shortens the refractory period of atrial and ventricular tissues while prolonging the refractory period and diminishing conduction velocity in the Purkinje fibers. Toxic doses of digoxin can result in ventricular arrhythmias (see discussion of digoxin on p. 326).

ADVERSE REACTIONS

Because of their narrow therapeutic index, antiarrhythmic agents are difficult to manage.

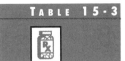

TABLE 15-3 Classification and Mechanism of Action of the Antiarrhythmics

ANTIARRHYTHMIC/CLASS		MECHANISM	EFFECT	COMMENT
IA	Quinidine, procainamide, disopyramide	Na^+ channel blocker (medium)	Blocks conduction; increases ERP	Decreases the rate of entry of Na^+ ions by slowing the rate of rise of the action potential that prolongs the duration of the action potential; depresses phase 0 and prolongs the action potential duration
IB	Lidocaine	Na^{++} channel blocker (fast)	Blocks conduction; decreases ERP	Shortens phase 3 repolarization; used to treat digitalis-induced arrhythmias (when blood level is too high)
IC	Flecainide, encainide, propafenone	Na^{++} channel blocker (slow)	Blocks conduction; little effect on ERP	Depresses phase 0 depolarization, resulting in a profound slowing of conduction; minimal effect on repolarization
II	Propranolol, esmolol, acebutolol	β-blockers	Decreases SA node automaticity	Reduces sympathetic activity, sympatholytic; depressed phase 4 depolarization, has been proved to reduce mortality Membrane-stabilizing agents that depress phase 0(?)
III	Bretylium and d-sotalol (non–β-blocking enantiomer) Amiodarone	K^+ channel blockers Na^+, Ca^{++}, K^+ channel blockers	Prolongs the action potential	Prolongs phase 3 (repolarization), delays repolarization
IV	Verapamil, diltiazem	Calcium channel blockers	Slows conduction velocity at AV node	Depresses phase 4 depolarization; lengthens phases 1 and 2 of repolarization without affecting the refractory period

ERP, Effective refractory period.

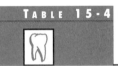

TABLE 15-4 Management of Dental Patients Taking Antiarrhythmics

ANTIARRHYTHMICS	IMPLICATIONS
All	Check for abnormal or extra beats when taking patient's blood pressure and pulse Record the type of arrhythmia and the drug therapy
Atrial fibrillation	Patient on warfarin—check INR
Amiodarone	Liver toxicity, blue skin discoloration, photosensitivity—dental light
Calcium channel blockers	Gingival enlargement (verapamil most reported)
Disopyramide	Anticholinergic—xerostomia
Procainamide	Reversible lupus erythematosus–like syndrome, 25%-30%; CNS depression, xerostomia
Quinidine	Nausea, vomiting, diarrhea; cinchonism—with large doses; atropine-like effect—xerostomia
Phenytoin	Gingival enlargement
β-Blockers, nonspecific	Drug interaction with epinephrine, limit to cardiac dose if patient's condition warrants

TABLE 15-5 Antianginal Preparations

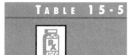

DRUGS	ROUTE(S)	ONSET (MIN)	DURATION (MIN)
ACUTE ATTACKS			
Nitrates			
Amyl nitrite	Inhalation	0.5	3-5
Short-acting nitrates			
Nitroglycerin (NTG, Nitrostat) (Nitrolingual)	Sublingual	1-3	30-60
	Oral spray		30-60
Isosorbide dinitrate	Sublingual	1-2	180-300
PROPHYLACTIC USE			(HR)
Long-acting nitrates			
Nitroglycerin (Nitro-Bid)	Sustained-release of oral tablets	20-45	3-8
(Nitro-Bid, Nitrol)	Ointment	30-60	2-12
(Nitro-Dur, Minitran)	Transdermal patches	30-60	to 24
Isosorbide dinitrate (Isordil, Sorbitrate)	Oral	20-40	4-6
Pentaerythritol tetranitrate (Peritrate)	Oral	30	to 12
β-Blockers*			
Propranolol	Oral	30	6-8
Calcium channel blockers*			
Verapamil (Calan, Isoptin)	Oral	30	6-8
Nifedipine (Procardia)	Oral, sublingual	20	3-6

*For a more complete listing see Box 15-4.

Therefore they are only used in patients with arrhythmias that prevent the proper functioning of the heart.

DENTAL IMPLICATIONS

The dental implications of the antiarrhythmic agents are summarized in Table 15-4.

ANTIANGINAL DRUGS

ANGINA PECTORIS

Angina—insufficient oxygen for body's demand

Angina pectoris is a common cardiovascular disease characterized by pain or discomfort in the chest radiating to the left arm and shoulder. Pain can also be reported radiating to the neck, back, and lower jaw. The lower jaw pain can be of such intensity that it may be confused with a toothache. Angina occurs when the coronary arteries do not supply a sufficient amount of oxygen to the myocardium for its current work. Anginal pain can be precipitated by the stress (increased workload on the heart) induced by physical exercise or emotional states such as the anxiety and apprehension generated by a dental appointment.

At one time the nitroglycerin-like compounds (Table 15-5) were the only class of drugs that could effectively relieve the symptoms of angina. More recently, the β-adrenergic blocking agents and the calcium channel blocking drugs have added a new dimension to drug therapy for angina.

The basic pharmacologic effect of drugs used to manage angina is reduction of the workload of the heart by decreasing the cardiac output, the peripheral vascular resistance, or both. The oxygen requirement of the myocardium is in turn reduced, which relieves the painful symptoms of angina. It is important, however, to keep in mind that these drugs are not curative and the dental team should be alert to the fact that an anginal episode could occur at any time. Appropriate emergency procedures to manage an acute anginal attack should be reviewed before treating a patient with angina (see Chapter 23). Table 15-5 lists the major antianginal drugs and some of their more pertinent characteristics.

NITROGLYCERIN-LIKE COMPOUNDS

Nitroglycerin [nye-troe-GLI-ser-in] (NTG) is by far the most frequently used nitrate for the management of acute anginal episodes. It is also used to manufacture dynamite. In addition to the long-acting **nitrates,** NTG is also used to prevent anginal attacks induced by stress or exercise. Box 15-3 provides guidelines for managing the patient taking nitroglycerin-like agents.

Mechanism. Nitroglycerin is a vasodilator. It releases free nitrite ion and nitric oxide. Nitric oxide, an even more potent vasodilator than nitrite,

---

| Releases NO = vasodilator |

---

activates guanylyl cyclase and increases cGMP, producing relaxation of vascular smooth muscle throughout the body. Indirectly, there is a reduction in work of the heart produced by the effect on both the venous and the arterial sides of the circulation. The venous dilation reduces the amount of blood returning to the heart (preload) and thereby reduces the heart's workload. The arterial dilation reduces the resistance against which the heart must pump (afterload). By reducing workload on the heart, NTG decreases the oxygen demand with relief or reduction of angina pain. Tolerance to these effects occurs, unless a nitrate-free period is observed daily.

Amyl nitrite is the only NTG-like agent that is not a nitrate—it is a nitrite. It is a volatile agent in a closed container. It is administered by crushing the container and inhaling the volatile fumes in an emergency situation (similar to the aromatic ammonia spirit inhalants ampules sniffed when one faints). Because amyl nitrite has no advantage over sublingual nitroglycerin and it has unapproved recreational uses, it is not frequently used.

Sublingual nitroglycerin is used to treat acute anginal attacks. It has a rapid onset (few minutes) by this route, and its effect can last up to 30 minutes. It is available as a sublingual tablet (Nitrostat) or spray used sublingually (Nitrolingual). Sublingual isosorbide dinitrate is also effective for an acute anginal attack. The dental office emergency kit should contain one of these products to manage acute anginal attacks. Dental patients with a history of angina should be asked to bring their NTG to each dental appointment.

Adverse reactions. Most adverse reactions associated with nitroglycerin occur because of its effect on vascular smooth muscle. Severe headaches are frequently reported (vasodilation) after the use of NTG. Flushing, hypotension, lightheadedness, and syncope (fainting) can also re-

---

BOX 15-3 MANAGEMENT OF THE DENTAL PATIENT TAKING NITROGLYCERIN-LIKE AGENTS

- Ensure availability before appointment begins
- Be seated before use
- Provide analgesic if headache occurs
- Watch for sycope, especially with rising
- Premedicate with anxiolytic or NTG
- Proper storage in dental office; avoid heat and moisture
- Watch expiration date
- Prepare office staff for an acute anginal attack

sult. Hypotension is enhanced by alcohol and hot weather. Sublingual NTG can produce a localized burning or tingling at the site of administration. The presence of stinging is not indicative of the potency of the NTG.

Storage. NTG is degraded by heat and moisture, but not by light. NTG should be stored in its original brown glass container and tightly closed, because it can be adsorbed by plastic. It should not be refrigerated because condensation of the moisture in the air produces moisture that can reduce its effectiveness.

If the original bottle is unopened, NTG is active until the expiration date printed on the bottle (assume average storage conditions). When the bottle is opened, the date opened should be written on the outside of the bottle. It should be discarded between 3 and 6 months (depending on the storage conditions). The NTG spray, because air does not enter the container with use, is effective until its expiration date is reached.

Various long-acting NTG-like products (see Table 15-5) such as isosorbide dinitrate [eye-soe-SOR-bide dye-NYE-trate] are available for prophylaxis of anginal attacks. The dosage forms available include tablets (swallowed) and topical (ointment and patch) products. With long-term,

regular use, tolerance to this effect develops. In fact, no difference can be detected between a long-acting nitrate and placebo when taken without a daily "vacation." To prevent tolerance, prophylactic nitrates should be given with at least an 8- to 12-hour "vacation" every day (often during sleeping, depending on symptom pattern).

CALCIUM CHANNEL BLOCKING AGENTS

Another group of drugs approved for use in angina pectoris is the calcium channel blockers (CCB) (see discussion in the section on hypertension). A few examples are verapamil [ver-AP-a-mil] (Calan, Isoptin), diltiazem [dil-TYE-a-zem] (Cardizem), and nifedipine [nye-FED-i-peen] (Procardia, Adalat) (Box 15-3).

The mechanism of action of CCBs for the treatment of angina pectoris is related to the inhibition of movement of

> Vasodilator decreases work of heart

calcium during the contraction of cardiac and vascular smooth muscle. Vasodilation and a decrease in peripheral resistance results, thereby decreasing the work of the heart. Some CCBs decrease myocardial contractility (negative ino-

TABLE 15-6 Calcium Channel Blocker Subgroups

Subgroups	Example	Mechanism	% AR	Comments
Diphenylalkylamines	Verapamil (only)	Least selective; affects both cardiac and vascular smooth muscle, vasodilator; direct effect on the myocardium (SA and AV nodes)	10	Inhibits P450 enzymes
Benzothiazepines	Diltiazem (only)	Less selective; affects both cardiac and vascular smooth muscle, vasodilator; direct effect on myocardium (depresses SA and AV nodes); less negative inotropic effect and better side effect profile than verapamil	2	Inhibits P450 enzymes
Dihydropyridines	Nifedipine and all others	Selective for vascular smooth muscle myocardium—primarily vasodilation; reflex tachycardia	20	

tropic effect), resulting in reduced cardiac output. Others increase coronary vasodilation. The choice of the specific CCB depends on the patient's cardiac disease.

In addition to their use in angina, these drugs are used in the treatment of cardiac arrhythmias and hypertension. Adverse effects include dizziness, weakness, constipation, and hypotension. Nifedipine has been associated with gingival enlargement and **dysgeusia.** The enlargement is similar to that produced by phenytoin. Dental patients receiving these drugs should be given additional oral hygiene instructions, and frequent dental appointments should be planned.

β-ADRENERGIC BLOCKING AGENTS

β-Adrenergic blocking drugs (see Box 15-3), such as propranolol [proe-PRAN-oh-lole] (Inderal), metoprolol [me-TOE-proe-lole] (Lopressor), and atenolol [a-TEN-oh-lole] (Tenormin) are used in the treatment of angina pectoris. These drugs block the β response to catecholamine stimulation, thereby reducing both the chronotropic and inotropic effects. The net result is a reduced myocardial oxygen demand. β-Adrenergic blockers are effective in reducing both exercise- and stress-induced anginal episodes. Adverse effects include bradycardia, CHF, headache, dry mouth, blurred vision, and unpleasant dreams. β-Adrenergic blocking drugs are discussed in the section on hypertension and in Chapter 5 in the section on sympathetic blockers.

DENTAL IMPLICATIONS

Treatment of an acute anginal attack. The dental team should be prepared to treat an acute anginal attack before treating any patient with a history of angina. The patient's personal nitroglycerin tablets or spray should be available and placed on the bracket table in case of an acute attack. Long-acting nitrates and topical products are not useful for the treatment of an acute anginal attack. For acute emergencies, the dental office should have a supply of sublingual NTG (see discussion of storage). The patient should be in the seated position before ingesting the NTG. One tablet can be administered at once, followed in 5 minutes by another, and in another 5 minutes by a third tablet. If these tablets do not stop the anginal attack, the patient should be taken to the emergency room. If using the spray, make sure that the patient does not inhale while spraying.

Prevention of anginal attack. Two methods to prevent an acute attack of angina include pretreatment with either an anxiolytic agent (e.g., benzodiazepine or N_2O) or with sublingual nitroglycerin.

ANXIOLYTICS Because anxiety produces stress and causes the heart to work harder, an antianxiety agent, or anxiolytic (benzodiazepine), may be prescribed to allay anxiety and prevent an acute anginal attack. Nitrous oxide–oxygen (N_2O-O_2) can also relax an anxious dental patient, and N_2O itself produces vasodilation.

NITROGLYCERIN Premedicating an anxious dental patient with sublingual nitroglycerin before any anxiety-provoking procedure can reduce the chance of an attack. For example, the patient can be given sublingual nitroglycerin a few minutes before a local anesthetic injection.

Myocardial infarction. A patient with symptoms of an anginal attack that is not relieved by three doses of nitroglycerin SL (0.04 mg) may be experiencing a myocardial infarction. If the patient who has not been previously diagnosed as having angina experiences chest pain, he or she should be taken to an emergency room for diagnosis. Occasionally, an anginal attack can proceed to an acute **myocardial infarction.** For this reason, the dental team should make sure any patient with an attack that is not relieved by NTG is accompanied by an employee to the hospital emergency room.

Storage of nitroglycerin. Because of NTG's instability, it must be properly stored in the dental office. Check the expiration date on the office supply regularly.

ANTIHYPERTENSIVE AGENTS

Hypertension is the most common of all cardiovascular diseases, affecting some 60 million Americans. Approximately 1 in 6 white and 1 in 4 black people are afflicted. Because blood pressure increases with age, by the age of 65, 2 in 5 whites and 1 in 2 blacks are affected. Statistically it is very likely that many of your dental patients will be suffering from hypertension.

The definition of hypertension is arbitrary and varies throughout the world; however, it has been defined as a blood pressure greater than 140/90 mm Hg. This value has been determined by clinical trials finding that blood pressures near these values are associated with an increase in both morbidity and mortality. Newer information suggests that even the blood pressures within the formerly "normal" blood pressure range is associated with an increase in morbidity. The most common symptoms associated with hypertension are—none. That is why hypertension is called the *"silent killer"*—it most commonly produces no symptoms. Often the use of the term *hypertension* gives patients the impression that it is related to stress or "tension." Patients need to be aware that high blood pressure occurs without regard to stress or "tension." Complications of hypertension affect organs such as the heart, kidney, and brain and the retina. After some damage has occurred, symptoms of malfunction become noticeable.

Eventually, a sustained elevated blood pressure damages the body's organs, so that untreated hypertensive patients are more likely to have kidney and heart disease and cardiovascular problems (myocardial infarction [MI], cerebro-

The silent killer . . . hypertension

vascular accident [CVA]). These complications are greatly increased with concomitant smoking.

Fortunately, early detection and treatment with drug therapy (Box 15-4) reduces the possibility of damage to vital organs (reduced morbidity) and extends the patient's lifetime (reduced mortality). Only about 50% of those with known hypertension are properly treated. If hypertensive patients are properly treated (blood pressure is normalized), their risk of complications is equal to that of the patient without hypertension. One wonders why more patients with hypertension do not comply with their drug therapy.

Hypertension is generally divided into the following categories based on the cause or progression of the disease:

- ***Essential hypertension.*** Approximately 85% to 90% of patients diagnosed with hypertension have *essential, idiopathic,* or *primary* hypertension. These terms all stand for hypertension from an unknown cause. Antihypertensive agents are used to control the hypertension in this group of patients. Essential hypertension is divided into stages depending on the severity of the elevation of the blood pressure (Table 15-7). This is the form usually seen in the dental office.

- ***Secondary hypertension.*** In approximately 10% of hypertensive patients, the cause can be identified and associated with (secondary to) a specific disease process involving the

TABLE 15-7 Stages of Hypertension

CATEGORY	SYSTOLIC (MM HG)		DIASTOLIC (MM HG)
Optimal	<120	and	<80
Normal	<130	and	<85
High normal	130-139	or	85-89
Stage 1	140-159	or	90-99
Stage 2	160-179	or	100-109
Stage 3	≥180	or	≥110

Box 15-4 Antihypertensive Agents

Diuretics

Thiazide

Bendroflumethiazide (Naturetin)
Benzthiazide (Exna)
Chlorothiazide (Diuril)
Hydrochlorothiazide (HCTZ, Esidrix)[a]
Hydroflumethiazide (Saluron, Diucardin)
Methyclothiazide (Enduron)
Polythiazide (Renese)
Trichlormethiazide (Naqua, Metahydrin)

Thiazide-Like

Chlorthalidone (Hygroton)
Indapamide (Lozol)
Metolazone (Zaroxolyn, Mykrox)

Loop

Bumetanide (Bumex)
Ethacrynic acid (Edecrin)
Furosemide (Lasix)[a]
Torsemide (Demadex)

Potassium-Sparing

Amiloride (Midamor)
Spironolactone (Aldactone)
Triamterene (Dyrenium)

Beta (β)-blockers

Nonspecific (Nonselective) β-Blockers $\beta_1 = \beta_2$

Carteolol (Cartrol)[b]
Carvedilol (Coreg)[c]
Levobunolol (Betagan)
Metipranolol (OptiPranolol)
Nadolol (Corgard)
Oxprenolol (Trasicor)
Penbutolol (Levatol)[c]
Pindolol (Visken)[c]
Propranolol (Inderal [LA])[a]
Timolol (Timoptic, Blocadren)

Specific (Selective) β-Blockers $\beta_1 > \beta_2$

Acebutolol (Sectral)[c] x
Atenolol (Tenormin)[a]
Betaxolol (Kerlone)
Bisoprolol (Zebeta)
Esmolol (Brevibloc)
Metoprolol (Lopressor)
Metoprolol (Toprol-XL)

α- and β-Blocker

Labetalol (Normodyne)

Calcium channel blockers (CCBs)

Diltiazem (Cardizem [SR], Dilacor [XR])[a]
Verapamil (Isoptin [SR], Calan [SR])[a]

Dihydropyridines

Amlodipine (Norvasc)
Bepridil (Vascor)
Felodipine (Plendil)
Isradipine (DynaCirc)
Nicardipine (Cardene [SR])
Nifedipine (Procardia [XL], Adalat [CC])[a]
Nimodipine (Nimotop)
Nisoldipine (Sular)

Calcium Channel (T) Blockers

Mibefradil (Posicor)[d]

Angiotensin-converting enzyme (ACE) inhibitors

Benazepril (Lotensin)
Captopril (Capoten)
Enalapril (Vasotec)
Fosinopril (Monopril)
Lisinopril (Zestril, Prinivil)[a]
Moexipril (Univasc)
Quinapril (Accupril)
Ramipril (Altace)
Trandolapril (Mavik)

BOX 15-4 ANTIHYPERTENSIVE AGENTS—CONT'D

Angiotensin-converting enzyme (ACE) inhibitors—cont'd

Angiotensin II Antagonists

Candesartan (Atacand)
Irbesartan (Avapro)
Losartan (Cozaar)
Telmisartan (Micardis)
Valsartan (Diovan)
Eprosartan (Tevetan)

α_1-Receptor Antagonists (Blockers)

Doxazosin (Cardura)[a,e]
Prazosin (Minipress)
Terazosin (Hytrin)[e]

Central adrenergic blockers

Clonidine (Catapres [TTS])[a]
Guanabenz (Wytensin)
Guanfacine (Tenex)
Methyldopa (Aldomet)

Peripheral Adrenergic Antagonists

Guanethidine (Ismelin)
Guanadrel (Hylorel)
Reserpine

Vasodilators (Direct)

Hydralazine (Apresoline)[f]
Minoxidil (Loniten)[g]

Combinations

Diuretic Combinations[h]

Thiazides + Potassium-sparing diuretics
Aldactazide
Dyazide
Maxzide[a]
Moduretic

β-Blockers + Diuretics
Corzide
Inderide
Lopressor HCT
Tenoretic
Timolide
Ziac

ACE Inhibitors + HCTZ

Capozide
Lotensin HCT
Vaseretic
Prinzide
Zestoretic
Uniretic

Calcium Channel Blocker + ACE Inhibitors

Lexxel
Lotrel
Tarka
Teczem

[a]Common example.
[b]Has intrinsic sympathetic activity (ISA) = β-agonist action.
[c]Has α_1-agonist action.
[d]Removed from market because it produced arrhythmias.
[e]Also indicated for BHP.
[f]Used in pregnancy.
[g]OTC for hair growth.

endocrine or renal systems. For example, renal hypertension can result from a narrowed renal **artery.** Drug therapy such as steroids, nonsteroidal antiinflammatory agents (NSAIAs), birth control pills, decongestants, and tricyclic antidepressants can also produce secondary hypertension. Secondary hypertension can be eliminated by removing the cause, that is, by surgically correcting the renal artery narrowing or discontinuing the offending drug.

* *Malignant hypertension.* In the third group of hypertensive patients, those with malignant hypertension, blood pressures are very high or rapidly rising and there is usually evidence of retinal and renal damage. The small number of patients in this group must be treated aggressively with antihypertensive agents. Malignant hypertension can develop in about 5% of patients with primary or secondary hypertension.

STEPPED-CARE REGIMEN

Pharmacologic management of hypertension involves the following stepped-care approach (Figure 15-4) as diastolic pressures become greater than 90 mm Hg:

* *Step 1.* In step 1, life-style changes are instituted. These include cessation of smoking (dental team can be involved; see Chapter 26), stress reduction, increased exercise, weight reduction, and salt restriction (10% to 50% of patients respond). The importance of sodium restriction depends on the individual patient.

On the other hand, sodium restriction stimulates the secretion of renin from the kidneys. Renin activates the production of angiotensin I, which then produces angiotensin II. This mechanism is used by the body to elevate blood pressure when blood volume is depleted.

Caffeine intake alone does not produce an increase in blood pressure, but when it is combined with smoking, elevation of the blood pres-

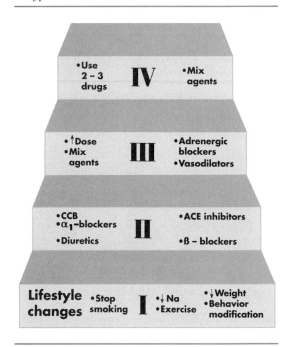

FIGURE 15-4 *Stepped-care approach to hypertension treatment.*

sure can occur. Calcium supplementation has variable results on blood pressure, depending on the specific patient. More research is needed in the field of blood pressure–lowering effects of many agents, including calcium and magnesium.

* *Step 2.* In step 2, therapy is initiated with any of the "Big 5" (Box 15-5). Sex, race, presence of diabetes or hyperlipidemia, and renin activity are taken into consideration (Table 15-8). Hypertensive patients may need to take several antihypertensive drugs (from different groups) for adequate management. By combining agents, the side effects of individual agents are less and the high blood pressure can be normalized. Diuretics are usually preferred in patients older than 50 years and in patients with complicating **peripheral vascular disease** or pulmonary disorders. β-Blockers are used frequently for those younger than age 50 and in patients with ischemic heart disease.

TABLE 15-8	Patient Characteristics That Determine Choice of Antihypertensives					
PATIENT CHARACTERISTICS	ACE INHIBITORS	DIURETICS	CLONIDINE	CALCIUM CHANNEL BLOCKERS	β-Blocker	α-Blocker
Black	Less	More		More	Less	
Diabetic	Y	N		Y	N	
Angina				Y	Y	
Hyperlipidemia	Y	N		Y	N	Y
Renal failure	N	Y		Y	Y	Y
Depression/confusion	Y	Y		Y	N	Y
Smoker			Y			
Asthma/COPD						
CHF	Y	Y		N—verapamil	N	Y
Sex problems	Y			Y		Y
PVD				Y	N	
Cost	$$$	¢	¢	$$$	¢	$$

CHF, Congestive heart failure, *COPD*, chronic obstructive pulmonary disease; *PVD*, peripheral vascular disease.

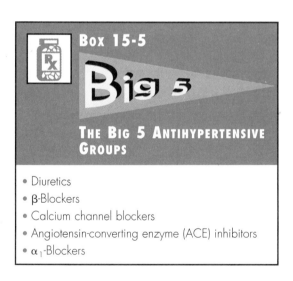

BOX 15-5

Big 5

THE BIG 5 ANTIHYPERTENSIVE GROUPS

- Diuretics
- β-Blockers
- Calcium channel blockers
- Angiotensin-converting enzyme (ACE) inhibitors
- α₁-Blockers

Table 15-9 lists some common antihypertensive agents and their various sites of action and side effects. The groups recommended for initial use include diuretics, β-blockers, angiotensin-converting enzyme inhibitors, CCBs, and α₁-blockers. A handy name for these five groups of antihypertensive drugs is the "Big 5." Antihypertensive products may contain one drug or be combinations of more than one drug (see Box 15-3). The combination products found in the Top 200 Drugs are listed in Appendix A. In step 3, the step 2 drugs are increased in dose, mixed together, or combined with other agents such as direct-acting vasodilators (hydralazine or minoxidil) or peripheral or central adrenergic blockers (clonidine). Step 4 care includes mixing two or three of the drugs already mentioned or the addition of a neuronal blocker such as guanethidine. The exact combination of drugs selected depends not only on the degree of hypertension but also on the patient's tolerance to the side effects.

The control of blood pressure is an interplay of many factors, and treatment of hypertension is directed at some of the forces that alter blood pressure. Figure 15-5 illustrates these factors. The cardiac output and peripheral resistance determine blood pressure. Other changes that affect blood pressure produce changes in these two factors. Because the sympathetic nervous

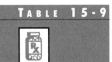

TABLE 15-9 Selected Antihypertensives, Their Mechanisms and Adverse Reactions

Group	Examples	Mechanism/Hypothesis	Dentally Important Comments
Thiazides	Hydrochlorothiazide	Initially reduces plasma and extracellular fluid volume; initially decreases cardiac output then returns to normal; decreases peripheral resistance by a direct effect on blood vessels	Hypokalemia
β-Blockers	Tenormin Lopressor	Reduces cardiac output, decreases sympathetic effect to blood vessels (blocks β stimulation), inhibits renin release	
ACE inhibitors	Lisinopril	Decreases conversion of angiotensin I to II (Inhibits ACE activity), decreases angiotensin II (action = vasoconstriction and increases plasma renin activity)	Dry, hacking cough
Calcium channel blockers	Verapamil Diltiazem Nifedipine	Inhibits calcium ion movement (arterial smooth muscle and cardiac muscle); relaxes arterial smooth muscle; decreases cardiac muscle cell contractility (a negative inotropic effect)	Gingival enlargement

FIGURE 15-5 *Factors controlling blood pressure.*

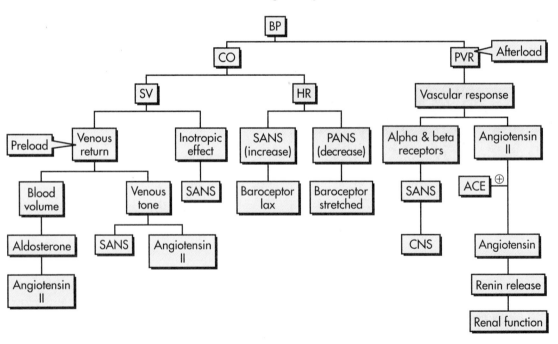

Factors affecting blood pressure

FIGURE 15-6 *Location of action of diuretics.*

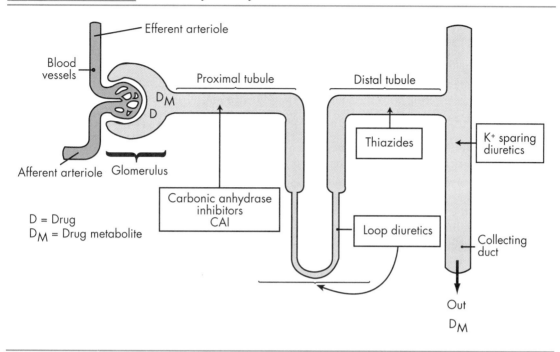

system can affect peripheral resistance, agents that block the sympathetic nervous system reduce blood pressure through their effect on peripheral resistance. Mechanisms of action of the antihypertensive agents attempt to lower blood pressure by their action on either cardiac output or total peripheral resistance.

Regardless of medication usage, the blood pressure of each hypertensive patient seen in the dental office should be measured and recorded. Only by recording successive blood pressures for an individual patient, can the patient's blood pressure control be evaluated and any abnormality for a particular patient noted. Also, because control of blood pressure is so important to patient health, patients should be questioned about compliance with their antihypertensive medication. Abrupt discontinuation of some blood pressure medicines may result in rebound hypertension. That means that the blood pressure

rises to a higher level than it was before treatment. Concern for patient total health is based on the fact that it is of little use for a patient to have clean and perfectly restored teeth if that patient has a fatal myocardial infarction resulting from untreated hypertension.

DIURETIC AGENTS

The three major types of diuretics are thiazides (-like), loop, and potassium (K)- sparing (Figure 15-6).

Thiazide diuretics. The thiazide diuretics are among the most commonly used agents for the treatment of hypertension. Hydrochlorothiazide [hye-droe-klor-oh-THYE-a-zide], abbreviated as *HCTZ*, is the most commonly used thiazide. Many patients with mild hypertension are treated solely with HCTZ. When other antihypertensive drugs are used, they are frequently combined with thiazides. Although a large number of thiazide and thiazide-like diuretics are currently available, these agents all have essentially the same pharmacologic effects. Even thiazide-like agents such as chlorthalidone [klor-THAL-i-doan] (Lozol) act by a similar mechanism—by interfering with the sodium reabsorption in the distal tubule.

MECHANISM OF ACTION The exact mechanism by which the thiazide diuretics lower blood pressure has not been determined (Table 15-10). The thiazides initially inhibit the reabsorption of sodium from the distal convoluted tubule and part of the ascending loop of Henle of the kidney. Water and chloride ions passively accompany the sodium, producing diuresis. Because more sodium is presented to the site of sodium-potassium exchange, there is also an increase in potassium excretion. If sodium intake is increased, the potassium loss is exacerbated.

The thiazides' effect on blood pressure may occur because of the following: Initially, thiazide diuretics reduce the extracellular fluid volume because of their natriuretic action. This volume reduction returns to normal with continued therapy, but a slight decrease in interstitial volume may remain. Other effects of the thiazides that may contribute to their antihypertensive effects include changes in sodium and calcium concentrations or a reduced sensitivity to the SANS.

ADVERSE REACTIONS Common adverse reactions associated with thiazides (Table 15-11) include hypokalemia (secondary to sodium-potassium exchange) and hyperuricemia (inhibits uric acid secretion). **Hyperglycemia, hyperlipidemia, hypercalcemia** (promote calcium reabsorption), and **anorexia** are other side effects. **Hyperuricemia** is of special concern when the patient has a history of gout. In the diabetic patient, hyperglycemia, or impaired glucose tolerance, must be managed by diet or insulin

alterations. There is a very small chance of cross-hypersensitivity (allergy) between the sulfonamide oral medicine (antimicrobial agents) and the thiazides because of the similarity in their structures. Oral adverse reactions include xerostomia and, rarely, oral lichenoid eruptions indistinguishable from lichen planus. This condition is reversible on discontinuation (with time).

The most important dental drug interaction with the thiazides is interaction with the non-steroidal antiinflam-

> NSAIAs reduce the antihypertensive effect of HCTZ.

matory agents (NSAIAs). NSAIAs can reduce the antihypertensive effect of the thiazide diuretics. This interaction takes a few days to develop, and therefore a few doses of an NSAIA can safely be used for acute pain control. A longer duration of use should be undertaken with blood pressure monitoring. Patients often have their own blood pressure monitoring systems at home. Patients are often taking thiazide diuretics for their blood pressure and NSAIAs for arthritis. With chronic use of both agents, their blood pressure medication is adjusted to account for the concurrent use of an NSAIA.

Thiazides can cause hypokalemia and can therefore sensitize the myocardium to developing arrhythmias. The potential for arrhythmias is exacerbated in patients taking digoxin, especially if digitalis toxicity is present. Epinephrine, as contained in local anesthetic mixtures, also has arrhythmogenic potential. So, in a dental situation in which a patient is taking thiazide diuretics and digitalis toxicity may be present, the epinephrine dose should be limited to the cardiac dose (0.04 mg, see Chapter 10). The thiazide diuretics potentiate the action of the other antihypertensives, increasing the potential for hypotension. This drug interaction is used to therapeutic advantage so lower doses of each drug are needed to control the patient's blood pressure.

TABLE 15-10 **Mechanism of Action of the Antihypertensive Agents**

Group	Subgroup, Example	Mechanism	Comments
Diuretics	Thiazide, Loop	Decreases PVR	Counteracts Na retention from other agents
ANS	β-Blockers	↓CO, ↓sympathetic outflow from CNS, reduces renin release	
	α₁-Adrenergic blockers	Blocks α₁; decreases peripheral vascular resistance; relaxes arterial and venous smooth muscles	First dose syncope; postural hypotension
Calcium channel blockers		Vasodilators; ↓TPR	
ACE inhibitors		Reduces PVR, decreases aldosterone secretion	Reduces rate of bradykinin (vasodilator) inactivation
Angiotensin II antagonists	Losartan	Vasodilation; decreases aldosterone secretion	
α₂-Adrenergic agonist, centrally acting	Clonidine	Reduces adrenergic outflow	Sedation, xerostomia
	α-Methyldopa	Reduces adrenergic outflow	
Vasodilators	Hydralazine	Direct vasodilation, arteries, and arterioles	Headache, nausea, sweating, lupus-like syndrome
	Minoxidil	Arteriole dilation	Na/H₂O retention, reflex ↓TPR ↑HR and CO, use with β-blocker and diuretic

ANS, Autonomic nervous system; *PVR*, peripheral vascular resistance; *TPR*, total peripheral resistance.

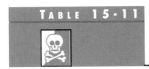

Adverse Reactions of the Thiazides		
PROBLEM WITH:	ADVERSE REACTION	DEFINE
Potentiate arrhythmias	Hypokalimia	↓ Potassium
Diabetes	Hyperglycemia	↑ Glucose
Hyperlipidemia	Hyperlipidemia	↑ Lipids
Gout	Hyperuricemia	↑ Uric acid, ↑ Calcium, ↓ Magnesium, ↑ Sodium

Loop diuretics. Loop diuretics can be considered the "strong cousins of the thiazides." Furosemide [fur-OH-se-mide] (Lasix), the most commonly used loop diuretic, is the prototype drug. Furosemide acts on the ascending limb of the loop of Henle and has some effect on the distal tubule. Like thiazides, loop diuretics inhibit the reabsorption of sodium with a concurrent loss of fluids (more loss than the thiazides; whereas thiazides filtrate 5%, the loop diuretics filtrate 25%). Furosemide's side effects are similar to those of the thiazides and include hypokalemia and hyperuricemia. Furosemide is used in management of hypertensive patients with CHF. Loop diuretics can be used when rapid diuresis is required. As occurs with thiazides, NSAIAs can interfere with furosemide's antihypertensive action (see comments on HCTZ).

Potassium-sparing diuretics. Potassium-sparing diuretics are "puny" diuretics with "potassium-catching" ability. Individual members of this group have different mechanisms of action, but all have weak diuretic action.

SPIRONOLACTONE Spironolactone [speer-on-oh-LAK-tone] (Aldactone) is chemically similar to aldosterone, but competitively antagonizes its action (aldosterone antagonist). The result is sodium excretion through diuresis and loss of fluid volume. However, potassium ion is conserved because some of the potassium is reabsorbed at the expense of sodium in the sodium-potassium exchange system in the distal tubule.

TRIAMTERENE Triamterene [trye-AM-ter-een] (Dyrenium), also a potassium-sparing diuretic, interferes with potassium/sodium exchange (active transport) in the distal and cortical collecting tubules and the collecting duct by inhibiting sodium-potassium-ATPase. The diuresis and potassium conservation that occurs resembles that of spironolactone.

The potassium-sparing diuretics act at different sites in the kidney than do the thiazide diuretics. These two types of diuretics have the opposite effect on potassium loss. A combination product is designed to reduce the amount of potassium loss and prevent hypokalemia. The combination of triamterene and hydrochlorothiazide (Dyazide, Maxzide) is one of the most frequently used preparations.

Potassium salts. Although the potassium salts are not cardiac drugs, lack of potassium caused

K^+ = potassium

by the diuretics must be managed, often with potassium supplementation. Potassium is involved in many important physiologic processes such as nerve impulses, contraction of smooth, cardiac, and skeletal muscles, and maintenance of normal renal function. It is indicated in the treatment of hypokalemia produced by diuretics. It is relatively contraindicated in patients with severe renal impairment or those receiving potassium-sparing diuretics (a few exceptions to this statement exist). The most common adverse reaction of potassium relates to the gastrointestinal tract and includes nausea and abdominal discomfort caused by gastrointestinal irritation. Patients taking potassium supplements should be questioned about their use of diuretics, and the possibility of cardiovascular disease should be explored when a drug history is taken. Examples of potassium supplements are K-Dur,

K-Tab, Micro-K, K-Lyte, K-Lor, and Klor-Con. Note the use of *K* (element symbol for potassium) in their names.

β-ADRENERGIC BLOCKING AGENTS

β-Adrenergic blockers, one group of adrenergic blocking agents, are used frequently to treat hypertension.

The adrenergic β-receptors are subtyped into β_1-receptors and β_2-receptors (there also may be a β_3-receptor). They have been shown in clinical trials to decrease both the morbidity and mortality related to hypertension.

β_1-Receptor stimulation is associated with an increase in heart rate, cardiac contractility, and AV conduction. Stimulation of β_2-receptors produces vasodilation in skeletal muscles and bronchodilation in the pulmonary tissues. These receptors are initially described in Chapter 5, which discusses the autonomic nervous system drugs.

Many β-adrenergic blocking drugs are approved for use in the management of hypertension (see Box 15-3). Nonselective or nonspecific β-adrenergic receptor blocking drugs, such as propranolol [proe-PRAN-oh-lole], the prototype, block both β_1- and β_2-receptors. In usual doses the selective, or specific, β-adrenergic receptor blocking drugs, such as metoprolol [me-toe-PROE-lole] block the β_1-receptors more than the β_2-receptors ($\beta_1 > \beta_2$). At larger doses, receptor selectivity disappears. Pindolol [PN-doe-lole] and acebutolol [a-se-BYOO-toe-lole] have partial agonist activity and cause some β-stimulation while blocking catecholamine action. The selective β-blockers ($\beta_1 > \beta_2$) have some advantages in patients who may have preexisting bronchospastic disease, such as asthma, because they do not block the airway's bronchodilating action (not as likely to result in bronchoconstriction). They are less likely to produce a drug interaction with epinephrine.

β-Adrenergic blockers lower blood pressure primarily by decreasing cardiac output. Other effects that may contribute to their antihypertensive effect include a lowering of plasma renin levels, a reduction in plasma volume and venous return, a decrease in sympathetic outflow from the central nervous system (CNS), and a reduction in peripheral resistance. These drugs are often used as step 2 drugs, either as a single drug or in combination with other antihypertensive drugs.

The side effects of the β-blockering agents include bradycardia, mental depression, and decreased sexual ability. CHF and CNS effects such as confusion, hallucinations, dizziness, fatigue have been reported. Gastrointestinal tract effects include diarrhea, nausea, and vomiting. β-Blockers can produce xerostomia (very mild) or worsen a patient's lipid profile. Exacerbations of asthma, angina, and peripheral vascular disease have been seen.

Suffix *-olol*

Dental drug interactions. Nonselective β-blockers can have a drug interaction with epinephrine. Patients pretreated with a nonspecific β-blocker such as propranolol and given epinephrine may have a two- to four-fold increase in vasopressor response (blood pressure goes up more in patients pretreated with β-blockers than in untreated patients), resulting in hypertension. The increased blood pressure triggers, via the **vagus** nerve, a reflex bradycardia.

The amount of caution required with this drug interaction depends on the patient's underlying cardiovascular disease, if any, and blood pressure and the dose of the β-blocker the patient is taking. In patients with cardiovascular disease or higher blood pressure the amount of epinephrine given to patients taking nonspecific β-blockers should be limited to the cardiac dose unless careful blood pressure monitoring accompanies the use of larger doses. Neither gingival retraction cord containing epinephrine nor

1:50,000 epinephrine should be used. Usual dental doses of epinephrine can be given to patients who are taking specific β-blockers (β$_1$-blockers) or α- and β-blockers. Box 15-3 separates the β-blockers into groups: specific and nonspecific.

α- And β-adrenergic blocking drug. Labetalol [la-BET-a-lole] (Trandate, Normodyne) is a nonselective β-adrenergic receptor blocking drug that also has α-receptor blocking activity. In addition to the typical β-adrenoceptor blocking effects, labetalol also reduces peripheral resistance through its α-blocking action. Labetalol is used either alone or in combination with the diuretics. Side effects and drug interactions are similar to the α- and β-adrenergic blockers.

CALCIUM CHANNEL BLOCKING AGENTS

Suffix: **-dipine**

The common calcium channel blockering agents (CCBs) include the drugs verapamil [ver-AP-a-mil] (Isoptin, Calan), nifedipine [nye-fed-i-peen] (Procardia, Adalat), and diltiazem [dil-TYE-a-zem] (Cardizem). Many CCBs (see Box 15-3) end in the suffix *dipine*. These agents are used to treat hypertension, as well as other cardiac conditions such as arrhythmias and angina.

Mechanism. CCBs inhibit the movement of extracellular calcium ions into cells, including those of the vascular smooth muscle and cardiac cells. The inhibition of calcium ion influx produces vasodilation, which produces coronary vasodilation and reverses vasospasms. By producing systemic vasodilation, the CCBs reduce the afterload on the heart (reduce the total peripheral resistance). These effects are useful in the treatment of both angina pectoris and hypertension.

At least four types of calcium channels, called *L*, *T*, *N*, and *P*, have been elucidated. The current CCBs are all of the L-type. A CCB of the T type (see Box 15-3) was available for a short time before it was removed from the market because of hepatotoxicity. L-type agents inhibit calcium-ion influx (slow channel blocking agents) in cardiac and smooth muscles. The binding sites are stereoselective (interact with only one enantiomer [optically active] of a drug), and binding gives rise to changes in conformation at the site.

CCBs inhibit the entry of calcium ions through voltage-sensitive areas termed *slow channels* across cell membranes. This blockade is similar to that produced by local anesthetics (block sodium channels) on the sodium channel. The decrease in transmembrane calcium current results in relaxation of vascular smooth muscle cells and reduction cardiac contractility and conduction. CCBs do not affect serum calcium levels, but there is some evidence that an increase in serum calcium may alter the therapeutic effect of the CCBs.

The L-calcium channel blockers are divided into three groups. Two of the groups only have one agent, whereas the third group includes all the other CCBs. Verapamil and diltiazem are each their own group. Nifedipine, a dihydropyridine, is representative of this group to which all the other CCBs belong.

Pharmacologic effects

SMOOTH MUSCLE Vascular smooth muscle is relaxed and dilation of coronary and peripheral arteries and arterioles occur, reducing preload. Other smooth muscle is relaxed but to a lesser extent. Orthostatic hypotension is uncommon. Some CCBs, such as nifedipine and its relatives, are more specific for this effect.

CARDIAC MUSCLE The effect of the CCBs on the heart may reduce its rate, decrease myocardial contractility (negative inotropic effect), and slow AV nodal conduction. Less specific CCBs have some of both effects.

Adverse reactions. Most side effects associated with the CCBs are merely extensions of their pharmacologic effects.

CENTRAL NERVOUS SYSTEM CCBs can produce excessive hypotension, which can cause dizziness and lightheadedness. Dental patients should be warned to rise from the dental chair slowly. Headache can occur in up to 10% to 20% of patients taking CCBs.

GASTROINTESTINAL Gastrointestinal side effects include nausea, vomiting, and constipation. Individual CCBs differ in the incidence of these various side effects.

CARDIOVASCULAR Because CCBs have a depressant effect on the heart, bradycardia and edema can result. Flushing as a result of vasodilation should not be confused with an allergic or adverse reaction. Peripheral edema has been reported.

OTHER Shortness of breath as a result of pulmonary edema has been reported. Nasal congestion and rhinitis may interfere with the administration of nitrous oxide–oxygen (N_2O-O_2) for analgesia and anxiety relief.

Gingival enlargement

Oral manifestations. The oral manifestations of the CCBs include xerostomia, dysgeusia, and gingival enlargement (formerly called *gingival hyperplasia*). Gingival enlargement has been reported most frequently with nifedipine, but diltiazem, verapamil, and other CCBs have been implicated.

Nifedipine's manufacturer originally reported the incidence of gingival enlargement as less than 0.5%. Manufacturers of both diltiazem and verapamil have mentioned gingival enlargement as an infrequently reported postmarketing event. Other studies have found the incidence for nifedipine to be 15% to 80% depending on the criteria used. In one study, diltiazem's incidence was determined to be 74%. These greatly varying rates of gingival enlargement may be the result of vastly differing criteria used in the studies (e.g., self-report by patients without prompting versus measuring gum changes in all patients). Studies with the highest rates evaluated the incidence of gingival enlargement versus a control group prospectively.

The gingival enlargement can begin 1 to several months after beginning therapy with a CCB. Some authors have found no relationship between the dose of the drug and the likelihood of a reaction occurring, whereas others indicate that higher doses produce more severe reactions. Like phenytoin enlargement, nifedipine enlargement begins as nodular and firm tissue that bleeds easily on probing. The enlargement begins in the anterior labial dental papillae and can proceed eventually to include the lingual and palatal gingiva. The hyperplastic interdental papillae can eventually extend onto crown surfaces, interfering with the ability to chew.

Detailed oral hygiene instructions and more frequent recall appointments to reduce plaque load have been said to reduce this enlargement, but no well-controlled studies have confirmed this suspicion. The patient may be told to maintain scrupulous oral hygiene until more information is available.

Upon discontinuation of the CCB or switching to a drug outside the CCB group, the gingival enlargement usually reverts to normal tissue and does not reappear. This may take weeks to months. If drug therapy cannot be discontinued because of the severity of the patient's cardiac condition, a gingivectomy or gingivoplasty may be required. Changing to another CCB does not appear to result in reversal of the enlargement.

Dental drug interactions. Carbamazepine (Tegretol), the drug of choice for the management of trigeminal neuralgia (tic douloureux), may occasionally be used by the dental profession. Both diltiazem and verapamil may increase serum levels of carbamazepine, resulting in toxicity. The CCBs are one of the few antihypertensive groups whose effect is not reduced by the NSAIAs.

Both nausea and constipation, side effects of the CCBs, could be additive with the side effects produced by NSAIAs (such as ibuprofen) (nausea) and the opioids (such as codeine) (constipation).

ANGIOTENSIN-RELATED AGENTS

There are two types of drugs whose mechanism involves angiotensin. One type, the angiotensin-converting enzyme (ACE) inhibitors (ACEIs), prevents the formation of angiotensin II. The other type, the angiotensin receptor antagonist, is more specific because it blocks the effect of angiotensin II at its receptor site.

Suffix: -pril

Angiotensin-converting enzyme inhibitors. The ACEI drugs are commonly used as antihypertensives. Examples include captopril [KAP-toe-pril] (Capoten), enalapril [e-NAL-a-pril] (Vasotec), and lisinopril [lyse-IN-oh-pril] (Prinivil, Zestril). Many ACEIs (see Box 15-3) end in the suffix *-pril*.

MECHANISM A complex but important homeostatic mechanism involved in maintaining blood pressure is the renin-angiotensin-aldosterone system. This system adjusts the quantity of sodium and water retained (circulatory volume) and the peripheral resistance (blood vessels). When the kidney senses a decrease in blood pressure or flow it releases renin, which catalyzes the conversion of angiotensinogen (inactive precursor) to angiotensin I. A second enzyme, ACE, converts angiotensin I to angiotensin II. This is the enzyme that is blocked by ACEIs (Figure 15-7). Angiotensin II produces vasoconstriction (increasing peripheral vascular resistance) and stimulates the adrenal cortex to release aldosterone, facilitating water retention. By blocking these events, the blood pressure is lowered. Cardiac output and heart rate are relatively unaf-

fected. ACEIs retard the progression of diabetic nephropathy whether hypertension is present or not.

ADVERSE REACTIONS The two most common kinds of adverse reactions associated with the ACEIs are those related to the CVS and CNS.

Cardiovascular Hypotension has produced dizziness, lightheadedness, and fainting. Tachycardia and chest pain have been noted.

Central nervous system Side effects may include dizziness, insomnia, fatigue, and headache.

Gastrointestinal Nausea, vomiting, and diarrhea can occur.

Respiratory An increase in upper respiratory symptoms, including a dry, hacking cough can occur. ACEIs can produce a dry cough that can occur within the first week of therapy and disappears after withdrawal of the drug. The cough begins as a tickle in the throat, leading to a dry, nonproductive, persistent cough that may be worse at night or in the supine position. It occurs because the ACE also inactivates bradykinin, a potent stimulator of allergic reactions, including cough. The blood levels of bradykinin rise because the ACEIs are blocking the enzyme that normally destroys bradykinin (Box 15-6).

Allergic-like reactions Allergic-like reactions including the following:
- **Angioedema.** Swelling of the extremities, face, lips, mucous membranes, tongue, glottis, or larynx can occur, especially following the initial dose. If airway obstruction is severe, it can impair breathing or swallowing and could be fatal.
- **Rash.**

Other Because teratogenicity can cause fetal and neonatal morbidity and mortality, ACEI should not be given to women who could be or become

FIGURE 15-7 *Site of action of ACE inhibitors.*

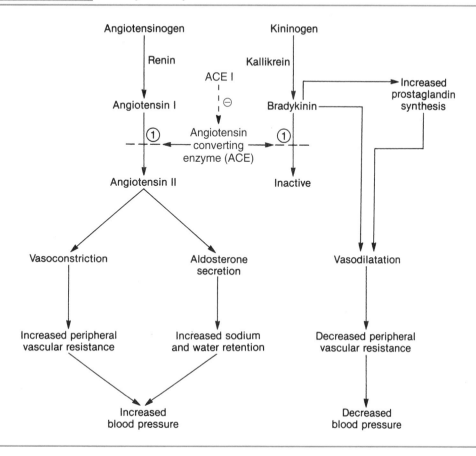

pregnant. Rarely, **pancreatitis,** with symptoms of abdominal pain, and abdominal distention have occurred. Proteinuria is more common in patients taking higher doses or who have renal impairment.

Oral adverse reactions Dysgeusia, an altered sense of taste, is a fairly common oral side effect of the ACEIs and is reported in about 6% of patients taking captopril. The incidence in patients taking other ACEIs is unknown. The loss of taste is usually reversible after a few months, even with continued drug treatment.

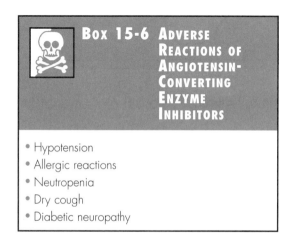

BOX 15-6 ADVERSE REACTIONS OF ANGIOTENSIN-CONVERTING ENZYME INHIBITORS

- Hypotension
- Allergic reactions
- Neutropenia
- Dry cough
- Diabetic neuropathy

Autoimmune oral lesions such as lichenoid or pemphigoid reactions may produce oral manifestations. This reaction may have a photosensitivity factor.

DENTAL DRUG INTERACTIONS The antihypertensive effectiveness of ACEI is reduced by administration of the NSAIAs. A few doses of an NSAIA are of little concern, but chronic administration for several days might result in an increase in the patient's blood pressure. The ACE inhibitors may be used alone as a step 2 drug or in combination with a β-blocker, thiazide diuretic, or CCB. These drugs are commonly prescribed, and the dental team will treat many patients taking one or more of these agents.

Angiotensin II receptor antagonists. The angiotensin II receptor antagonists act by attaching to the angiotensin II receptor and blocking the effect of angiotensin II. One example, losartan {loe-SAR-tan] (Cozaar), is the prototype. Losartan has a high affinity and selectivity for the AT_1 receptor. It blocks the vasoconstrictor and aldosterone-secreting effects of angiotensin II. An increase in plasma renin level follows.

ADVERSE REACTIONS Because angiotensin II receptor antagonists work by blocking angiotensin II at its receptor, they are more specific than ACEIs and may be expected to have fewer adverse reactions.

Central nervous system CNS effects can include dizziness, fatigue, insomnia, and headache.

Upper respiratory infections Upper respiratory infections occur more frequently in patients taking losartan. A dry cough and nasal congestion can also occur.

Gastrointestinal Losartan can produce diarrhea.

Pain Both muscle cramps and leg and back pain have been reported with losartan.

Angioedema Rarely, angioedema can occur.

Teratogenicity Fetal and neonatal morbidity and mortality can occur if losartan is administered to a pregnant woman.

DENTAL DRUG INTERACTIONS NSAIAs may antagonize the antihypertensive effect of losartan by inhibiting renal prostaglandin synthesis or causing sodium and fluid retention

α_1-ADRENERGIC BLOCKING AGENTS

The adrenergic blockers include the α-blockers and β-blockers, which were discussed earlier. Two α-receptor subtypes, α_1 and α_2, have been identified (see Box 15-3). Doxazosin [doks-AYE-zoe-sin] (Cardura) and terazosin [ter-AY-zoe-sin] (Hytrin) are selective α_1-adrenergic blocking drugs.

Mechanism. The α_1-receptors, located on postsynaptic receptor tissues, produce vasoconstriction and increase peripheral resistance when stimulated. The α_1-blocking agents produce peripheral vasodilation in the arterioles and venules that decreases peripheral vascular resistance. They have little effect on cardiac output or renal blood flow. They are more effective when combined with diuretics or β-blockers.

α_1-Adrenergic blockers result in a reduction in urethral resistance and pressure, bladder outlet resistance, and urinary symptoms. This effect accounts for their use in management of older males who have an enlarged **prostate gland.** Surgery can often be avoided in these patients who are managed by drug therapy. If a man has both hypertension and BPH, then one can "kill two birds with one stone."

Adverse reactions

ORTHOSTATIC HYPOTENSION Orthostatic hypotension can result in dizziness or syncope. A "first-dose orthostatic hypotensive reaction" sometimes occurs with the initial dose or with changes in the dose of doxazosin. Syncope is more likely to occur when the patient is volume-depleted or sodium-restricted. Both exercise and alcohol may exaggerate the effect.

CENTRAL NERVOUS SYSTEM α_1-Adrenergic blockers can cause CNS depression, producing either drowsiness or excitation and headache. Caution should be exercised when doing anything requiring alertness until the patient's response can be evaluated.

CARDIOVASCULAR Tachycardia, arrhythmias, and **palpitations** can occur. Peripheral edema is another side effect related to the cardiovascular system.

Dental drug interactions

THE NONSTEROIDAL ANTIINFLAMMATORY AGENTS The nonsteroidal antiinflammatory agents (NSAIAs), especially indomethacin, can reduce the antihypertensive effect of the α_1-blockers (Box 15-7). They produce this effect by inhibiting renal prostaglandin synthesis or causing sodium and fluid retention.

EPINEPHRINE The sympathomimetics can increase the antihypertensive effects of doxazosin. The α_1-blockers prevent the α_1-agonist effects (vasoconstriction) of epinephrine, leaving the β_1- and β_2-agonist effects (vasodilation) to predominate. The combined vasodilation can result in severe hypotension and reflex tachycardia.

Uses. In addition to being indicated for the treatment of hypertension, both doxazosin and terazosin are indicated for the management of benign prostatic hypertrophy (BPH). Difficulty in urination is reduced by taking these agents.

OTHER ANTIHYPERTENSIVE AGENTS

These other antihypertensive agents are used less than those previously described because they generally have more or less tolerated adverse reactions. Clonidine is used in some patients in whom the above antihypertensives are ineffective.

Clonidine. Clonidine [KLON-i-deen] (Catapres) is a CNS-mediated (centrally acting) antihypertensive drug. Clonidine reduces peripheral resistance through a CNS-mediated action on the α-receptor. Stimulation of presynaptic central α_2-adrenergic receptors results in decreased sympathetic outflow. Thus clonidine reduces heart rate, cardiac output, and total peripheral resistance. It is indicated for the management of essential hypertension and can be administered orally or by a transdermal patch (Catapres-TTS).

ADVERSE EFFECTS Adverse effects include a high incidence of sedation and dizziness. Rapid elevation of blood pressure has occurred with abrupt discontinuation. CNS depressants employed in dental conscious-sedation techniques may contribute to postural hypotension when used in a patient taking clonidine.

ORAL EFFECTS The oral effects of clonidine include a high incidence of xerostomia (40%), parotid gland swelling, and pain. Another side effect is dysgeusia (unpleasant taste), whose

---

> **BOX 15-7 MANAGEMENT OF DENTAL PATIENTS TAKING α_1-BLOCKING AGENTS**
>
> - Orthostatic hypotension—dizziness, lightheadedness, or syncope
> - Drowsiness or nervousness
> - NSAIAs interfere with the antihypertensive effect of α_1-blockers
> - Epinephrine (sympathomimetics)—don't use to treat hypotension

mechanism is unknown but may be related to xerostomia.

OTHER CENTRALLY ACTING ANTIHYPERTENSIVE AGENTS Two other centrally acting antihypertensive drugs, methyldopa [meth-ill-DOE-pa] (Aldomet) and guanabenz [GWAHN-a-benz] (Wytensin), are also available. Adverse effects and indications for use are similar to those of clonidine. The centrally acting antihypertensive drugs may be combined with diuretics in essential hypertension management.

Guanethidine. Guanethidine's [gwahn-ETH-i-deen] (Ismelin) severe adverse reactions severely limit its use. It acts by blocking the release of norepinephrine from the sympathetic nerve endings. It also depletes the amount of norepinephrine stored in synaptic vesicles. Both actions decrease the amount of norepinephrine that can be released with sympathetic stimulation, thereby reducing sympathetic nervous system tone and decreasing blood pressure (see Figure 15-5). Guanethidine has a delayed onset of action, and its effects can persist for at least 2 weeks after it is discontinued.

Guanethidine causes severe postural and exertional hypotension, which is exacerbated by anything that causes vasodilation, such as warm weather, ingestion of alcohol, or exercise. Hypotension is most severe after the patient has spent several hours in a supine position, such as in the dental chair. Other adverse reactions include diarrhea, interference with ejaculation, and cardiac problems. Muscle weakness has also been reported.

Reserpine. Originally employed as a tranquilizer, reserpine [re-SER-peen] is currently used in low doses as an antihypertensive agent. Like guanethidine, reserpine depletes norepinephrine from the sympathetic nerve endings and can accumulate in the body. Adverse reactions include diarrhea, bad dreams, sedation, and even psychic depression leading to suicide. Reserpine in-

creases the production of stomach acid and aggravates peptic ulcers. It can also produce galactorrhea, breast engorgement, and **gynecomastia.**

Hydralazine. Hydralazine [hye-DRAL-a-zeen] (Apresoline) exerts its antihypertensive effect by acting directly on the arterioles to reduce peripheral resistance (vasodilation). At the same time a rise in heart rate and output occurs. Propranolol is often administered concurrently to reduce the reflex tachycardia and increased cardiac output. Hydralazine is often used in combination with the thiazides or other antihypertensive agents. Both diastolic and systolic blood pressures are reduced proportionately, and there is little orthostatic hypotension. The most commonly reported side effects associated with hydralazine are cardiac arrhythmias, angina, headache, and dizziness. A serious toxic reaction produces symptoms like those of systemic lupus erythematosus (lupuslike reaction). Hydralazine is the drug of choice for the treatment of a pregnant hypertensive woman.

MANAGEMENT OF THE DENTAL PATIENT TAKING ANTIHYPERTENSIVE AGENTS

Although the antihypertensive drugs cause a variety of adverse reactions, many of them exert similar actions that can alter dental treatment (Box 15-8). Because the hypertension of patients taking antihypertensive medications may or may not be controlled, the blood pressure of each patient should be measured on each visit to the dental office. Not uncommonly, a patient whose blood pressure is "normal" on one visit might be found to be hypotensive or hypertensive on a subsequent visit.

Adverse effects

XEROSTOMIA Dry mouth is an adverse reaction associated with several of the antihypertensives. If the dental health care worker notices this effect, it is imperative to discuss with

BOX 15-8 MANAGEMENT OF THE DENTAL PATIENT TAKING ANTIHYPERTENSIVES

- Check for xerostomia and its management.
- If on CCB, check for gingival enlargement.
- Check blood pressure before each appointment.
- Avoid dental agents that add to side effects, such as opioids (sedation and constipation).
- If on diuretics, check for symptoms of hypokalemia, which may exacerbate arrhythmias from epinephrine.
- If on ACE inhibitors, check for symptoms of neutropenia.

the patient methods used to alleviate this discomfort.

DYSGEUSIA With some antihypertensives, an altered sense of taste may occur, which may be related to xerostomia.

GINGIVAL ENLARGEMENT CCBs can produce gingival enlargement. Meticulous oral hygiene and frequent recall appointments may minimize this effect.

ORTHOSTATIC HYPOTENSION When a patient has been in a supine position and suddenly rises to an upright position, a sudden fall in blood pressure may occur. This side effect is called **orthostatic hypotension.** Patients taking antihypertensive agents who have been supine for some time should be slowly raised from that position. They should dangle their legs over the side of the chair and wiggle them before rising to the standing position. The patient should be supported for a few steps to prevent syncope. Guanethidine causes this problem frequently; other agents produce variable amounts of orthostatic hypotension.

CONSTIPATION Some antihypertensive agents can cause constipation, which could be additive with the constipation produced by the opioids. An increase in **dietary fiber,** a bulk laxative, or a stool softener may be considered if an opioid is prescribed for a patient receiving a constipation-producing antihypertensive medication.

CENTRAL NERVOUS SYSTEM SEDATION Several antihypertensives can produce sedation, which is additive with other CNS depressants such as opioids or benzodiazepines. The psychic depression generated by the older antihypertensive agents could lead to suicide attempts, so the dosage of potentially lethal medication prescribed in the dental office should be limited if depression is evident. With the newer antihypertensives in use today, this effect does not occur.

ANTIHYPERLIPIDEMIC AGENTS

Hyperlipidemia and hyperlipoproteinemia are elevations of plasma lipid concentrations above accepted normal values. These metabolic disorders include elevations in cholesterol and/or triglycerides and are associated with the development of arteriosclerosis, although the exact correlation is unknown. There are many different types of hyperlipoproteinemias that result in elevations of chylomicrons, very-low-density lipoproteins (VLDLs), low-density lipoproteins (LDLs), or combinations of these.

Foam cells, more prevalent in uncontrolled diabetes, become filled with cholesterol esters. Accumulation of these esters leads to deposition of lipids in the arteries. Collagen and fibrin also accumulate, occluding the vessels. Atherosclerosis can lead to coronary artery disease, myocardial infarction, and cerebral arterial disease. The endothelium over the plaques activates platelets, leading to the formation of thrombi and clinical symptoms. Additional risk factors for development of complication include untreated hypertension, smoking, **obesity,** and alcohol use.

LDL = Bad cholesterol
HDL = Good cholesterol

Cholesterol and other plasma lipids are transported in the blood in the form of protein complexes (lipoproteins) to make them more soluble in plasma. LDLs are referred to as "bad cholesterol" because they carry the greatest concentration of cholesterol and are considered to be the most dangerous. **High-density lipoproteins (HDLs)** are referred to as "good cholesterol" because they have the lowest cholesterol content and are considered to be beneficial (they carry cholesterol away from the blood vessels).

The first line of treatment of hyperlipoproteinemia is increasing exercise and decreasing saturated fat and cholesterol from the diet. Depending on the severity of the condition and the success of the patient in making permanent lifestyle changes, drug therapy may be considered.

Therapy of hyperlipoproteinemia is directed at lowering the level of LDL cholesterol. Drugs are available that reduce hyperlipoproteinemias, some more specific for cholesterol and some more specific for the triglycerides. Antihyperlipidemic drugs include the bile acid–binding resins, niacin, gemfibrozil, and HMG Co-A reductase inhibitors (Table 15-12). The HMG Co-A reductase inhibitors are the most commonly used antihyperlipidemics.

HMG Co-A Reductase Inhibitors

Suffix: *-statins*

The HMG Co-A reductase inhibitors are often referred to as the "statins" because their generic names end in that suffix. Their side effect profile is more desirable than any of the other drugs used to treat hyperlipidemias.

Lovastatin [LOE-va-sta-tin] (Mevacor) is one example of the "statins." Atorvastatin [a-TORE-va-sta-tin] (Lipitor), the newest member of this

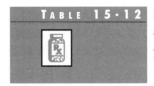

TABLE 15-12 Effect of Antihyperlipidemic Agents on Serum Lipids

	Chol	TGD	VLDL	LDL	HDL
HMG-CoA reductase inhibitors ("-statins")					
Atorvastatin (Lipitor)					
Cerivastatin (Baycol)					
Fluvastatin (Lescol)	−	−	—	—	+
Lovastatin (Mevacor)	−	−	—	—	+
Provastatin (Pravachol)	−	−	—	—	+
Simvastatin (Zocor)	−	−	—	—	+
Bile acid sequestrants					
Cholestyramine (Questran, Prevalite)	−	±	±	—	±
Colestipol (Colestid)	−	±	+	−	±
Miscellaneous					
Clofibrate (Atromid-S)	−	−	—	=,−	±
Dextrothyroxine (Choloxin)	−	=	=	—	=
Fenofibrate (Lipidil, Tricor)					
Gemfibrozil (Lopid)	−	−	—	=,−	+
Nicotinic acid (Niacin)	−	−	—	−	+

Chol, Cholesterol; *HDL*, high-density lipoproteins; *LDL*, low-density lipoprotein; *TGD*, triglycerides; *VLDL*, very-low-density lipoproteins.

family, is the most potent HMG Co-A reductase inhibitor; with a direct-to-patient advertising campaign, it has become popular. It lowers triglycerides more than the other HMG Co-A reductase inhibitors. The statins lower cholesterol levels by inhibiting HMG-CoA reductase, the rate-limiting enzyme in cholesterol synthesis. They may work because they are structural analogues of HMG Co-A reductase and thereby inhibit that enzyme. Another possible mechanism of the HMG Co-A reductase inhibitors may relate to the increase in the number of low-density lipoprotein receptors that occurs. The effectiveness of the HMG Co-A reductase inhibitors should be monitored by a lipid panel repeated once or twice a year.

Adverse effects. Adverse effects of HMG Co-A reductase inhibitors include gastrointestinal complaints such as stomachache, constipation, diarrhea, and gas. Other side effects are **my-ositis**, skin rash, **impotence**, hepatotoxicity, blurred vision, and lens (in the eye) opacities. Myositis results in complaints of muscle pain. Liver function tests should be performed because of the small potential for hepatotoxicity. These agents can increase the anticoagulant effect of warfarin.

NIACIN

Niacin [NYE-a-sin] (nicotinic acid) is a B vitamin (discussed in Chapter 14). In larger doses, niacin produces a therapeutic effect. It lowers cholesterol levels by inhibiting the secretion of VLDLs without accumulation of triglycerides in the liver. This reduces LDL synthesis. At these larger doses, niacin commonly produces cutaneous flushing (especially the face and neck) and a sensation of warmth after each dose. The prostaglandin-mediated flushing is blocked by pretreatment with 0.3 gm of aspirin taken one-half hour before taking niacin or by taking 1 tablet of ibuprofen daily. This side effect can be minimized by beginning with low doses of niacin and slowly increasing the dose over a period of weeks. Increasing the dose of niacin enough to produce a decrease in lipids without having intolerable adverse effects is challenging. Hyperuricemia can occur and can be treated with allopurinol. Allergic reactions, cholestasis, and hepatotoxicity have been reported.

Dental implications. Hypotension may occur as a result of the vasodilation, especially in patients taking antihypertensives. Rising from the dental chair should be attempted slowly to prevent orthostatic hypotension.

CHOLESTYRAMINE

The bile acid–binding resins, cholestyramine [koe-less-TIR-a-meen] (Questran) and colestipol [koe-LES-ti-pole] (Colestid), lower cholesterol concentrations because cholesterol is a pre-cursor that is required for the synthesis of the new bile acids. When the resins bind with the bile acids they produce an insoluble product that is lost through the gastrointestinal tract. The bile acids, which must be replaced, use up cholesterol, thereby reducing cholesterol levels. Adverse reactions relate to the gastrointestinal tract and include constipation and bloating, but serious side effects are infrequent. These drugs are poorly tolerated because of their effects on the gastrointestinal tract and patients often abandon their use.

GEMFIBROZIL

Gemfibrozil [gem-FI-broe-zil] (Lopid) is used to treat hyperlipidemias, especially when triglycerides are elevated. It works by increasing lipolysis of triglycerides, decreasing lipolysis in adipose tissue, and inhibiting secretion of VLDLs from the liver. This drug causes fewer gastrointestinal complaints than the bile acid–binding drugs, but it can promote gallstone formation (cholelithiasis). Taste perversion and hyperglycemia have been reported. Hematologic and liver function should be monitored routinely.

DENTAL IMPLICATIONS

Patients who take antihyperlipidemic agents have a higher risk of arteriosclerosis and are therefore at increased risk for

> Take BP and HR at each appointment.

cardiovascular emergencies. These patients are at increased risk for myocardial infarctions and cardiac arrest. Dental health care workers should be prepared to handle such emergencies. The patient's blood pressure and pulse rate should be taken before each appointment and recorded in the dental chart. If an emergency occurs, it is important to know the preemergency blood pressure and heart rate so that these can be compared with the current measurements. Because gastrointestinal and liver abnormalities are side effects associated with many of these drugs, their tolerance to the agents taken should be determined before dental drugs are prescribed or suggested. The small possibility of liver abnormalities requires laboratory testing for abnormal liver function.

DRUGS THAT AFFECT BLOOD COAGULATION

ANTICOAGULANTS

Anticoagulants are drugs that in some way interfere with coagulation. The first anticoagulant was discovered when cows that ingested spoiled sweet clover silage became hemorrhagic. The toxic agent in the clover was found to be dicum-

arol, and warfarin is a close relative. Warfarin has been used as a rodenticide. When the rats eat the warfarin they begin to bleed and eventually die. Therapeutically, anticoagulants are administered in an attempt to prevent clotting. Examples of indications for warfarin are after a myocardial infarction or thrombophlebitis. Warfarin (Coumadin) is the most important oral anticoagulant and is the one used almost exclusively in therapy.

Hemostasis. Hemostasis is a normal mechanism in the body that is designed to prevent the loss of blood after injury to a blood vessel. The leaking vessel is plugged by a complicated process of clot formation. In the presence of a vascular injury the entire clotting mechanism is initiated. Thromboplastin, factors V, VII, and X, and calcium ions form prothrombin, thrombin, and finally fibrinogen and fibrin (Figure 15-8). The fi-

FIGURE 15-8 *Intrinsic and extrinsic systems of blood coagulation. The boxed clotting factors (II [prothrombin], VII [extrinsic], IX [intrinsic], and X) are dependent on vitamin K for their synthesis. Warfarin inhibits these four clotting factors.*

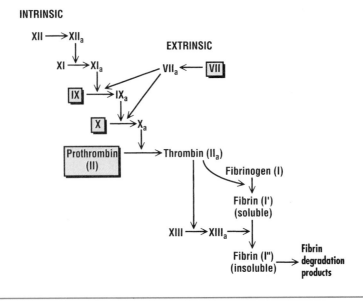

brin, along with vascular spasms, platelets, and red blood cells, quickly forms the clot.

If the blood vessel's interior remains smooth, circulating blood does not clot. However, if internal injury to the vessel occurs and a roughened surface develops, intravascular clotting will take place. This process involves an intrinsic prothrombin activator that includes a platelet factor, factor V, factors VIII through XII, and calcium ions. The prothrombin activator, which was formerly called *thromboplastin*, converts prothrombin to thrombin. Thrombin then converts fibrinogen to fibrin, and clot formation occurs.

Many of the factors required in the clotting process are synthesized in the liver. Prothrombin (II) and factors VII, IX, and X require vitamin K for synthesis. Because warfarin antagonizes vitamin K, it interferes with the synthesis of four clotting factors to produce an anticoagulant effect.

In certain diseases, intravascular clots can form. These clots, or thrombi, may break off, forming **emboli** that lodge in the smaller vessels of major organs such as the heart, brain, and lungs, producing severe and even fatal thromboembolic disease. Anticoagulant therapy attempts to reduce intravascular clotting and prevent life-threatening situations. Each person's anticoagulant therapy must be adjusted to suit his or her needs. If the dose of the anticoagulant is too large, hemorrhage may occur. If the dose is too small, the danger of **embolism** remains.

Warfarin. Warfarin [WAR-far-in] (Coumadin) is an oral anticoagulant (interferes with coagulation). It blocks γ-carboxylation of glutamate residues in the synthesis of factors VII, IX, and X, prothrombin (II), and endogenous anticoagulant protein C. Instead of forming the factors, incomplete and inactive molecules are formed that do not function properly. Warfarin also prevents the metabolism of the inactive vitamin K epoxide back to its active form.

Warfarin's pharmacologic effect is delayed when therapy begins and ends. This latent period in the onset of action of warfarin occurs for the following two reasons:

1. The blood level of the warfarin accumulates over time until it plateaus or reaches steady state. The maximum effect for one dose occurs after 5 half-lives = 5 × 42 hr = 210 hr [9 days])

2. Endogenous clotting factors II, VII, IX, and X have half-lives that are 60, 6, 24, and 40 hours, respectively. They must become depleted before the anticoagulant effect is maximized.

When reducing the dose of warfarin or discontinuing it, there will be a delay in the change in the effect because the drug must be metabolized to inactivate it and the clotting factors must be synthesized again.

MONITORING Warfarin's effect is monitored using the International Normalized Ratio (INR). The INR is a function of the **prothrombin time (PT)** of the patient, PT of control, and the **International Sensitivity Index (ISI)**. The ISI is a number that is a function of the potency of the specific (human or rabbit) thromboplastin used in the particular laboratory. The advantage of the INR over the PT ratio is that the INR value from any laboratory in the world can be compared, whereas the PT ratio varies among laboratories. The formula for the INR is as follows:

$$INR = \left[\frac{PT_{patient}}{PT_{control}} \right]^{ISI}$$

The therapeutic target INR (number at which the provider is trying to keep the patient's INR) for most indications such as thrombophlebitis or atrial fibrillation is between 2 and 3. For patients with a prosthetic heart valve, the target INR is between 2.5 and 3.5. The INR can range from 1 (INR without drug effect) to 4, although with overdose it can reach higher levels.

In the past, the laboratory test that was used to monitor warfarin was the prothrombin time ratio. The prothrombin time ratio (PT_r) is the ratio of the $PT_{patient}/PT_{control}$. Some laboratories are still reporting the PT_r. Prothrombin time ratios range from 1 (PT_r without drug) to 2.5 or higher. The target numbers for the PT_r and the INR are *not* interchangeable.

Because warfarin is orally effective and less expensive than heparin, it is used in long-term treatment of thromboembolic diseases such as thrombophlebitis and myocardial infarction.

ADVERSE REACTIONS The most common adverse effects associated with the oral anticoagulants are various forms of bleeding, including hemorrhage. Because of its narrow therapeutic index and because of numerous drug interactions, serious reactions can easily occur. Look for petechial hemorrhages on the hard palate. Ecchymoses can occur, even without concomitant trauma. With mild trauma, these effects may be seen in the oral cavity. Studies compared effects of lower and higher doses of warfarin in clot prevention. They found no advantage in use of higher doses, but found an increase in adverse reactions. Dosing of warfarin is now titrated to a lower INR than in the past.

Aspirin The most serious drug interaction of warfarin is with aspirin (Table 15-13). Patients taking warfarin should not be given aspirin or aspirin-containing products ("cold preparations") because bleeding episodes or fatal hemorrhages can result. Aspirin interacts with warfarin in several ways. First, aspirin causes hypoprothrombinemia and alters platelet adhesiveness (see Chapter 6). These effects in themselves reduce clotting ability. Aspirin can also irritate the gastrointestinal tract, which might bleed more in a patient taking warfarin. Another factor in the aspirin-warfarin interaction is related to protein binding of drugs. Warfarin is

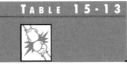

TABLE 15-13	Drug Interactions Between NSAIAs and Warfarin
SEVERITY	**DRUG EXAMPLES**
Major	Aspirin
Moderate	Indomethacin
	Meclofenamate
	Piroxicam
	Sulindac
Minor	Diclofenac
	Fenoprofen
	Ibuprofen
	Naproxen
None	Nonacetylated salicylates
	Acetaminophen (small)

more than 99% bound to plasma proteins and about 1% free drug. Only the free drug (less than 1%) exerts the pharmacologic effect of decreased clotting. Because warfarin and aspirin compete for the same plasma protein–binding site, aspirin displaces the bound warfarin, thereby increasing the proportion of free (unbound) warfarin and, hence, potentiating its activity. Only the free drug in the blood exerts a pharmacologic effect. The bound drug is merely a reservoir for the drug. Even a small increase in free warfarin can lead to a large increase in effect, leading to dire consequences, including hemorrhage. If an NSAIA is to be used in a patient taking warfarin, ibuprofen or naproxen should be prescribed. These agents have only a minor interaction with warfarin, and a few doses can be given in the patient with an INR within the therapeutic target. The nonacetylated salicylates do not have an effect on platelets.

Acetaminophen Acetaminophen and its effect on warfarin was prospectively analyzed. Hylek[1] studied patients taking warfarin in an attempt to identify factors that were associated with an INR above 6 (therapeutic INR = 2 to 3.5). A statistically significant association was found between

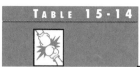

TABLE 15-14	Warfarin and Antiinfective Drug Interactions	
MOST	SOME	LEAST
Metronidazole	Tetracycline	Clindamycin
Erythromycin	Doxycycline	
Ketoconazole (-azole antifungals)	Penicillin, ampicillin, amoxicillin, dicloxacillin	
Cephalosporins	Quinolones	

BOX 15-9 MANAGEMENT OF THE DENTAL PATIENT TAKING WARFARIN (COUMADIN)

- Obtain prothrombin time (PT) or international normalized ratio (INR) and history to establish bleeding potential
- For PT or INR greater than 2 × normal, request reduction in dose
- Since latent time to onset and recovery allow several days for change in effect if dose of warfarin changed.
- Check with physician regarding resuming dose
- Avoid aspirin and aspirin-containing compounds
- Acetaminophen and opioids OK
- Oral hygiene with subgingival calculus removal can produce bleeding (oozing); use local pressure
- Determine underlying disease of patient
- May have atrial fibrillation
- Patient should be free of infection before scaling/root planning
- Some suggest prophylactic antibiotics after surgery
- Check with patient regarding healing

acetaminophen use and the abnormal elevation of the INR. With higher doses of acetaminophen (9 gm/wk) there was a 10-fold increase in the likelihood of presenting with an abnormal INR. Whether there is a causal relationship between acetaminophen use and warfarin toxicity has not been proved. Managing patients taking warfarin who need analgesics may require more frequent monitoring of the INR, especially with intermittent use.

Antibiotics Antibiotics can also potentiate the effect of warfarin. Antibiotics reduce the bacterial flora in the gastrointestinal tract that normally synthesize vitamin K. This results in a decrease in vitamin K absorbed. Because warfarin also inhibits vitamin K–dependent factors, there is an added anticoagulant effect. If an antibiotic is to be used with warfarin (Table 15-14), clindamycin has no effect, doxycycline, tetracycline, and amoxicillin have small effect, and erythromycin and metronidazole have the greatest effect on altering warfarin's anticoagulant action. If the antibiotic is used for prophylaxis before a dental procedure (1 dose) the interaction would not have a chance to develop.

Induction of the microsomal enzymes increases warfarin's metabolism and reduces its effect. Phenobarbital induces the liver microsomal enzymes that would normally destroy the anticoagulant. Alcohol's effect on warfarin depends on the pattern of alcohol use. With chronic alcohol ingestion, the metabolism of warfarin is stimulated. Acute alcohol intoxication inhibits the metabolism of warfarin. Other agents that inhibit the metabolism of warfarin include cimetidine, disulfiram, and metronidazole.

MANAGEMENT OF THE DENTAL PATIENT TAKING WARFARIN See Box 15-9 for a summary of the management of dental patients taking warfarin.

Most dental procedures require no change in dose of warfarin.

Bleeding Before any dental procedure is begun, the patient should be interviewed to determine

TABLE 15-15   **Safety of Outpatient Dental Treatment for Patients Receiving Warfarin (Coumadin) Anticoagulant Therapy**

	INTERNATIONAL NORMALIZED RATIO [INR][a]					
				MECHANICAL HEART VALVES[b]		OUT OF RANGE
	SUBOPTIMAL RANGE		NORMAL TARGET INR[c]			
DENTAL TREATMENT	<1.5	1.5 TO <2.0	2.0 < 2.5	2.5 TO 3.0	>3.0 TO 3.5	>3.5
Examination, radiographs, study models						
Simple restorative dentistry, supragingival prophylaxis						[e]
Complex restorative dentistry, scaling and root planing, endodontics					Probably safe[f]	
Simple extraction, curettage, gingivoplasty				Local measures[g]	Local measures[g]	
Multiple extractions, removal of single bony impaction			Local measures[g]	Local measures[g]	Local measures[g]	
Gingivectomy, apicoectomy, minor periodontal flap surgery, placement of single implant	Probably safe (IR)[h]	Probably safe[f]	Probably safe[f]			
Full-mouth/full-arch extractions	Probably safe[f]	Local measures[g]				
Extension flap surgery, extraction of multiple bony impactions, multiple implant placement	Probably safe[f]					
Open-fracture reduction, orthognathic surgery						

Modified from Herman WW, et al: Current perspectives on dental patients receiving coumarin anticoagulant therapy, *JADA* 128(3):327-35, 1997.

[a]INR is this ratio: $[PT(patient)/PT(control)]^{ISA}$.

[b]INR 2.5 to 3.5 = therapeutic range for mechanical prosthetic heart valves.

[c]INR 2 to 3 = therapeutic range for venous thrombosis, pulmonary embolism, systemic embolism (myocardial infarction, valvular, atrial fibrillation).

[d]White boxes indicate that it is safe to proceed in a routine manner (local factors such as periodontitis or gingival inflammation can increase the severity of bleeding; the clinician should consider all factors when making a risk assessment).

[e]Diagonal shading indicates procedure not advised at current INR level; refer to physician for adjustment.

[f]Probably safe, can perform procedure with care.

[g]Use local measures: Increased need for sutures, oxidized cellulose hemostat, topical thrombin and tranexamic acid.

[h]*IR,* Insufficient research, but research data available for other similar procedures.

whether any symptoms relating to bleeding have been noted. Many surgical procedures can be carried out on a patient receiving therapeutic doses of anticoagulants (Table 15-15). Check with the prescribing physician to obtain the patient's INR or PT_r and the date the blood for the test was drawn. A higher INR can be tolerated if local measures are added.

Whenever a decision is being made to change the dose of warfarin the *risk* of lowering the dose of warfarin must be weighed against the *benefit* of lowering the dose of warfarin (Box 15-10). Discontinuing warfarin for a few days without knowledge of the patient's INR could expose the patient to an increased risk of clotting. If the patient does not need the anticoagulant, then it can be permanently discontinued. If the patient needs anticoagulation, then the risk of intravascular clotting in these patients should not be underestimated.

Box 15-10 WARFARIN—TO CLOT OR BLEED: THAT IS THE QUESTION

Point-Counterpoint. The **risk** of clotting if the dose of warfarin is reduced must be weighed against the **benefit** of reduced oral cavity bleeding from lowering the dose of warfarin. *Perspective makes the difference.*

From the dental health care worker's perspective, the important risk is related to excessive bleeding. From the provider's viewpoint, the important risk is intravascular clotting. The INR value and the indication for the use of warfarin will determine what would be best for the patient. Often patients will be subtherapeutic and may have even taken the warfarin for the necessary time, but it had not been discontinued.

Analgesics Aspirin and aspirin-containing products are absolutely contraindicated in patients taking warfarin unless the patient is taking one aspirin tablet daily for its anticoagulant effect. In this case, the monitoring of warfarin effect is done while the patient is taking aspirin. Acetaminophen or any opioid alone or together may be substituted if analgesia is desired. A few doses of ibuprofen or naproxen may be safely used if there is no other contraindication to their use.

Heparin. Heparin [HEP-a-rin] is one of the most commonly employed anticoagulant agents in hospitalized patients. Because it must be given by injection and cannot be used orally, its outpatient use is essentially nonexistent. Newer heparins, termed *low-molecular-weight heparins*, are being used, but until an oral dosage form is developed, use of these heparins will be limited. Because its effect begins quickly, heparin is the first anticoagulant given to hospitalized patients with excessive clotting. Patients who might receive heparin are those with myocardial infarction, stroke (embolism), or thrombophlebitis. When the heparin is started (ASAP), warfarin is also begun. Because warfarin's effect has a latent period, the heparin can provide immediate anticoagulant effect while the warfarin is building up. The effect of an overdose of heparin is antagonized by protamine sulfate, which immediately reverses its anticoagulant effects.

Ticlopidine. The drug ticlopidine [tye-KLOE-pi-deen] (Ticlid) is an irreversible inhibitor of ADP-induced platelet aggregation, which results in prolonged bleeding time. Ticlopidine is indicated to decrease thrombotic stroke in patients with previous stroke. It is used in patients who are intolerant of aspirin. Its major side effect, neutropenia, is monitored by appropriate blood tests. An increase in infections could signal neutropenia. It does not alter the PT or INR.

Ticlopidine is taken with food because it can produce diarrhea, nausea, and vomiting. Patients taking ticlopidine have increased bleeding after trauma or surgery. It takes 10 to 14 days to eliminate the bleeding effect. Bleeding can lead to ecchymoses, epistaxis, and perioperative bleed. For emergency surgery, injectable methylprednisolone can reverse the prolonged bleeding to normal in a few hours. Nonsteroidal anti-inflammatory agents should be avoided because gastrointestinal bleeding can result. Patients taking this drug should be carefully managed in the dental office, but no laboratory tests are used to monitor ticlopidine.

Streptokinase and alteplase (tPA). Enzymes, called "clotbusters," such as streptokinase [strep-toe-KYE-nase] (Streptase, Kabikinase), and the recombinant tissue-type plasminogen activator, alteplase [AL-ti-plase] (tPA, Activase), are sometimes used in the therapy of deep vein thrombosis, arterial thrombosis, pulmonary embolism, and acute coronary artery thrombosis associated with myocardial infarction. These may appropriately be termed *thrombolytic drugs* because they promote the conversion of plasminogen to plasmin, the natural clot-resolving enzyme. They are usually administered by direct vessel perfusion to the clot site. Considerable technical skill and immediate treatment of the thrombus is required for satisfactory results. Because streptokinase is a protein, allergic reactions can occur. Hemorrhage may result from the use of any of these drugs and they are contraindicated in patients at risk for hemorrhage.

Dipyridamole. The drug dipyridamole [dye-peer-ID-a-mole] (Persantine) is used to prolong the life of platelets in patients with prosthetic heart valves. The artificial valves cause premature death of the platelets because of their mechanical effect (trauma) on the blood cells passing through the valves. Dipyridamole does not add any additional anticlotting benefit over the use of aspirin and/or warfarin. It does not affect bleeding related to dental treatment.

Pentoxifylline. Pentoxifylline [pen-tox-IF-i-lin] (Trental) is a dimethylxanthine that improves blood flow by its hemorrheologic effects, which include lowering blood viscosity and improving the flexibility of red blood cells. It is indicated for intermittent claudication produced by chronic occlusive artery disease of the limbs. Side effects associated with pentoxifylline include cardiovascular and gastric symptoms. Dry mouth, bad taste, excessive salivation, and swollen neck glands have infrequently been reported. Pentoxifylline does not alter blood clotting.

DRUGS THAT INCREASE BLOOD CLOTTING

Hemostatic agents (fibrinolytic inhibitors). Aminocaproic acid (EACA) and its analogue, tranexamic acid (Cyklokapron), are similar to the amino acid lysine, and they inhibit plasminogen activation (synthetic inhibitor of fibrinolysis).

Aminocaproic acid and tranexamic acid are used intravenously, orally, or topically. Adverse effects include intravascular thrombosis, hypotension, and abdominal discomfort. Some literature recommends the use of topical tranexamic acid before dental procedures in patients taking warfarin who are at risk of bleeding. It is indicated in the treatment of hemorrhage following dental surgery.

Reference

1. Hylek EM et al: Acetaminophen and other risk factors for excessive warfarin anticoagulation, *JAMA* 279:657, 1998.

REVIEW QUESTIONS

1. State the best way to prevent actinic lip changes.
2. Describe the treatment of a patient with acute necrotizing ulcerative gingivitis.
3. Describe the appropriate treatment for herpes labialis. State what has been proved to be effective in the treatment of recurrent herpes labialis in a nonimmunocompromised patient. Write a prescription for two different antiherpes agents.
4. Describe two appropriate treatments for recurrent aphthous stomatitis (RAS). Write a prescription for one agent.
5. State three drugs used for oral candidiasis and discuss when each agent would be appropriate.
6. Name two ways to reduce alveolar osteitis. Write a prescription for two agents, one topical and one systemic, used to treat oral candidiasis.
7. Describe three causes of xerostomia and state several drugs that can produce this effect.
8. Explain the management of xerostomia. Include preventive measures to be included.

Anticonvulsants

EPILEPSY

Epilepsy comprises a group of disorders that involve a chronic stereotyped recurrent attack of involuntary behavior or experience or changes in neurologic function caused by electrical activity in the brain that can be recorded via an electroencephalogram (EEG). This activity can be localized or generalized. Each episode is termed a *seizure*. The seizure may be accompanied by motor activity such as convulsions or by other neurologic changes (e.g., sensory or emotional).

Because seizure disorders are estimated to affect approximately 1% of the population, the dental team is likely to encounter a patient with epilepsy. Because these anticonvulsant agents are used chronically, one must consider potential adverse reactions that might alter dental treatment.

There are many etiologies for epilepsy, including infection, trauma, toxicity to exogenous agents, genetic or birth influences, circulatory disturbances, meta-

Idiopathic epilepsy (cause unknown)

365

bolic or nutritional alterations, **neoplasms,** hereditary factors, fevers, and degenerative diseases. The majority of epileptic patients have *idiopathic epilepsy;* this term is used when the cause is unknown.

Epilepsy has been classified based on causes, symptoms, duration, precipitating factors, postictal state, and **aura.** Currently, The International Classification of Epileptic Seizures (Figure 16-1) divides seizures into two major groups and a miscellaneous group. The two major groups are partial and generalized seizures. **Partial seizures** are divided into simple and complex attacks. The most common generalized seizures are (1) tonic-clonic and (2) absence seizures. The miscellaneous group consists of seizures that are not classified as either partial or generalized (Box 16-1).

GENERALIZED SEIZURES

Generalized seizures are divided into two large groups: absence and tonic-clonic types. Consciousness is lost in both types. Whereas little movement occurs in absence seizures, in tonic-clonic seizures, major movement of large muscle groups occurs. Management of seizures is discussed at the end of this chapter.

Absence seizures (petit mal). The symptoms of absence seizures include a brief (few seconds) loss of consciousness with characteristic EEG waves and little movement. Absence seizures usually begin during childhood and disappear in middle age. The patient is usually unaware that these seizures are occurring

Absence—Petit mal

FIGURE 16-1   *The International Classification of Epileptic Seizures: Status epilepticus; elementary motor (Jacksonian) autonomic seizures; temporal lobe (psychomotor) seizures; secondarily generalized seizures; partial seizures; unilateral seizures; generalized seizures; tonic-clonic seizures; myoclonic seizures; akinetic seizures; unclassified seizures. Seizure type patterns: same pattern indicates that same group of drugs are usually effective.*

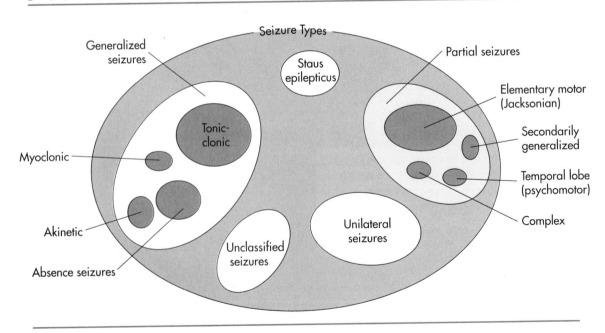

and body tone is not lost. There is no aura or postictal state, and the patient quickly returns to normal activity. The drug of choice in the treatment of typical absence seizures is either ethosuximide or valproic acid (Table 16-1).

Management of absence seizures poses no problems for the dental team. The team's main concern when treating patients with absence seizures is the adverse reactions that can occur from long-term administration of the drugs used to treat the disease.

Tonic-clonic—Grand mal

Tonic-clonic seizures. The generalized tonic-clonic (**grand mal**) seizures include longer periods of loss of consciousness and major motor activity of the large muscles of the body. The seizure begins by the body becoming rigid and the patient falling to the floor. Urination, apnea, and a cry may be present. Tonic rigidity is followed by clonic jerking of the face, limbs, and body. The patient may bite the cheek or tongue. Finally, the patient becomes limp and comatose. Consciousness returns gradually, with postictal confusion, headache, and drowsiness. Some patients experience prodromal periods of varying durations, but a true aura does not occur. Because this seizure type involves the violent movement of major muscle groups, it is more likely to result in serious injury to the patient. Valproic acid, phenytoin, phenobarbital, and carbamazepine are used to treat tonic-clonic seizures.

Status epilepticus. Status epilepticus seizures are continuous tonic-clonic seizures that last longer than 30 minutes or reoccur before the end of the postictal period of the previous seizure. This is an emergency situation, and rapid therapy is required, especially if the seizure activity has produced hypoxia. Parenteral benzodiazepines such as diazepam (Valium) are the drugs of choice to control this seizure type (see Chapter 11).

PARTIAL (FOCAL) EPILEPSIES

Partial epilepsies involve activation of only part of the brain, and the location of the activity determines the clinical manifestation. When con-

Box 16-1 SEIZURE CATEGORIES

Partial

Simple
Complex
Secondarily generalized
Psychomotor
Temporal-lobe

Generalized

Tonic-clonic (grand mal)
Absence (petit mal)
Tonic
Atonic
Clonic/myoclonic

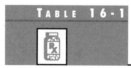

| TABLE 16-1 | **Anticonvulsant Drugs of Choice** | |

| | DRUGS | |
SEIZURE DISORDER	FIRST CHOICE	ALTERNATIVES
GENERALIZED SEIZURES		
Tonic-clonic (grand mal)	Phenytoin Divalproex	Phenobarbital Lamotrigine Topiramate
Absence (petit mal)	Ethosuximide Divalproex	Lamotrigine Topiramate Felbamate
Atonic Myoclonic	Divalproex	Lamotrigine Topiramate Felbamate
Status epilepticus	Diazepam (Valium) IV Phenytoin (Dilantin) IV Phenobarbital (Luminal) IV	
PARTIAL SEIZURES		
Simple Complex Secondarily generalized	Phenytoin Carbamazepine Divalproex	

sciousness is not impaired, the attack is called an *elementary* (simple) *partial attack*. When consciousness is impaired, the attack is termed a *complex partial attack*. Complex seizures are also called *psychomotor* or *temporal-lobe seizures*. In contrast to absence seizures that last a few seconds, these complex partial seizures last several minutes. Some patients with complex partial seizures have an aura, and full consciousness is slow to return. For the partial epilepsies carbamazepine, phenytoin, phenobarbital, and primidone are used.

DRUG THERAPY OF PATIENTS WITH EPILEPSY

| Dosing anticonvulsants difficult | Drug therapy of the patient with epilepsy has variable efficacy, from complete control of all seizures to |

reducing the frequency of seizures. Anticonvulsant agents may be used singly or in combination. The goal is to control seizures and minimize potential adverse reactions. Some newer anticonvulsants are able to treat previously untreatable seizures, but more serious side effects can accompany them. General principles on the management of the dental patient taking any anticonvulsant agents are listed in Box 16-2.

Anticonvulsant agents are central nervous system (CNS) depressants that attempt to prevent epileptic seizures without causing excessive drowsiness. Although their exact mechanisms of action are unknown, these agents prevent the spread of abnormal electric discharges in the brain.

The anticonvulsant drug used to treat a specific patient depends on the type of seizures the patient has. Because these agents are usually taken for life, their chronic toxicity becomes an important consideration in choosing a particular anticonvulsant agent and determining the drug's dental implications.

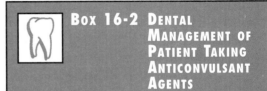

BOX 16-2 DENTAL MANAGEMENT OF PATIENT TAKING ANTICONVULSANT AGENTS

- Review emergency management of epileptic patients (remove hands and dental instruments from mouth, turn head to side)
- Take a thorough medical and drug history including medications and frequency of seizures
- Additive CNS depression—use additional CNS depressants cautiously
- Additive gastrointestinal adverse reactions—use drugs that are gastric irritants cautiously (e.g., NSAIAs)
- Drug interactions—induction of hepatic microsomal enzymes, metabolizes certain drugs more quickly (lowers blood level and effect) Dental drugs affected—propoxyphene, doxycycline

GENERAL ADVERSE REACTIONS TO ANTICONVULSANT AGENTS

Several factors make dosing with anticonvulsants more difficult than with other drugs. First, the anticonvulsants have a narrow therapeutic index so the dose must be carefully titrated to obtain the desired blood levels. It cannot be too low or too high. Second, most anticonvulsants stimulate liver microsomal enzymes that metabolize both themselves as well as other anticonvulsants. When a second anticonvulsant is added to the first, it changes the metabolism of both anticonvulsants. The third effect, which may be even more important than the others, is that the metabolism of the anticonvulsants can saturate the liver microsomal enzymes. With low doses, the metabolism is first order and the drug is being removed from the body. At some point, when the enzymes become saturated, the metabolism converts to zero-order kinetics and the drug level can increase abruptly. At the point of saturation, a very small change in the dose can lead to a large increase in the blood level of the drug.

The dental team must be aware of the side effects of the anticonvulsant agents that might influence dental treatment.

The anticonvulsant drugs possess a unique set of adverse reactions. Adverse reactions that the anticonvulsants have in common are discussed first.

Central nervous system depression. Depressed CNS function is a common side effect of the anticonvulsant agents. Tolerance often develops to these sedative effects while the anticonvulsant effect persists. Impaired learning and cognitive abilities occur in some patients. Behavior alterations reported include both hyperactivity and sedation. Another CNS side effect is exacerbation of a seizure type that is not being treated. This CNS depression is additive with other CNS depressants such as the opioids. If another CNS drug is given to the patient, the dose should be reduced.

Gastrointestinal tract. Gastrointestinal distress, including anorexia, nausea, and vomiting, can occur with most anticonvulsants. These effects can be minimized by taking the drug with food. Agents with adverse reactions related to the gastrointestinal tract, for example the NSAIAs or opioids, should be prescribed cautiously.

Anticonvulsant drug interactions

Drug interactions. Many drug interactions can occur with the anticonvulsants. They may interact with themselves, with each other, or with other drugs. The mechanisms of drug interactions include altering absorption or renal excretion and inducing or inhibiting metabolism. The outcome may alter the levels of the inducing drug itself, another concomitant anticonvulsant, or some other drug that is extensively metabolized by the liver microsomal enzymes.

The most important drug interaction of the anticonvulsants involves stimulation of the hepatic microsomal enzymes. Inducing these enzymes results in a reduction in the blood level of the affected drugs (those metabolized by the liver enzymes). Figure 2-23 shows the normal, unaffected enzyme situations (A). When the enzymes are stimulated (B) the level of the affected drug (D) is reduced because it is being metabolized more quickly, producing its metabolite (D_M).

Drug interactions with the anticonvulsants are more significant than with other drug groups because of their narrow therapeutic indexes. If the level of an anticonvulsant is altered sufficiently by a drug interaction, either toxicity (level too high) or loss of seizure control (level too low) can result. Before any changes or additions are made to a patient's therapy, the possibility of drug interactions should be considered.

IDIOSYNCRATIC REACTIONS A wide range of idiosyncratic reactions occur with the anticonvulsants. Dermatologic side effects include rash, Stevens-Johnson syndrome, exfoliative dermatitis, and erythema multiforme. Drug-induced systemic lupus erythematosus and hematologic effects have also been reported with most of these agents.

TERATOGENICITY/GROWTH Reports have associated the anticonvulsant agents with alteration in growth, with profound effects on fetal development and children receiving anticonvulsant medications during growth and development. The teratogenic potential of the anticonvulsants has been documented. Several have been implicated in the production of fetal anomalies.

WITHDRAWAL Abrupt withdrawal of any anticonvulsant medication can precipitate seizures. Although many patients require medication for life, certain seizure types tend to disappear as the patient grows older. In these patients, gradual withdrawal of their seizure medication under controlled conditions can be undertaken after an appropriate interval of drug use.

OTHER Another adverse reaction resulting from suppression of ADH is dilutional hyponatremia. Renal toxicity or failure, paresthesias, and thrombophlebitis have also been recorded.

CARBAMAZEPINE

Carbamazepine for trigeminal neuralgia

Structurally related to the tricyclic antidepressants, carbamazepine [kar-ba-MAZ-e-peen] (Tegretol) is used to treat convulsions. It is of special interest in dentistry because of its use in the treatment of trigeminal neuralgia (tic douloureux). It is also indicated in the treatment of bipolar depression. In fact, several anticonvulsants are used to manage chronic pain syndromes.

Pharmacologic effects. Carbamazepine has the following properties: anticonvulsant, anticholinergic, antidepressant, sedative, and muscle relaxant. It also has antiarrhythmic, antidiuretic, and neuromuscular transmission-inhibitory actions. Its mechanism of action involves blocking sodium channels, which blocks the propagation of nerve impulses. Other effects of carbamazepine include inhibition of high-frequency repetitive firing in neurons and decrease in synaptic transmission presynaptically.

Adverse reactions. Carbamazepine can have many types of adverse reactions, some quite serious, but most patients seem to tolerate it well. CNS depression and gastrointestinal tract problems are most common.

CENTRAL NERVOUS SYSTEM Carbamazepine can produce dizziness, vertigo, drowsiness, fatigue, ataxia, confusion, headache, nystagmus, and visual (diplopia) and speech disturbances. Activation of a latent psychosis, abnormal involuntary movements, depression, and peripheral neuritis occur rarely.

GASTROINTESTINAL Gastrointestinal side effects include nausea, vomiting, and gastric distress. Abdominal pain, diarrhea, constipation, and anorexia have also been noted. Taking carbamazepine with food can reduce its chance of producing nausea and vomiting.

HEMATOLOGIC Fatal blood dyscrasias, including aplastic anemia and agranulocytosis, have been reported related to carbamazepine therapy. It usually occurs within 4 months and has been reported in elderly patients taking carbamazepine for trigeminal neuralgia (may be caused by the higher doses used). Thrombocytopenia and leukopenia have also been reported. Because of the hematologic adverse effects, it is necessary to perform laboratory tests to follow these patients. Patients should be made aware of the symptoms of blood dyscrasias and warned to stop the drug and report any of the symptoms immediately. The dental team should observe the oral cavity of patients taking carbamazepine with these side effects in mind (look for petechiae or signs of infection).

DERMATOLOGIC Rashes, urticaria, photosensitivity reactions, and altered skin pigmentation can occur. Erythema multiforme, erythema nodosum, and aggravation of systemic lupus erythematosus have been reported. **Alopecia** can also occur.

ORAL Dry mouth, glossitis, and stomatitis can sometimes be seen in patients taking carbamazepine. A child who is taking chewable carbamazepine, often 4 times daily, will be exposed to a sugar for an extended period of time (sticks to teeth). The pediatric dosage form of carbamazepine contains 63% sugar in its chewable tablet. The mother should be questioned concerning the child's medication usage and the oral hygiene methods being used.

OTHER Cardiovascular side effects include congestive heart failure and alterations in blood pressure. Abnormal liver function tests and cholestatic jaundice have been reported. Urinary frequency and retention, oliguria, and impotence have been reported with carbamazepine use. Elevated blood urea nitrogen levels, albuminuria, and glycosuria have been seen. Lymphadenopathy, aching joints, and punctate lens opacities have occurred rarely.

Drug interactions. Carbamazepine has many drug interactions. Like many of the other anticonvulsants, it can induce liver microsomal enzymes, altering the metabolism of many drugs, including carbamazepine itself. Carbamazepine can decrease the effect of doxycycline, warfarin, theophylline, and oral contraceptives. Carbamazepine's effect may be increased by erythromycin, isoniazid, propoxyphene, and calcium channel blockers. The dental management of patients taking carbamazepine is discussed in Box 16-3.

VALPROATES

A group of anticonvulsant agents that are not structurally related to any other

> Valproate used—divalproex (Depakote)

anticonvulsants are the valproates, which include valproic [val-PRO-ik] acid, valproate [val-PRO-ate] sodium, and divalproex [dye-VAL-pro-ex] sodium. The term *valproate* is used here to refer to all of these agents. Divalproex sodium is a 1 to 1 ratio of valproic acid and valproate sodium. The mechanism of action of valproate may be its effect on sodium or potassium channels, a reduction in aspartate levels, or an increase in the inhibitory neurotransmitter, γ-aminobutyric acid (GABA) [evidence is mounting against this as the only mechanism].

Adverse reactions

GASTROINTESTINAL Indigestion, nausea, and vomiting are the most frequent adverse effects associated with valproate. These can be minimized by giving the drug with meals or increasing the dose very gradually. Divalproex sodium may have fewer adverse gastrointestinal effects than its components. Other gastrointestinal side effects include hypersalivation, anorexia, increased appetite, cramping, diarrhea, and constipation.

CENTRAL NERVOUS SYSTEM Sedation and drowsiness have been reported with valproate. Rarely, ataxia, headache, and nystagmus have been noted. Some children exhibit hyperactivity, aggression, and other behavioral disturbances. Weight gain and an increase in appetite have been reported.

HEPATOTOXICITY The idiosyncratic toxicity of valproate is hepatotoxicity. Dose-related changes in liver enzymes frequently occur in these patients. Deaths caused by hepatic failure have also been reported. Because valproic acid can produce serious hepatotoxicity, hepatic function tests should be performed.

BOX 16-3 DENTAL MANAGEMENT OF PATIENT TAKING CARBAMAZEPINE (TEGRETOL)

- Check for dry mouth, glossitis, and stomatitis
- Additive bleeding—use drugs that can alter coagulation cautiously
- Look for symptoms of blood dyscrasias
- Drug interactions—doxycycline (reduced doxycycline effect) and erythromycin (increased carbamazepine)
- Perform appropriate laboratory testing (if being prescribed by dentist for trigeminal neuralgia):
  Hematologic tests
  Ophthalmologic examination
  Complete urinalysis
  Liver function tests
- For a child using chewable carbamazepine tablets, the large amount of sugar could predispose the child to a higher caries rate—emphasize oral hygiene

Platelet aggregation inhibited

BLEEDING Valproate inhibits the second phase of platelet aggregation; therefore bleeding time may be prolonged. Thrombocytopenia, petechiae, bruising, and hematoma have been reported. Platelet counts, bleeding time, and coagulation studies should be performed before surgical procedures.

TERATOGENICITY Several reports suggest an association between the use of valproate in pregnant women and an increase in birth defects (particularly neural tube defects).

Drug interactions. Other drugs that are CNS depressants can have an additive CNS depressant effect when used with valproate. Valproate inhibits the metabolism of phenobarbital, producing excessive sedation. Valproate has also been associated with drug interactions with phenytoin—resulting in decreased action of valproate and increased phenytoin action. Because valproate can affect bleeding, other drugs that affect bleeding should be used cautiously. Box 16-4 summarizes the management of dental patients taking valproic acid.

PHENOBARBITAL

The most common barbiturate used in the treatment of epilepsy is phenobarbital [fee-noe-BAR-bi-tal]. The barbiturates are discussed in detail in Chapter 11. Primidone [PRYE-mih-done] (Mysoline) differs from phenobarbital by one functional group and mephobarbital [me-foe-BAR-bi-tal] (Mebaral) is metabolized to phenobarbital in the body, so both have actions similar to phenobarbital. Because these agents are similar in their action, phenobarbital is discussed as the prototype for this group.

Phenobarbital is used alone and in combination with other anticonvulsants such as phenytoin. It is used to treat tonic-clonic and partial seizure types (see Table 16-1). Other anticonvulsants are often used first.

The most common side effect associated with phenobarbital is sedation. With continued use, tolerance to the drowsiness but not the anticonvulsant effect often develops. In children, excitement and hyperactivity are often produced. The elderly sometimes exhibit confusion, excitement, or depression.

Skin reactions occur in 1% to 3% of patients. Rarely, exfoliative dermatitis, erythema multiforme, or Stevens-Johnson syndrome have been reported. Stomatitis may herald the onset of cutaneous reactions, some of which have been fatal. The barbiturates should be discontinued if any skin reactions occur.

PHENYTOIN

Because phenytoin [FEN-i-toyn] (Dilantin), formerly called *diphenylhydantoin (DPH)*, is the most commonly used hydantoin, it is discussed as the prototype for the hydantoin group. Because phenytoin is associated with gingival enlargement, the dental team plays an integral role in the management of these patients.

Phenytoin is used to treat both tonic-clonic and partial seizures with complex symptomatology. It is not useful in the treatment of pure absence seizures, but may be used in combination with other agents indicated for absence seizures to control combined seizure types. It has also been used to treat trigeminal neuralgia. In addition to its anticonvulsant properties,

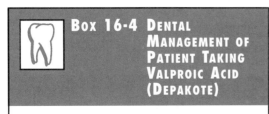

BOX 16-4 DENTAL MANAGEMENT OF PATIENT TAKING VALPROIC ACID (DEPAKOTE)

- Additive bleeding—use drugs that can alter coagulation cautiously
- Look for signs of hepatotoxicity

phenytoin has quinidine-like antiarrhythmic properties.

Adverse reactions The adverse reactions associated with phenytoin are frequent, affect many body systems, and may, rarely, be serious. Because of phenytoin's narrow therapeutic index, adverse reactions associated with elevated blood levels can occur. The chance for toxicity is also increased because phenytoin's metabolism is a saturable process. Phenytoin has a propensity for drug interactions because of its enzyme stimulating property.

GASTROINTESTINAL Gastrointestinal adverse reactions are not uncommon. Taking the medication with food can reduce these side effects. Other drugs with the potential for adverse gastrointestinal tract effects, such as NSAIAs or opioids, should be used carefully.

CENTRAL NERVOUS SYSTEM The CNS effects that can occur with phenytoin include mental confusion, nystagmus, ataxia, slurred speech, blurred vision, diplopia, amblyopia, dizziness, and insomnia. Because these effects are dose related, they can often be controlled by reducing the dose of phenytoin.

DERMATOLOGIC Skin reactions to phenytoin range from rash to, rarely, exfoliative dermatitis, lupus erythematosus, or Stevens-Johnson syndrome. Some patients experience irreversible hypertrichosis or hirsutism (excessive hairiness) on the trunk and face. This is one reason why alternative drugs are often selected, especially in the young female patient.

VITAMIN DEFICIENCY Deficiency produced by phenytoin may involve vitamin D and folate. Osteomalacia may result from phenytoin's interference with vitamin D metabolism. The first symptoms of folate deficiency may be oral mucosal changes such as ulcerations or glossitis. Treatment involves administering folic acid.

TERATOGENICITY/GROWTH *Fetal hydantoin syndrome* is the term given to the congenital abnormality associated with maternal ingestion of phenytoin. It includes craniofacial anomalies, microcephaly, nail/digit hypoplasia, limb defects, growth deficiency, and mental retardation. Thickening of facial structures and coarsening of facial features have been noted.

GINGIVAL ENLARGEMENT Another adverse reaction to phenytoin, gingival enlargement (previously referred to as *gingival hyperplasia*) occurs in approximately 50% of all chronic users. The name change is the result of an increased understanding of the nature of the enlargement. In about 30% of affected patients, gingival enlargement is severe enough to require surgical intervention.

> Gingival enlargement

Symptoms The clinical symptoms that occur with gingival enlargement may appear as little as a few weeks or as long as a few years after initial drug therapy. It often begins as a painless enlargement of the gingival margin. The gingiva is pink and does not bleed easily unless other factors are present. With time, the interproximal papillae become involved and finally coalesce to cover even the occlusal surfaces of the teeth. The hyperplasia is more commonly located in the anterior rather than the posterior surfaces, and the buccal rather than the lingual surfaces. The affected areas of the mouth in order of severity are the maxillary anterior facial, mandibular anterior facial, maxillary posterior facial, and mandibular posterior facial areas. In the affected patient, both normal and abnormal tissue may be found. Edentulous areas are rarely involved.

The better the patient's oral hygiene, the less likely the lesions are to occur or the less severe they will be if they do occur. Younger patients are more likely to experience this adverse reaction. Controversy exists on the contribution of dose and duration of therapy to the risk for the development of gingival enlargement.

Etiology The cause of phenytoin gingival enlargement is unknown. Many causes have been investigated, including alteration in the function of the adrenal gland, hypersensitivity or allergic reaction, immunologic reaction, and vitamin C or folate deficiency. Because it is known that phenytoin may be found in the saliva, some investigators suggest a local etiology.

Management The management of phenytoin-induced gingival enlargement requires consultation between dental personnel and the patient's physician. Some possible alternatives are as follows:

- *Alter the drug.* Choosing another effective antiepileptic drug is one method of handling the gingival enlargement produced by phenytoin.
- *Use.* Ethotoin [ETH-oh-toyn]. Another hydantoin, related to phenytoin, has traditionally been said to have less seizure control efficacy, but other authors attribute this reduced efficacy to inadequate doses. [Translation: We don't know.] Some patients with gingival enlargement from phenytoin have experienced a regression in the gum hypertrophy when ethotoin was substituted for phenytoin.
- *Discontinue phenytoin.* Patients who have discontinued phenytoin will experience a decrease in gingival enlargement over a 1-year period. Surgical intervention should wait until at least 18 months after cessation of therapy because some patients experience additional reduction in the enlargement after the 1-year period.
- *Improve oral hygiene.* Scrupulous oral hygiene may delay the onset or reduce the rate of formation of enlargement. Avoiding irritating restorations may also reduce enlargement. Even with ideal oral hygiene,

enlargement is not always totally preventable, and once it has formed is not easily reversed.

- *Gingivectomy.* When gingival enlargement interferes with plaque control, esthetics, or mastication and when oral hygiene has not been successful in controlling enlargement, surgical elimination is indicated. It is not a permanent solution because if the patient continues on phenytoin, enlargement quickly returns in most cases and can progress to the presurgical level in a short period.
- *Other drugs.* Although many types of drugs, such as diuretics, corticosteroids, mouthwashes, vitamin C, folic acid, and antihistamines, have been tried in the treatment of this condition, none has been shown to be effective in controlled trials.

Box 16-5 summarizes the management of dental patients taking phenytoin.

MISCELLANEOUS ANTICONVULSANT AGENTS

Ethosuximide. The drug of choice for the treatment of absence seizures (see Table 16-1) is ethosuximide [eth-oh-SUX-i-mide] (Zarontin). Its mechanism of action may involve inhibiting the T-type calcium channels. It is ineffective in partial seizures with complex symptoms or

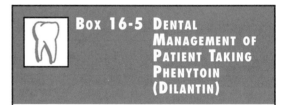

BOX 16-5 DENTAL MANAGEMENT OF PATIENT TAKING PHENYTOIN (DILANTIN)

- If patient has nausea, avoid drugs that are gastric irritants
- Monitor for gingival enlargement
- Provide extensive oral hygiene instruction
- Schedule more frequent oral prophylaxis

in tonic-clonic seizures. In the treatment of mixed seizures, agents effective against tonic-clonic seizures must be used in addition to ethosuximide.

Gastrointestinal adverse effects include anorexia, gastric upset, cramps, pain, diarrhea, and nausea and vomiting. CNS adverse effects include drowsiness, hyperactivity, headache, and hiccups. Ethosuximide has been associated with blood dyscrasias, a positive direct Coombs' test, systemic lupus erythematosus, Stevens-Johnson syndrome, and hirsutism. Oral effects reported with ethosuximide include gingival enlargement and swelling of the tongue.

Benzodiazepines. Benzodiazepines such as clonazepam [kloe-NA-ze-pam] (Klonopin) and clorazepate [klor-AZ-e-pate] (Tranxene) are used orally as anticonvulsant adjuvants. Diazepam (Valium), lorazepam (Ativan), and midazolam (Versed) are used parenterally to treat recurrent tonic-clonic seizures or status epilepticus.

Clonazepam is used as an adjunct to treat absence seizures not responsive to ethosuximide. Drowsiness and ataxia occur frequently. Behavioral disturbances and adverse neurologic effects can occur. Other side effects reported relate to the gastrointestinal tract and to the dermatologic and hematologic systems. Oral manifestations include increased salivation, coated tongue, dry mouth, and sore gums. It is also used as an adjunct in the treatment of certain mental illnesses.

NEW ANTICONVULSANT AGENTS

The newer anticonvulsants are listed in Table 16-2. Because gabapentin is gaining in popularity, it is discussed separately.

Felbamate [fel-BA-mate] (Felbatol) is a newer anticonvulsant that has been associated with serious toxicities. Aplastic anemia and acute hepatic failure have been reported. This agent should be reserved for use only if the seizures are refractory to other anticonvulsant agents.

Gabapentin. *Gabapentin* [GA-ba-pen-tin] (Neurontin), an analog of GABA, is effective as an adjunct against partial and generalized tonic-clonic seizures. Its mechanism of action is unknown, but it is not a GABA agonist. Like other anticonvulsants, it can cause CNS effects such as somnolence, dizziness, tremor, and ataxia. Gastric complaints include dyspepsia, nausea, and vomiting. It can increase the blood pressure and produce edema. There is an increase in rhinitis, pharyngitis, and cough. Ophthalmic adverse reactions include diplopia (6%) and amblyopia (4%). Myalgia and back pain have been reported. Hypersensitivity reactions have included skin rash and pruritus. Oral manifestations of gabapentin include mucositis, hiccups, and nasal obstruction.

One major advantage of gabapentin over the other anticonvulsant agents is that it is not metabolized. Because it does not affect the hepatic microsomal enzymes, it lacks of significant drug interactions, which gives it a distinct advantage over the other anticonvulsants.

DENTAL TREATMENT OF THE PATIENT WITH EPILEPSY

The dental team should not treat a patient who has a history of seizure disorders without reviewing the management of the patient with epilepsy, including the procedures for handling a patient experiencing tonic-clonic seizures. Preventive measures include a detailed seizure history, treatment planning to avoid excessive stress and missed medications, and education of the entire dental office staff. The management of the patient experiencing tonic-clonic seizures should include moving the patient to the floor if possible, tilting the patient's head to one side to prevent aspiration, and removing objects from the patient's mouth before the seizure to prevent fractured teeth. The use of tongue blades is not recommended because the blades may split and produce additional trauma in the oral cavity.

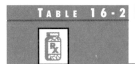

TABLE 16-2	**Newer Anticonvulsants**		
DRUG	MECHANISM	INDICATIONS	ADVERSE REACTIONS
Gabapentin (Neurontin)	GABA analogue, but does not interact with GABA receptor	Partial/generalized tonic-clonic seizures	Somnolence, dizziness, tremor, ataxia; good effect; may increase norethindrone level not metabolized and does not affect liver enzymes, antacids reduce effect, cimetidine increase
Topiramate (Topamax)	Blocks Na channels, potentiates GABA at different site from other drugs	Partial/generalized tonic-clonic seizures	No effect on metabolism, some DI, BCP less effective
Tiagabine (Gabitril)	Inhibitor or GABA uptake	Adjunct, partial seizures	Dizziness, nervousness, tremor, depression; rash idiosyncratic
Lamotrigine (Lamictal)	Inactivates sodium channels	Partial/secondary generalized seizures; adjunct or monotherapy for several types of convulsions	Dizziness, headache, nausea, somnolence, diplopia, headache; rash/hypersensitivity [? GE]
Vigabatrin (γ-vinyl GABA) (Sabril)	Irreversible inhibitor of GABA aminotransferase (enzyme that destroys (GABA)	Partial seizures	Agitation, confusion, psychosis
Felbamate (Felbatol)	Antagonist to glycine (stimulant neurotransmitter)	Adjunct for partial seizures	Bone marrow depression (agranulocytosis, aplastic anemia), severe hepatitis, monitor LFTs, third-line drug
Fosphenytoin (Cerebyx)	Stabilizes neuronal membranes	Acute seizures	Parenteral use

BCP, Birth control pill; *DI,* drug interaction; *GE,* gingival enlargement; *LFTs,* liver function tests.

NONSEIZURE USES OF ANTICONVULSANTS

Neurologic pain. Several anticonvulsants are used to manage chronic pain syndromes. An example is carbamazepine, which is used to treat trigeminal neuralgia and atypical facial pain. Phenytoin has also been used to treat neurologic pain. Valproic acid has been used for **migraine headache** prophylaxis.

Psychiatric use. Carbamazepine, valproic acid, clonazepam, and gabapentin have been used in the treatment of certain mental disorders (see Chapter 17). They are sometimes called "mood stabilizers" in this context. They can be used to "level out," or stabilize, the mood in patients with **bipolar disorder.** Thus a patient taking an anticonvulsant drug may or may not have a seizure disorder.

> Anticonvulsants for bipolar disorder

REVIEW QUESTIONS

1. Briefly describe the most common seizure types, including the following:
   a. grand mal (tonic-clonic)

b. absence (petit mal)

c. status epilepticus

2. State the general measures with which the dental team should be familiar before treating a patient with epilepsy.

3. Explain the major adverse reactions associated with these anticonvulsants:

a. phenytoin

b. phenobarbital

c. carbamazepine

d. valproic acid

e. gabapentin

4. Describe a few major adverse reactions caused by the less frequently used anticonvulsants.

5. Discuss the gingival enlargement associated with phenytoin, including its incidence, cause, minimization, and treatment. Explain the dental team's essential role in preventing and treating this condition.

6. Describe a dental-related use of carbamazepine and name what laboratory test monitoring is involved.

7. Enumerate the adverse reactions associated with many anticonvulsants. State how to minimize these with patients with epilepsy who are taking several medications.

8. Explain uses of the anticonvulsants for conditions other than seizures.

Psychotherapeutic Agents

Many drugs have the ability to affect mental activity. Some of these drugs are used in the treatment of psychiatric disorders. The dental health care worker is most likely to encounter the use of these agents in dental patients who have had them prescribed by psychiatrists or other physicians. Because these agents are so widely prescribed and can alter the patient's dental treatment, the dental health care worker must understand their pharmacologic effects, adverse reactions, and dental implications.

Agents used in the treatment of the major psychiatric disorders are discussed in this chapter. Those used to treat anxiety are discussed in Chapter 11. The anticonvulsants used as "mood stabilizers" are discussed in Chapter 16.

Because the psychotherapeutic drugs are classified by their therapeutic use, a brief discussion of the common psychiatric illnesses follows.

PSYCHIATRIC DISORDERS

There are many psychiatric disorders. They may be divided into types such as organic and functional or primary and secondary, depending on their suspected cause. Organic illness is congenital or caused by an injury or a disease. Functional disorders are partially of psychogenic origin, without evidence (yet) of structural or biochemical abnormality (Figure 17-1). The naming and categorization of different mental disorders changes as more information becomes available. Functional disorders include the following categories:

- Psychoses
- Affective disorder
- Neuroses (anxiety)

The psychoses are discussed first. Schizophrenia, the most common type of psychosis, is an extensive disturbance of the patient's personality function with a loss of perception of reality. Schizophrenia is derived from the word meaning "splitting," and in context it refers to patients splitting from reality (not into multiple personalities). The patient's ability to function in society is impaired because of altered thinking. The impaired thinking of these patients may be so detached from reality and their delusions or paranoia (e.g., someone is out to get me) so severe that their illness could lead committing of serious crimes, including assassination attempts or murders. Patients may suffer from hallucinations, delusions, or agitation. The positive symptoms of psychosis include agitation, extrapyramidal symptoms, and auditory hallucinations. Other patients may be introspective and uninvolved. The negative ef-

> Loss of reality

F I G U R E   1 7 · 1   *Classification of common mental illnesses.*

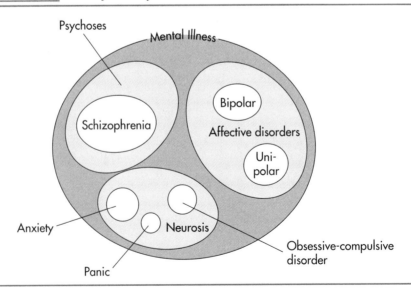

fects of psychosis include flat affect and apathy (Box 17-1).

The etiology of schizophrenia is not specifically known, but a familial pattern is often seen. The biochemical actions of the brain and even brain anatomy have been demonstrated to be different from findings in normal individuals in some patients with schizophrenia.

Affective disorders include endogenous and exogenous unipolar depression and bipolar depression **(mania).** The condition in patients who exhibit only depression is termed *unipolar depression.* Endogenous (involutional) depression seems to be unrelated to external events, whereas exogenous (reactive) depression appears to be related to specific external events. Whether there are actually two types of depression separated by circumstances of occurrence is

questionable. Theories for several different types of depression based on the biochemical situation in the brain have been hypothesized, but no one has been able to show different groups. Patients who exhibit alternating periods of depression and excitation (mania, elation) have bipolar (*bi*, two) depression.

Neuroses are less severe than psychoses but can also be helped by drug therapy. Examples include anxiety, panic disorder, **phobias,** and obsessive-compulsive disorder. Psychophysiologic (somatic) disorders are those that have an emotional origin but manifest by physiologic symptoms. Personality disorders include sexual deviation, alcoholism, and drug dependence. Although many of these conditions are managed using the antidepressants and/or antipsychotics, the anxiety-related problems sometimes require the use of the benzodiazepines. The most common benzodiazepine used for psychiatric conditions is clonazepam. Divisions of these different mental disorders have been and are continually changing to reflect either an increased knowledge or a political or "fad" perspective. [What is "normal" anyway?]

This presentation is an oversimplification of the classifications of psychiatric disorders. The drug groups discussed in this chapter include antipsychotic agents, used to treat psychoses; antidepressant agents, used to treat affective disorders; and lithium, used to treat bipolar disorder. The minor tranquilizers, used to manage various neuroses, are discussed in Chapter 11.

Before the antipsychotic drugs were introduced into the management of psychiatric disorders, many physical methods were employed to treat patients. Only electroconvulsive therapy (ECT, shock therapy) is still used in the treatment of depression. With the use of neuromuscular blocking agents, the use of ECT therapy has become much safer. ECT produces the fastest results of any treatment for depression. It is reserved for patients who are refractive to anti-

---

Box 17-1 SYMPTOMS OF PSYCHOSES

Positive

Hallucinations, auditory
Delusions
Unwanted thoughts
Disorganized behavior
Agitation
Distorted speech, communication

Negative

Flat affect
Unemotional
Apathetic, passivity
Abstract thinking difficult
Spontaneity and goals lacking
Thought and speech impaired
Lack of pleasure
Social withdrawal

depressants. Some memory loss occurs during the treatment (several sessions).

When treating patients with mental disorders, the following general precautions should be observed by the dental health care worker:

> **Watch verbal interaction with patient**

- *Communication.* Patients with various mental disorders may perceive comments or movement from dental health care workers as threatening. Even normal office discussions may be perceived differently than they are intended. For example, small talk with a peer may be interpreted as a conspiracy by the patient. What you say around and to the patient should be carefully monitored. [I once asked a patient "How are you?" and the patient replied with a loud and angry voice, **"Why are you asking me that question!"**]

- *Compliance.* Patients undergoing drug therapy for the treatment of psychoses often do not take their medication as prescribed. A thorough health history including the patient's medication and its dosage should be obtained.

- *Suicide.* Depressed patients may attempt suicide. Therefore the amount of any drug prescribed at one time should not exceed the amount required for a lethal dose (usually a 1-week supply). When patients are severely depressed they have no motivation and usually do not act on any irrational thoughts of suicide. After beginning to take an antidepressant, partial improvement gives them the motivation to attempt suicide before the full antidepressant effects have developed. In a suicide attempt, drugs are often combined. For example, a patient may mix an opioid analgesic given for the relief of a toothache, a sedative-hypnotic prescribed for dental anxiety, and an antidepressant medication prescribed by the patient's physician.

ANTIPSYCHOTIC AGENTS

The antipsychotic agents are divided into several classes depending on their chemical structure. Until the last few years, the phenothiazines [FEE-noe-THYE-a-zeens] were the most frequently used group of antipsychotics. Table 17-1 lists some phenothiazines and other agents with antipsychotic action and their usual adult daily dose for **outpatient treatment.** More patients are now being treated with the newer antipsychotics referred to as the "atypical" antipsychotics.

The atypical antipsychotics—so named because they were unlike the phenothiazines—have different receptor activities and adverse reaction profiles. As a group, these agents have more nausea and less anticholinergic and sedative effects than occur with the traditional antidepressants.

The actions of the antipsychotic agents are diverse. Of the older antipsychotics, no single agent is clearly superior in its antipsychotic action. But, with the advent of the "atypical" antipsychotics, patients who were previously resistant to typical antipsychotic agents have been adequately managed with these new drugs. Antipsychotics that act on several receptors have a broader range of action and can be used in more difficult cases. Clinical judgment and the drug's side effect profile in a particular patient determine which agent is used. In general, the lower-potency agents such as chlorpromazine [klor-PROE-ma-zeen] (Thorazine) have more sedation, more peripheral side effects, and more autonomic effects (e.g., dry mouth), whereas the higher-potency agents such as haloperidol [ha-loe-PER-i-dol] have more extrapyramidal effects and less sedation. Other common phenothiazines include thioridazine [thye-oh-RID-a-zeen] (Mellaril) and trifluoperazine [trye-floo-oh-PAIR-a-zeen] (Stelazine). Because the phenothiazines have been the most frequently used antipsychotic agents, they are discussed as the prototype. Most nonphenothiazine antipsychotic agents have effects similar to that of the

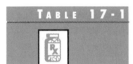

TABLE 17-1 Antipsychotic Agents

DRUG GROUP	DRUG NAME GENERIC (TRADE)	EQ DOSE (MG)*	DAILY DOSE (MG)†	SIDE EFFECTS‡			
				SED	EP	AC	OH
PHENOTHIAZINES							
Aliphatic	Chlorpromazine (Thorazine)	100	30-800	3	2	2	3
	Promazine (Sparine)	200	40-1200	2	2	3	2
	Triflupromazine (Vesprin)	25	60-150	3	2	3	2
Piperozine	Trifluoperazine (Stelazine)	5	2-40	1	3	1	1
	Prochlorperazine (Compazine)	15	15-150	2	3	1	1
	Perphenazine (Trilafon)	10	12-64	2	2	1	1
	Fluphenazine (Prolixin)	2	0.5-40	1	3	1	1
	Acetophenazine (Tindal)	20	60-120	2	3	1	1
Piperidine	Thioridazine (Mellaril)	100	150-800	3	1	3	3
	Mesoridazine (Serentil)	50	30-400	3	1	3	2
OTHERS							
	Haloperidol (Haldol)	2	1-15	1	3	1	1
	Thiothixene (Navane)	4	8-30	1	3	1	2
	Chlorprothixene (Taractan)	100	75-600	3	2	2	2
	Molindone (Moban)	10	15-225	2	2	1	1
	Loxapine (Loxitane)	15	20-250	1	2	1	1
	Clozapine (Clozaril)§	50	300-900	3	1	3	2
	Pimozide (Orap)‖	0.3-0.5	1-10	2	3	2	1
ATYPICAL ANTIPSYCHOTICS							
	Risperidone (Risperdal)		4-16	1	1-2	0	1
	Olanzapine (Zyprexa)		5-20	3	1	3	2
	Quetiapine (Seroquel)		50-800	2	1	0	2
	Sertindole (Serlect)		4-24	½	½	½	1

*Equivalent dose (to other agents).
†Usual oral dosage range for outpatient treatment in milligrams; inpatient treatment uses higher doses.
‡*Sed*, Sedation; *EP*, extrapyramidal; *AC*, anticholinergic; *OH*, orthostatic hypotension.
§Agranulocytosis, weekly WBC lab needed.
‖Only for severe tics associated with Tourette's disorder unresponsive to standard treatment.

phenothiazines. Newer "atypical" antipsychotic agents have quite different adverse reaction profiles.

PHARMACOLOGIC EFFECTS

Phenothiazines. When phenothiazines are used for treatment of psychoses, any effects other than the antipsychotic effect could be considered an adverse reaction. When used as an antiemetic, other actions would be adverse reactions, such as sedation. The pharmacologic effects of the antipsychotic agents include the following.

ANTIPSYCHOTIC All phenothiazines possess antipsychotic effects associated with slowing of the psychomotor activity in an agitated patient and calming of emotion with suppression of hallucinations and delusions. These agents are active against the positive effects of psychosis, but have little effect on the negative effects. Newer agents differ in that they are effective against both the positive and negative symptoms of schizophrenia. There is also a lack of response without a loss of intellectual function.

ANTIEMETIC The phenothiazines' antiemetic effect is due to depression of the chemoreceptor trigger zone, an area in the brain that causes nausea and vomiting. These agents are very useful in the symptomatic treatment of certain types of nausea and vomiting. Historically, prochlorperazine (Compazine) has been the phenothiazine used for this effect.

POTENTIATION OF OPIOIDS When phenothiazines are combined with central nervous system (CNS) depressants, such as opioids, they potentiate the action of the depressants. When phenothiazines are added to opioids, the dose of the opioid used should be decreased by half.

Atypical antipsychotic agents. There are several differences between the older antipsychotic agents and the newest, or atypical, antipsychotic agents. The older antipsychotic agents were pri-

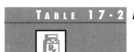

TABLE 17-2 Antidepressants

Drug Name Generic (Trade)	Dose[a] Range (mg)	$t_{1/2}$ (hr)	Side Effects AC[b]	Sed[c]	OH[d]	Wt+[e]	N, D[f]	Blocks Reuptake NE[g]	Sert[h]
TRICYCLIC—TERTIARY AMINES									
Amitriptyline (Elavil)	50-300	31-46	4	4	2	4	0	2	4
Clomipramine (Anafranil)[i]	25-250	19-37	3	3	2	4	1	2	5
Doxepin (Adapin, Sinequan)	25-300	8-24	2	3	2	4	0	1	2
Imipramine (Tofranil)	30-300	11-25	2	2	3	4	1	2	4
Trimipramine (Surmontil)	50-300	7-30	2	3	2	4	0	1	1
TRICYCLIC—SECONDARY AMINES									
Amoxapine (Asendin)	50-600	8	3	2	1	2	0	3	2
Desipramine (Norpramin, Pertofrane)	25-300	12-24	1	1	1	1	0	3	2
Nortriptyline (Pamelor, Aventyl)	50-150	18-44	2	2	1	1	0	2	3
Protriptyline (Vivactil)	15-60	67-89	3	1	1	0	0	4	2
SEROTONIN-SPECIFIC REUPTAKE INHIBITORS (SSRI)									
Fluoxetine (Prozac)	20-80	1-16 days	0-1	0-1	0-1	0	3	0-1	5
Sertraline (Zoloft)	50-200	1-4	0	0-1	0	0	3	0-1	5
Paroxetine (Paxil)	10-50	10-24	0	0-1	0	1	3	0-1	5
Citalopram (Celexa)	20-60	33	0	0	0	3	0	0	5
OTHERS									
Trazodone (Desyrel)	50-600	4-9	1	4	2	2	1	0	3
Bupropion (Wellbutrin)	200-450	8-24	2	2	1	0	1	0-1	0-1
Maprotiline (Ludiomil)	50-225	21-25	2	2	1	2	0	3	0-1
ATYPICAL 3RD/4TH GENERATION									
Mirtazapine[j] (Remeron)	15-45	20-40	2	3	2	0	3	3	3
Venlafaxine (Effexor)[k]	75-225	5-11	1	0	0	0	3	3	3
Nefazodone (Serzone)[l]	200-600	2-4	1	2	1	0	1	0-1	3
Fluvoxamine (Luvox)[l]	50-300	15.5	0-1	0-1	0	1	3	0-1	5

[a]Usual adult daily dose (mg).
[b]*AC*, Anticholinergic.
[c]*Sed*, Sedation.
[d]*OH*, Orthostatic hypotension.
[e]*Wt+*, Weight gain.
[f]*N, D*, Nausea and diarrhea.

[g]*NE*, Norepinephrine reuptake inhibitors.
[h]*Sert*, Serotonin reuptake inhibitors.
[i]Used for OCD.
[j]Antagonizes α_2-adrenergic receptors.
[k]In divided doses.
[l]Used primarily for OCD.

marily dopamine antagonists. The atypical agents have action at more than one receptor, for example, the dopamine, serotonin, and norepinephrine receptors, which results in the improved efficacy of these agents. The side effects of the atypical antipsychotics are less than the older antipsychotics. Like the other phenothiazines, the atypical antipsychotics are effective against the positive effects associated with psychoses. But, unlike the older antipsychotics, the atypical antipsychotic agents are effective against the negative effects. Table 17-1 lists the common antipsychotic agents and some atypical antipsychotic agents.

ADVERSE REACTIONS

Table 17-1 lists the side effects of the older antipsychotic agents, and Figure 17-2 demonstrates the relative side effects of several antipsychotic agents. Management of patients taking these agents involves minimizing the troubling side effects in each patient.

Sedation. Phenothiazines differ in the degree of sedation and drowsiness they produce. The degree of sedation is one factor that determines which antipsychotic agent is prescribed. In contrast to the sedative-hypnotic agents, with higher doses the phenothiazines do not produce

anesthesia and the patient is easily aroused. Tolerance develops to the sedative effect but not to the antipsychotic effect.

Extrapyramidal effects. The most common type of adverse reactions associated with these agents results from stimulation of the extrapyramidal system. All phenothiazines produce this effect, although the incidence of the reaction varies. The following types of extrapyramidal effects can occur:

- Acute dystonia consisting of muscle spasms of the face, tongue, neck, and back
- Parkinsonism with symptoms of resting tremor, rigidity, and akinesia
- Akathisia, or increased, compulsive motor activity
- Tardive dyskinesia, an irreversible dyskinesia involving the tongue, lips, face, and jaw.

Tardive dyskinesia is typically seen in women patients who are more than 40 years old and have been taking large doses of the phenothiazines for a minimum of 6 months to 2 years or as long as 20 years. The onset is gradual and the movements are coordinated and rhythmic. This effect is exacerbated by drug withdrawal. The involuntary movements, especially those involving the face, jaw, and tongue, can make home care difficult if not impossible. Performing oral

FIGURE 17-2 *Comparison of selected antipsychotic adverse reactions.*

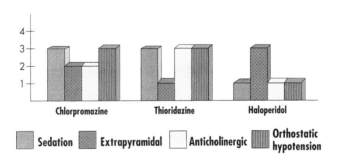

prophylaxis is difficult because of the strength of the oral facial and tongue muscles.

The dental health care worker should discuss the patient's side effects with his or her physician if oral prophylaxis cannot be performed. A dosage or drug change may be instituted by the patient's psychiatrist. With the availability of the atypical agents, extrapyramidal side effects can be greatly minimized.

The extrapyramidal side effects of phenothiazines can cause severe intermittent pain in the region of the temporomandibular joint (TMJ). This pain is produced by a spasm of the muscles of mastication. In an acute attack it becomes difficult or impossible to open or close the jaw. Should muscle spasm be present, force should not be exerted to open the patient's mouth for dental treatment because dislocations of the **mandible** can occur.

Treatment of an acute spasm of the mandible must be undertaken after consultation with the patient's prescribing physician. Alternatives may include decreasing the dose of the patient's medication, adding an anticholinergic medication to counteract the spasm, or changing the patient's antipsychotic medication to one that produces fewer extrapyramidal effects. The anticholinergics used to counteract the extrapyramidal side effects of the antipsychotics include benztropine (Cogentin) and trihexyphenidyl (Artane).

Orthostatic hypotension. Because these agents depress the central sympathetic outflow and block the peripheral adrenergic receptors (α-sympathetic blockers) they can produce orthostatic hypotension that is additive with other CNS depressants. When a patient rises rapidly from the supine position, a compensatory tachycardia can accompany the orthostatic hypotension.

Seizures. Because phenothiazines lower the convulsion threshold, seizures may be more easily precipitated in a patient taking these agents, especially if a previous history of epilepsy exists.

Bupropion (Zyban) can produce seizures, and therefore patients on phenothiazines may not be candidates for its use. Consultation with the patient's psychiatrist would be warranted.

Anticholinergic effects. The anticholinergic effects of phenothiazines produce blurred vision, xerostomia, and constipation. This is especially significant because the anticholinergic effects of other medications the patient may be taking are additive. The anticholinergics, such as benztropine, used to treat the extrapyramidal symptoms are additive, too. The dental health care worker should be aware of the presence of xerostomia and question patients regarding their method of managing this problem.

> Xerostomia with older antipsychotics

Other effects. As previously mentioned, phenothiazines have many adverse effects, including blood dyscrasias, cholestatic jaundice, skin eruptions, and photosensitivity reactions that are exaggerated by sunlight or even by the light from the dental unit.

Agranulocytosis. An antipsychotic unrelated to the others, clozapine [KLOE-za-peen] (Clozaril), is very useful to improve certain patients with refractory schizophrenia. Because it produces potentially life-threatening agranulocytosis, clozapine should be tried only after several trials of other agents have failed. Frequent white blood cell counts with differential are required during therapy. With the release of new atypical antipsychotic agents, use of this agent becomes less needed.

DRUG INTERACTIONS

Central nervous system depressants. Phenothiazines interact in an additive or even potentiating fashion with all CNS depressants, including barbiturates, alcohol, general anesthetics, and opioid analgesics. Sedation and respiratory depression can occur.

Epinephrine. Epinephrine, used as a vasoconstrictor in local anesthetic solutions, can be safely used in patients taking phenothiazines. But, because the phenothiazine agents are α-adrenergic blockers, epinephrine should not be used to treat vasomotor collapse (acute drop in blood pressure) because it could cause a further decrease in blood pressure. This occurs because of the predominant β-agonist (vasodilating) activity of epinephrine in the presence of the phenothiazines (α-blockers). However, using epinephrine-containing local anesthetics in patients taking antipsychotics is acceptable in dentistry.

Anticholinergic agents. To control excessive extrapyramidal stimulation, phenothiazine therapy often must be combined with antiparkinson medication of the anticholinergic type, for example, benztropine (Cogentin). This combination is bound to exacerbate antimuscarinic peripheral effects such as xerostomia, urinary retention, bowel paralysis, and inhibition of sweating.

Uses

Antipsychotic effects. Antipsychotics are the drugs of choice for treatment of schizophrenia. Long-acting injectable phenothiazines, such as fluphenazine (Prolixin), are available for patients with schizophrenia who fail to take their oral medication.

Antiemetic effects. Because phenothiazines prevent or inhibit vomiting, they are useful in the treatment of some types of nausea and vomiting. The drug prochlorperazine [proe-klor-PAIR-a-zeen] (Compazine) has traditionally been used.

Other. Intractable hiccups and certain drug withdrawals have been successfully treated with phenothiazines. Use of these agents as chemical restraints in nursing homes is unethical.

DENTAL IMPLICATIONS

The dental management of patients taking antipsychotics is summarized in Box 17-2.

Sedation. Sedation, an adverse reaction of the phenothiazines, is additive with that of other sedating agents.

Anticholinergic effects. Phenothiazines are additive with other agents with atropine-like effects; this combination can lead to toxic reactions, including tachycardia, urinary retention, blurred vision, constipation, and xerostomia. The dental health care worker should be aware that patients may use sugar-containing candy to counteract xerostomia. Use of sugarless products or artificial saliva (Orex, Xero-Lube, Moi-Stir) should be encouraged.

Orthostatic hypotension. Orthostatic hypotension effect can be minimized by raising the dental

---

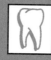

BOX 17-2 MANAGEMENT OF THE DENTAL PATIENT TAKING ANTIPSYCHOTIC AGENTS

- Use caution with patient interactions (patient may misinterpret your verbal or nonverbal actions).
- Check for xerostomia and its management.
- Emphasize oral hygiene instruction.
- Extrapyramidal dyskinesia may make oral hygiene more difficult.
- Check the TMJ for extrapyramidal side effects (mouth may be difficult to open, do not force).
- Sedation is additive with other agents with sedative effects.
- Epinephrine can be safely used in a dental local anesthetic.
- Encourage patient to rise slowly from the dental chair to minimize orthostatic hypotension.
- Disease may cause difficulty in following an oral care program (depends on disease severity).

chair slowly and assisting the patient's first few steps.

> Can use epinephrine with antipsychotics

Epinephrine. Epinephrine should be avoided in the management of an acute hypotensive crisis in patients taking antipsychotics. It may be safely used in local anesthetic solutions for dental patients.

Temporomandibular joint pain. As a result of the phenothiazines' extrapyramidal effects, the muscles of mastication may be in spasm.

Tardive dyskinesia. Tardive dyskinesia is irreversible and should be reported to the patient's physician.

Other antipsychotic drugs. The other older antipsychotic drugs have essentially the same pharmacologic effects, adverse reactions, and dental implications as the phenothiazines. They differ only in the relative degree of these effects. In general, an inverse relationship exists between the sedative and extrapyramidal effects. The antipsychotics that have low potency (require higher doses) tend to be more sedating. For example, haloperidol has more extrapyramidal side effects but less sedative effect than chlorpromazine (Figure 17-3).

ANTIDEPRESSANT AGENTS

Antidepressant agents are used not only to manage depression but also for a variety of other uses such as chronic pain adjuvant or migraine headache prophylaxis. Question the patient to determine the indication for which a tricyclic antidepressant is being prescribed. Do not assume that the patient is being treated for depression. Until the late 1950s, there was no widely accepted pharmacologic treatment for depression. Forms of mild depression were treated with psychotherapy, and severe depression was treated with ECT. Several classes of antidepressants are currently available, including tricyclic antidepressants (TCAs) and serotonin-specific reuptake inhibitors (SSRIs). Several new, atypical antidepressants, some with unique properties, have been recently released. ECT is still used in the treatment of severely suicidal patients and those resistant to antidepressants. In the case of suicidal thoughts, ECT works faster than any antidepressant drug.

The antidepressants may block norepinephrine (NE) and/or serotonin (5-HT) reuptake (see Table 17-2), produce sedation, and have anticholinergic side effects. One theory of their mechanism of action involves blocking reuptake of NE and/or 5-HT. Another involves down-regulation of the β-adrenergic receptors.

TRICYCLIC ANTIDEPRESSANTS

The TCAs are structurally similar to the phenothiazines. They are sometimes referred to as the *first-generation antidepressants* because they

F IGURE 1 7 - 3 *Relationship among potency, dose, and side effects of antipsychotic agents.*

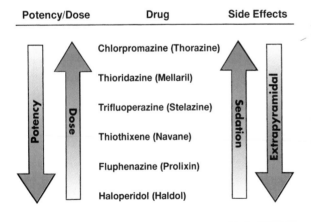

were developed and marketed before the second-generation agents. Table 17-2 lists the antidepressants with their usual adult outpatient daily dose in milligrams. All older TCAs are similar in their antidepressant effectiveness, differing only in their side effect profile.

Pharmacologic effects. The action of TCAs on normal and depressed patients is somewhat different. In the normal patient, an undesirable sedation and fatigue and strong atropine-like side effects are noted. In the depressed patient, a feeling of well-being, elevation of mood, and a dulling of depressive ideation are noted. Sedation occurs frequently, but tolerance to this effect often develops. Increased ability to concentrate and improvement in sleep is seen with the TCAs. Their antidepressant action can take up to 1 month to 3 to 6 weeks to maximize.

Adverse reactions. Some of the widely diverse adverse reactions associated with the tricyclic antidepressants resemble those of the antipsychotic agents (see Table 17-2, Figure 17-4).

CENTRAL NERVOUS SYSTEM Almost all of the TCAs induce some degree of sedation, and some of them can produce **tremors.** The latter effect is not caused by extrapyramidal stimulation and therefore does not respond to antiparkinsonian medication. It consists of a fine tremor in the upper extremities (arms or hands) and occurs in at least 10% of the patients treated with these drugs.

AUTONOMIC NERVOUS SYSTEM The peripheral effects of TCAs are primarily on the autonomic nervous system. These agents possess distinct anticholinergic effects resulting in xerostomia, blurred vision, tachycardia, constipation, and urinary retention. Some tolerance can develop with continued use. Although TCAs initially produce orthostatic hypotension like the phenothiazines, tolerance to this effect occurs.

TCAs = xerostomia

CARDIAC The most serious peripheral side effect associated with the TCAs is cardiac toxicity. Myocardial infarction and congestive heart failure have occurred during the course of treatment. Arrhythmias and episodes of tachycardia can be caused by the antimuscarinic (anticholinergic, atropine-like) effects of the TCAs. New antidepressants do not cause this reaction.

DEPENDENCE OR WITHDRAWAL Rarely, TCAs have been found to produce psychic or physical dependence. Slight withdrawal effects

FIGURE 17-4 *Relative side effects of antidepressants.*

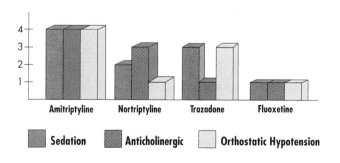

after abrupt discontinuation have been reported. Tolerance develops to many of the side effects, although not to the antidepressant effect.

Drug interactions. Unlike phenothiazines, TCAs potentiate the behavioral actions of the amphetamines and other CNS stimulants. TCAs potentiate the pressor effect of injected sympathomimetics. These agents also interact with monoamine oxidase inhibitors, resulting in severe toxic reactions. TCAs may be displaced from plasma protein–binding sites by phenytoin. TCAs may be metabolized more quickly because of induction of hepatic microsomal enzymes by barbiturates, carbamazepine, and cigarette smoking. They may interfere with the antihypertensive effects of guanethidine and clonidine. Additive anticholinergic effects are seen if they are administered with other agents with anticholinergic action.

Poisoning. Accidental poisoning with TCAs has become more common, and such an overdose can be lethal. The effects of acute poisoning are severe hypertension, cardiac arrhythmias, hyperpyrexia, convulsions, coma, and respiratory failure. Survivors may have permanent myocardial damage. The treatment is symptomatic and should be conservative in view of the interactions with other CNS vasopressor agents. Activated charcoal or gastric lavage may be helpful. Physostigmine has been reported to be effective in treating mild poisoning by tricyclic antidepressants.

Uses. TCAs can be used alone or in combination with phenothiazines or ECT in the treatment of depression. In patients who are suicide risks, the long onset of action of the TCAs (several weeks) requires the use of ECT during the initial phase of drug treatment. These agents, after several weeks are allowed for the development of their effects, can prevent relapse and thus provide long-term control of depression.

When sedation is desired, amitriptyline [a-mee-TRIP-ti-leen] (Elavil) is used. When less sedation is needed, nortriptyline [nor-TRIP-ti-leen] (Pamelor, Aventyl) or protriptyline [proe-TRIP-ti-leen] (Vivactil) can be tried.

TCAs are often combined with one of the phenothiazines in the treatment of patients with both psychoses and depression. One example is a combination of perphenazine and amitriptyline (Triavil, Etrafon). Comments relating to the dental implications of both TCAs and phenothiazines apply to patients taking this type of product. Certain antidepressants are used for specific indications. For example, imipramine [im-IP-ra-meen] (Tofranil) is used to control nocturnal **enuresis** (incontinence) in children. Clomipramine [cloe-MIP-ra-meen] (Anafranil) is used only in the treatment of obsessive-compulsive disorder. Patients with obsessive-compulsive disorder repeatedly perform certain rituals such as hand washing. Doxepin [DOX-e-pin] (Adapin, Sinequan) is used when an anti-anxiety effect is desired.

Dental implications. The management of dental patients taking antidepressants is summarized in Box 17-3.

SYMPATHOMIMETIC AMINES Vasoconstricting drugs (sympathomimetic amines) in the local anesthetic solution must be administered with caution to patients taking TCAs. They may potentiate vasopressor (increased blood pressure) response to epinephrine. In the usual cardiac dose (0.04 mg), the sympathomimetic amines present in a local anesthetic solution can be safely administered to patients without preexisting arrhythmias.

XEROSTOMIA The anticholinergic effect of sympathomimetic amines is additive with that of other agents that produce dry mouth. The dental health care worker should question patients about the products used to alleviate this trouble-

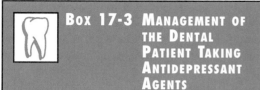

BOX 17-3 MANAGEMENT OF THE DENTAL PATIENT TAKING ANTIDEPRESSANT AGENTS

- Use caution in patient interactions.
- Drug used for other than depression; ask patient why he or she is taking the drug.
- Check for xerostomia and its management.
- Epinephrine may cause an increased vasopressor response (blood pressure response). Limit dose of epinephrine to 0.04 mg if blood pressure is a concern.
- Limit total amount of any potentially lethal drugs prescribed if patient is depressed.
- Increase motivation for good oral hygiene (usually improves with treatment of depression).

some side effect and suggest alternatives such as artificial saliva or sugarless gum.

TREMORS The fine tremors associated with use of the TCAs may make it difficult for patients to maintain good oral hygiene.

SECOND-GENERATION ANTIDEPRESSANTS

Second-generation antidepressants (see Table 17-2) are newer antidepressants that possess fewer side effects than the tricyclic antidepressants. For example, they have fewer anticholinergic effects and less cardiotoxicity, and some have less sedation effect. The choice of antidepressant is based on the adverse reaction profile and the individual patient's response to the agent.

Trazodone. Trazodone [TRAZ-oh-done] (Desyrel) is an antidepressant unrelated chemically to TCAs. It appears to have antidepressant ef-

fects equivalent to those of TCAs. Its advantages include that it has fewer anticholinergic effects (e.g., xerostomia) and is less cardiotoxic even in toxic doses. Its disadvantages include that it is highly sedative and has been associated with painful priapism requiring surgical intervention and leaving some patients permanently impotent.

SEROTONIN-SPECIFIC REUPTAKE INHIBITORS

A newer group of antidepressants, the serotonin-specific reuptake inhibitors (SSRI), have specific action on inhibiting the reuptake of serotonin. Fluoxetine [floo-OX-uh-teen] (Prozac) was the first member of this group and others have followed. Sertraline [SER-tral-leen] (Zoloft), paroxetine [pa-ROKS-e-teen] (Paxil), and fluvoxamine [floo-VOX-a-meen] (Luvox) are other members of this group. Their antidepressant action is equivalent to that of TCAs. Their advantage lies in their adverse reaction profile, which differs from that of TCAs (see Table 17-2).

Central nervous system. Unlike many of the TCAs, the serotonin reuptake inhibitors tend to produce CNS stimulation (activation) rather than CNS depression. Headache, dizziness, tremor, agitation, sweating, and insomnia are side effects associated with stimulation. Weight loss or weight stabilization occurs more frequently than the weight gain that occurs with TCAs. Somnolence and fatigue have also been reported.

Gastrointestinal. Nausea and diarrhea occur in about 15% to 30% of patients. Anorexia, dyspepsia, and constipation have been reported.

Oral. Oral side effects include xerostomia (10% to 15%), taste changes, aphthous stomatitis, **glossitis,** and, rarely, increased salivation, salivary gland enlargement, and tongue discoloration or edema. The SSRIs have little differences in the incidence of the side effects.

Other. The SSRIs frequently produce anorgasmia. The incidence varies but may be more than 50% with some agents. Sertraline is a substrate and an inhibitor of cytochrome P-450 2D6 enzymes. Excessive sweating is another common side effect. Palpitations have been reported.

BUPROPION

Bupropion [byoo-PROE-pee-on] (Wellbutrin [SR]) has been on the market and then off the market; in 1993 it was back on the market with increased warnings. About 0.4% of patients treated with bupropion have experienced seizures. This incidence may be 4 times greater than with the TCAs and as much as 10 times greater with TCAs at higher doses. Because of its seizure potential, it is reserved for patients who are not responsive to other agents. Gastrointestinal effects such as constipation, nausea, and vomiting occur in about 20% of patients. Neurologic effects such as dry mouth (28%), headache (25%), excessive sweating, and tremors have been reported. Agitation (32%) and dizziness (22%) occur frequently. Divided doses, slow titration of doses, and careful patient selection can minimize seizure risk.

| Zyban helps in tobacco cessation |

Recently, bupropion has been released under another trade name, Zyban, which is indicated as an adjuvant in a smoking cessation program (see Chapter 26). The only difference between Zyban and Wellbutrin is the imprint on the tablet.

ATYPICAL ANTIDEPRESSANT AGENTS

Nefazodone [nef-AY-zoe-done] (Serzone) and venlafaxine are examples of atypical antidepressants. They are indicated for the treatment of depression and are effective in obsessive-compulsive disorder. They both inhibit serotonin and norepinephrine reuptake, but nefazodone has α_1-antagonist action and venlafaxine is a weak inhibitor of dopamine reuptake. The incidence of xerostomia is greater than 10%, and sexual dysfunction frequently occurs. Venlafaxine is a weak inhibitor of cytochrome P-450 2D6 isoenzymes. Nefazodone increases the serum levels of alprazolam, triazolam, and digoxin. Other important drug interactions will continue to be identified.

MONOAMINE OXIDASE INHIBITORS

Monoamine oxidase inhibitors (MAOIs) include a large variety of drugs that have the ability to

| MAOI—many drug interactions |

inhibit monoamine oxidase. Because MAOs are not responsible for metabolism of endogenous amines, MAOIs do not alter significantly their effects. One MAOI, pargyline (Eutonyl) is used to treat hypertension. MAOIs possess many adverse effects, and an overdose can lead to a severe toxic reaction. Because the enzymes inhibited by the MAOIs inactivate many endogenous amines, the action of any exogenous sympathomimetic amine is potentiated (i.e., it is not metabolized as quickly). The MAOIs interact with many drugs, such as amphetamines, and with foods such as cheeses, wines, and fish, precipitating a hypertensive crisis and even death. Patients taking MAOIs have detailed food prohibitions because of the chance of drug-food interactions. Because of the potential for life-threatening situations, MAOIs are used as drugs of last choice. Patients taking MAOIs should not be given any drug unless the prescriber has first consulted a reference source on drug interactions.

DRUGS FOR TREATMENT OF BIPOLAR DEPRESSION

Until fairly recently, lithium was the major drug used in the treatment of bipolar depression. Other agents commonly used today include a variety of anticonvulsants, including carbamazepine, valproate, and gabapentin. These agents are often referred to as "mood stabilizers."

LITHIUM

Lithium [LITH-ee-um] (Eskalith, Lithobid) is used in the treatment of bipolar (manic) depression, which is characterized by cyclic recurrence of mania alternating with depression. The side effects, which can be minimized by monitoring serum lithium levels, include polyuria, fine hand tremor, thirst, and, in more severe cases, slurred speech, ataxia, nausea, vomiting, and diarrhea. Patients undergoing lithium therapy should be observed for signs of overdose toxicity, which may be exhibited by CNS symptoms including muscle rigidity, hyperactive deep reflexes, excessive tremor, and muscle fasciculations. Because lithium is handled in the body like sodium, changes in sodium levels can affect lithium levels. Salt intake and sweating can also change lithium levels. Some nonsteroidal antiinflammatory agents can decrease lithium clearance, leading to an increase in lithium levels (Box 17-4). A patient's serum lithium levels before, during, and after taking naproxen are illustrated in Figure 6-11.

ANTICONVULSANTS

In the treatment of bipolar depression (mania), several anticonvulsant agents have been used. The manic phase has been treated with anticonvulsants such as carbamazepine, valproate, and gabapentin. These agents are usually reserved for lithium-resistant cases. Occasionally, lithium and the anticonvulsants are used concomitantly.

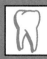

BOX 17-4 MANAGEMENT OF THE DENTAL PATIENT TAKING LITHIUM

- Monitor toxicity related to lithium levels; sweating and salt intake can alter levels.
- Tremors may interfere with oral hygiene.
- Drowsiness additive with other CNS depressants.
- Xerostomia or excessive salivation reported.
- Naproxyn (other NSAIAs) can produce lithium toxicity.

REVIEW QUESTIONS

1. Explain the difference between the neuroses and the schizophrenias.
2. Name three commonly used phenothiazines.
3. State the major pharmacologic effect of the phenothiazines.
4. State the adverse reactions attributable to the phenothiazines.
5. Describe the following adverse reactions, including methods of recognition in the dental office:
   a. orthostatic hypotension
   b. extrapyramidal symptoms
   c. tardive dyskinesia
   d. anticholinergic effects
6. Name three uses for the phenothiazines.
7. List four ways in which you would handle a patient taking antipsychotic agents differently from a nonmedicated patient.
8. Explain the drug interactions between epinephrine and the phenothiazines and epinephrine and the tricyclic antidepressants. State which is clinically significant.
9. Describe two advantages of the atypical antipsychotics.
10. List three adverse reactions associated with the tricyclic antidepressants.

11. Describe two ways in which you would treat a patient taking antidepressants differently from a nonmedicated patient.
12. State the agent used in the treatment of poisoning by tricyclic antidepressants.
13. Name two second-generation antidepressants and describe two advantages and one disadvantage of each.
14. State the advantages and disadvantages of the SSRIs over the TCAs.
15. Describe two advantages of the atypical antidepressants over the TCAs.
16. Name the agent used to treat bipolar affective disorders and describe its effect on saliva.
17. Describe the effect of the NSAIAs on lithium.

CHAPTER 18

Autacoids and Antihistamines

The term **autacoids** is a word derived from the Greek *autos* ("self") and *akos*, ("remedy"). Although the agents in this class possess widely differing pharmacologic actions, they all occur naturally in the body, are produced by many tissues, and are formed by the tissues on which they act.

The autacoid agonists or antagonists include the H_1- and H_2-receptor antagonists (H_1-RA) or blockers, the eicosanoids (prostaglandins [PGs], thromboxanes [TXs], and leukotrienes [LTs]), serotonin agonists, angiotensin inhibitors, and cytokinins. As research on these agents continues, the agonists and their potential antagonists hold great promise for future therapy in many different areas. In fact, leukotriene antagonists (see Chapter 23) are new drugs used for the management of asthma.

HISTAMINE

Histamine is a rather ubiquitous biogenic amine. Although many of its peripheral actions are well known, its precise physiologic function, particularly in the central nervous system (CNS), is not clear. The structure of histamine is as follows:

$$H-N \diagdown\diagdown \quad CH_2 \diagdown CH_2 \diagdown NH_2 \quad N$$

Almost all mammalian tissues contain or can synthesize histamine. In humans, histamine is stored in the **mast cells** in the intestinal mucosa and in the CNS. When an allergic reaction occurs, the mast cells degranulate and histamine is released.

Histamine is released from the tissues in the body by normal reactions, abnormal reactions, or the administration of certain drugs. The amount of histamine released in these reactions determines the effects seen in the patient.

PHARMACOLOGIC EFFECTS

In humans, histamine causes the following effects:

H_1-agonist effects:
* Vasodilation
* Increased capillary permeability
* Bronchoconstriction
* Pain or itching in cutaneous nerve endings

H_2-agonist effects:
* Increased gastric acid secretion

With the synthesis of agents that can block some of the effects of histamine, new pharmacologic agents have been developed. The histamine receptors are termed H_1 and H_2. Some evidence of an H_3-receptor exists. The H_1-receptors are primarily related to vasodilation, increased capillary permeability, bronchoconstriction, and pain or itching at the nerve endings (the first four items on the preceding list). The H_2-receptors are responsible for stimulating gastric acid secretion (the last item on the preceding list). The action of the H_3-receptor is unknown.

Histamine's actions are mediated by activation of H_1-receptors, H_2-receptors, or other receptors. Agents that block or antagonize the effects of histamine at the H_1-receptors are referred to as H_1-*blockers* or H_1-*receptor antagonists (H_1-RA)* and at the H_2-receptors they are **H_2-blockers** or H_2-*receptor antagonists (H_2-RA)*.

ADVERSE REACTIONS

When an allergic reaction occurs, an antigen-antibody reaction causes the release of histamine and other autacoids. Anaphylaxis is a serious and sometimes fatal reaction to a foreign protein or drug introduced into the body. Difficulty in breathing, convulsions, lapses into unconsciousness, and death can ensue. The predominant feature in this syndrome is bronchoconstriction.

In addition to bronchoconstriction, the action of histamine during an anaphylactic reaction includes vasodilation and increased capillary permeability, both of which lead to decreased blood pressure followed by shock and cardiovascular collapse. Other symptoms of anaphylaxis include apprehension, paresthesia, urticaria, edema, choking, cyanosis, coughing, and wheezing. Fever, shock, loss of consciousness, coma, convulsions, and death may result.

Although the treatment of anaphylaxis is described in Chapter 23, it is discussed here in relation to its cause. The drug of choice for anaphylaxis is parenteral epinephrine, a physiologic antagonist (epinephrine dilates bronchioles via the β_2 receptors) rather than an antihistamine, which is a pharmacologic antagonist (antihistamine blocks the bronchoconstriction produced by histamine at the same H_1-receptor). The reason for this is that antihistamines antagonize only some of the effects of histamine, and they work competitively, whereas epinephrine acts as a direct β_2-agonist.

USES

Histamine's only clinical use is in the diagnosis of achlorhydria and pheochromocytoma.

ANTIHISTAMINES (H_1-RECEPTOR ANTAGONISTS)

Antihistamines = H_1-RA

The common term *antihistamine* refers to agents that are H_1-receptor antagonists or H_1-blockers. They are widely used drugs, and dental practitioners should be familiar with them for the following reasons:

- Many patients have seasonal allergic reactions (e.g., hay fever) that make dental treatment difficult. The dentist may prescribe or the patient may self-medicate with antihistamines before a dental procedure to reduce the symptoms of hay fever and make it easier for the patient to breathe.
- A mild allergic reaction to a drug may be treated with antihistamines in the dental office. If the allergic reaction is severe, epinephrine is the drug of choice.
- Patients taking antihistamines may experience side effects such as xerostomia, but the newer nonsedating antihistamines have less anticholinergic effect.

- Antihistamines interact with many other drug groups and are additive with other CNS depressants.

PHARMACOLOGIC EFFECTS

The older H_1-receptor antagonists, also called H_1-*blockers*, have several pharmacologic effects, including antihistaminic, anticholinergic, antiserotonergic, and sedative effects. Because they have a chemical structure similar to that of histamine, they can bind with the H_1-receptor and prevent or block the action of histamine (if it is released). Table 18-1 gives the chemical groups of various antihistamines, some examples of each group, and the properties of each group.

Figures 18-1 and 18-2 compare the relative sedative, antihistaminic, anticholinergic, and antiemetic effects of four common antihistamines: diphenhydramine [dye-fen-HYE-dra-meen] (Benadryl), chlorpheniramine [klor-fen-EER-a-meen] (Chlor-Trimeton), promethazine [proe-METH-a-zeen] (Phenergan), and loratidine [lor-A-ti-deen] (Claritin). Note that some H_1-RAs are effective for nausea and that some have more anticholinergic effects (more xerostomia).

The pharmacologic effects of antihistamines can be divided into those caused by blocking histamine at the H_1-receptor and those independent of this effect.

H_1-receptor blocking effects. These drugs, which are H_1-antagonists, competitively block or antagonize histamine's effect at the following sites:

Counteracts histamines effects

- *Capillary permeability.* By blocking capillary permeability produced by histamine, less tissue edema occurs from the transport of the serum into the intracellular spaces.
- *Vascular smooth muscle (vessels).* The anti-

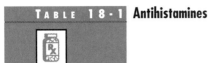

TABLE 18-1 Antihistamines

DRUG NAME	SINGLE ADULT DOSE (mg)	DOSING INTERVAL (HRS)	SEDATIVE EFFECTS*	ANTIHISTAMINIC ACTIVITY*	ANTICHOLINERGIC ACTIVITY*	ANTIEMETIC EFFECTS*
ETHANOLAMINES						
Diphenhydramine (Benadryl)†	25-50	6-8	+++	+/++	+++	++/+++
Carbinoxamine (Clistin)	4-8	6-8	++	+/++	+++	++/+++
Clemastine (Tavist)	1	12	++	+/++	++	++/+++
ETHYLENEDIAMINES						
Tripelennamine (PBZ)	25-50	4-6	++	+/++	+	—
Pyrilamine (various)†	25-50	6-8	+	+/++	+	—
ALKYLAMINES						
Chlorpheniramine† (Chlor-Trimeton)	4	4-6	+	++	++	—
Dexchlorpheniramine (Polaramine)	2	4-6	+	+++	++	—
Brompheniramine (Dimetane)†	4-8	4-6	+	+++	++	—
Triprolidine (Actidil)†	2-5	4-6	+	++/+++	++	—
PHENOTHIAZINES						
Promethazine (Phenergan)	12.5-25	6-24	+++	+++	+++	++++
Trimeprazine (Temaril)	2.5	6	++	++/+++	+++	++++
Methdilazine (Tacaryl)‡	8	6-12	+	++/+++	+++	++++
PIPERIDINES						
Cyproheptadine (Periactin)	4	8	+	++	++	—
Azatadine (Optimine)	1-2	12	++	++	++	—
Diphenylpyraline (Hispril)	5	12	+	++	++	—
Phenindamine (Nolahist)†	25	4-6	—	++	++	—
PIPERAZINES						
Hydoxyzine (Vistaril, Atarax)	25-100	4-8	++/+++	++	+++	
NONSEDATING ANTIHISTAMINES						
Terfenadine (Seldane)‖	60	12	±	++/+++	±	—
Astemizole (Hismanal)‖	10	24	±	++/+++	±	—
Loratidine (Claritin)‖	10	24	±	++/+++	±	—

*++++, Very high; +++, high; ++, moderate; +, low.
†Available OTC.
‡No longer available.

histamines block the dilation of the vascular smooth muscle that histamine produces.

- **Nonvascular (bronchial) smooth muscle.** Because other autacoids are also released in an anaphylactic reaction, antihistamines are not effective in counteracting all the bronchoconstriction present during that reaction.
- **Nerve endings.** Antihistamines can suppress the itching and pain associated with this histamine-mediated reaction at the cutaneous nerve endings.

Other effects (unrelated to H$_1$-blocking effects)

CENTRAL NERVOUS SYSTEM The antihistamines produce varying degrees of CNS depression. Because diphenhydramine produces a high degree of sedation, it is the principal agent used in over-the-counter (OTC) sleep aids (Sominex, Nytol). It is less expensive as an antihistamine than as a sleep aid.

ANTICHOLINERGIC An anticholinergic effect (cholinergic blockade), weaker than but similar

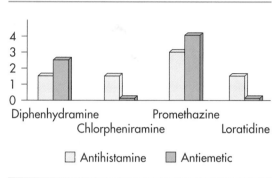

FIGURE 18-1 *Antihistamine pharmacologic effects.*

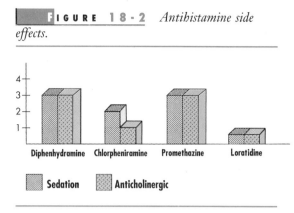

FIGURE 18-2 *Antihistamine side effects.*

to that of atropine, can be used to "dry up" secretions when treating the symptoms of certain upper respiratory diseases (allergies, "cold"). A potential disadvantage with the anticholinergic effect is that secretions may be "dried up" and more difficult to clear.

ANTIEMETIC Some antihistamines, such as meclizine (Dramamine, Bonine), have pronounced antiemetic or antimotion sickness activity. These agents are also effective in controlling the dizziness and labyrinthine-induced nausea and vomiting that occurs with **Meniere's syndrome** (inner ear).

Antihistamines with antiemetic effects may be useful in dentistry to manage postoperative nausea and vomiting, especially when opioid agents have been used. The antihistamines that have phenothiazine-like action, such as promethazine, are the most effective antiemetics.

LOCAL ANESTHESIA Although antihistamines are not as effective as the other local anesthetics, they can be administered topically or by injection to provide some local anesthesia. They are similar in structure to the local anesthetics and have a similar effect (Structure Activity Relationship [SAR]).

ADVERSE REACTIONS

Like the pharmacologic effects of the antihistamines, the adverse reactions vary in relative amounts among the different agents. Figures 18-1 and 18-2 show how adverse reactions, as well as pharmacologic effects, vary among antihistamines.

Central nervous system depression. This effect can be either a pharmacologic effect (you want the effect) or an adverse reaction (you do not want the effect), depending on the use. Sedation is the most common side effect associated with the older antihistamines, and it may be accompanied by dizziness, tinnitus, incoordination, blurred vision, and fatigue. Patients who are given antihistamines should be warned against operating a motor vehicle or signing important documents. Sedation with antihistamines is additive with that caused by other CNS depressant drugs.

As with all drugs that depress the CNS, stimulation or excitation can occur in a few cases. Symptoms include restlessness, excitation, and, in severe cases, convulsions. It is more common in children, elderly patients, and those who use a larger dose than prescribed. The newer nonsedating H_1-blockers such as loratadine (Claritin) produce less sedation because they do not penetrate the brain as easily, they produce less sedation.

When antihistamines are combined with decongestants (adrenergic agents) the antihistamine-related CNS depression is counteracted by the CNS stimulation of the decongestants. The planned result is for each agent's CNS effects to cancel out the others.

Many antihistamine-decongestant combinations are marketed for treatment of colds or sinus problems. They are available over the counter and by prescription (e.g., Naldecon, Claritin D).

Gastrointestinal. The gasrointestinal complaints commonly associated with the antihistamines include anorexia, nausea, vomiting, and constipation. Xerostomia is categorized as an anticholinergic adverse reaction. The H_2-blockers (see Chapter 22), not the H_1-blockers, antagonize histamine's effect on the secretion of stomach acid.

Anticholinergic = xerostomia

Anticholinergic. The H_1-receptor antagonists have varying anticholinergic effects. The importance to the dental health care worker is that anticholinergic effects lead to xerostomia and xerostomia leads to numerous dental problems. Xerostomia can cause an increased caries rate in patients taking antihistamines on a long-term basis. In patients taking chronic antihistamines, the mouth should be observed for symptoms of xerostomia and counseling about techniques to manage it (see Chapter 5) should be presented.

The nonsedating antihistamines have much less anticholinergic effect and are less likely to produce xerostomia. Loratidine (Claritin) is a heavily advertised nonsedating antihistamine.

Toxicity

Antihistamine poisoning has become more common in recent years because of the easy accessi-

bility of the agents in OTC preparations promoted as sleep aids. Excitation predominates in small children, and sedation can occur in adults. Death usually results from coma with cardiovascular and respiratory collapse. The treatment is conservative and directed at specific symptoms.

Uses

Allergic reactions. Certain allergic reactions such as allergic rhinitis and seasonal hay fever can be controlled by antihistamines. With continued use, tolerance can develop to the effects of a particular antihistamine. Changing to an agent in another chemical group can often restore the effects desired. These agents are less useful in the treatment of the common cold. Some people like the anticholinergic effect on secretions and want all their secretions to stop.

Acute urticarial attacks can be treated with antihistamines to relieve itching, edema, and erythema. In the treatment of anaphylaxis, the physiologic antagonist epinephrine rather than the antihistamines is indicated first. The xanthines (aminophylline) are also more effective than the antihistamines in producing bronchodilation in acute anaphylaxis. Because antihistamines produce some local anesthetic effect when applied topically, certain painful oral lesions can be treated with topical antihistamines. For example, with discomfort the patient may swish and swirl diphenhydramine liquid inside the mouth.

Nausea and vomiting. Because of the antiemetic action of some antihistamines, they are used to prevent and treat motion sickness and to control postoperative vomiting and vomiting induced by radiation therapy. The nausea and vomiting associated with pregnancy should *not* be treated with antihistamines because of these agents' alleged potential for fetal harm.

Preoperative sedation. The use of the older H_1-antihistamines in dentistry is primarily based on their CNS effects. They are employed for preoperative sedation because of their sedative and antiemetic effects. Hydroxyzine and promethazine are useful for this purpose (see Table 18-1). Their antiemetic actions can be helpful to counteract the adverse effect of the opioids.

Over-the-counter sleep aids. Diphenhydramine (Nytol) is used in products that are sold as OTC sleep aids.

Local anesthesia. Although not as effective as the local anesthetics usually employed, an antihistamine such as diphenhydramine (Benadryl) can be used by injection to provide some local anesthesia. This may be necessary when patients have exhibited allergies to the normally used local anesthetic agents.

PERIPHERAL (NONSEDATING) H₁-RECEPTOR ANTAGONISTS

Chemically, members of the nonsedating H₁-receptor antagonists do not have any common denominator. They are quite different in origin, chemical structure, solubility, and metabolic effects. They all share the specific blocking action of peripheral H₁ receptors. Because they do not cross the blood-brain barrier in usual therapeutic doses, they do not produce sedation [Really, they are less likely to produce sedation]. Table 18-1 lists the nonsedating antihistamines. Two members of this group are fexofenadine (Allegra) and loratadine (Claritin). These new antihistamines are much more expensive than the older antihistamines.

FEXOFENADINE

Fexofenadine [feks-oh-FEN-a-deen] (Allegra) is an active metabolite of terfenadine (Seldane) and was developed by the manufacturer of terfenadine (Seldane) to replace it. Terfenadine was found to be responsible for cardiac arrhythmias and changes in the EKG secondary to other drugs that inhibited its metabolism. Terfenadine has been recalled from the market.

Because fexofenadine does not cross the blood-brain barrier to any appreciable degree, the potential for sedation is greatly reduced. Side effects include drowsiness and viral infections. It has little of the anticholinergic effects exhibited by the traditional H₁ blockers. Both erythromycin and ketoconazole increase the level of fexofenadine (by inhibiting its metabolism), but no clinical manifestations have been noted. Whether interactions will occur with other imidazoles or macrolides (clarithromycin, azithromycin) must be determined. Its onset of action is about 1 hour, and its time to peak serum concentration is 2.6 hours. Its duration of action is at least 12 hours, and its half-life is 14.4 hours. About 20% is metabolized in the liver and excreted in the urine, while 80% is excreted in the feces. Its dose is 60 mg twice a day.

ASTEMIZOLE

Astemizole [a-STEM-mi-zole] (Hismanal) is a nonsedating antihistamine. It must be taken on an empty stomach (food reduces absorption 60%). Its very long half-life of 7 to 11 days makes it useful only for chronic conditions. The onset of its antihistaminic effect takes several days. Because astemizole's metabolism is inhibited by erythromycin and ketoconazole, it has recently been removed from the market.

LORATIDINE

Loratidine [lor-AT-i-deen] (Claritin), another nonsedating antihistamine, has similar action to the other drugs in this group. Its onset is 1 to 3 hours, its peak effect is 8.4 to 28 hours, its duration of action is 24 hours, and its half-life is 12 to 15 hours. It is extensively metabolized to an active metabolite. Adverse reactions include headache, somnolence (less than 10%), fatigue, and xerostomia.

CETIRIZINE

Cetirizine [se-TI-ra-zeen] (Zyrtec) is the most recently released nonsedating H_1-receptor blocker. Its onset of action is usually less than ½ hour and it peaks in about 1 hour. Its half-life is 8 hours. The intense competition among the companies selling nonsedating antihistamines is brutal. Because there are few important differences, advertising emphasizes supposed "differences" such as chewable tablets.

Peripheral (nonsedating) antihistamines have become valuable adjuncts in the therapy of seasonal and perennial rhinitis, as well as certain forms of urticaria. It is likely that these agents will eventually replace the older H_1-receptor antagonists for these conditions. In the treatment of dental patients, however, the place of the older H_1-receptor blockers is assured because these compounds are used as much for their side effects (sedation, potentiation of opioids, reduced nausea) as for their antihistaminic action.

Completing the histamine antagonists are the H_2-blocking agents, such as cimetidine (Tagamet), which inhibit the action of histamine at the H_2-receptors. Because they are used to treat gastrointestinal problems, they are discussed in Chapter 22.

OTHER AUTACOIDS

PROSTAGLANDINS AND THROMBOXANES

The prostaglandins and thromboxanes are members of a group of biologically active agents termed *eicosanoids*. Other members of this group include the leukotrienes, lipoxins, hydroperoxyeicosatetraenoic acids (HPETEs), hydroxyeicosatetraenoic acids (HETEs), and epoxyeicosatetraenoic acids (EETEs). The prostaglandins and thromboxanes have been found in most body tissues and fluids. They are produced in the body in response to many dif-

FIGURE 18-3   *Prostaglandin nomenclature*

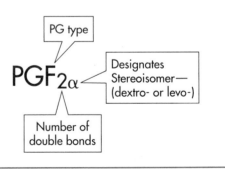

ferent stimuli, and small quantities produce a large spectrum of effects on many different body systems.

The family of prostaglandins is divided into six main series of agents, A, B, C, D, E, and F, of which the last two (E and F) are predominant. These main groups are further subdivided and give rise to an extensive and complicated series of compounds. The subscript numbers (1, 2, and 3) following the letters indicate the degree of saturation. The α or β refers to the spatial configuration of the carbon 9 hydroxyl group (e.g., $PGF_{2\alpha}$) (Figure 18-3).

Until recently, PGEs and PGFs were the most abundant and most intensively studied prostaglandins. Now many new prostaglandins (e.g., PGG and PGH), thromboxanes (e.g., TXA and TXB), and prostacyclin (PGI) have become of central interest.

Pharmacologic. The pharmacologic effects of the prostaglandins encompass many diverse actions. Not only is there a wide spectrum of action but different prostaglandins have different activities in different tissue. As prostaglandin agonists or antagonists are identified, the number and range of actions in the body will be increased. Some currently known effects of the prostaglandins include the following.

SMOOTH MUSCLE Vascular smooth muscle may be either relaxed (vasodilation) or stimulated (vasoconstriction) depending on the specific prostaglandins. The effect of prostaglandins on the gastrointestinal tract is to produce cramping (increased motility). Their effect on the uterus is to cause contraction, especially in the near-term uterus. This effect has led to the development of a therapeutic product (see discussion of uses).

PLATELETS Another example of the opposing actions of different prostaglandins is thromboxane and prostacyclin. Thromboxane, produced by platelets, stimulates platelet aggregation and is a vasoconstrictor, whereas prostacyclin, produced by the vessel walls, inhibits platelet aggregation and is a vasodilator. Very fine gradations of action in the body can be elicited using this mechanism where two different chemicals produce the opposite effect. If secretion of one of the paired autacoids is increased, then the desired action is produced. Conversely, secretion of the other autacoid produces the opposite effect. In addition, antagonists to these autacoids block their normal effects. For adjusting one particular effect, there may be both agonist and antagonist effects for each autacoid. This "system" to modulate adequate coagulation can be modified by adding a drug. Adding of aspirin can alter the clinical outcome. Even altering the dose of aspirin can produce different effects (low dose and high dose).

REPRODUCTIVE ORGANS Prostaglandins are abundant in the **semen,** but their role is unknown. Both PGE and PGF have oxytocic (uterine contraction) action, making them useful as abortifacients in the second trimester and as inducers of labor at full term.

CENTRAL NERVOUS SYSTEM Prostaglandins increase body temperature by releasing interleukin-1, which promotes the release and synthesis of PGE. PGEs stimulate the release of hormones such as growth hormone, prolactin, TSH, ACTH, FSH, and LH. The interdependence of the autacoids is demonstrated.

OTHER EFFECTS These include increased heart rate and cardiac output, increased capillary permeability, increased renal blood flow, sedation, and stimulation of pain fibers.

Because the individual prostaglandins have many activities, it is unlikely that they have a single receptor. They are released by mechanical, thermal, chemical, bacterial, or traumatic injuries. Their role is more important in chronic inflammation, and this effect may account for their importance in the etiology of periodontal disease.

Dentistry. The prostaglandins are important in dentistry because they have been implicated in periodontal disease.

> Prostaglandins are related to periodontal disease.

At least two stages of periodontal disease may involve prostaglandins. The first is the inflammation of the gingiva with its resultant erythema, edema, and increase in gingival exudate. Prostaglandins, thought to be mediators of the inflammatory response in oral soft tissues, may be involved in this initial stage of periodontal disease. The second is the resorption of alveolar bone with tooth loss. Prostaglandins also prevent the synthesis of new bone by inhibiting osteoblastic activity. This explains the reason the use of NSAIAs in the management of periodontal disease is being explored.

Newer research concerning the etiology of periodontal disease has been discovering more correlations among different factors. Certainly several autacoids have been found to be involved in the production of periodontal disease—prostaglandins, leukotrienes, and cytokines, for example.

Uses. One therapeutic use of the prostaglandins is inducing midtrimester abortions. Prostaglandins are administered by intraamniotic injection (a salt of PGF) or vaginal suppository (PGE analogue). For very early abortions, PGE analogues are combined with antiprogestins (RU-486) in an oral dosage form currently available in France. A prostaglandin agonist (misoprostol [Cytotec]) is available for the prevention of NSAIA-induced ulcers. PGE is cytoprotective at low doses. Currently, prostaglandins are being studied in the treatment of bronchial asthma and hypertension.

Prostaglandin antagonists. The administration of prostaglandin antagonists may prove useful in the treatment of certain pathologic conditions. This seems reasonable in view of the many effects of the prostaglandins in the body. For example, aspirin can inhibit platelet aggregation by blocking thromboxane (which promotes aggregation). Indomethacin, an NSAIA, blocks the effect of the prostaglandins on the ductus arteriosus (prostaglandins keep the ductus arteriosus open). After birth, if the ductus arteriosus does not close, indomethacin (given intravenously) can close the ductus, thereby making open heart surgery unnecessary. There is also some evidence that certain phenolic compounds such as eugenol (clove oil), dentistry's poultice, inhibit prostaglandin. Because prostaglandins are involved in inflammation, agents that inhibit the prostaglandins may be useful in the treatment of inflammation.

LEUKOTRIENES

Leukotrienes are another complex group of autacoids that are also derived from arachidonic acid. They were formerly called *slow-reacting substance(s) of anaphylaxis (SRS-A).* Although they show considerable species variation, their dom-

Leukotrienes—role in allergy and inflammation

inant action in humans is powerful bronchoconstriction. In that effect, leukotrienes are far more potent than histamines. They also contract other smooth muscle such as the uterus and gastrointestinal tract. Extensive research is devoted to these substances and great progress can be expected, potentially in the treatment of asthma and other forms of bronchoconstriction.

KININS

Kinins are polypeptides that are distributed in a great variety of body tissues. Two members of this group, kallidin and bradykinin, are found in plasma and may play a role in dental diseases. These agents are formed by the action of certain proteolytic enzymes (kininogenases) such as kallikrein on their common precursor, kininogen. Other kininogenases include trypsin, plasmin, and certain snake venoms. There are at least two receptors for bradykinin: the B_1-receptor and the B_2-receptor. The *B* in these receptors stands for *bradykinin;* they are not to be confused with the β-adrenergic receptors present in the sympathetic autonomic nervous system.

The plasma kinins may be involved in shock and acute or chronic allergic or inflammatory conditions such as anaphylaxis and arthritis. Their effects on the body include vasodilation, increased capillary permeability, edema, pain resulting from action on nerve endings, and contraction or relaxation of nonvascular smooth muscles. The kinins apparently mediate pulpal pain and are implicated in the control of the synthesis of endogenous analgesics, particularly the endorphins, during caries formation. It is possible that inhibitors of kinins may be useful dental therapeutic aids in the future.

Although no specific antagonists of the kinins are yet available, some drugs are known to inhibit kinin-evoked responses. For example, salicylates (aspirin) and glucocorticoids (steroids) inhibit kallikrein activation and may play a role in future therapy. The synthesis of antagonists to the autacoid kinins and their possible clinical use are currently being investigated.

SUBSTANCE P

Substance P is a peptide thought to function as a neurotransmitter in the CNS and a local hormone in the gastrointestinal tract. It is a vasodilator and produces hypotension. It increases the action of the intestinal and bronchial smooth muscle. It also causes secretion in the salivary glands and an increase in sodium and water excretion from the kidney. Substance P may be a transmitter that is released from unmyelinated fibers that respond to pain. It is also involved in many other functions because it is present in areas of the brain that are not involved in pain.

REVIEW QUESTIONS

1. Define the term *autacoid*.
2. Name the major pharmacologic effects of histamine.
3. Describe the effects of stimulation of histamine and H receptors.
4. Explain why the older antihistamines are called *H antagonists* or *H blockers*.
5. Explain the pharmacologic effects of the older antihistamines.
6. Describe the effects of the antihistamines that are related to their action on the CNS.
7. Explain the major adverse reactions associated with antihistamines.
8. Discuss the therapeutic uses of all antihistamines. Name a specific use for the antihistamines in dentistry.
9. Name a nonsedating antihistamine and explain one advantage and disadvantage it possesses.
10. Name two therapeutic uses for the prostaglandins.
11. Describe why the prostaglandins have taken on increased importance to the dental profession.
12. Name two types of drugs that inhibit the synthesis of prostaglandin and give one example of each type. Explain how this action is used therapeutically.
13. State two eicosanoids and their relationship to dentistry.

CHAPTER 19

Adrenocorticosteroids

The term *adrenocorticosteroids* [a-dree-noe-KOR-ti-KO-ster-oids] (adrenal corticosteroids, adrenocorticoids, corticosteroids, steroids) refers to a group of agents secreted by the adrenal cortex. The dental team should be aware of the effects, adverse reactions, and dental implications of these agents for at least the following reasons:

- **Use in dentistry.** These compounds are used topically or systemically for the treatment of oral lesions associated with inflammatory diseases.

• **Long-term therapy.** The adrenocorticosteroids, or *steroids* as they are commonly called, are prescribed for many patients with chronic systemic diseases such as asthma or arthritis. If taken chronically in high enough doses, these agents can cause a variety of adverse reactions that may influence the patient's dental treatment.

MECHANISM OF RELEASE

| Negative feedback mechanism |

The adrenocorticosteroids are naturally occurring compounds secreted by the adrenal cortex.

FIGURE 19-1 CRF, *Corticotropin releasing factor*; ACTH, *adrenocorticotropic hormone*; Ach, *acetylcholine pathways*; NE, *norepinephrine pathways*.

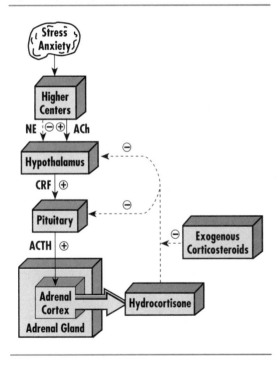

Their release is triggered by a series of events (Figure 19-1). First a stimulus such as stress (1) causes the hypothalamus (2) to release corticotropin releasing factor (CRF) (3), which acts on the pituitary gland (4). Under the influence of CRF the pituitary gland secretes adrenocorticotropic hormone (ACTH) (5), which stimulates the adrenal cortex (6) to release hydrocortisone (7). Hydrocortisone then acts on both the pituitary (8) and the hypothalamus (9) to inhibit the release of CRF and ACTH, respectively. This mechanism is called *negative feedback*. Exogenous steroids act in the same way as hydrocortisone (10); that is, they inhibit the release of CRF and ACTH. With long-term administration of steroids, ACTH release is suppressed and the adrenal gland atrophies. If the administration of exogenous steroid is then abruptly stopped, a relative steroid deficiency results. This can cause severe problems, including adrenal crisis.

CLASSIFICATION

The adrenocorticosteroids can be divided into two major groups: the glucocorticoids, which affect intermediate

| Glucocorticoids, mineralocorticoids |

carbohydrate metabolism, and the mineralocorticoids, which affect the water and electrolyte composition of the body. The major glucocorticoid present in the body is cortisol (hydrocortisone). Without stress, the normal adult secretes about 20 mg of hydrocortisone daily. A 10-fold increase can occur with stress. Maximal secretion occurs between 4 AM and 8 AM in people with a normal schedule. The chemical structures of the synthetic agents and the naturally occurring adrenocorticosteroids such as hydrocortisone are similar. Many chemical modifications have been made in an attempt to produce synthetic glucocorticoids with fewer adverse reactions and more specific activity.

Although the term *adrenocorticosteroids* refers

to those steroids secreted by the adrenal cortex and includes both the glucocorticoids and the mineralocorticoids, this chapter discusses primarily the action of glucocorticoids because of their more frequent use.

DEFINITIONS

The following terms are used in this chapter:
- *Addison's disease:* Disease/condition produced by a deficiency of adrenocorticosteroids
- *adrenocorticosteroids/corticosteroids/steroids:* Steroidal components released from the adrenal cortex, including glucocorticoids and mineralocorticoids
- *adrenocorticotropic hormone (ACTH):* Agent secreted by the pituitary that causes the release of hormones from the adrenal cortex
- *Cushing's syndrome:* Disease/condition produced by an excess of adrenocorticosteroids
- *glucocorticoids:* Adrenocorticosteroids that primarily affect carbohydrate metabolism
- *mineralocorticoids:* Adrenocorticosteroids that affect the body's sodium and water balance (fluid levels)

ROUTES OF ADMINISTRATION

Glucocorticoids are available in a wide variety of dosage forms. They are routinely used topically, orally, intramuscularly, and intravenously. Systemic effects are commonly obtained when the drug is administered orally or parenterally, but topical administration may rarely cause systemic effects. If a large quantity of a steroid is applied topically, especially if the skin is denuded or an occlusive dressing such as plastic wrap is applied, systemic effects can occur. Table 19-1 shows the relative potency of selected topical corticosteroid products.

MECHANISM OF ACTION

The mechanism of action of the steroids involves binding to a specific receptor and forming

> Effect has lag time

a steroid-receptor complex. The complex then translocates into the nucleus and alters gene expression (turn genes on or off), resulting in the regulation of many cellular processes. Because of

TABLE 19-1 Relative Potency of Selected Topical Corticosteroid Products

POTENCY (I TO VII)	POTENCY (7 TO 1)	DRUG GENERIC (TRADE)	DOSAGE FORM	STRENGTH
VII	1	Clobetasol propionate (Temovate)	Cream, ointment	0.05%
VII	2	Fluocinolone acetonide (Lidex)	Cream	0.2%
III	4	Triamcinolone acetonide (Aristocort, Flutex, Kenalog)	Ointment	0.1%
III	5	Betamethasone valerate (Valisone)	Cream	0.1%
II	4	Flucinolone acetonide (Synalar)	Cream, ointment	0.025%
II	5	Triamcinolone acetonide (Aristocort)	Cream, ointment, lotion Cream, ointment, lotion Cream, ointment	0.025% 0.1% 0.5%
I	7	Hydrocortisone (Cortaid, Anusol, Hytone, Dermacort, Penecort, Cetacort)	Lotion Cream, ointment, lotion, aerosol Solution Aerosol Cream, ointment, lotion	0.25% 0.5% 0.5% 1% 2.5%

the mechanism, a lag time exists in the action of the steroids and the relationship between their effects and blood level is poor. Other effects of glucocorticoids are mediated by catecholamines producing vasodilation or bronchodilation.

| Many effects |

The antiinflammatory action of glucocorticoids results from their profound effects on the number, distribution, and function of peripheral leukocytes and to their inhibition of phospholipase A. The use of steroids results in an increase in the concentration of neutrophils and a decrease in the lymphocytes (T and B cells), monocytes, eosinophils, and basophils. Steroids induce the synthesis of a protein that inhibits phospholipase A, decreasing the production of both prostaglandins and leukotrienes from arachidonic acid.

These agents, responsible for the delayed phase of acute inflammation, act synergistically. Steroids also inhibit interleukin-2, migration inhibition factor, and macrophage inhibition factor. These antiinflammatory effects not only serve therapeutic uses but also produce many of these agents' most severe adverse effects.

PHARMACOLOGIC EFFECTS

The pharmacologic effects and the adverse reactions of corticosteroids are closely related. The effects for which they are used include their antiinflammatory action and suppression of allergic reactions. They also suppress the immune response. Corticosteroids are palliative rather than curative. The glucocorticoid effects and the mineralocorticoid effects are listed below. Many of these effects produce adverse reactions and are discussed in the following section.

- *Glucocorticoid effects*
  - ◆ Broad
    Carbohydrate metabolism
    Antiinflammatory
    Antiallergenic
    Enzyme action
    Membrane function
    Nucleic acid synthesis
  - ◆ Specific
    Catabolic
    Increase gluconeogenesis
    Decrease glucose use
    Inhibit protein synthesis
    Increase protein catabolism
    Decrease growth
    Decrease bone density
    Decrease resistance to infection
- *Mineralocorticoid effects*
  - ◆ Increase sodium retention
  - ◆ Increase potassium loss
  - ◆ Edema and hypertension

ADVERSE REACTIONS

The adverse reactions of corticosteroids are proportional to the dosage, frequency and time of administration, and duration of treatment. With prolonged therapy and sufficiently high doses the following side effects occur.

Metabolic changes. Moon face (round), buffalo hump (fat deposited on back of the neck), truncal obesity, weight gain, and muscle wasting give patients the Cushing's syndrome appearance. Hyperglycemia (diabetes-like) may be aggravated or initiated, especially in prediabetic patients. More antidiabetic medication may be required.

Infections. Corticosteroids decrease resistance to infection. Because of their antiinflammatory action, they may also mask its symptoms. Patients taking long-term glucocorticoid therapy are given isoniazid, an antituberculosis agent, to prevent tuberculosis.

Central nervous system effects. Changes in behavior and personality, including euphoria (with increasing dose), agitation, psychoses, and depression (with decreasing dose), can occur.

Peptic ulcer. Because corticosteroids stimulate an increase in production of stomach acid and pepsin they may exacerbate peptic ulcers. Healing is impaired, and the ulcer may perforate.

Impaired wound healing and osteoporosis. The catabolic effects of steroids that result from impaired synthesis of college can impair wound healing. This same process can cause osteoporosis or impair growth in children. If the osteoporosis affects alveolar bone, it could result in tooth loss. Thinning bones can also result in fractures in patients on chronic steroids without trauma. Muscle wasting, bruising, and abdominal striae are other symptoms associated with catabolism.

Ophthalmic effects. Because corticosteroids can increase intraocular pressure, glaucoma may be exacerbated. Cataracts are also associated with steroids.

Electrolyte and fluid balance. Glucocorticoids that possess some mineralocorticoid action can produce sodium and water retention. Hypertension or congestive heart failure may be exacerbated. Hypokalemia may also result.

Adrenal crisis. With prolonged use, adrenal suppression can occur. If a very stressful situation arises, the adrenal gland cannot respond adequately. Symptoms of adrenal crisis include weakness, syncope, cardiovascular collapse, and death.

Dental effects. Oral tissue changes may occur in patients taking corticosteroids. Their mucosal surfaces heal more slowly, are more likely to have infection, and are more friable. With the use of oral steroid inhalers for asthma, oral candidiasis may result. This may be prevented by rinsing the mouth after inhaler use.

USES

MEDICAL USES

There are many conditions for which corticosteroids may be administered (Box 19-1). Patients with these conditions should be questioned concerning past use of systemic steroids.

BOX 19-1 CONDITIONS FOR WHICH CORTICOSTEROIDS MAY BE USED

If patient using steroids, patient may be at risk.

Corticosteroid abnormalities

Addison's disease (deficiency of steroids)
Cushing's disease (excess steroids)

Autoimmune diseases

Arthritis, rheumatoid
Collagen diseases
    Pemphigus vulgaris
    Psoriasis
    Systemic lupus erythematosus
    Scleroderma

Gastrointestinal disease

Chron's disease
Ulcerative colitis
Inflammatory bowel disease (IBD)

Others

Hematologic
Hypercalcemia
Organ transplants
With chemotherapy (antiemetic)
Asthma

Replacement. Patients with hypofunction of the adrenal cortex (Addison's disease) need replacement of glucocorticoid and mineralocorticoid activity. Usually, hydrocortisone is used to restore glucocorticoid activity and desoxycorticosterone is used to restore mineralocorticoid activity. Patients with a hyperfunctioning adrenal cortex (Cushing's syndrome) may have a majority of the gland removed surgically. In this case replacement therapy is needed.

Emergencies. Corticosteroids are used in emergency situations for the treatment of shock or adrenal crisis, as discussed in Chapter 23.

Inflammatory/allergic. The most extensive use of the corticosteroids in both medicine and dentistry is in the treatment of a wide variety of inflammatory and allergic conditions. These agents are not curative but merely ameliorate symptoms because of their antiinflammatory activity. Some conditions that have been treated with corticosteroids are rheumatoid arthritis, rheumatic fever, systemic lupus erythematosus, scleroderma, inflammation of the joints and soft tissues, acute bronchial asthma, severe and acute allergic reactions, and severe allergic dermatoses. Prednisone [PRED-ni-sone] is the most common corticosteroid used orally.

Topical corticosteroids are used for a variety of skin conditions, which involve various dermatoses or "irritations." The steroids can be divided into several classes depending on their relative maximum potency*—the least efficacious to the most efficacious and in between. An example of the weakest is hydrocortisone [hyedroe-KOR-ti-sone]), an example of an "in between" is triamcinolone [trye-am-SIN-oh-lone] acetonide, and an example of the most potent is

| Topical steroids |

*Using the strict definition of potency and efficacy, the term *potency* as used to refer to topical steroids is really efficacy.

augmented betamethasone [bay-ta-METH-a-sone] dipropionate). Fluocinonide [floo-oh-SIN-oh-nide] is classified as less potent.

DENTAL USES

Because of the adrenocorticosteroids' antiinflammatory action, they are administered topically, intraarticularly, or orally in several dental situations. Although the use of steroids in dentistry has had mixed success, double-blind controlled studies are needed to determine unequivocally their proper place in the therapeutic armamentarium.

Oral lesions. Systemically administered steroids are often effective in the treatment of oral lesions associated with noninfectious inflammatory diseases, including erythema multiforme, lichen planus, pemphigus, desquamative gingivitis, and benign mucous membrane pemphigoid. It is imperative that an infectious etiology, such as herpes, be ruled out.

Aphthous stomatitis. The evidence for the benefit of adrenocorticosteroids in the treatment of aphthous stomatitis seems clear. Triamcinolone acetonide (Kenalog in Orabase) has been advocated. Orabase is a mineral oil gel base that sticks to the oral mucosa forming a plasticlike surface. Other topical steroids, such as fluocinonide and fluocinolone [floo-oh-SIN-oh-lone], can be used topically.

Temporomandibular joint (TMJ). The TMJ affected with arthritis (inflammation) also responds to the systemic administration of steroids. If only this joint is affected, an intraarticular injection can often decrease the pain and improve the joint movement.

Uses in oral surgery.

The adrenocorticosteroids have been used in oral surgery

| Weigh pro vs. con |

to reduce postoperative edema, trismus, and pain. Although the decrease in edema with steroid use can be easily documented, the magnitude of the benefit must be weighed against the potential risk of infection and decreased healing. The safety and effectiveness of these agents have not been proved in controlled double-blind studies.

Pulp procedures. The adrenocorticosteroids have been used in pulp capping, pulpotomy procedures, and the control of hypersensitive cervical dentin. Their use in these situations is currently empirical or experimental.

CORTICOSTEROID PRODUCTS

Selected synthetic corticosteroids are arranged in Table 19-2 according to their duration of action—short, intermediate, and long. The relative antiinflammatory and salt-retaining activity and equivalent oral dose are given, with hydrocortisone arbitrarily assigned the value of 1 for each activity. The other agents are then given values in relation to those of hydrocortisone. For example, prednisone, with an antiinflammatory activity of 4, has 4 times as much antiinflammatory action as hydrocortisone. Therefore, only ¼ as much prednisone is required to produce the same effect produced by hydrocortisone. The mineralocorticoid, or salt-retaining, prop-

erties of the glucocorticoids are also compared with that of hydrocortisone. For example, triamcinolone does not increase salt retention, whereas hydrocortisone does.

Table 19-2 lists the equivalent oral dose in milligrams based on 20 mg of hydrocortisone, the amount normally secreted daily by an adult without stress. One can see that 0.75 mg of dexamethasone or 5 mg of prednisone is approximately equivalent to 20 mg of hydrocortisone.

DENTAL IMPLICATIONS

Box 19-2 summarizes the management of dental patients taking steroids. Because steroids suppress immune reaction, with chronic administration of steroids, infections are more likely to occur and healing is delayed. These factors are important in dental patients, especially if a surgical procedure is to be performed. Since the symptoms of infection may be masked, the wound site should be carefully examined.

ADVERSE REACTIONS

Gastrointestinal effects. Adrenocorticosteroids stimulate acid secretion; patients taking these agents should be given other ulcerogenic medications such as the salicylates or the nonsteroidal antiinflammatory agents with caution.

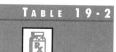

TABLE 19-2 **Selected Corticosteroids, Oral**

Group	Drug name	Activity		Equivalent oral dose (mg)
		Anti-inflammatory	Salt retention	
Short acting	Hydrocortisone (Cortisol)	1	1	20
	Prednisone (Deltasone)	4	0.3-0.5	5
	Methylprednisolone (Medrol)	5	0.3-0.5	4
Intermediate acting	Triamcinolone	5	0	4
	Prednisolone	4	0	5
Long acting	Dexamethasone	30	0	0.75
	Betamethasone	25	0	0.6-0.75

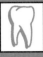

Box 19-2 MANAGEMENT OF DENTAL PATIENT TAKING/HAS TAKEN CORTICOSTEROIDS

Most dental patients taking steroids having normal dental treatment rendered DO NOT need additional corticosteroids. Supplemental steroids may be required if patient has severe dental fears or for major surgical procedures.

Precautions to avoid stress

Obtain good anesthesia
Check blood pressure
Provide postoperative analgesics (prn)

No supplementation

Stop using >1 year ago
Dose <20 mg/d HC or 5 mg/d prednisone
Dose >40 mg/d HC or 10 mg/d prednisone
Duration of therapy <1 mo
Every other day therapy
Topical use—rash, asthma inhaler, nose spray

May need supplementation

Dose 20-40 mg HC or 5-10 mg prednisone/d
Duration >2 wks
Topical (above) in very large doses or over entire body
If supplementing—different regimens
• Double normal dose morning of appointment
• Double normal dose the day before, the day of, and 2 days after (depends on stress/pain level) appointment

HC, Hydrocortisone.

Blood pressure. The blood pressure of patients taking corticosteroids should be measured, because these agents can exacerbate hypertension. The more mineralocorticoid action, the more likely the agent is to raise blood pressure.

Glaucoma. Other agents that can induce or exacerbate glaucoma, such as the anticholinergics, should be used with caution in patients taking adrenocorticosteroids.

Behavioral changes. A patient's bizarre behavior may be explained by the presence of, or withdrawal from, adrenocorticosteroids. Psychosis, euphoria, or depression might be seen.

Osteoporosis. Dental radiographs may demonstrate osteoporosis in patients taking long-term adrenocorticosteroids. More than 50% bone loss is required to observe osteoporosis (radiographically). These patients are more likely to suffer fractures either with or without trauma.

Infection. Because of the antiinflammatory activity of the adrenocorticosteroids, they may mask the symptoms of an infection. They decrease a patient's ability to fight infection by suppression of migration of polymorphonuclear leukocytes reducing lymph system action.

Delayed wound healing. Because the adrenocorticosteroids cause delayed wound healing, special precautions should be taken when surgical procedures are performed in the oral cavity. Friability of the tissue also requires special care when closing wounds and extra sutures may be required.

Adrenal crisis. The body releases corticosteroids and epinephrine from the adrenal gland when

Only with *severe stress*

people experience stress. Under normal conditions, when the body sends a message (ACTH) to the adrenal gland it is stimulated and secretes hydrocortisone. Because the adrenal gland of a normal person is regularly stimulated when the person experiences stress, the adrenal gland stays ready for a message to put out hydrocortisone. The body does not differentiate between the hydrocortisone (endogenous) it secretes and the hydrocortisone or prednisone (exogenous) given to a patient by any route. When a patient is taking chronic prednisone, the steroid provides negative feedback to the hypothalamus (reduces release of CRF) and the pituitary (reduces release of ACTH). With prolonged administration of steroids, suppression of the hypothalamic-pituitary-adrenal axis occurs. With suppression, the body does not quickly respond to stress with release of hydrocortisone. Suppression is proportional to the potency of the agent, the dose of the agent, and the duration of administration. The longer the duration, the higher the dose, and the greater the potency of the steroid, the quicker the suppression occurs. Once suppression occurs, it can take weeks or months for the adrenal gland to respond normally. Without the proper response to stress, adrenal crisis is possible. The crisis occurs because of a relative lack of corticosteroids during stress, such as a dental appointment for a patient with dental phobia. It may be necessary to administer adrenal steroids before a stressful dental procedure to prevent crisis. A consultation with the patient's physician is helpful. Generally, low and very high (mega) doses do not present problems; problems may occur with mid-range doses.

Periodontal disease. Steroids have actions that can contribute to periodontal disease. First, they interfere with the body's response to infection (inflammatory mediators are inhibited). Second, steroids can produce osteoporosis which may reduce the bony support for the teeth.

STEROID SUPPLEMENTATION

Maybe 5 to 10 mg prednisone/day

There are many ways of using supplemental steroids in patients who use chronic steroids and are to undergo a very stressful dental procedure. One approach to determine if additional steroids are needed is diagrammed in Figure 19-2. With both low (<20 mg hydrocortisone or 5 mg prednisone)

and very high doses (immunosuppressive; >40 to 60 mg hydrocortisone/day or 10 to 15 mg prednisone/day) no additional steroid supplementation is needed. With some intermediate doses of steroids (estimated to be between 20 to 40 mg/day hydrocortisone or 5 to 10 mg prednisone/day), additional steroids may be indicated if the procedure will produce severe stress. After consultation with the patient's physician, one suggested regimen is to administer 2 to 3 times the patient's usual daily dose of steroids the day of the procedure and 1 hour before the surgery or procedure. If pain is expected to persist into the next day, then 2 times the usual daily dose of steroids should also be given the following day. Some authors state that steroid supplementation is only needed if severe stress is expected (evaluate dental anxiety and dental procedure severity). The patient should be evaluated for likelihood to experience stress based on the patient's degree of anxiety, not the specific procedure planned. Administering additional steroids for 1 or 2 days poses no additional risk above that produced by chronic use of steroids.

RULE OF TWOS

The Rule of Twos is a *very* conservative approach and is *not* recommended. It states that adrenal suppression may occur if a patient is taking more than 20 mg of cortisone (or equivalent) daily, for 2 weeks within 2 years of dental treatment. Another suggestion includes doubling the dose of steroids for patients taking 20 to 40 mg of hydrocortisone (or equivalent) and giving the usual daily dose for patients taking more than 40 mg daily. Because a one-time increase in steroid dose produces no additional risk over the usual chronic doses, it may be better to err on the side of administering additional steroids.

TOPICAL USE

Steroids are used in dentistry to manage certain oral conditions, such as aphthous stomatitis, related to inflammatory or immune mechanisms.

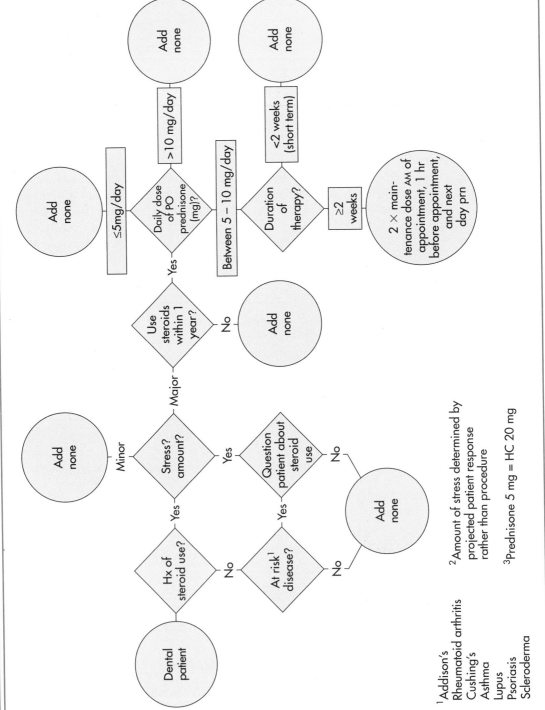

FIGURE 19-2   *Steroid decision tree.*

[1]Addison's
Rheumatoid arthritis
Cushing's
Asthma
Lupus
Psoriasis
Scleroderma

[2]Amount of stress determined by
projected patient response
rather than procedure

[3]Prednisone 5 mg = HC 20 mg

Both topical and systemic steroids are used in these instances (see Chapter 14). The relative potencies of selected topical glucocorticoids are listed in Table 19-1.

REVIEW QUESTIONS

1. Compare and contrast the activity of the glucocorticoids and mineralocorticoids.
2. Explain the relative salt-retaining, antiinflammatory, and topical activity of the steroids.
3. Describe the calculations used to determine relative potency.
4. List and explain the routes of administration for the steroids used in dentistry.
5. Enumerate the major pharmacologic effects and adverse reactions associated with the glucocorticoids.
6. Describe the three major uses of the steroids in medicine.
7. List the contraindications and cautions associated with the adrenocorticosteroids and explain how these adverse effects are related.
8. Describe how the adverse effects of the adrenocorticosteroids can be minimized or treated. Include the rationale for the administration of isoniazid and antacid.
9. Explain how to evaluate a patient undergoing steroid therapy and how to determine whether the patient's physician should be consulted. State what problems could arise from dental treatment and how these adverse effects could be monitored.
10. Compare and contrast the glucocorticoids available, and state the agent used for various dental conditions.
11. Define the terms *Cushing's syndrome* and *Addison's disease*.
12. Explain the relationship between hydrocortisone and prednisone in terms of the minimum dose of agents that can cause Cushing's syndrome. Explain what effect 100 mg of hydrocortisone or its equivalent can produce.
13. Describe the decision tree that determines whether a dental patient should receive supplemental steroids before a dental appointment. State the pertinent factors.

Other Hormones

CHAPTER OUTLINE

Hormones are secreted by **endocrine glands** and transported by the blood to target organs, where they are biologically active. Endocrine glands include the pituitary, thyroid, **parathyroids, pancreas,** adrenals, gonads, and placenta. They help maintain homeostasis by regulating body functions and are controlled themselves by feedback systems. In most of these systems, the hormone released has a negative feedback effect on the secretion of the hormone stimulating substance. Patients being treated in the dental office may be taking these hormones to treat various diseases.

Drugs that affect the endocrine system include the hormones secreted by the endocrine glands, synthetic hormone agonists and antagonists, and substances that influence the synthesis and secretion of hormones. The most important clinical application of these drugs is their use in replacement therapy, such as in the treatment of diabetes mellitus (insulin) and hypothyroidism (levothyroxine). Additional applications include diagnostic procedures, contraception, and the treatment of glandular hyperfunction, cancer, and other systemic disorders.

PITUITARY HORMONES

Pituitary = master gland

The pituitary gland (hypophysis) is a small endocrine organ located at the base of the brain. It has been called the "master gland" because of its regulatory effect on other endocrine glands and organs of the body. It secretes peptide hormones that regulate the thyroid, adrenal, and sex glands; the kidney and uterus; and growth.

In addition to their regulatory effect, the pituitary hormones have a trophic effect that is necessary for the maintenance of many systems. For example, without the gonadotropins, the entire reproductive system fails; without growth hormone and thyrotropin, normal growth and development are impossible.

The secretion of pituitary hormones is influenced by peripheral endocrine glands via hormonal feedback mechanisms and by neurohumoral substances from the hypothalamus. When the hypothalamus releases specific hormone-releasing substances, the specific pituitary hormone is released.

Pituitary deficiency (hypopituitarism) can produce a loss of secondary sex characteristics, decreased metabolism, dwarfism, diabetes insipidus, hypothyroidism, Addison's disease, loss of pigmentation, thinning and softening of the skin, decreased libido, and retarded dental development. Hypersecretion of pituitary hormones can produce sexual precocity, goiter, Cushing's disease, acromegaly, and giantism. There are two parts to the pituitary gland, the anterior lobe (adenohypophysis) and the posterior lobe (neurohypophysis).

ANTERIOR PITUITARY

The anterior lobe of the pituitary gland secretes growth hormone, or somatotropin; **luteinizing hormone** (LH);

Anterior pituitary—gland-stimulating hormones

follicle-stimulating hormone (FSH); thyroid-stimulating hormone (TSH), or thyrotropin; adrenocorticotropic hormone (ACTH), or corticotropin; and prolactin (Figure 20-1). β-Lipotropin, secreted by the pituitary, is a precursor to β-endorphin (see Chapter 9).

Genetic engineering has been able to produce human growth hormone since 1987. Human growth hormone is used medically to treat children who lack it and illicitly by body builders and weight lifters to develop muscles. [Some say that in athletic events at which the contestant's urine is tested, for example, the Olympics, growth hormone cannot be detected as easily as the androgenic steroids.]

Pharmaceutical gonadotropin-releasing hormone (GnRH) is a synthetic analogue. One

FIGURE 20-1 *Pituitary hormones. Hormones and actions are not all-inclusive.* ANT PIT, *Anterior pituitary;* POST PIT, *posterior pituitary;* GH, *growth hormone;* ACTH, *adrenocorticotropic hormone;* TSH, *thyroid-stimulating hormone;* FSH, *follicle-stimulating hormone;* LH, *luteinizing hormone;* PRO, *prolactin;* VAS, *vasopressin;* OXY, *oxytocin.*

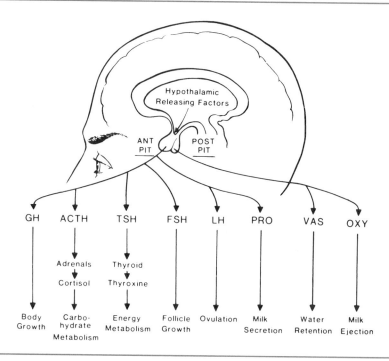

example, leuprolide, stimulates the pituitary function and is used to treat infertility. GnRH agonists are used to treat prostate cancer and endometriosis. The secretions from the anterior pituitary that stimulate other glands are used to test the function of the stimulated glands.

FSH-like products, which stimulate follicle growth, and LH-like products, which induce **ovulation,** are used in the treatment of infertility. Although LH itself is not available, human chorionic gonadotropin (hCG), which is almost identical in structure, can be used as an LH substitute for deficiency. Human menopausal gonadotropin (hMG) contains FSH and LH and is commercially available as menotropin (Pergo-

nal). This preparation is used in infertility to stimulate ovarian follicle development. When follicular maturation has occurred, the hMG is discontinued and hCG is given to induce ovulation. [Bang, septuplets!]

Bromocriptine. Bromocriptine [broe-moe-KRIP-teen] (Parlodel), an ergot derivative, inhibits pituitary function. Although not a hormone, it is a dopamine agonist that suppresses prolactin levels. It is used to treat prolactin-secreting adenomas producing (hyperprolactinemia), acromegaly, and Parkinson's disease. In the past it was used to dry up the milk in a woman who did not want to nurse. It is no longer used for this purpose.

POSTERIOR PITUITARY

Posterior—vasopressin/oxytocin

The posterior pituitary gland secretes two hormones: they are vasopressin (antidiuretic hormone [ADH]) and **oxytocin.** Vasopressin [vay-soe-PRES-in] (Pitressin) has vasopressor and antidiuretic hormone activity and is used for treatment of transient diabetes insipidus. Synthetic analogues of vasopressin (desmopressin [DDAVP, Stimate] and lypressin [Diapid]) are used for chronic treatment of pituitary diabetes insipidus and to treat certain clotting disorders (hemophilia A and von Willebrand's disease). Available as nasal solutions, these two analogues have the same action as vasopressin, but are longer acting.

Oxytocin [oks-i-TOE-sin] (Pitocin, Syntocinon) either by injection or intranasally, is used to induce labor, control postpartum hemorrhage, and induce postpartum lactation.

THYROID HORMONES

The thyroid gland secretes two iodine-containing thyroid hormones: triiodothyronine (T_3) and tetraiodothyronine (T_4, thyroxine). Calcitonin, another hormone secreted by the thyroid, regulates calcium metabolism. Thyroid hormones act on virtually every tissue and organ system of the body and are important for energy metabolism, growth, and development. Vulnerability to stress, altered drug response, and altered orofacial development are all possible manifestations of thyroid dysfunction. The head and neck examination performed by dental practitioners can identify some thyroid abnormalities. Swallowing can accentuate the thyroid to allow palpitation. The consistency of the gland varies with the abnormality.

Thyroid hormones are synthesized from iodine and tyrosine and stored as a complex protein until TSH stimulates their release. The actions of the thyroid hormones include those on growth and development, calorigenic effects, and metabolic effects. In frogs, thyroid hormone can transform a tadpole into a frog.

IODINE

Iodine deficiency—goiter

Normal function of the thyroid gland requires an adequate intake of iodine (approximately 50 to 125 mg per day). Without it, normal amounts of thyroid hormones cannot be made, TSH is secreted in excess, and the thyroid hypertrophies. This thyroid hypertrophy is called *simple* or *nontoxic* goiter. Because iodine is not abundant in most foods, simple goiter is quite prevalent in some areas of the world. Marine life is the only common food that is naturally rich in iodine. Use of iodized salt (contains potassium iodide [KI]) has decreased the incidence of simple goiter in many countries. Iodine is currently used in conjunction with an antithyroid drug in hyperthyroid patients preparing for surgery.

Iodide in high concentrations suppresses the thyroid in a still poorly understood manner. It may produce gingival pain, excessive salivation, and sialadenitis as side effects.

HYPOTHYROIDISM

↓ Thyroid: child = cretinism
adult = myxedema

In the small child, hypofunction of the thyroid is referred to as *cretinism*. In the adult this condition is called *myxedema* or *simple hypothyroidism.* The main characteristics are mental and physical retardation. Such patients are usually drowsy, weak, and listless and exhibit an expressionless, puffy face with edematous tongue and lips. Oral findings in children usually include delayed tooth eruption, malocclusion, and increased tendency to develop periodontal disease. The teeth are usually poorly shaped and carious.

The gingiva is either inflamed or pale and enlarged. The cretin is often uncooperative and difficult to motivate for plaque control. Diagnostic radiographs and routine dental prophylaxis in these patients may require special assistance.

Hypothyroid patients have difficulties withstanding stress and tend to be abnormally sensitive to all central nervous system (CNS) depressants, including the opioids and sedatives. If opioid analgesics are used, their dosages should be reduced. Hypothyroid pregnant women tend to produce offspring with large teeth.

Thyroid hypofunction is rationally and effectively treated by oral administration of exogenous thyroid hormones. The most common thyroid hormone used for replacement therapy is levothyroxine [lee-voe-thye-ROX-een]. Box 20-1 lists preparations used for thyroid **hormone replacement therapy.**

Box 20-1 Thyroid and Antithyroid Agents

Thyroid replacements

- Levothyroxine sodium (L-T_4) (Synthroid)
- Liothyronine sodium (L-T_3) (Cytomel)
- Liotrix (T_3 + T_4) (Euthroid, Thyrolar)
- Thyroglobulin (Proloid)
- Thyroid (Desiccated Thyroid, Armour Thyroid)

Antithyroid drugs

- Iodine
- Propylthiouracil (PTU)
- Methimazole (Tapazole)

HYPERTHYROIDISM

↑ Thyroid: Graves'
Plummer's
Hashimoto's

Diffuse toxic goiter (Graves' disease) and toxic nodular goiter (Plummer's disease) are the two forms of thyroid hyperfunction. Diffuse toxic goiter is characterized by a diffusely enlarged, highly vascular thyroid gland. It is common in young adults and is considered to be a disorder of the immune response. Toxic nodular goiter is characterized by nodules within the gland that spontaneously secrete excessive amounts of hormone while the rest of the glandular tissue is atrophied. It occurs primarily in older patients and usually arises from long-standing nontoxic goiter.

Hashimoto's disease, a chronic inflammation of the thyroid associated with an autoimmune response, produces hyperthyroidism. Antithyroglobulin antibody can be detected. It occurs in middle-age women and often occurs concomitantly with other autoimmune diseases.

Excessive levels of circulating thyroid hormone produce thyrotoxicosis. The adverse effects include excessive production of heat, increased sympathetic activity, increased neuromuscular activity, increased sensitivity to pain, ophthalmopathy, exophthalmos (protruding eyes), and anxiety. Oral manifestations include accelerated tooth eruption, marked loss of the alveolar process, diffuse demineralization of the jawbone, and rapidly progressing periodontal destruction.

The cardiovascular system is especially hyperactive because of a direct inotropic effect, increased peripheral oxygen consumption, and increased sensitivity to catecholamines. Epinephrine is relatively contraindicated in these patients. The potentiating effects of excess thyroid hormone and epinephrine on each other could result in cardiovascular problems, such as angina, arrhythmias, and hypertension. β-Blockers such as propanolol are used to counteract the tachycardia.

In addition to their increased sensitivity to pain, hyperthyroid persons have an increased tolerance to CNS depressants. They may require higher than usual doses of sedatives, analgesics, and local anesthetics.

No treatment should be begun for any patient with a visible goiter, exophthalmos, or a history of taking antithyroid drugs until approval is obtained from the patient's physician. Medical management of the condition is important before any elective surgery is performed. A surgical procedure or an acute oral infection could precipitate a crisis. Hydrocortisone should be administered IV and cold towels placed on the patient. The use of epinephrine should be avoided in poorly treated or untreated thyrotoxic patients. The cardiac dose of epinephrine can be used, carefully. Even in controlled patients who are considered to be euthyroid, stress should be kept at a minimum, preoperative sedation should be considered, and the dental team should be alert for signs of hypothyroidism or hyperthyroidism.

Treatment of hyperthyroidism usually includes one of the following:
Drugs
 • Iodide

 Antithyroid drugs
 • Radioactive iodine (iodine-131 [^{131}I])
   Partial thyroidectomy

The two most common treatments are ^{131}I and thyroidectomy. ^{131}I is usually the drug of choice for patients over 21 years old. It is taken internally and sequestered by the gland; localized destruction of thyroid tissue results. Thyroidectomy is the surgical approach to hyperthyroidism. Both radioactive iodine and thyroidectomy usually result in hypothyroidism because a dose that produces an inadequate effect would require repeating the procedure. If a patient has been adequately treated for hyperthyroidism either with radioactive iodine or thyroidectomy and is taking supplemental thyroid (prn), then that patient may be treated like a euthyroid patient.

Antithyroid agents. Antithyroid drugs, such as propylthiouracil (PTU) and methimazole (Tapazole), are used in patients who cannot tolerate surgery or treatment with ^{131}I. These drugs interfere directly with the synthesis of thyroid hormones by inhibiting the iodination of tyrosine moieties and the coupling of the iodotyrosines. Adverse reactions associated with PTU include fever, skin rash, and leukopenia. The most serious adverse reaction is agranulocytosis, which can lead to poor wound healing, oral ulcers or necrotic lesions, and oral infections. Paresthesia of facial areas and loss of taste are also seen. Not only are antithyroid drugs used over prolonged periods to bring a hyperactive thyroid to the euthyroid state but they are also given before thyroidectomy to reduce the possibility of thyroid storm, a life-threatening acute form of thyrotoxicosis.

Propranolol, a β-blocker, is often given concomitantly with antithyroid agents. The β-blocker prevents the tachycardia and tremors.

PANCREATIC HORMONES

Two primary hormones secreted by the islets of Langerhans of the pancreas are insulin and glucagon. Insulin promotes fuel storage [pack the bags—glucose out of blood], whereas glucagon promotes fuel mobilization [empty the bags—glucose into blood] in the body. Other hormones secreted by the pancreas are islet amyloid polypeptide (IAPP, amylin) and pancreatic peptide. Their functions have not yet been elucidated.

DIABETES MELLITUS

Diabetes mellitus (DM) is manifested by abnormal carbohydrate metabolism and inappropriate hyperglycemia. It is thought that the hyperglycemia leads to the many complications of diabetes. DM is currently classified (Table 20-1) as type I (insulin-dependent [IDDM]), type II (**non–insulin-dependent**

TABLE 20-1   Types I and II Diabetes

Properties	IDDM	NIDDM*
Synonym	Type I	Type II
Age of onset	Juvenile	Adult
Onset of symptoms	Acute	Gradual
Incidence	10%	90%
Etiology	Autoimmune reaction	Fat, sugar—pooped out pancrease
Genetics	Just a little	Quite a bit
Receptors	Normal	Defective
Plasma insulin	No	Normal or elevated then over time reduced
Ketoacidosis	Yes	No

IDDM, Insulin-dependent diabetes mellitus; *NIDDM*, non–insulin-dependent diabetes millitus.
*May still require insulin after the pancrease is "pooped out."

[NIDDM]), or type III (e.g., drug induced) diabetes.

Symptoms and complications result, usually from inadequate or poorly timed secretion of insulin from the pancreas, and/or insulin resistance of the cells. The new criteria for the diagnosis of DM is two consecutive fasting blood sugars of greater than 126 mg/dL. This will simplify the diagnosis of DM and add many patients to the ranks of people with diabetes.

> FBS > 126 mg/dL

Diabetes is primarily characterized by hyperglycemia and glycosuria. Other characteristics include hyperlipemia, azoturia, ketonemia, and, when the deficiency is severe, ketoacidosis. Patients usually experience general weakness, weight loss, polyphagia, polydipsia, and polyuria.

Types of diabetes

TYPE I Type I (previously called *juvenile-onset*) diabetes usually develops in persons younger than 30 years (juveniles) and results from an autoimmune destruction of the pancreatic β cells. There is some genetic predisposition to this immune response, but type II diabetes has a much greater genetic component. The type I autoimmune response may be in response to an infection, a slow virus, environmental insults, or some as yet unknown factor. It is associated with a complete lack of insulin secretion, increased glucagon secretion, rapid onset of disease, ketosis, and severe symptoms. Without insulin, type I DM is fatal. Type I must be treated with injections of insulin because the pancreas does not produce any insulin. Some oral agents may be combined with the insulin in patients with type I diabetes who have poor control of blood sugar.

TYPE II Type II (previously called *maturity-onset*) **diabetes** usually develops in persons older than 40 years. It is associated with the ability of the pancreas to secrete enough insulin to prevent ketoacidosis, but not enough to normalize plasma glucose. The insulin secreted does not reduce the glucose levels in the serum to normal levels. This problem may be due to some of the following:

1. β cells in the pancreas have a reduced or delayed response to glucose.
2. Secretion of insulin is delayed so that blood glucose levels are elevated.

3. Because cells in the body have insulin resistance (are not as sensitive to insulin as normal cells), more that the usual amount insulin is required to produce a response. An immune response is associated with the insulin resistance.

4. "Pooped out" pancreas (P^3) [a euphemism, of course]. Because of the delay in insulin secretion and insulin resistance, the insulin released from the pancreas does not effectively lower the blood sugar. The pancreas is working overtime secreting a lot of insulin, but without producing the desired results (decrease in blood sugar). Over time, the pancreas cannot continue to supply this increased production to keep up with the need for insulin. Either a relative (as a result of resistance) or absolute lack of insulin occurs.

5. Adipose tissue is "antiinsulin."

Because of prolonged hyperglycemia and resulting hyperinsulinemia, insulin resistance develops and the overworked pancreas gives out. Type II diabetes involves a slower onset of disease, less severe symptoms, and lack of ketoacidosis. Tissue insensitivity to insulin, a deficiency of the pancreas' response to glucose, and obesity results in impaired insulin action. In the presence of hyperglycemia, the resistance of the tissues to insulin and the impaired β cells' response are exaggerated. Normal serum glucose levels improve these parameters toward normal.

Type II diabetes is treated first with diet and exercise, then with orally acting agents and, if these modalities fail, with insulin. Therefore patients with type II diabetes may be taking insulin either with or without oral agents. Because of the etiology of the hyperglycemia in patients with type II diabetes, moderate improvement of the diet and/or an increase in exercise can produce a large improvement in the glucose levels. Exercise increases the sensitivity of the cells to insulin. Unfortunately, these behavior modifications are difficult to carry out on a routine basis for almost all patients.

Complications of diabetes. Uncontrolled diabetes produces a pronounced susceptibility to dental caries. This is caused mainly by decreased salivary flow (xerostomia) related to fluid loss. The loss is secondary to an increase in urination that occurs because of poor use of carbohydrates and the glucose that is excreted via the kidneys (water follows glucose). The complications of xerostomia are due to the lack of its normal functions: lubrication, cleansing, regulating pH, destroying microorganisms and their products, and maintaining the integrity of the oral structures. A dry, cracking oral mucosa with the presence of mucositis, ulcers, infections, and an inflamed painful tongue may result. Any change in glucose in saliva probably contributes little to the increased caries rate.

XEROSTOMIA The small increase (maybe) in parotid saliva glucose would appear to have little effect on the incidence of caries. In Finland, a recent study was conducted to determine the relationship between dental caries and NIDDM and its control. Over a 15-year period, 25 patients were monitored. The metabolic control of the diabetes was unrelated to dental caries. There was no increase in caries in NIDDM over control patients. A relationship was found between a reduction in salivary flow and an increase in dental caries. The most important risk factor was shown to be the best predictor of prevalence of caries.

DM mellitus can affect the dental development of children. Diabetic children have been shown to differ from normal children in the median ages at which they lose their deciduous teeth and gain their permanent teeth.

PERIODONTAL DISEASE Patients with uncontrolled or undiagnosed diabetes are more prone to periodontal disease. However, the periodontal status of the patient with well-controlled diabetes has been somewhat more controversial. Despite the fact that some investigators reported a lack of correlation between diabetes and increased periodontal disease, many other studies have resulted in the opposite conclusion. [My guess is that if control is very good, then there is hardly any effect, whereas if control is poor, then there is a greater effect.] In the population of Southwestern Native American over 35 years old, the incidence of type II diabetes is very high.

Periodontal findings include inflammatory and degenerative changes ranging from mild gingivitis to painful periodontitis with a widened periodontal ligament, multiple abscesses, putrescent exudates from periodontal pockets, and increased tooth mobility caused by destruction of supporting alveolar bone. Even though it may be more severe, diabetic periodontal disease appears to be similar to that found in nondiabetics. The diabetic state probably serves as a predisposing factor that can accelerate the periodontal destruction originated by microbial agents. The proposed etiology for the periodontal changes seen in the patient with diabetes includes microangiopathy of the tissues, thickening of capillary basement membranes, changes in glucose tolerance factor (more glucose), altered polymorphonuclear leukocyte function, and enhanced collagenase activity.

| AGE—accumulation partially accounts for complications |

AGEs Many of the complications that occur with diabetes are now thought to be produced by an accumulation of advanced glycation end-products (AGEs). When blood glucose is higher, there is an increase in AGEs. Collagen becomes crossed-linked under the influence of AGEs. Thickening of blood vessels is associated with elevated AGEs. The vessels of the eye, just like those of the retina and kidney, are thickened by AGEs.

Dental appointments should not interfere with meals and should involve minimal stress. In patients with controlled diabetes, oral surgical procedures should be performed 1.5 to 2 hours after the patient has eaten normal breakfast and taken regular antidiabetes medication. Following surgery, the patient should receive an adequate caloric intake to prevent hypoglycemia. With general anesthesia, patients are often kept NPO (nothing by mouth) and should take half of their usual dose of insulin and receive intravenous D_5W (5% glucose in distilled water).

Patients with diabetes have fragile blood vessels, delayed wound healing, and a tendency to develop infections; therefore surgical therapy should be approached with caution. Sealing and soft tissue curettage usually are tolerated well. The bulk of the literature suggests that prophylactic use of antibiotics should be avoided even though many practitioners routinely use antibiotics. If infection is present or if infection ensues, it should be aggressively treated. Measures to reduce the possibility of infection should be used (sterilize instruments, rinse mouth before procedures). The oral complications of diabetes are summarized in Table 20-2.

Cautions and contraindications. Drugs that may decrease insulin release or increase insulin requirements, such as epinephrine, glucocorticoids, or opioid analgesics, should be used with caution in patients with diabetes. Caution should also be exercised with general anesthetics because of the possibility of acidosis. If diabetes is in good control, then these drugs can be used.

Systemic complications of diabetes. The systemic complications of diabetes include actions affecting almost all the body tissues and organs.

CARDIOVASCULAR SYSTEM The incidence of cardiovascular problems is higher in patients with diabetes. Both macroangiopathy and microangiopathy, as well as hyperlipidemia, are common. Atherosclerosis is also more common in these patients.

RETINOPATHY Because microvascular disease affects the blood supply to the retina, the func-

▮ᴛᴀʙʟᴇ 20-2   Oral Complications of Diabetes Mellitus

Manifestation	Comment	Outcome
Xerostomia	Saliva lubricates, cleanses regulate acidity; has electrolytes, glycoproteins, antimicrobial enzymes	Increase in aries Problem with tasting Problem swallowing Wetting food difficult Problem with mastication Mucositis, ulcers, desquamation Painful tongue
Slightly elevated sugar	In parotid saliva	Not clinically significant
Caries rate	Some say less Some say more	Result of diabetic diet Glucose in saliva
Microvascular disease—small blood vessel disease	Less blood flow to oral cavity	Infection more difficult to treat (antibiotic can not reach site)
Altered immunity/white blood cell abnormality	Less ability to fight microorganisms	Get infections more easily Periapical abscesses Periodontal abscesses
Regulate acidity	Oral infection reduces DM control, need more insulin Oral infection after surgery	Infection treated, better insulin control (need less)
Neuropathy	From diabetes	Numbness, burning, tingling, pain in nerves
Infections	Candidiasis Mucormycosis	Fungal infections more likely
Symptoms	Burning mouth syndrome	Unknown cause
Delayed, impaired healing	With oral trauma	Collagen poorly formed

All complications worsen with hyperglycemia, either acute or chronic. Acute fasting glucose (mg/dL) measured by glucose monitor are reflective of glucose *at that moment,* and chronic glucose levels measured by HgA$_{1c}$ are reflective of glucose control *over the previous 2-3 months.*

Oral complications are xerostomia, infection, poor healing, increased caries, candidiasis, gingivitis, periodontal diseases, periapical abscess, and burning mouth syndrome.

---

tioning of the retina is impaired. In fact, diabetes is the major cause of blindness in adults.

Neuropathy Neuropathy is another complication of diabetes. It leads to reduced and sometimes absent feelings, especially in the lower extremities. A variety of sensations, including pain and burning, have been reported. The oral complaints of pain and discomfort related to the tongue and other oral structures are related to diabetic neuropathy. Drugs used to manage this problem include amitriptyline, carbamazepine, phenytoin, and capsaicin (made from hot peppers). The neurologic problems of diabetes can produce atony of the gastrointestinal tract (diabetic gastroparesis). Metoclopramide and cisapride are used to manage this complication.

Infections Gangrene can occur in the peripheral extremities, especially the feet and legs. This occurs because of the deficiencies of diabetes, depressed immunity, less effective white blood cells, microvascular changes (less blood), and neuropathy (can't feel the problem).

HEALING Slower healing must be taken into account so that precautions during surgery are taken. Related to this problem is the likelihood of infection, which exacerbates the healing problem.

Summary. A patient with diabetes has reduced blood flow to the feet because of microvascular disease and reduced sensation because of peripheral neuropathy. The patient has reduced ability to fight infection as a result of altered leukocyte chemotactic properties. The blood does not get to the extremities as easily, so even when antiinfective agents are present in the blood the antibiotics have difficulty reaching the site of action. Neuropathy occurs in the extremities, and these patients cannot easily feel their feet. Because there is lack of feeling, trauma or infections of the feet go unnoticed. Poor circulation, lack of feeling, and inability to fight infection lead to infection of extremities. Couple that with the fact that the patient with diabetes cannot see as well and the pathway to disaster becomes evident!

Amputations often begin with the toes, progress to ankles and knees, and finally result in amputation of the entire leg. At the same time, microvascular disease reduces the blood supply to the kidneys, producing an increase in protein loss in the urine. Additional reduction in renal function may require dialysis or a kidney transplant. Many of the dialysis beds are filled with patients with diabetes.

Effect of drugs on complications of diabetes. The
Diabetes Control and Complications Trial (DCCT)[2] was a randomized, controlled clinical trial conducted at 26 centers, primarily in the United States. The intensive intervention included additional interactions with a health care provider. Data were collected from patient notifications of events and from quarterly interviews. The 1441 volunteers had IDDM for 1 to 15 years. The average length of follow-up was 6.5 years. Subjects were randomly assigned to conventional or intensive diabetes treatment. Intensive therapy included three or more insulin injections daily or a continuous subcutaneous infusion of insulin (insulin pump) guided by four or more glucose tests per day. Conventional therapy included one or two insulin injections daily. This study demonstrated that intensive treatment of patients with IDDM can substantially reduce the onset and progression of diabetic retinopathy, nephropathy, and neuropathy. The major risk associated with the intensive treatment is recurrent hypoglycemia that was 3 times higher than those with conventional therapy. Another disadvantage was that the intensive therapy resulted in a larger gain in weight.

Comparing the intensive therapy with traditional therapy resulted in both "good news" and "bad news:"

- Good news: The complications of diabetes were decreased or delayed in onset of effect (60% reduction!).
- Bad news: The risk of hypoglycemia increased 3 times, and the increase in weight gain tended to be greater.

Evaluation of the dental patient with diabetes.
Asking a patient "How well is your diabetes controlled" does not often produce useable information. In my experience the answer patients give to this question does not relate to the actual control of the patient's diabetes. Some questions for the patient that might provide useful information are "What numbers have you been getting for your blood sugar? What was your test this morning? When did you last test your blood glucose? What were the results?" No matter what the number is, do not be judgmental.

Both the oral and systemic complications of diabetes are exacerbated by poor glucose control. There are two laboratory tests useful to evaluate a patient's glucose control: serum glucose and glycosylated hemoglobin (Table 20-3). Serum glucose is a measure of the patient's glu-

TABLE 20-3   Test Results for Average and Diabetic Patient

	NORMAL	GOAL	TAKE ACTION
Fasting plasma glucose (mg/dL)	<115	80-120	<80/>140
Glycosylated hemoglobin (HbA$_{1c}$)(%)	<6	<7	>8

cose control *at the time that the blood is sampled*. It does not reflect the patient's overall glucose control. The second test is the glycosylated hemoglobin (HbA$_{1c}$). Because this test reflects the glucose control over a 2- to 3-month period, it more accurately measures the patient's overall serum glucose control. Of course, a relationship exists between all the blood glucose levels and the glycosylated hemoglobin.

Treatment of hypoglycemia. Prevent hypoglycemia by remembering that "An ounce of prevention is worth a pound of cure." It is very easy to question patients concerning their insulin use and dietary intake. The treatment of hypoglycemia depends on whether a patient retains the swallowing reflex. In the early stages, when the patient is awake, the treatment consists of any of the following: fruit juice, cake icing, glucose gel, or soluble carbohydrates. If the patient is unconscious and lacks a swallowing reflex, treatment consists of intravenous dextrose (50%). Intravenous glucose fluids can be given, as well as glucagon. Since changes in behavior and in vital signs occurs with hypoglycemia, dental teams should be able to use an oral product to manage their hypoglycemic patients. One of these items should be readily available in the dental office for emergencies.

Clinically, it is often difficult to distinguish an insulin reaction—hypoglycemia (low glucose) from hyperglycemia (high glucose). It is useful to give a patient sugar for two reasons. First, the small amount of sugar used to treat hypoglycemia will produce little additional harm if hyperglycemia is present. Second, the dental office is not equipped to treat hyperglycemia. Insulin should not be administered in a dental office emergency; the patient should be immediately taken to a hospital emergency room.

Drugs used to manage diabetes

INSULINS Insulin [IN-su-lin] is usually administered by subcutaneous injection because its large molecular size prevents it from being absorbed from the gastrointestinal tract. The major difference among the currently used types of insulin is their duration of action. The older preparations were prepared from beef or pork pancreases, but human insulin is now used exclusively. Human insulin is produced by two different processes: through recombinant DNA synthesis and by modifying porcine (pig) insulin. Both compounds are identical to the human insulin secreted by people. Recombinant deoxyribonucleic acid (DNA) synthesis produces human insulin by gene splicing carried out by *Escherichia coli*. The processing of pork insulin involves transpeptidation of the pork insulin until it is the same as human insulin. Pig insulin has only two amino acids that are different from those in human insulin.

Table 20-4 lists insulin preparations, their peak effect, and their duration of action. The most common insulins used in clinical practice are human regular and NPH* (isophane insulin suspension) insulin (Figure 20-2). Lispro, a new insulin, is made by exchanging two amino acids in the structure of human insulin. This change results in an insulin with a faster onset of action. The use of lispro insulin to obtain tighter con-

---

NPH, Neutral protein Hagedorn.

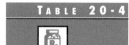

TABLE 20-4 **Insulin Preparations**

Action	Preparation	Onset (hr)	Peak (hr)	Duration (hr)
Rapid	Insulin injection (Novolin R*, Humulin R*)	0.5-1	5-10	18-12
	Prompt insulin zinc suspension (Semilente)	0.5-1.5	5-10	12-16
	Insulin lispro (Humalog)	0.25	0.25-1.25	6-8
Intermediate	Isophane insulin suspension (NPH, Humulin N†, Insulatard NPH*, Novolin N†)	1-1.5	4-12	24
	Insulin zinc suspension (Lente, Humulin L‡)	1-2.5	7-15	24
Long	Protamine zinc insulin suspension (PZI)	4-8	14-20	36
	Insulin-zinc suspension, extended (Ultralente, Humulin U§ Ultralente)	4-8	16-18	>36
Mixed	Isophane insulin suspension and insulin injection (Humulin 70/30†, Mixtard)	1	4-8	24

*R = regular
†70% NPH, 30% regular.

FIGURE 20-2 *Serum levels of insulin and its effect on plasma glucose (milligrams per deciliter) levels.*

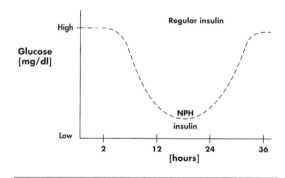

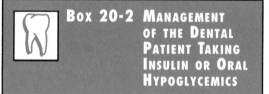

BOX 20-2 MANAGEMENT OF THE DENTAL PATIENT TAKING INSULIN OR ORAL HYPOGLYCEMICS

- Hypoglycemia—Question patient regarding last meal ingested.
- Infection more likely—Monitor closely and give antibiotics if needed (treat aggressively).
- Healing prolonged—Follow patient with any surgical procedure.
- Drug interactions—Large doses of salicylates may produce hypoglycemia.
- Appoint patient in morning after breakfast and insulin or oral hypoglycemic agent.
- Provide quick glucose source for hypoglycemia (cake icing).
- Check for oral complications related to diabetes.
- Ask patient what the results of their blood glucose monitoring has been (if checked).

trol of blood glucose is being used in highly motivated patients.

ADVERSE REACTIONS The most common adverse reaction associated with insulin is hypoglycemia.

The dental health care worker should be most concerned about a hypoglycemic reaction (Box 20-2) in the diabetic dental patient on insulin. This can be caused by an unintentional insulin overdosage (insulin shock), failure to eat, or increased exercise or stress. Symptoms that can be explained by an increased release of epinephrine from the adrenals include sweating, weakness, nausea, and tachycardia. Symptoms caused by glucose deprivation of the brain include head-ache, blurred vision, mental confusion, incoherent speech, and, eventually, coma, convulsions, and death.

Another side effect associated with insulin is an allergic reaction, usually caused by noninsulin contaminants. Lipodystrophy at the injection site produces atrophy of the subcutaneous fatty tissue. The incidence of these reactions has decreased because the newer insulin preparations are purer.

Oral antidiabetic agents. There are currently four groups of oral agents used to treat diabetes, referred to as *oral antidiabetics*. Each group works by a different mechanism and has a different adverse reaction profile. The oldest group of oral antidiabetic agents, the sulfonylureas, are also known as *oral hypoglycemic agents*. The other three groups are more precisely referred to as the *antihyperglycemic agents* because they lower an elevated blood sugar but do not produce hypoglycemia by themselves.

SULFONYLUREAS For many years, the sulfonylureas (Table 20-5) were the only orally active agents used to manage diabetes. There are

three major groups: first-generation, second-generation, and third-generation sulfonylureas. Their actions are similar, but the second-generation agents are more potent than the first-generation agents, so their doses are smaller. Glyburide, one of the most commonly used oral sulfonylureas, is discussed as the prototype.

The mechanism of action of the sulfonylureas includes stimulation of the release of insulin from the β cells of the pancreas, reduction of glucose from the liver, reduction in serum glucagon levels, and increasing the sensitivity of the target tissues to insulin (probably secondary to reduced hyperglycemia).

Sulfonylureas are indicated for the treatment of patients with NIDDM who cannot be treated with diet and exercise alone and/or who are unable or unwilling to take insulin. These agents are most often used in patients older than 50 years of age.

Adverse reactions of the sulfonylureas include blood dyscrasias, gastrointestinal disturbances, cutaneous reactions, and liver damage. Because sulfonylureas are used only to treat type II diabetes, the likelihood of hypoglycemia is much less than in patients with either type I or II diabetes who are using insulin.

TABLE 20-5 Antidiabetic Agents—Sulfonylureas

Drug	Total Daily Dose; How Divided (mg)	$T_{1/2}$ (hrs)	Onset (hr)	Peak (hr)	Duration (hr)
FIRST GENERATION					
Acetohexamide (Dymelor)	250-1500 bid	6-8*	1	1.5-2 [2-6]†	12-24
Chlorpropamide (Diabinese)	100-500 qd	36	1	2-4	up to 60
Tolazamide (Tolinase)	100-1000 qd or bid	7	4-6	3-4	12-24
Tolbutamide (Orinase)	500-2000 bid	4.5-6.5	1	3-4	6-10
SECOND GENERATION					
Glyburide (DiaBeta, Micronase) = nonmicronized	1.25-20 qd or bid	6-10	2-4	3.4-4.5	12-24
Glyburide (Glynase PresTab) = micronized	0.75-12 qd or bid	4	1	2.3-3.5	24
Glipizide (Glucotrol)‡	2.5-40 qd or bid	2-4	1-1.5	1-3	10-24
Glipizide (Glucotrol-XL)‡	5-10 qd	2-4	—	6-12	24
Glimepiride (Amaryl)	1-4 qd	2-4	0.5-1.5	2-3	12-24

*Parent drug and metabolite.
†$t_{1/2}$ of metabolite.
‡Take ½ hour before meals.

Aspirin can interact with the sulfonylureas, producing a decrease in serum glucose levels. This is not clinically significant unless the diabetic patient is especially brittle. Table 20-5 lists the first generation and second generation sulfonylureas, their average daily dose, and their duration of action. Tolbutamide [tole-BYOO-ta-mide] is an older first-generation sulfonylurea that was once popular, but most patients currently take a second-generation sulfonylurea.

The first line of treatment of type II diabetes usually involves a sulfonylurea or a biguanide. These two agents can be used together to lower the blood level more than either one individually.

In addition to the biguanides, there are two other new antihyperglycemic* drug groups that have become available for the management of diabetes. It has been suggested that rather than being called *oral hypoglycemic agents* they should be called *euglycemic agents.* They work to lower blood glucose and glycosylated hemoglobin by different mechanisms. In some instances, combining agents from more than one group can produce a greater reduction in blood glucose than either agent used alone. Table 20-6 lists some properties of these three groups of antihyperglycemic agents.

BIGUANIDES Metformin [met-FOR-min] (Glucophage) is a member of the biguanide group. It lowers blood glucose but used alone does not produce hypoglycemia. The action of metformin involves inhibiting the production of glucose from the liver by reducing hepatic gluconeogenesis. Other proposed mechanisms of action include stimulation of glycolysis, slowing of glucose absorption from the gastrointestinal

tract, and reduction of plasma glucagon levels. Other hypotheses include decreasing production and increasing uptake of insulin, potentiating the effects of insulin, increasing peripheral glucose uptake and utilization; increasing sensitivity at receptor and postreceptor binding sites, increasing glucose uptake, increasing hepatic glycogen stores, decreasing intestinal glucose absorption, and reducing fatty acid oxidation and acetyl CoA formation (through noninsulin mechanism).

Metformin may be used alone, in combination with a sulfonylurea, or with insulin for management of type II diabetes.

Adverse reactions of metformin are primarily related to the gastrointestinal tract (30%) and include anorexia, dyspepsia, flatulence, nausea, and vomiting. It can produce headache and interfere with B_{12} absorption. It accumulates in renal and hepatic impairment. Lactic acidosis, its most serious side effect, is rare. Predisposing factors to lactic acidosis include alcoholism, binge drinking, and renal or hepatic dysfunction. Metformin is contraindicated in patients with these conditions, or who are fasting, because they predispose a patient to lactic acidosis. Oral manifestations include a metallic taste. The dose ranges from 500 mg to 2550 mg divided into 2 or 3 daily doses.

α-Glucosidase inhibitors. Acarbose (Precose) is an α-glucosidase inhibitor. Simply, it slows the breakdown of ingested fat so that postprandial hyperglycemia is reduced. It is a competitive, reversible inhibitor of gastrointestinal tract enzymes—intestinal α-glucosidase and pancreatic α-amylase. The intestinal glucosidases hydrolyze saccharides to glucose or other monosaccharides that can be absorbed. The pancreatic amylase hydrolyzes complex starches to oligosaccharides in the intestine. By inhibiting these enzymes, glucose availability and therefore absorption are delayed and postprandial hyperglycemia is lowered. The result is that the blood levels of both glucose and glycosylated

---

Antihyperglycemic refers to agents that prevent an elevation in the blood glucose, whereas *hypoglycemic* refers to agents that lower blood glucose (sometimes grouped with sulfonylureas as oral hypoglycemic agents). Note that the former does not produce hypoglycemia, whereas the latter may.

TABLE 20-6 Oral Antidiabetic Agents (*Not* Sulfonylureas)

Drug	Dose (mg)	Mechanism	Adverse Reactions	Oral/DDI	ADME* (hr)	Comments
BIGUANIDES						
Metformin (Glucophage)	500/850 bid-tid; max 2550	Decreases production of insulin; ↑ effects of insulin†	GI (30% increase): anorexia, dyspepsia, flatulence, nausea, vomiting. CNS: headache; lactic acidosis (serious), interferes with B_{12} absorption; accumulates with renal and hepatic impairment	Metallic taste. DI-EtOH acute/chronic, elevates lactate concentration, especially without food	Peak 2 hr, $t_{1/2}$: 18	With or without sulfonylureas, increases effect of sulfonylureas 20%
α-GLUCOSIDASE INHIBITORS						
Acarbose (Precose)	50 tid with first bite of meal	Delays digestion (breakdown) of ingested carbohydrate so delays glucose absorption‡ producing a smaller rise in BG	GI: abdominal pain, flatulence (77%) diarrhea, pain		Not metabolized	Alone and with sulfonylureas
Miglitol (Glyset)	50-100 tid	Same as above	GI: flatulence (42%), diarrhea, abdominal pain, PGB, no hypoglycemia alone	No dental drug interactions	Peak 2-3, $t_{1/2}$: 2. No metabolites	
GLITAZONES						
Troglitazone (Rezulin)	400-600 mg qd, with food (increases absorption)	Decreases insulin resistance, improves insulin sensitivity	Induces and inhibits P450 3A4, decreases Hgb, decreases Hct, LFT changes		Peak 2-3. $t_{1/2}$ 16-34; food ↑ absorption 50%	Type II on insulin >30 U/day in multiple injections, and HgA_{1c} >8.5%

*$t_{1/2}$, Peak, duration (hr).

†Does not stimulate pancreatic β cells, decreases hepatic glucose production, increases peripheral glucose uptake and utilization; increases sensitivity at receptor and post-receptor binding sites, increases glucose uptake, increases hepatic glycogen stores, decreases intestinal glucose absorption, reduces fatty acid oxidation and acetyl CoA formation (through non-insulin mechanism).

‡Does not produce hypoglycemia alone, reduces the insulinotropic and weight-increasing effects of sulfonylureas.

BG, Blood glucose; *CNS,* central nervous system; *GI,* gastrointestinal; *LFT,* liver function test.

hemoglobin decrease. This agent is not effective in patients on a low fat diet. (This drug is saving us from ourselves.) The patient's dose of insulin can sometimes be decreased.

Acarbose can be used alone or with other agents, including insulin, sulfonylureas, and biguanides. Both IDDM and NIDDM can benefit from use of acarbose, but it is not effective in all patients. It is slightly less effective than either biguanides or sulfonylureas. Its major adverse effect is flatulence (77%), which is produced by bacteria acting on the undigested carbohydrates and producing gas. Other gastrointestinal tract adverse reactions include diarrhea, abdominal pain, and distension. These effects are often tolerated if the dose of the drug is increased slowly and after using the drug for sometime. Anemia and elevated transaminase levels have been reported. The dose of acarbose is 50 to 100 mg 2 or 3 times daily, given with the first bite of food. New α-glucosidase inhibitors are being developed and released (see Table 20-6).

Whether these agents will catch on for use in diabetics is unknown, but the gastrointestinal tract adverse reactions may limit their widespread use.

Thiazolidinediones.

Reduces insulin resistance

The drug troglitazone [TROE-gli-to-zone] (Rezulin) is the first member of a new class of antihyperglycemic agents, the thiazolidinediones, that reduce insulin resistance and improve insulin sensitivity. Blood sugar is lowered by decreasing hepatic glucose output and increasing glucose uptake by skeletal muscle.

Troglitazone's unique mechanism of action is dependent on the presence of insulin. Troglitazone decreases hepatic glucose output and increases insulin-dependent glucose disposal in skeletal muscle and possibly liver and adipose tissue. Unlike sulfonylureas, troglitazone does not produce an increase in insulin secretion.

Troglitazone is indicated in the treatment of patients with type II diabetes currently on insulin who have been inadequately controlled (HbA 1C > 8.5%) although using more than 30 units of insulin per day. Administering troglitazone to patients with type II diabetes who are using insulin has resulted in a decrease in the HbA_{1c}, leading to a decrease in the insulin dose and number of daily injections. Some patients (15%) were even able to discontinue using insulin.

Troglitazone's absorption is increased 30% to 85% by ingestion with food, so it is taken with food. The maximum serum level is achieved in 2 to 3 hours. Troglitazone is metabolized to several metabolites with varying actions; 85% is excreted in the feces. It inhibits hepatic microsomal isoenzymes CYP 3A4, 2C9, and 2C19 (a total of seven isoenzymes are affected, so before prescribing drugs metabolized by these isoenzymes, check for significant drug interactions). Its half-life is 16 to 34 hours, so steady state is reached within a few days.

Adverse reactions associated with troglitazone were similar to those with placebo. It decreases blood glucose and **hematocrit** and can produce LFT changes. It was removed from the market in Europe because of the LFT changes. Used with insulin, troglitazone can produce hypoglycemia.

Glucagon.
Glucagon is a polypeptide hormone produced by the α cells of the pancreas. It increases liver glycogenolysis by stimulating cyclic AMP synthesis and increasing phosphorylase kinase activity. It increases the breakdown of glycogen to glucose, elevating blood glucose.

Glucagon stimulates hepatic gluconeogenesis by promoting the uptake of amino acids and converting them to glucose precursors. Lipolysis in the liver and adipose tissue is enhanced (via adenyl cyclase activation), liberating free fatty acids and glycerol to further stimulate ketogenesis and gluconeogenesis.

Glucagon's role is as an antagonist to insulin. Higher levels of glucagon are present in the blood of patients with diabetes, even when normal blood glucose levels are maintained. Glucagon may be used parenterally for the emergency treatment of hypoglycemia, but glucose is usually preferred.

FEMALE SEX HORMONES

There are both male and female sex hormones. However, most sex hormones occur in both sexes but in different proportions.

The two major female sex hormones are the estrogens [ES-troe-jenz] and progestins [proe-JES-tins] (e.g., **progesterone** [proe-JES-te-rone]). Products containing these hormones are listed in Table 20-7. They are secreted primarily by the **ovaries** but also by the testes and placenta. They are largely responsible for producing the female sex characteristics, developing the reproductive system, and preparing the reproductive system for conception.

Estrogen and progesterone levels vary daily. These changes are dependent on the pituitary gonadotropic hormones FSH and LH. The interrelationship among these hormones during the female sexual cycle is as follows: On day 1 of an average 28-day cycle, when the menstrual flow begins, the secretions of FSH and LH begin to increase. This release is caused by a reduction in the blood levels of estrogen and progesterone, which normally inhibit their release. In response to increased FSH, an ovarian egg matures, and the follicle in which it is contained grows in size and begins to produce and secrete estrogen. For reasons not entirely understood, on approximately day 12 the rate of secretion of FSH and LH increases markedly to cause a rapid swelling of the follicle that culminates in ovulation on day 14.

Following ovulation, LH causes the secretory cells of the follicle to develop into a corpus luteum that secretes large quantities of estrogen and progesterone. This causes a feedback de-

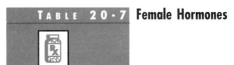

TABLE 20-7 Female Hormones

HORMONES	EQUIVALENT DOSE
ESTROGENS	
Conjugated estrogens (Premarin)	0.3-1.25 mg/d
Esterified estrogens (Estratab, Menest)	0.3-1.25 mg/d
Estradiol transdermal system (Estraderm)	Patch 0.025-0.1 mg/d
Estradiol (Estrace, Estraderm)	Patch 0.1 mg/d
Ethinyl estradiol (Estinyl)	0.025-0.05 mg/d
Diethylstilbestrol (DES)	0.25-0.5 mg/wk
PROGESTINS	
Medroxyprogesterone	2.5-10 mg
Contraceptive progestins	
Parenteral	
Depo-Provera: IM	150 mg q 3 mo
Norplant: implant	36 mg
Minipills	0.35 mg
Norethindrone (Micronor)	0.075 mg
Norgestrel (Ovrette)	

crease in the secretion of both FSH and LH. On approximately day 26, the corpus luteum completely degenerates. The resultant decrease in estrogen and progesterone leads to menstruation and increased release of FSH and LH. The FSH initiates growth of new follicles to begin a new cycle.

ESTROGENS

In addition to their role in the female sexual cycle, estrogens are largely responsible for the changes that take place at puberty in girls. They promote the growth and development of the vagina, uterus, fallopian tubes, breasts, and axillary and pubic hair. They increase the deposition of fat in subcutaneous tissues and increase the retention of salt and water. They also cause increased osteoblastic activity and early fusion of the epiphyses.

The most potent endogenous estrogen is 17β-estradiol. The liver readily oxidizes it to estrone, which in turn can be hydrated to estriol. Because synthetic estrogens can be administered orally, they are used for therapy and contracep-

██ **T**ABLE **2 0 - 8** **Oral Contraceptive Ingredients**		
ORAL CONTRACEPTIVE NAME(S)	ESTROGEN	PROGESTIN
Genora 1/50, Norinyl 1/50, Ortho-Novum 1/50	Mestranol	Norethindrone
Desogen, Ortho-Cept	Ethinyl estradiol	Desogestrel
Demulen 1/35, 1/50; Zovia 1/35	Ethinyl estradiol	Ethynodiol
Levlen, Tri-Levlen, Levora, Nordette, Triphasil	Ethinyl estradiol	Levonorgestrel
Brevicon; Loestrin 1/20, 1.5/30; Modicon; Ovcon 35/50; Tri-Norinyl; Genora 1/35, Norinyl 1/35, Ortho-Novum 1/35	Ethinyl estradiol	Norethindrone
Ortho-Cyclen, Ortho-Tri-Cyclen	Ethinyl estradiol	Norgestimate
Lo/Ovral, Ovral	Ethinyl estradiol	Norgestrel

tion. Table 20-8 lists some estrogens and progestins used for birth control.

In addition to their presence in oral contraceptives, estrogens are used to treat menstrual disturbances (dysmenorrhea, dysfunctional uterine bleeding), osteoporosis, atrophic vaginitis, nondevelopment of the ovaries, hirsutism, cancer, and symptoms of **menopause** (particularly vasomotor instability [hot flashes and night sweats]). Estradiol transdermal system (Estraderm) is applied to the skin twice a week to treat the vasomotor symptoms of menopause.

In the past, diethylstilbestrol (DES) was used as a postcoital or "morning-after" pill. Currently, 2 tablets of norgestrel (nor-JES-trel] (Ovral) every 12 hours for 2 doses are used in place of DES. These preparations have side effects but are useful in emergencies such as after cases of rape or incest.

The most common side effects of estrogen therapy are nausea and vomiting. With continued treatment, tolerance develops and these symptoms usually disappear. Other side effects include uterine bleeding, vaginal discharge, edema, thrombophlebitis, weight gain, and hypertension. Estrogen therapy may also promote endometrial carcinoma in postmenopausal women. This risk may be cancelled out by administration of a progestin (e.g., medroxyprogesterone [Provera]) for the last 10 days of the cycle. A small increase in risk of breast cancer has been demonstrated, but the unusual form is more easily "cured" than the usual breast cancer. The incidence of vaginal and cervical carcinoma has been shown to increase in the female offspring of women given DES.

Effect on oral tissues. Estrogens influence the gingival tissues. For example, changes in sex hormone levels during the life of the female are related to the development of gingivitis at puberty (puberty gingivitis), during pregnancy (pregnancy gingivitis), and after menopause (chronic desquamative gingivitis). Conscientious plaque control helps to minimize these conditions. The increase in gingival inflammation may occur even with a decrease in the amount of plaque. This may be a result of increased levels of prostaglandin E (PGE), estradiol, and progesterone in the saliva.

Other side effects of estrogens are discussed in the section on oral contraceptives.

PROGESTINS

The corpus luteum is the primary source of progesterone during the normal female sexual cycle. Progesterone promotes secretory changes in the endometrium and prepares the uterus for implantation of the fertilized ovum. If implantation does not occur by the end of the menstrual cycle, progesterone secretion declines, and the onset of menstruation occurs. If implantation takes place, the developing trophoblast secretes chorionic gonadotropin, which sustains the corpus luteum, thus maintaining progesterone and estrogen levels and preventing menstruation. Other effects of progesterone include suppression of uterine contractility, proliferation of the acini of the mammary gland, and alteration of transplantation immunity to prevent immunologic rejection of the fetus.

Medroxyprogesterone [me-DROKS-ee-proe-JESS-ter-one] (Provera), a progestin, is used orally by postmenopausal women in conjunction with estrogens. It prevents the increase in the risk of uterine cancer that can occur with unopposed estrogen. Women who have had a hysterectomy do not need to take medroxyprogesterone with estrogens.

Progestins alone are used in a variety of dosage forms. Parenteral medroxyprogesterone (Depo-Provera) is administered every 3 months as a contraceptive. Progestin-only **"minipills"** (see Table 20-7) are used orally for contraception in patients in whom estrogens are contraindicated. They must be taken each day of the month and are slightly less effective than the combination oral contraceptive products. They are very infrequently used.

A progestational agent can be administered in the form of an **intrauterine device (IUD)** impregnated with a progestational agent (Progestasert) or an implant placed under the skin on the arm (levonorgestrel [Norplant]). Norplant provides contraception for at least 5 years. These implants can produce prolonged, spotty, and irregular bleeding, or amenorrhea; however, many women find them convenient and problem free. The problem with Norplant seems to be that removing the five containers in which the drug was contained has proved very difficult.

The primary use of the progestins is as one of the ingredients in almost all oral contraception combinations. The second most common use is in combination with estrogen for postmenopausal women. Other uses of the progestational agents include the treatment of endometriosis, dysmenorrhea, dysfunctional uterine bleeding, and premenstrual tension.

ORAL CONTRACEPTIVES

Oral contraceptives consist of estrogens and progestins, in various combinations. These are the most common birth control pills and are more than 99% effective (if patient compliance is perfect). Preparations that contain a progestin alone (the minipill) are slightly less effective and produce less regular menstrual cycles, but do not have most of the side effects of the estrogen contained in the combination preparation (Box 20-3).

The compounds most commonly found in oral contraceptives are the estrogens, ethinyl estradiol and mestranol, and the progestins norgestrel, norethindrone, and norethynodrel. The combination type of oral contraceptive is taken for 21 days of each month. With a 28-day pack, the 7 pills in the fourth week contain no active ingredient, but remind the patient to take a pill every day. After the third week, the menstrual cycle occurs. At least three different formulations exist: the fixed combination, the biphasic (two different strengths of tablets), and the triphasic (three different types of tablets with varying amounts of the estrogenic and progestogenic component). The biphasic and triphasic agents are said to mimic the "natural" hormones more closely. No documented advantage has been demonstrated between these three combinations.

Oral contraceptives interfere with fertility by inhibiting the release of FSH and LH and therefore preventing ovulation. Early follicular FSH and midcycle FSH and LH increases are not seen. In addition, these contraceptive agents interfere with impregnation by altering the endometrium and the secretions of the cervix.

The side effects associated with oral contraceptives include increased tendency to clot (produces thrombophlebitis and thromboembolism) and carcinogenicity. The minor side effects of nausea, dizziness, headache, weight gain, and breast discomfort resemble those during early pregnancy and are mainly attributable to the estrogen in the preparation. These effects usually last only several weeks. Other side effects include blood pressure elevation and liver damage.

The hormones in oral contraceptives increase gingival fluid, stimulate gingivitis, and are associated with gingival inflammation similar to, but not as prominent as that seen in pregnancy. Others have not shown any significant differences between the plaque scores, gingival scores, or loss of attachment when comparing users and nonusers of oral contraceptives. This discrepancy may be based partly on differences in dose between studies. Also, this effect may not be evident in all users but may be of clinical significance only in those persons who are highly susceptible to oral soft tissue disorders. In any case the dentist and dental hygienist should be aware that oral contraceptives do have the potential to cause or aggravate gingival inflammation.

Oral contraceptives are also associated with a significant increase in the frequency of dry socket after extractions. This risk can be minimized by performing extractions during days 23 through 28 of the tablet cycle. Contraindications for the use of oral contraceptives include thromboembolic disorders, significant dysfunction of the liver, known or suspected carcinoma of the breast or other estrogen-dependent neoplasm, and undiagnosed genital bleeding.

In light of the increased use of antibiotics in periodontal therapy, the importance of the antibiotic–oral contraceptive interaction must be mentioned (Table 20-9). Certain antibiotics have been said to reduce the effectiveness of oral contraceptives. They are thought to do so, indirectly, by suppressing the intestinal flora and thus diminishing the availability of hydrolytic enzymes to regenerate the parent steroid molecule. Consequently, plasma concentrations of the steroids are said to be abnormally low, and the steroid is cleared more rapidly from the body than under normal circumstances. Some recom-

---

BOX 20-3 MANAGEMENT OF THE DENTAL PATIENT TAKING ORAL CONTRACEPTIVES (OC)

Estrogen-related

Increased incidence of post-extraction dry socket
Chloasma, melasma, watch dental light
Increased susceptibility to candida, check oral cavity, check after antibiotic therapy
Decreased glucose tolerance, blood glucose level if needed
Increased thromboembolytic disease, for long appointments, give break
Antibiotics said to reduce OCs' effectiveness

OCs can produce an increase in blood pressure
Gingivitis and periodontitis; check; more frequent recall appointments if found
May be taking calcium supplementation for bones, avoid taking concomitantly with tetracycline or doxycycline

Progestin-related

Melasma or chloasma, watch dental light
Thrombophlebitis

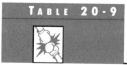

TABLE 20-9	Oral Contraceptive–Dental Drug Interactions
Penicillin	Decreased effectiveness of OC*
Tetracyclines	Decreased effectiveness of OC
Acetaminophen	OC increased hepatotoxicity of acetaminophen
Benzodiazepines	OC increased clearance of benzodiazepines

*OC, Oral contraceptive.

mend that the patient might want to use an additional method of contraception until the end of her cycle. Other suggestions include the substitution of topical for systemic antibiotics, if possible, and the use of oral contraceptives with higher levels of the estrogen component. The latter suggestion should only be undertaken by the patient's physician. Although all antibiotics have been implicated in this drug interaction, the incidence is indeed rare. If the patient is in the last week (week 3) or the placebo week (week 4), the chances of oral contraceptive therapy failure is even slimmer. In our litigation-conscious society, there should be documentation in the dental chart that the patient was informed about the rare chance of a drug interaction between oral contraceptives and antibiotics (see Table 20-9).

MALE SEX HORMONES

ANDROGENS

The main androgen, testosterone, has both androgenic and anabolic effects. Because there is overlap between androgens and **anabolic steroids,** separating them is difficult. Table 20-10 lists the male hormones and their antagonists and the female hormone antagonists. Androgens are responsible for the development of secondary male sex characteristics. Their anabolic action results in an increase in tissue protein and nitrogen retention in the body. Other actions of the androgens include increased osteoblastic activity, epiphyseal closure (can't grow any taller), and an increase in sebaceous gland activity (increased acne).

TABLE 20-10   **Male Hormones, Agonists, and Antagonists; Female Hormone Antagonists**

Drug Group	Examples	Indications
MALE REPRODUCTIVE SYSTEM		
Androgens	Testosterone	Deficiency of testosterone, estrogen-dependent
	Methyltestosterone	malignancy
Anabolic agents	Methandrostelone (Dianabol)	Body builders use illicitly
	Nandrolone	
	Stanozolol	
Antiandrogens	Cyproterone acetate	Female hirsutism
	Flutamide (Eulexin)	Advanced or metastatic prostate carcinoma in
	Nilutamide (Nilandron)	males
	Bicalutamide (Casodex)	
	Finasteride (Propecia, Proscar)	Inhibits 5-α-reductase; baldness, benign prostatic hypertrophy
FEMALE REPRODUCTIVE SYSTEM		
Gonadotropin-releasing hormone	Gonadorelin (Factrel)	Stimulates release of FSH and LH
Nonpituitary chorionic gonadotropin	Gonadotropin, chorionic (APL, Pregnyl)	
Menotropins	Menotropins (Pergonal)	Infertility; like FSH and LH
Antiestrogens	Danocrine (Danazol)	Endometriosis
	Tamoxifen (Nolvadex)	Advanced breast cancer
	Raloxifen (Evista)	Prevents breast cancer in selected high-risk populations of women
	Clomiphene (Clomid, Serophene)	Infertility; increases FSH and LH
	Nafarelin (Synarel)	Endometriosis; gonadotropin-releasing hormone agonist; stimulates LH and FSH
Progestin antagonist	Mifepristone (RU-486)	Fetal abortion, used with prostaglandin E

Puberty gingivitis can occur related to hormonal changes. Androgenic steroids are used medically in the treatment of breast cancer or for replacement therapy. Treatment includes subgingival debridement and oral hygiene instructions (Box 20-4)

Androgens are used illicitly by body builders, weight lifters, and other athletes for muscle mass gain. Some athletic events now test the urine for the presence of anabolic steroids. Because of their abuse, androgenic steroids are Schedule III controlled substances (same category as Tylenol #3). The side effects of androgenic steroids include nausea, cholestatic jaundice, hepatocellular neoplasms, increased serum cholesterol, habituation, and depression and excitation. In females, virilization (acne, hirsutism, deepening voice, clitoral enlargement, malelike baldness) occurs. Considering the potential for side effects, the illicit use of these agents is difficult to understand.

OTHER AGENTS THAT AFFECT SEX HORMONE SYSTEMS

Other agents that affect sex hormones may either act like the hormones or they may inhibit the action of the naturally occurring sex hormones (Table 20-11). Hormones from the opposite sex are often used to manage prostate, breast, and uterine cancers because the cancer is often stimulated by the patient's own sex hormones. For example, prostate cancer is often stimulated by testosterone, so men with prostate cancer are given estrogens to inhibit the cancer's growth.

BOX 20-4 ANDROGENIC AND ANABOLIC STEROIDS

Androgenic/anabolic steroid indications

- Testosterone deficiency: androgen replacement therapy in the treatment of delayed male puberty, postpartum breast pain and engorgement, inoperable breast cancer, male hypogonadism
- Methyltestosterone (Metandren, Android): hypogonadism, delayed puberty, impotence and climacteric symptoms
- Female: palliative treatment of metastatic breast cancer; postpartum breast pain and/or engorgement
- Used with estrogen is postmenopausal women (?)
- *Nandrolone (Androlone, Deca-Durabolin) metastatic breast cancer, anemia of renal insufficiency
- Oxymetholone (Anadrol): anemias caused by antineoplastics
- Danazol (Danocrine): endometriosis, hereditary angioedema
- Stanozolol (Winstrol): hereditary angioedema
- Fluoxymesterone (Halotestin)
- Methandrostenolone (Dianabol)

Antiandrogen indications

- Bicalutamide (Casodex), nilutamide (Nilandron): in combination therapy with LHRH agonist analogues—prostatic carcinoma
- Finasteride (Proscar): benign prostatic hyperplasia (BPH), prostatic cancer; alopecia

---

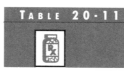

TABLE 20-11   Other Agents That Affect Sex Hormone Systems

DRUG	ACTION	INDICATION
Clomiphene (Clomid, Serophene)	Estrogen antagonist and agonist	Infertility
Lupron injections		Infertility
Tamoxifen (Nolvadex)	Estrogen agonist-antagonist Antiestrogen	Breast cancer
Toremifene (Fareston)		
Danazol (Danocrine)	Estrogen antagonist Antiestrogen	

CLOMIPHENE

Clomiphene [KLOE-mi-feen] (Clomid, Serophene) has the ability to induce ovulation in some anovulatory women. Clomiphene reduces the number of estrogenic receptors (antiestrogen) by binding to them. The hypothalamus and pituitary then falsely interpret the situation as estrogen levels that are low and increase their secretion of LH, FSH, and gonadotropins. Because clomiphene is a partial estrogen agonist it acts as a competitive inhibitor of endogenous estrogen. Ovarian stimulation then results. Its side effects include hot flashes, eye problems, headaches, and constipation. Other side effects result from the symptoms of ovulation. Clomiphene is used to treat infertility in females and has been used experimentally for males also. The chance of multiple pregnancies increases about 6 times with clomiphene treatment. Female dental patients being treated with clomiphene should be considered to be pregnant, unless known to be not pregnant.

LEUPROLIDE

Leuprolide [loo-PROE-lide] (Lupron) is a gonadotropin-releasing hormone analog used intramuscularly in the management of endometriosis and to treat fertility. It suppresses production of male and female steroids as a result of a decreased level of LH and FSH.

TAMOXIFEN

Tamoxifen [ta-MOKS-i-fen] (Nolvadex) is a competitive inhibitor of estradiol at the receptor. It is indicated in the palliative treatment of advanced breast cancer in postmenopausal women. A large study recently published determined that the use of tamoxifen as a prophylactic (preventive) for primary breast cancer in women at increased risk reduced the risk by about 50%. A similar new drug is raloxifene (Evista).

DANAZOL

Danazol [DA-na-zole] (Danocrine) possesses weak progestational and androgenic action. It suppresses ovarian function and prevents LH and FSH midcycle surge. Its side effects include an increase in weight, decrease in breast size, acne, increased hair, lowered voice, headache, and hot flushes. It is used to treat endometriosis and fibrocystic breast disease in women.

References

1. Collin HL et al: Caries in patients with NIDDM, *Oral Surg Oral Med Oral Pathol Oral Radiol Endodon*, 85(6): 680-685, 1998.
2. Crofford OB: Diabetes control and complications, *Annu Rev Med* 46:267-279, 1995.

REVIEW QUESTIONS

1. List one drug group (for each) to which patients with hypothyroidism (uncontrolled) and hyperthyroidism (poorly controlled) may have an altered response.
2. Describe these diseases:
   a. cretinism
   b. myxedema
   c. dwarfism
   d. Addison's disease
   e. acromegaly
   f. giantism
   g. Graves' disease
   h. Plummer's disease
3. Compare and contrast types I and II DM.
4. Describe the two situations that can occur when insulin, glucose, and exercise are not in balance in the diabetic patient.
5. Explain the oral manifestations of diabetes and explain their causes.
6. Describe the two commonly used types of insulin and state their most common usage pattern. Describe the best use of insulin to minimize the complications of diabetes.

7. Name four oral hypoglycemic agents (from different groups) and state two side effects of this group of drugs.

8. State what two drug groups are combined to produce the common birth control pill. State what dental drugs have been thought to reduce their efficacy (they probably do not).

9. State the relationship between birth control pills, their oral manifestations, and the incidence of postextraction dry socket.

10. Discuss the potential problems with the use of anabolic steroids for body building.

11. State a use for tamoxifen, clomiphene, and danazol.

CHAPTER 21

Antineoplastic Drugs

Antineoplastic agents are so named because these agents were designed to treat malignancies. A relatively new use of these agents is in the management of diseases with an inflammatory component, such as psoriasis, rheumatoid arthritis, and systemic lupus erythematosus. Depending on their usage, these agents are prescribed by oncologists and rheumatologists, as well as oral pathologists, for oral conditions related to systemic autoimmune diseases. For treating malignancies, the dental health care worker should be aware of the relationship between the timing of the treatments and the effects on the bone marrow. The dental health care worker should be familiar with the side effects of these agents, especially their oral manifestations.

Current research is elucidating many different mechanisms involved in the etiology of cancer, including genetics, viruses, deleted or damaged tumor suppressor genes, specific oncogenes, and changes in both ribonucleic acid (RNA) and deoxyribonucleic acid (DNA) that affect the growth of cells. Many animal carcinogens have been identified, but proving carcinogenic potential in humans is much more difficult.

Many human carcinogens are environmental carcinogens, for example, polychlorinated biphenyls (PCBs) from transformers. Other known carcinogens include second-hand tobacco smoke, aflatoxins (produced by moldy peanuts), sunlight (increase in malignant **melanoma** and squamous cell carcinoma), and benzene. Most believe that the herpes and papilloma

Environmental carcinogens

viruses have a potential for producing cancerous changes. Patients with a history of certain diseases such as hepatitis have a higher incidence of liver cancer than normal patients.

Normal cells have a mechanism to turn off cell growth under certain signals. With cancer, a change in the cells occur so that they continue to grow. With a lack of control (switch does not turn off), the abnormal neoplastic cells continue to grow. The cell surface antigens appear similar to the normal fetal types, so the body does not mount an immune response. The tumor stem cells have chromosomal abnormalities, repetitions, and select subclones. With repeated cycles the cells can migrate to distant sites and metastases form colonies. For example, cancer that begins in the breast may spread to the bone or liver.

USE OF ANTINEOPLASTIC AGENTS

Antineoplastic agents, sometimes called *cancer chemotherapeutic agents*, are used clinically to interfere with the neoplastic cells. The antineoplastic agents interfere with some function of the malignant cells. They suppress the growth of the cells and attempt to destroy and prevent the spread of malignant cells. These agents are used either alone or in combination or with radiation or surgery, depending on the type of malignancy being treated. Each type of malignancy may be more or less sensitive to each of the three modalities—drugs, radiation, and surgery.

> Drugs effective for some cancers

For treatment of certain malignancies, for example, the leukemias, choriocarcinoma, multiple **myeloma,** and Burkitt's **lymphoma,** drugs are considered the primary choice. Often combinations of several antineoplastic agents, used in conjunction with surgery and/or irradiation, may effect a cure that each procedure alone could not. Certain cancers are relatively insensitive to antineoplas-

tic agents. These cancers are treated with either radiation and/or surgery. Box 21-1 lists malignancies and their likelihood of sensitivity to cancer chemotherapy agents.

The current philosophy for the use of the antineoplastic agents involves treating the initial stages of disease very aggressively. This approach promises more chance of controlling and curing the disease, but also involves many severe

---

BOX 21-1 SENSITIVITY OF NEOPLASTIC DISEASES TO CHEMOTHERAPY

High activity

Acute lympho-cytic leukemia	Hodgkin's disease
Acute myelocytic leukemia	Oat cell
Breast cancer	Burkitt's lymphoma
Ewing's sarcoma	Wilm's tumor

Moderate activity

Head and neck, squamous	Endometrial
	Prostate
Neuroblastoma	Chronic lympho-cytic leukemia
Bladder	Chronic myelocytic leukemia
Colorectal	Kaposi's sarcoma (AIDS)
Cervix	
Ovary	

Least activity

Liver	Pancreatic
Lung	Renal
Melanoma	

side effects, including some that affect the oral cavity. The treatment of some cancers involves the removal of cells from the bone marrow before administering the chemotherapy or radiation. In the past, the dose administered would have been fatal. But, after treatment is complete, the cells taken from the bone marrow are returned to the patient's body and they begin making the blood elements that are made in bone marrow. Gene therapy is being used, and many advances are continuing to be made. New research is attempting to use the body's immune system to fight the cancer cells. Endocrine agonists and antagonists are useful in treatment of endocrine-stimulated neoplasias.

MECHANISMS OF ACTION

The efficacy of antineoplastic agents is based primarily on their ability to interfere with the metabolism or reproductive cycle of the tumor cells, thereby destroying them. The reproduc-

tive cycle of a cell is considered to consist of the following four stages (Figure 21-1):
1. **G_1 ("gap" 1),** which is the postmitotic or pre-DNA synthesis phase
2. **S,** which is the period of DNA synthesis
3. **G_2 ("gap" 2),** which is the premitotic or post-DNA synthesis phase
4. **M,** which is the period of mitosis

Cells in a resting stage that are not in a process of cell division are described as being in the G_0 stage. Cells enter the cycle from the G_0 stage. In some tumors a large proportion of the cells may be at the G_0 level. These cells are difficult to reach and destroy.

Most of the antineoplastic agents are labeled as being either *cell-cycle specific* (Table 21-1), indicating that they are effective only at specific phases of cellular growth, or *cell-cycle nonspecific,*

Cell-cycle specific/nonspecific

FIGURE **2 1 · 1**   *Cell cycle.*

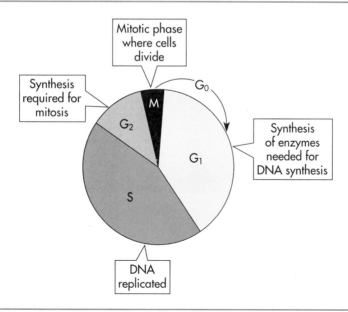

indicating that they are effective at all levels of the cycle (effective both in the resting and the proliferating cells). For example, the alkylating agents interfere with the malignant cells during all phases of the reproductive cycle, as well as the resting stage (G_0) and therefore are classified as cycle independent.

A major problem with treating neoplastic cells is that the cell growth is exponential. Before diagnosis is made, a large cell load must be present. If 10^{12} cells are present and 99.9% of the cells are killed, 10^9 cells would remain; if 99.9% of those cells were killed, 10^6 cells would still be present. Mixing several chemotherapeutic agents can increase the chance of killing more cells because they work by different mechanisms and have different adverse reactions.

Resistance to chemotherapy occurs by either of the following methods:

- ***de novo resistance:*** The neoplasm was always resistant to the chemotherapeutic agents.
- ***acquired resistance:*** Resistance occurs through the natural selection of mutations.

CLASSIFICATION

The antineoplastic agents are divided into groups depending on their mechanism and site of action (Figure 21-2). Box 21-2 lists some antineoplastic agents by classification.

> Groups divided by how they work

The alkylating agents contain alkyl radicals that react with DNA in all cycles of the cell, preventing reproduction. The antimetabolites attack the cells in the S period of reproduction by interfering with purine or pyrimidine synthesis. They incorporate the drug into a compound or inhibit an enzyme from functioning and are more effective on rapidly proliferating neoplasms. Plant alkaloids are mitotic inhibitors and act by arresting cells in metaphase. Because of their low bone marrow toxicity, they are often used in combination with other agents with

TABLE 21-1 Classification of Antineoplastic Drugs

Cell-Cycle Specific	Cell-Cycle Nonspecific
Antimetabolites	Alkylating agents
Bleomycin	Antibiotics
Vinca alkaloids	Cisplatin
Podophyllin	Nitrosoureas

FIGURE 21-2 *Location of action of some antineoplastic agents. The synthesis of proteins can be interfered with at the purine/pyrimdine, DNA, or RNA level.*

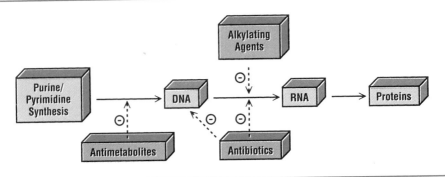

more bone marrow toxicity. Antibiotics are cell-cycle nonspecific and are effective for solid tumors. Other agents include hormones, such as prednisone, which interrupt the cell cycle at the G stage. Steroids are used to suppress lymphocytes in leukemias and lymphomas and in combination therapies. Estrogens are used for palliation in inoperable breast cancer. Tamoxifen, an antiestrogenic substance, is used to manage breast cancer. It has also recently been shown to prevent breast cancer when used in high-risk women. Cisplatin, a heavy metal complex of platinum, is cell-cycle nonspecific. Hydroxyurea inhibits ribonucleotide reductase, which interferes with RNA synthesis. Procarbazine produces chromosomal breakage.

 BOX 21-2 ANTINEOPLASTIC AGENTS BY GROUP

Alkylating agents

Nitrogen Mustard

Mechlorethamine (Mustargen)
Cyclophosphamide (Leukeran)
Chlorambucil (Leukeran)
Melphalan (Alkeran)
Uracil mustard
Ifosfamide (Ifex)

Nitrosoureas

Carmustine (BCNU, BiCNU)
Lomustine (CCNU, CeeNU)
Semustine (Methyl-Cee NU)
Streptozocin (Zanosar)
Estramustine (Emcyt)

Miscellaneous

Busulfan (Myleran)
Pipobroman (Vercyte)
Thiotepa
Cisplatin (Platinol)
Carboplatin (Paraplatin)

Antimetabolits

Folic Acid Analog

Methotrexate (Amethopterin)

Pyrimidine Analog

Fluorouracil (5-FU)
Floxuridine (FUDR)
Cytosine arabinoside (ARA-C, Cytosar-U)
Azacitidine

Purine Analog

Mercaptopurine (6-MP, Purinethol)
Thioguanine (6-TG)
Cladribine (Leustatin)
Fludarabine (Fludara)
Pentostatin (Nipent)

Miscellaneous antineoplastics

Plant Alkaloids

Vinblastine (Velban)
Vincristine (Oncovin)

Antibiotics

Dactinomycin (Actinomycin-D, Cosmegen)
Doxorubicin (Adriamycin)
Bleomycin (Blenoxane)
Mitomycin-C (Mutamycin)
Plicamycin (Mithramycin, Mithracin)
Daunorubicin (Cerubidine)

Hormones

Adrenocorticosteroids (prednisone)
Androgen
    Testolactone (Teslac)
    Fluoxymesterone (Halotestin)
Antiandrogen
    Flutamide (Eulexin)
    Nilutamide (Nilandron)
    Bicalutamide (Casodex)
Estrogen
    Diethylstilbestrol
    Ethinyl estradiol (Estinyl)

Hormones

Antiestrogen
    Tamoxifen (Nolvadex)
Progestin
    Medroxyprogesterone
    Megestrol (Megace)
Goserelin (Zoladex)
Leuprolide (Lupron)

Immune Modulators

Levamisole (Ergamisol)
Interferon α-n3 (Alferon N)
Interferon α-2b (Intron A)
Interferon α-2a (Roferon-a)

Podophyllotoxin Derivatives

Etoposide (VePesid)
Teniposide (Vumon)

Other

L-Asparaginase (Elspar)
Hydroxyurea (Hydrea)
Procarbazine (Matulane)
Paclitaxel (Taxol)
Altretamine (Hexalen)

TABLE 21-2 Selected Adverse Reactions of Some Antineoplastic Agents

Drug	Adverse Reaction
Methotrexate (MTX)	GI, BMS, leukovorin rescue; used for severe arthritis and psoriasis
5-Fluorouracil	GI, BMS, topical for superficial basal cell carcinoma
Dactinomycin	GI, **BMS**
Doxorubicin	GI, BMS, **cardiotoxicity**
Mechlorethamine	Nitrogen mustard during WWI (chemical warfare); vomiting, BMS, bifunctional (binds at two sites)
Cyclophosphamide	BMS, **hemorrhagic cystitis** (Tx: ↑ H_2O + mannitol + topical in bladder [MESNA]), ↑ ADH (Tx: furosemide)
Nitrosoureas	**Hematopoietic depression,** phenobarbital reduces cytotoxicity
Vinblastine	**BMS**
Vincristine	**Peripheral neuropathy** (foot drop)
Tamoxifen (Nolvadex)	Increased pain if bone metastasis
Cisplatin	Platin complex, persistent vomiting, **nephrotoxicity** (Tx: ↑ H_2O + mannitol); ↓ Ca, ↓ Mg, ototoxicity, paresthesias
Procarbazine	**BMS,** psychic disturbances, MAO inhibitor interactions with food
Asparaginase	**Hypersensitivity,** reduced clotting, liver toxicity, pancreatitis, seizures

Bold face, Toxicity usually dose limiting; *GI,* gastrointestinal tract toxicity; *BMS,* bone marrow suppression; *MAO,* monoamine oxidase, *Tx,* treatment.

ADVERSE DRUG EFFECTS

Rapidly growing cells, such as neoplastic cells, are more susceptible to inhibition or destruction by antineoplastic agents. The most serious difficulty encountered in antineoplastic therapy stems from the lack of selectivity between tumor tissue and normal tissue. Some normal cells exhibit a faster reproduction cycle than do slowly growing tumor cells. In an effort to eradicate a malignancy, certain normal cells are also destroyed, resulting in adverse effects. Because the cells of the gastrointestinal tract, bone marrow, and hair follicles are among the faster growing normal cells, the early side effects are associated with these tissues.

Table 21-2 lists the most common adverse reactions associated with some antineoplastic agents. These are the more common or agent-specific reactions associated with the drugs listed. The principal adverse effects are as follows.

Bone marrow suppression (BMS). The bone marrow is suppressed because it is a tissue that is rapidly turning over. Inhibition of the bone marrow results in leukopenia or agranulocytosis, thrombocytopenia, and anemia. The degree of cytopenia that results depends on the drugs being employed, the condition of the bone marrow at the time of administration, and other contributing factors. Symptoms of this adverse reaction may include susceptibility to infection, bleeding, and fatigue. The rise and fall in hematologic effects are related to location in the cycle of administering the drug.

Gastrointestinal effects. Gastrointestinal problems are common because the gastrointestinal tract is a tissue that is rapidly turning over. The sloughing of the gastrointestinal mucosa can produce many symptoms. Clinically, these disturbances are expressed as nausea, stomatitis, oral ulcerations, vomiting, and hemorrhagic diarrhea. Nausea and vomiting may be treated using phenothiazines (prochlorperazine [Compazine]), cannabinoids (dronabinol [Marinol] and nabilone [Cesamet]), metoclopramide (Reglan), cisapride (Propulsid) and scopolamine.

Dermatological effects. Cutaneous reactions vary from mild erythema and maculopapular eruptions to exfoliative dermatitis and Stevens-Johnson syndrome. Alopecia is frequent, but the hair usually regrows when therapy is discontinued.

Hepatotoxicity. Liver problems occur principally with the antimetabolites (e.g., methotrexate), but may occur with other agents as well.

Neurologic effects. Neurotoxic effects such as peripheral neuropathy, ileus, inappropriate antidiuretic hormone secretion, and convulsions have been associated primarily with vincristine or vinblastine administration.

> Allopurinol prevents hyperuricemia

Nephrotoxicity. The renal tubular impairment that occurs secondary to hyperuricemia is caused by rapid cell destruction and the release of nucleotides. The treatment of leukemias and lymphomas often results in rapid tumor destruction with a consequent high uric acid level. Allopurinol (Zyloprim) is a xanthine oxidase inhibitor used in the management of gout. It blocks the production of uric acid by blocking its synthesis. Before the initiation of a regimen of antineoplastic agents that release purines and pyrimidines, allopurinol is administered to prevent hyperuricemia. Allopurinol can prolong the action and increase the toxicity of cyclophosphamide and the thiopurines (azathioprine and mercaptopurine).

Immunosuppression. Because the antineoplastic agents have an **immunosuppressant** effect, enhanced susceptibility to infection or a second malignancy may occur after treatment.

Germ cells. Inhibition of spermatogenesis and oogenesis is frequent, at least temporarily. Mutations within the germ cells may occur. The menstrual cycle may also be inhibited. Recovery occurs after discontinuation of the drug.

Oral effects. Adverse effects on the oral tissue are primarily those of discomfort, sensitivity of the teeth and gums, mucosal pain and ulceration, gingival hemorrhage, dryness, and impaired taste sensation. Infection of the oral mucosa from leukopenia and bleeding (petechiae on the hard palate) from thrombocytopenia can occur. Appropriate maintenance of the oral cavity (Box 21-3) should be undertaken even before and certainly during antineoplastic therapy.

Patients taking antineoplastic agents may experience inflammation of the mouth, xerostomia, or glossitis. In these cases the dental health care worker should not recommend any products containing alcohol (such as elixirs), because alcohol is drying to the oral mucosa.

COMBINATIONS

Agents of widely differing mechanisms of action are often employed together to inhibit the reproduction of neoplastic cells in all phases and to gain therapeutic advantage for the host. Mixtures of these agents may act synergistically, leading to enhanced cytotoxicity with fewer side effects. This is the rationale for combination drug therapy.

USE IN TREATMENT OF INFLAMMATORY PROCESSES

Antineoplastic drugs are used in lower doses to manage diseases associated with inflammation or autoimmune conditions and transplants. Examples include azathioprine (Imuran), methotrexate (MTX; Rheumatrex), and cyclosporin

(Sandimmune). Diseases that are treated with these agents include rheumatoid arthritis, systemic lupus erythematosus, pemphigus vulgaris, and psoriasis.

The doses of these agents used to treat diseases with an autoimmune component is often lower than the doses used to treat cancer. Some drug interactions that would be important with higher doses are often safe in the lower doses used for autoimmune diseases. With organ transplants, immunosuppressives are used to prevent rejection of the foreign tissue.

DENTAL IMPLICATIONS

Dental patients who are to take cancer chemotherapy agents should optimize their oral health before antineoplastic agents are begun (ideal conditions). However, often the dental health care worker has less than a day in which to attempt to attain this degree of dental health.

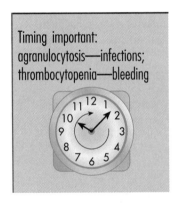

Timing important: agranulocytosis—infections; thrombocytopenia—bleeding

If oral hygiene or dental procedures are to be performed on a patient who is taking antineoplastic agents, the procedures should be planned to coincide with the presence of the highest level of formed blood elements. That time would be either just before treatment or on the first few days of treatment (drug does not immediately depress the bone marrow maximally).

After a cycle of drugs is completed, the effect on the bone marrow increases until the maximum effect is obtained. During this time, dental treatment should be avoided. The white blood cell count is often too low (agranulocytosis) and the chance of infection is great. The platelets may also be low (thrombocytopenia) and bleed-

ing can occur. The optimal time for performing dental procedures will vary with each drug or drug regimen. Proper oral management of the patient receiving chemotherapy is given in Box 21-3. The general dental implications of the antineoplastic agents are listed in Box 21-4.

Box 21-3 ORAL CARE FOR PATIENTS ON ANTINEOPLASTIC AGENTS

Before chemotherapy

Eliminate and/or manage infection
Control periodontal disease (include prophylaxis)
Provide oral hygiene instruction

During chemotherapy

Schedule appointment just before next chemotherapy
Consult with oncologist before any procedure
Document hematologic status (lab test)
Treat only if neutrophil count is ≥1000/mm
Give endocarditis antibiotic prophylaxis if venous catheter present
Institute oral hygiene program—brush properly, rinse with baking soda/saline and/or chlorhexidine (avoid mouthwash), soda/saline after emesis, no dentures at night, topical fluoride if prolonged xerostomia
Culture lesions for infection

After chemotherapy

Follow and maintain oral health

BOX 21-4 MANAGEMENT OF THE DENTAL PATIENT TAKING ANTINEOPLASTIC AGENTS

• Maximize oral hygiene before chemotherapy
• Hygiene instructions to match patient's symptoms
• Potential for infection; watch for symptoms
• Check neutrophil count before treatment
• Check thrombocytes for adequate clotting
• Rinse with soda/saline and/or chlorhexidine

REVIEW QUESTIONS

1. Describe the different stages in the reproductive cycle of a cell. State their importance to antineoplastic drug therapy.

2. State the major classifications of the antineoplastic agents, and give one example of each.

3. Explain the adverse effects associated with the antineoplastic agents, and state the symptoms associated with each effect.

4. Explain oral care for patients receiving chemotherapy. Explain the importance of factors such as white blood cell count. State agents to use or to avoid to alleviate oral discomfort.

5. Describe two or three cancers that are amenable to drug treatment. State two that are usually not.

CHAPTER 22

Respiratory and Gastrointestinal Drugs

CHAPTER OUTLINE

FIGURE **2 2 - 1**   *Respiratory and gastrointestinal drug groups.*

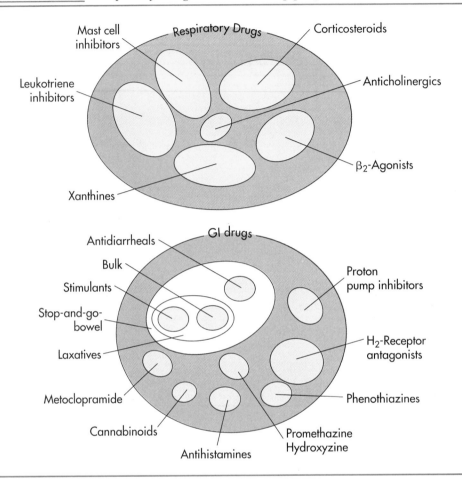

Diseases of the respiratory and gastrointestinal tracts are common, so dental health care workers are sure to encounter patients taking drugs for these diseases (Figure 22-1). Because the medications given to treat these diseases can affect dental treatment, the dental health care worker should be aware of the effects of these drugs on the patient and how these drugs can alter the dental treatment plan.

RESPIRATORY DRUGS

Diseases that are treated with respiratory drugs include asthma, chronic obstructive pulmonary disease (COPD), and upper respiratory tract infections (Figure 22-2). Respiratory drugs include a wide range of drug groups, from adrenergic drugs for bronchodilation to corticosteroids for reducing inflammation. Drugs that increase expectoration and reduce coughs are also included in this discussion. Many drugs used to treat re-

FIGURE 22-2 *Respiratory diseases.*

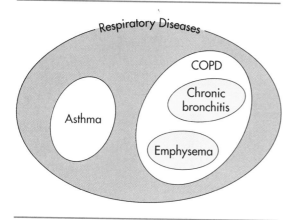

spiratory problems are administered topically via the lungs by the use of a metered-dose inhaler (MDI).

RESPIRATORY DISEASES

Noninfectious respiratory diseases are divided into two groups, asthma and chronic obstructive pulmonary diseases (COPD) (see Figure 22-2). COPD is further divided into chronic bronchitis and emphysema. Other respiratory problems are related to respiratory infections, such as viral or bacterial.

Asthma—reversible airway obstruction with inflammation

Asthma. One common respiratory disease is asthma. It is characterized by reversible airway obstruction and is associated with reduction in expiratory airflow. A few hours later, inflammation occurs resulting in an increase in secretions in the lungs and swelling in the bronchioles. When asthma is treated, both components of the disease must be addressed. Asthma may be precipitated by allergens, pollution, exercise, stress, or upper respiratory infection (allergic reaction to viruses). In status asthmaticus, patients have persistent life-threatening bronchospasm despite drug therapy. The large increase in asthma, seen especially in inner city children, may be due to the allergenicity of cockroach feces (like dust mite feces). Environmental pollution may also play an important role in the increase in asthma. The dental health care worker should treat dental patients with asthma so that minimal stress is induced. Patients should bring their fast-acting β_2-agonist inhalers to be used prophylactically or in the management of an acute asthmatic attack in the dental office. Signs of asthma include shortness of breath and wheezing. Observation and questioning of the patient for asthma control before the dental appointment by the dental health care worker can prevent an acute attack. β-Adrenergic agonists, xanthines, cromolyn, corticosteroids, leukotriene-altering agents, and anticholinergics are used to treat this disease.

Chronic obstructive pulmonary disease. COPD is characterized by irreversible airway obstruction, which occurs with

COPD—irreversible airway obstruction

either chronic bronchitis or emphysema. Smoking is associated with almost all COPD. Chronic bronchitis is a result of chronic inflammation of the airways and excessive sputum production. Emphysema is characterized by alveolar destruction with airspace enlargement and airway collapse. The anticholinergics are the first-line treatment, but β-adrenergic agonists and xanthines are also used to produce bronchodilation in these patients. Experimental surgery involving removing the most severely affected lung tissue has been tried experimentally, but more studies are needed before any conclusions can be made. Both conditions are associated with an increase in the incidence of bronchospasm and with fixed airway obstruction. Patients with upper respiratory tract infections frequently take adrenergic agonists for nasal congestion or bronchoconstriction, antihistamines to reduce secretions, **expectorants** to thin sputum, and antitussives to control coughing. Each drug group is discussed separately.

In the normal person, the drive for ventilation (breathing) is stimulated by an elevation in the partial pressure of carbon dioxide ($PaCO_2$). The partial pressure of oxygen (PaO_2) can vary widely without stimulating ventilation in the normal patient. Patients with COPD, because their ventilation is compromised, experience a gradual rise in $PaCO_2$ over time. Because this mechanism becomes resistant to this stimulus, a new stimulus emerges—the partial pressure of PaO_2. The patient's ventilation is then driven by a decrease in PaO_2. If a patient with COPD is given oxygen and the PaO_2 rises, the stimulant to breathing is removed and there is the possibility of inducing apnea. For patients with COPD ASA III and IV, it is suggested that oxygen be limited to less than 3 L/minute. Other literature recommends that in severe COPD oxygen by nasal cannula be used during a dental appointment, especially if pain or stress is expected (increased oxygen demand).

DRUGS USED TO TREAT RESPIRATORY DISEASES

SYMPATHOMIMETIC AGENTS

Sympathomimetic or adrenergic agonists produce bronchodilation by stimulation of the β-receptors in the lungs. β-Receptor activation results in accumulation of cyclic adenosine monophosphate (cAMP) in the smooth muscles, producing a reduction in cytoplasmic calcium concentration and thereby relaxing the smooth muscle (Figure 22-3). Chapter 5 discussed the presence of β-receptors in the heart (tachycardia) and lungs (bronchodilation). With the development of selective β_2-agonists ($\beta_2 > \beta_1$), bronchodilation with fewer cardiac side effects can be

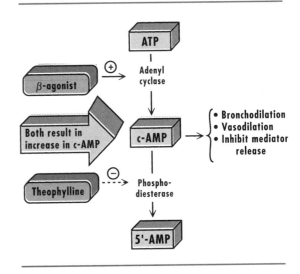

FIGURE   **2 2 - 3**   *Effect of β-agonists and theophylline on cAMP and bronchodilation.*

achieved. The selective β_2-agonists, used orally, by inhalation, and parenterally, are currently one of the mainstays of respiratory therapy.

Nonselective (nonspecific) β-adrenergic agonists. Both epinephrine, an α- and a β-agonist, and isoproterenol, a nonspecific β-agonist, can produce bronchodilation by stimulation of the β_2-receptors in the lungs. Parenteral epinephrine is still used to treat acute asthmatic attacks. Isoproterenol (nonselective β-agonist) has been used, but selective β_2-agonists are preferred because they produce fewer side effects.

Selective (specific) β_2-agonists. The selective β_2-agonists have specificity for the respiratory tree.

Albuterol = β_2-agonist

Like epinephrine, they do produce side effects, but they do so to a lesser extent. Side effects include nervousness, tachycardia, and insomnia. β_2-Agonists, such as albuterol, may be administered by inhalation (metered dose or nebulization with an air compressor), or orally (tablet or liquid). They differ in their duration of action and preparations available. Table 22-1 lists some selective β₂-agonists and their routes of administration. The first line of treatment for mild occasional asthma is a selective β₂-agonist. The selective β₂-agonists are the drugs of choice for the emergency treatment of an acute attack of asthma. Recent studies have found that the overuse of these agents results in airway hyperresponsiveness and a decrease in the lung's response to them. Therefore these agents should be used primarily for the treatment of acute problems, not for the management of normal breathing function. One major mistake that many asthmatics make is to rely on the albuterol inhaler and omit using the steroid inhaler. The reason this occurs is because the albuterol gives an immediate response

Sustained β-agonists. A newer β₂-agonist inhalant is salmeterol [sal-MET-er-ole] (Serevent). Its onset is delayed and its duration of action is sustained, lasting approximately 12 hours. It is important that this inhaler is *not* used for management of an acute asthmatic episode. The onset of action is 10 to 20 minutes, and the peak is 2 to 4 hours.

METERED-DOSE INHALERS

The metered-dose inhaler (MDI) (Figure 22-4), developed in the 1950s, provides a useful method to administer certain medications to the respiratory tree. Its advantages include the following:

Inhalers—quick onset, low toxicity

- It delivers the medication directly into the bronchioles, thereby keeping the total dose low and side effects minimal.
- The bronchodilator effect is greater than a comparable oral dose.

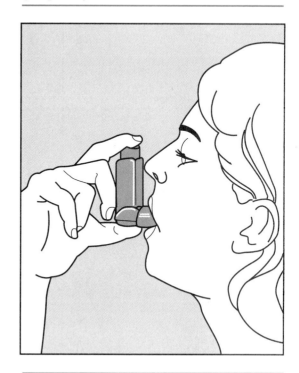

FIGURE 22-4 *Inhaler for treatment of respiratory conditions.*

- The inhaled dose can be accurately measured.
- The onset of action is rapid and predictable (versus unpredictable response with orally administered agents).
- MDIs are compact, portable, and sterile, making them ideal for the ambulatory patient.

Disadvantages of MDIs are that they are difficult to use properly (particularly for children) and they can be abused, with a resultant decrease in response. Additional patient education is required to get the most from this dosage form. Sometimes a "spacer" is placed between the MDI and the mouth to optimize use of the medicine. Medications currently available in MDIs include β-agonists, both specific and nonspecific, corticosteroids, cromolyn, and ipratropium and leukotriene-blocking drugs.

TABLE 22-1   Drugs Used to Manage Asthma

Group	Drug Example(s)	Mechanism of Action	Adverse Reactions	Dental Drug Implications
ADRENERGIC AGONISTS (INHALER)				
α-, β-Agonist	Epinephrine (Primatene, Bronkaid)	Stimulates α and β (β$_1$ and β$_2$) receptors	Tachycardia, tremors, anxiety	Additive with epinephrine-containing local anesthetic agents Xerostomia
β-Agonist	Isoproterenol (Isuprel, Medihaler-Iso)	Stimulates β$_1$ and β$_2$ receptors		
β$_2$-Agonist	Albuterol (Proventil, Ventolin)* Metaproterenol (Alupent, Metaprel) [IH] Salmeterol (Serevent)†	Stimulates β$_2$ receptors (bronchodilation)		Use for acute asthmatic attack Slow onset, long duration
CORTICOSTEROIDS (INHALER)				
Corticosteroids, topical	Triamcinolone (Azmacort) Beclomethasone (Beclovent, Vanceril) Flunisolide (Aerobid [M], Nasarel) Fluticasone (Flovent) Budesonide (Pulmicort, Rhinocort)	Reduces inflammation, inhibits release of inflammatory substances	Cough, dysphonia (hoarseness)	Oral candidiasis (rinse mouth to prevent), unpleasant taste, xerostomia
Corticosteroids, oral	Prednisone (Deltasone, Meticorten) [PO]	Reduces or prevents inflammatory processes	Hyperglycemia, osteoporosis, fluid retention	Suppresses adrenal gland Healing slower Infection more likely, symptoms masked
OTHERS				
Anticholinergics	Ipratropium (Atrovent) [IH]	Blocks muscarinic receptors, inhibits brochiolar secretions	URI (13%) epistaxis, hypersensitivity reactions, bronchitis; cross-hyperreactivity with peanut/soybean allergies	Xerostomia (3%),

LEUKOTRIENE ANTAGONISTS

Leukotriene pathway antagonist	Zafirlukast (Accolate) [PO]		Nausea, CNS depression, increase in LFTs, myalgia	Erythromycin lowers zafirlukast levels (40%); inhibitor of CYP 3A 3/4; Aspirin raises zafirlukast levels (45%) [PO 20 bid]
Leukotriene pathway (synthesis inhibitor) [LPI]	Zileuton (Zyflo) (Leutrol) [PO]	Inhibits 5-lipoxygenase that catalyzes production of LTs (LTD_4 and LTE_4)		

MAST CELL DEGRANULATION INHIBITORS

	Cromolyn (Intal) (Nasalcrom) IH; Nedocromil (Tilade) IH—see benefit in 2 weeks	Mast cell stabilizer (degranulation inhibitor); affects cells of inflammation	URI, nausea, HA, cough, epistaxis
(Methyl) Xanthines	Theophylline‡ (Theo-Dur, Slo-Bid) [PO]; Aminophylline-theophylline ethylene diamine	Direct smooth muscle relaxant (inhibition of PDEs, adenosine receptor antagonism)	Gastric reflux, headache, tachycardia, insomnia, nausea trembling, nervousness
Local anesthetic	Lidocaine 2% aerosolization (experimental)	Blocks nerve impulses by decreasing neuronal permeability to sodium ions (propagated action potential blocked)	Localized burning, sensitivity reaction

Disease: avoid AM appointment, more allergenic potential, hypersensitivity to aspirin, nonsteroidal antiinflammatory agents, sulfites; more common, especially with nasal polyps.

BP, Blood pressure; *CNS,* central nervous system; *LFTs,* liver function tests; *LTs,* leukotrienes; *PO,* by mouth.
*Use as emergency treatment.
†Do not use in an emergency, delayed onset > 1 hour, prolonged effect (12 hours).
‡Relative of caffeine found in coffee and cola beverages

CORTICOSTEROIDS

First used for the treatment of arthritis, the corticosteroids were soon employed for the treatment of asthma. As their side effects became evident (see Chapter 19), physicians began limiting corticosteroid therapy to only those patients who were refractory to other treatments. In 1975, however, aerosol preparations containing corticosteroids were introduced. The typical side effects associated with corticosteroid therapy do not occur with topical aerosol administration.

Steroid inhaler— for inflammation

Several aerosolized corticosteroids are marketed in the United States for the therapy of asthmatic patients (see Table 22-1). Common inhalers contain beclomethasone [be-kloe-METH-a-sone], triamcinolone [trye-am-SIN-oh-lone], and fluticasone (Flovent). Patients taking these corticosteroids have a significant improvement in pulmonary function with a decrease in wheezing, tightness, and cough. The topical inhalation corticosteroids are especially useful in reducing inflammation and therefore the secretions and swelling that occur within the lungs after an asthma attack occurs. Because inhalation of β_2-agonists produces bronchodilation, they should be used before using an aerosolized corticosteroid.

Inhalation corticosteroids are usually added to the treatment regimen when the asthmatic patient uses more than three inhalations of albuterol weekly. Although the steroids produce no immediate benefit in an acute asthmatic attack, they hasten recovery and decrease morbidity in these patients. They also reduce hyperreactive airway.

The side effects of steroids vary depending on the route of administration, frequency of intake, duration of intake, total dose, and preexisting diseases a patient may have.

Chronic oral corticosteroids, such as pred-nisone, may be necessary in some severely asthmatic patients and even in patients with moderate asthma, especially during respiratory infections. Prolonged systemic use can result in adrenal suppression, poor wound healing, and immunosuppression. Supplemental steroids may need to be considered if adrenal suppression has occurred (see Chapter 19).

Candidiasis of the oral cavity can result from the chronic use of an inhalation corticosteroid. When the dental health professional performs an oral examination of any patient using steroid inhalers, any symptoms of candidiasis should be noted and treated. Patients using oral corticosteroid inhalers should be advised to rinse the mouth and gargle with water after using the inhaler to minimize the chance of candidiasis.

Steroids are also available as sprays for nasal stuffiness. An example is beclomethasone (Beconase, Vancenase). It reduces the stuffiness by reducing inflammation within the nasal canal.

LEUKOTRIENE-PATHWAY INHIBITORS

Leukotrienes (LTs) are synthesized by the enzyme 5-lipoxygenase from arachidonic acid. They are synthesized from arachidonic acid that also produces prostaglandins. These LTs are produced by cells of inflammation and produce bronchoconstriction, increased mucous secretion, mucosal edema, and increased bronchial hyperreactivity. The LT pathway inhibitors block the effects of the release of LTs. They are used to manage patients with asthma that is not controlled by β_2-agonists and corticosteroid inhalers.

Zileuton (Zyflo) is a 5-lipoxygenase inhibitor that works by preventing the synthesis of the LTs. Zafirlukast (Accolate) is an LT (LTD_4) receptor antagonist (LTRA). It works by blocking the receptors for LT_4. They are not as effective as the corticosteroid inhalers. Both are effective taken orally. Some patients respond better than others, but who will respond cannot be predicted. In patients with aspirin hypersensitivity, the LT pathway inhibitors significantly reduce the reaction to aspirin. This effect fits in with the theory that the hyperreactivity to aspirin and the NSAIAs, which is not allergic in nature, is due to a shunting of the precursors of PG synthesis (inhibited by aspirin and NSAIAs) to LT synthesis.

The adverse reactions of these agents include irritation of the stomach mucosa, headache, and alteration of liver function tests. Zafirlukast has a drug interaction with erythromycin and aspirin. Zafirlukast increases the effect of warfarin. Caution should be exercised when giving to patients taking drugs metabolized by 2C9 (tolbutamide, phenytoin, carbamazepine) or 3A4 (dihydropyridines, cyclosporin, astemizole, cisapride). Erythromycin lowers the level of zafirlukast by about 40%. Aspirin raises zafirlukast levels by about 50%. Zafirlukast has recently been found to increase the level of theophylline in the blood. This may be explained by the fact that zafirlukast is an inhibitor of cytochrome P-450 3A3/4 isoenzymes and is a substrate for cytochrome P-450 isoenzyme 2C9.

Inhibits mast cell degranulation

Cromolyn. An agent that is effective only for the prophylaxis of asthma and not for treatment of an acute attack is cromolyn [KROE-moe-lin] (Intal, Nasalcrom). It has no intrinsic bronchodilator, antihistaminic, or antiinflammatory action. Cromolyn prevents the antigen-induced release of histamine, leukotrienes, and other substances from sensitized mast cells. It appears to do this by preventing the influx of calcium provoked by immunoglobulin E antibody–antigen interaction on the mast cell. This effect accounts for the group name that these drugs have been given—mast cell degranulation inhibitors. Cromolyn is the least toxic of all asthma medications. It is currently available in a metered dose form like the other inhalation agents. Nedocromil (Tilade) is similar in action to cromolyn.

The advantage of cromolyn is its safety. It may be used prophylactically by patients with chronic asthma or taken before exercise-induced asthma. Intranasal cromolyn (Nasalcrom) is available over the counter (OTC) for allergic rhinitis.

METHYLXANTHINES

The xanthines and methylxanthines consist of theophylline [thee-OFF-i-leen] (Theo-Dur, Slo-Bid), caffeine, and theobromine. Theophylline, used as a bronchodilator, can be combined with ethylenediamine to produce aminophylline [am-in-OFF-i-leen], which is more soluble. Theophylline is used to treat chronic asthma and the bronchospasm associated with chronic bronchitis and emphysema. Bronchodilation is the major therapeutic effect desired. The mechanism of action of the xanthines is complex. It involves antagonism of the receptor-mediated action of adenosine, inhibition of cyclic nucleotide phosphodiesterase (the effect on this enzyme that metabolizes cAMP is probably not important to theophylline's mechanism of action), mobilization of intracellular calcium pools, protein kinase activity modulation, and inhibition of prostaglandins.

Side effects associated with the methylxanthines include central nervous system (CNS) stimulation, cardiac stimulation, increased gastric secretion, and diuresis. [Think of drinking a few cups of coffee.] Patients often complain of nervousness and insomnia. Erythromycin can increase the serum levels of theophylline, and toxicity may result.

Intravenous aminophylline and rapidly absorbed oral liquid preparations are used to manage acute asthmatic attacks and status asthmaticus. To manage chronic asthma, sustained-release preparations in tablet or capsule form are used. Patients on chronic theophylline may have blood levels drawn to determine if the dose they are taking is appropriate. Current literature suggests that the use of theophylline should be limited to patients whose asthma is not controlled with other agents. When the chance of theophylline toxicity is weighed against the potential therapeutic benefit, theophylline is often omitted from an asthmatic's therapeutic regimen.

ANTICHOLINERGICS

Ipratropium—1st choice for emphysema

Atropine is an old remedy for asthma, although its side effects limit its usefulness. There are newer anticholinergic drugs that have fewer side effects. An example is ipratropium [i-pra-TROE-pee-um] (Atrovent), which is available for inhalation. It has several advantages over atropine. Its low lipid solubility limits its bioavailability and makes it bronchoselective with minimal side effects. Side effects, including dry mouth and bad taste, are minimized with administration by inhalation. Its bronchodilating effect is additive with that of the β-agonists. It is the drug of choice for long-term management of COPD. Other indications include the patients with poorly controlled asthma or those who do not tolerate the side effects of the β-agonists.

AGENTS USED TO MANAGE UPPER RESPIRATORY INFECTIONS

Nasal decongestants. Nasal decongestants are β-adrenergic agonists that act by constricting the blood vessels of the nasal mucous membranes (α effect). Some examples of these include phenylpropanolamine [fen-ill-proe-pa-NOLE-a-meen] (in Entex LA, Naldecon, and Tavist-D), pseudoephedrine [soo-doe-e-FED-rin] (Sudafed, Sucrets, in Actifed), and phenylephrine [fen-ill-EF-rin] (Neo-Synephrine, Sinex, Allerest). Many nasal decongestants are available OTC for both local and systemic use (see also Table 5-7). Chronic topical use of decongestants may result in rebound swelling and congestion. Therefore decongestant nose sprays

should not be used for more than a few days. Unwanted side effects of adrenergic stimulation may occur. Phenylephrine (Neo-Synephrine) is used topically as a nasal spray, and phenylpropanolamine is used systemically as a decongestant (α-agonist action). Pseudoephedrine, both an α-adrenergic agonist and a β-adrenergic agonist, is used systemically as a nasal decongestant.

Expectorants and mucolytics. Expectorants are drugs that promote the removal of exudate or mucus from the respiratory passages. Liquefying expectorants are drugs that promote the ejection of mucus by decreasing its viscosity. Mucolytics destroy or dissolve mucus.

Some expectorants act by their ability to cause reflex stimulation of the vagus, which increases bronchial secretions. Guaifenesin [gwye-FEN-e-sin], the most popular expectorant, is contained in a variety of OTC products mixed with other active ingredients. Robitussin is available as guaifenesin alone (Robitussin plain) and mixed with an antitussive agent (Robitussin DM).

Mucolytics are enzymes that are able to digest mucus, decreasing its viscosity. Acetylcysteine (Mucomyst) is a mucolytic used to loosen secretions in pulmonary diseases, including cystic fibrosis. It is also used orally as an antidote for acetaminophen toxicity.

Antitussives. Antitussives may be opioids or related agents used for the symptomatic relief of nonproductive cough. Opioids are the most effective, but because of their addicting properties, other agents are often used. Codeine-containing cough preparations are commonly employed, but their histamine-releasing properties may precipitate bronchospasm.

Dextromethorphan [dex-troe-meth-OR-fan] (the *DM* in cough medicines such as Robitussin DM), an opioid-like compound, suppresses the cough reflex by its direct effect on the cough center. It does not cause the release of histamine. It may potentiate the effects of CNS depressants. It is available both alone and in combination with other ingredients. By impairing coughing, dextromethorphan may not allow the secretions to be cleared from the lungs.

DENTAL IMPLICATIONS OF THE RESPIRATORY DRUGS

About 10% of the population has some pulmonary disease, so patients taking medications for asthma, emphysema, or chronic bronchitis are frequently encountered. With severe COPD, a patient can develop pulmonary hypertension, increasing the risk for cardiac arrhythmias. Stress should be minimized and adrenal supplementation instituted if the patients are taking certain doses of steroids and the procedure is likely to produce severe stress. Patients prone to developing respiratory failure, if given oxygen (either alone or with nitrous oxide) or CNS depressants, may manifest acute respiratory failure. Aspirin should be avoided in pa-

tients with asthma, and erythromycin may alter the metabolism of theophylline (Box 22-1). Emergency equipment and medications should be available when treating these patients (see Table 23-1 and Box 23-3).

GASTROINTESTINAL DRUGS

There are many drugs, both over-the-counter and on prescription, that are used for gastrointestinal diseases. Some are used to treat specific gastrointestinal diseases, and others are used to provide symptomatic relief.

GASTROINTESTINAL DISEASES

Ulcers and gastroesophageal reflux disease are common gastrointestinal tract diseases. With the discovery of the etiology of ulcers, the incidence of ulcers in the population has decreased substantially. Nonspecific complaints of GERD include burping, cramps, flatulence, fullness, and congestion in the stomach. The gastrointestinal tract is highly susceptible to emotional changes because it is innervated by the vagus nerve associated with the automatic nervous system.

Gastroesophageal reflux disease. Gastroesophageal reflux disease (GERD), or **"heartburn,"** is the

GERD = heartburn

most prevalent gastrointestinal disease in the U.S. population. In this condition, the stomach contents, including the acid, reflux, or flow backward through the cardiac sphincter, up into the esophagus. Because the esophagus is not designed to endure the stomach's acid, irritation, inflammation, and erosion can occur. The pain from the inflamed esophagus may be severe and located in the middle of the chest, causing it to be interpreted as a heart attack and trigger an emergency room visit. The main problem is the lack of adequate function of the cardiac sphinc-

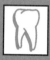

BOX 22-1 MANAGEMENT OF THE DENTAL PATIENT WITH ASTHMA

- Watch analgesic use—avoid aspirin, NSAIAs, and strong opioids; weaker opioids, acetaminophen probably OK
- Watch sulfiting agents in local anesthetic agents with vasoconstrictor → bronchoconstriction
- Avoid erythromycin with theophylline → toxicity
- Review emergency treatment of asthma with staff
- Have patient's inhaler available for use—albuterol
- Watch for oral candidiasis—inhaled steroid; rinse mouth to prevent
- Patients on long-term PO steroids may need supplemental steroids for severe stress
- Patient management—reduce stress
- Use N_2O with caution if needed for sedation

ter, allowing backflow to occur. The symptoms of GERD are exacerbated by eating large meals (blowing up a balloon [stomach] increases the back pressure) and by assuming the supine position (gravity no longer helping).

Life-style changes that can reduce symptoms include avoiding eating for 4 hours before bedtime, eating smaller meals more frequently, and raising the head of the bed with bricks or using several pillows. If untreated, some patients may have such severe symptoms that they cannot sleep lying down (sit in a chair).

GERD is treated in two ways: one is to decrease the acid in the stomach and the other is to constrict the cardiac sphincter (the muscle between the stomach and the esophagus). If the sphincter is tighter, it is less likely that the contents will flow back into the esophagus. The H_2-blockers and the proton pump inhibitors reduce or eliminate the stomach's acid. The gastrointestinal stimulants act by increasing the tone in the cardiac sphincter. Sometimes both of these approaches are required to make the patient asymptomatic. Antacids are used for acute relief of symptoms.

Ulcers. Ulcers may occur in the stomach or small intestine. In the past, it was thought that ulcers were caused by "too much acid." However, in the last decade it has been determined that most ulcers are related in some way to the presence of the organism *Helicobacter pylori*. Many ulcers can now be cured by using a combination of one or more antibiotics and an H_2-blocker or a proton pump inhibitor to reduce the acid in the stomach. Some ulcers, especially in the elderly, are secondary to the chronic use of the nonsteroidal antiinflammatory agents (NSAIAs). NSAIA-induced ulcers occur because NSAIAs inhibit synthesis of prostaglandins, which are cytoprotective to the stomach. Based on this specific mechanism of the NSAIA-induced ulcers, the treatment of NSAIA-related ulcers is quite specific, in fact, using a prostaglandin ($PGE_{2\alpha}$) misoprostol (Cytotec).

DRUGS USED TO TREAT GASTROINTESTINAL DISEASES

HISTAMINE$_2$-BLOCKING AGENTS

Histamine$_2$ (H_2)–receptor antagonists block and inhibit basal and nocturnal gastric acid secretion by competitive inhibition of the action of histamine at the histamine H_2-receptors of the parietal cells. They also inhibit gastric acid secretion stimulated by other agents such as food and caffeine. All the members of this group, which are now available OTC, are listed in Table 22-2. Cimetidine [sye-MET-i-deen] (Tagamet) is discussed as the prototype.

Uses. This group is indicated for the treatment of ulcers and the management of the symptoms of ulcers and gastroesophageal reflux disease (GERD). Combining H_2-blockers with antacids has no therapeutic advantage; in fact, antacids inhibit their absorption and should not be administered within 1 hour of H_2-blockers. H_2-blockers should be administered with meals and at bedtime. For maintenance, if only 1 dose is needed daily, the bedtime dose is most effective.

Cimetidine is also used as an adjunct in the management of urticaria.

Because smoking increases acid production and reduces the effect of the H_2-blockers, smoking cessation assistance should be offered to dental patients who smoke. Cimetidine blocks H_2-receptors, which in part are responsible for the inflammatory response, in the cutaneous blood vessels of humans.

Adverse reactions. The side effects of cimetidine include CNS effects such as slurred speech, delusions, confusion, and headache. Because cimetidine binds with the androgen receptors it produces antiandrogenic effects such as gynecomastia, reduction in sperm count, and sexual dysfunction (e.g., impotence). Unlike cimetidine, neither ranitidine nor famotidine has been

TABLE 22-2 **Gastrointestinal Drugs**

Drug Group	Subgroup	Examples
Acid reducers	H$_2$-Blockers	Cimetidine (Tagamet [HB])
		Famotidine (Pepcid [AC]) Ranitidine (Zantac [75])
		Nizatidine (Axid)
	Proton pump inhibitors	Omeprazole (Prilosec)
		Lansoprazole (Prevacid)
GI stimulant	Dopamine antagonists	Metoclopramide (Reglan)
		Cisapride (Propulsid)
Antacids	Systemic	Sodium bicarbonate
	Nonsystemic	Magnesium hydroxide
		Aluminum hydroxide
		Calcium carbonate
Laxatives	Bulk	Psyllium seed (Metamucil)
		Carboxymethylcellulose
		Methylcellulose
		Polycarbophil (FiberCon)
	Stool softeners, emollient	Docusate (dioctyl sodium sulfosuccinate, DSS, Colace)
	Stimulants	Milk of magnesia (MOM)
		Bisacodyl (Dulcolax)
		Cascara sagrada
		Senna
		Casanthranol
		Castor oil
		Phenolphthalein
	Hyperosmotic	Glycerin
		Lactulose
		Salts (magnesium citrate, hydroxide, oxide, or sulfate; sodium phosphate)
Prostaglandins	Misoprostol (Cytotec)	
Antiflatulents	Simethicone (Mylicon, Gas-X)	
Antidiarrheals	Opioid-like agents	Loperamide (Imodium)
		Diphenoxylate (in Lomotil)
	Adsorbents	Kaolin and pectin (Kaopectate)
Emetics	Ipecac	
	Apomorphine	
Antiemetics	Phenothiazines	Prochlorperazine (Compazine)
	Antihistamines	Meclizine (Bonine)
		Dimenhydrinate (Dramamine)
		Trimethobenzamide (Tigan)
	Cannabinoids	Dronabinol (Marinol)
		Nabilone (Cesamet)
Agents used in treatment of inflammatory bowel disease	Release 5-ASA	Sulfasalazine (Azulfidine [EN])
		Mesalamine (Rowasa, Pentasa, Asacol)
		Olsalazine (Dipentum)
	Prednisone	
	Immune modifiers	Cyclosporin
		Azathioprine
		6-Mercaptopurine
	Antibiotics	Metronidazole

found to possess antiandrogenic activity. Famotidine has been associated with dry mouth and taste alterations. Cimetidine's hematologic effects include granulocytopenia, thrombocytopenia, and neutropenia. Reversible hepatitis and abnormal liver functions tests have been reported with all of the H_2-blockers.

Cimetidine inhibits liver microsomal enzymes responsible for the hepatic metabolism of some drugs (cytochrome P-450 oxidase system), resulting in a delay in elimination and an increase in serum levels of some drugs, possibly producing toxicity. Ranitidine inhibits the P-450 enzymes much less than does cimetidine, and the other H_2-blockers have no effect on the P-450 enzymes. A few examples of drugs that are metabolized by the P-450 pathway include warfarin, metronidazole, lidocaine, phenytoin, theophylline, diazepam, and carbamazepine.

Dental drug interactions. The metabolism of the following drugs occasionally used in dentistry may be reduced by the administration of cimetidine:

- *Ketoconazole and itraconazole.* Toxic levels of these antifungal agents may be produced if they are used continuously for the management of chronic fungal infections. H_2-receptor antagonists may increase gastrointestinal pH. Concurrent administration with H_2-receptor antagonists may result in a marked reduction in absorption of itraconazole or ketoconazole. Patients taking itraconazole or ketoconazole should take H_2-receptor antagonists at a different time.
- *Alcohol.* The blood alcohol levels of persons who have ingested alcoholic beverages may be higher if the patient has been taking cimetidine.
- *Benzodiazepines.* The metabolism of the benzodiazepines such as diazepam and midazolam may be slower. The recovery from use of these drugs might be slower.

OTHER H_2RECEPTOR ANTAGONISTS The other H_2-blockers are unlikely to produce important dental drug interactions. Because the H_2-blockers reduce some inflammatory actions, skin tests may produce false-negative reactions. H_2RA should be discontinued before skin tests are performed.

PROTON PUMP INHIBITORS (PPI)

Omeprazole. Omeprazole [om-PRAY-zole] (Prilosec) was the first proton pump inhibitor marketed, and it is discussed as the prototype drug. It is a potent inhibitor of gastric acid secretion, is effective (in combination with the antibiotics) in healing both gastric and duodenal ulcers, and is now approved to treat and maintain GERD. Omeprazole's mechanism of action involves inhibition of the H/K ATPase enzyme system at the surface of the gastric parietal cell and is called a *gastric acid (proton) pump inhibitor.* Side effects of omeprazole include headache and abdominal pain. In rats, omeprazole produced an increase in gastric carcinoid tumors, but it has now been determined that this is unlikely to occur with use in humans. Therefore the original limit on the duration of use of omeprazole has been lifted. Although it is unknown whether a relationship exists between omeprazole and mucosal atrophy of the tongue and dry mouth, these side effects have been reported. Another PPI released on the market is lanosprazole.

MIXED ANTIINFECTIVE THERAPY FOR ULCER TREATMENT

Ulcers are closely related to the organism *Helicobacter pylori.* To treat ulcers, a combination of two or three antiinfective agents—tetracycline, metronidazole, or amoxicillin; an acid reducer; an H_2-blocker or a proton pump inhibitor; and bismuth subsalicylate (Pepto-Bismol) may be used. Newer combinations often use one antibiotic and a proton pump inhibitor such as omeprazole and clarithromycin. These agents are used for 2 weeks and result in a cure in many patients.

ANTACIDS

Antacids are used to treat a variety of gastric conditions, by both self-medication and recommendation of the patient's prescriber. Acute gastritis and symptoms of ulcers are sometimes managed with antacids. Acute gastritis, the most common type of gastric distress, is termed "heartburn" or "upset stomach." The symptoms include epigastric discomfort or a burning feeling. The symptoms of gastric ulcers can be managed with antacids.

Antacids are drugs that partially neutralize hydrochloric acid in the stomach. By raising the pH to 3 or 4, the erosive effect of the acid is decreased and pepsin activity is reduced. Antacids are classified as systemic or nonsystemic, depending on the amount of absorption from the gastrointestinal tract (see Table 22-2).

Sodium bicarbonate, the only systemic antacid, rapidly neutralizes gastric acid. Its major disadvantage is that alkalosis can occur. It also contains sodium and is contraindicated in cardiovascular patients who are to minimize sodium intake. For these reasons it is not recommended, although it is still used by the lay public.

The active ingredients in nonsystemic antacids, the preferred antacids, include calcium carbonate, aluminum and magnesium salts, and magnesium-aluminum hydroxide gels. Calcium salts may result in acid-rebound, constipation, or hypercalcemia. Aluminum salts can produce constipation. Magnesium salts produce osmotic diarrhea. Hypermagnesemia has been reported in patients with renal disease. Drug interactions with the antacids include altering the absorption of other drugs from the gastrointestinal tract. Drugs whose absorption is inhibited include tetracyclines, digitalis, iron, chlorpromazine, and indomethacin. Conversely, levodopa's absorp-

tion is increased because stomach emptying time is shortened. By mixing aluminum and magnesium salts in a single preparation, the effects on the bowel can be balanced.

MISCELLANEOUS GASTROINTESTINAL DRUGS

Misoprostol. Misoprostol [mye-soe-PROST-ole] (Cytotec) is the prostaglandin $PGE_{2\alpha}$ and is indicated in the management of NSAIA-induced ulcers. Both H_2-blockers and proton pump inhibitors reduce the symptoms of NSAIA-induced ulcers but do not prevent the ulcers. Misoprostol increases gastric mucus and inhibits gastric acid secretion. Its side effects include stomach distress and diarrhea (caused by prostaglandins). Its FDA pregnancy category is X because it stimulates uterine contractions.

Sucralfate. Sucralfate [soo-KRAL-fate] (Carafate), a complex of aluminum hydroxide and sulfated sucrose (a polysaccharide with antipeptic activity), is used to treat duodenal ulcers. In the stomach, the aluminum ion splits off, leaving an anion that is essentially nonabsorbable. Sucralfate combines with proteins, forming a complex that binds preferentially with the ulcer site. It can be thought of as a "bandage" for ulcers. It inhibits the action of pepsin and absorbs the bile salts. Its acid-neutralizing capacity does not contribute to its antiulcer action. Constipation is the most frequent side effect reported (2.2%). Other side effects (less than 0.3%) include dry mouth, nausea, rash, and dizziness. It must be taken on an empty stomach and can inhibit the absorption of tetracycline.

Metoclopramide. The drug metoclopramide [met-oh-KLOE-pra-mide] (Reglan) is a dopaminergic antagonist. It blocks the action of dopamine, and that action facilitates cholinergic effects within the gastrointestinal tract. Metoclopramide stimulates the motility of the upper gastrointestinal tract without stimulating secretions and relaxes smooth muscle innervated by dopamine. It relaxes the pyloric sphincter and increases peristalsis in the duodenum. This results in an accelerated gastric emptying time. It also increases the tone of the lower esophageal sphincter. Its antiemetic property is the result of its antagonism of dopamine receptors both centrally and peripherally.

Metoclopramide is indicated for the relief of symptoms associated with diabetic gastroparesis (gastric stasis) and improves delayed gastric emptying time. Another indication is short-term therapy for gastroesophageal reflux with symptoms. The most common CNS side effects are restlessness, drowsiness, and fatigue and occur in 10% to 25% of patients. Parkinson-like reactions can occur in up to 10% of patients. Gastrointestinal side effects include nausea and diarrhea. Additive CNS depression may occur when other CNS depressants are used concomitantly.

Cisapride, another dopamine antagonist, is similar to metoclopramide.

Simethicone. Simethicone (Mylicon, Gas-X) is an agent used to relieve flatulence (gas). It lowers the surface tension and breaks up gas pockets so they can be expelled.

LAXATIVES AND ANTIDIARRHEALS

Laxatives. Self-medication with laxatives is a common practice among the lay public. Although a few indications for the use of laxatives exist, overuse is common and habituation can result. The myth that "regular" bowel habits are essential has led to this practice. Abuse of these substances occurs in bulimic patients. Short-term, occasional use for constipation and use before diagnostic procedures (barium enema) are legitimate indications. The types of laxatives (see Table 22-2) are as follows:

• *Bulk laxatives.* Bulk laxatives are preferred because they are the safest and act most like the normal physiology of humans. They contain polysaccharides or cellulose derivatives that combine with intestinal fluids to form gels. This increases peristalsis and facilitates movement through the intestine. Patients with problems with constipation can increase their intake of fiber or use any bulk laxative daily without problems.

• *Lubricants.* Mineral oil, a lubricant that was previously frequently used, is no longer recommended. It can be absorbed if used over a long period and can interfere with the absorption of the fat-soluble vitamins (A, D, E, K).

• *Stimulants.* These laxatives act by producing local irritation of the intestinal mucosa. Because of their potent effect, intestinal cramping can result. Bisacodyl, a member of this group, is frequently used before bowel surgery or radiologic examinations, but should not be used for simple constipation.

• *Stool softeners (emollients).* Dioctyl sodium sulfosuccinate, an anionic detergent, wets and softens the stool by accumulating water in the intestine. These agents should be limited to short-term use, even though they are termed *nontoxic.*

• *Osmotic (saline) laxatives.* Magnesium sulfate or phosphate produces its laxative effect by osmotically holding water. It should be used with caution in patients with renal impairment.

Antidiarrheals. Drugs used to treat diarrhea are either adsorbents or opioid-like in action. Antidiarrheals are used to minimize fluid and electrolyte imbalances. In certain poisonings or infections, antidiarrheals are contraindicated. The most common adsorbent combination used to treat diarrhea is kaolin and pectin (Kaopectate). The opioids, such as diphenoxylate with atropine (Lomotil) and loperamide (OTC Imodium), are the most effective antidiarrheal agents. They decrease peristalsis by acting directly on the smooth muscle of the gastrointestinal tract.

EMETICS AND ANTIEMETICS

Drugs used to induce vomiting and to prevent vomiting are used for certain gastrointestinal tract problems.

Emetics. Ipecac is an emetic used to treat persons who have ingested an overdose of drugs that could be harmful. It has been abused by individuals with bulimia. Over time, with chronic use, the body becomes resistant to the emetic effect and the ipecac is absorbed. The cardiac toxicity produced by the retained ipecac has been fatal to patients with bulimia.

Antiemetics Vomiting may occur because of a variety of situations such as motion sickness, pregnancy, drugs, infections, or radiation therapy. Choice of the drug to treat vomiting depends to some extent on the cause of the vomiting.

PHENOTHIAZINES Phenothiazines (e.g., prochlorperazine [Compazine]) are used to control severe nausea. Their side effects include sedation and extrapyramidal symptoms, including tardive dyskinesia (see Chapter 17). Promethazine (Phenergan), a phenothiazine with antihistaminic and anticholinergic properties, is used in dentistry to treat nausea and vomiting associated with surgery and anesthesia. It also has sedative and antisialagogue action. It is sometimes used concurrently with opioids to minimize the nausea they produce.

ANTICHOLINERGICS Anticholinergics can be used for the nausea and the vomiting associated with motion sickness and labyrinthitis. Both dimenhydrinate (Dramamine) and meclizine (Bonine) possess antiemetic, antivertigo, and antimotion sickness action. Because they have antihistaminic action, sedation is a side effect. A scopolamine transdermal patch (Transderm-Scop) is placed postauricularly (behind the ear) and releases medication over a 3-day period. It is used for motion sickness on ships and boats. It is contraindicated whenever anticholinergics are

used (see Chapter 5). Idiosyncratic reactions, dry mouth, blurred vision, sedation, and dizziness have been reported.

ANTIHISTAMINES The agent diphenhydramine (Benadryl), an antihistamine with antiemetic properties, commonly produces sedation. Hydroxyzine (Atarax) is used in dentistry as an antiemetic or antianxiety agent.

TRIMETHOBENZAMIDE The drug trimethobenzamide (Tigan) has an antiemetic effect that is mediated through the chemoreceptor trigger zone. It produces sedation, agitation, headache, and dry mouth. It is available orally or as a suppository that contains 2% benzocaine (avoid in patients allergic to ester local anesthetics).

METOCLOPRAMIDE Metoclopramide (Reglan) can control the nausea and vomiting of patients receiving cancer chemotherapeutic agents. It acts both centrally (dopamine antagonist) and peripherally (stimulates release of acetylcholine). It is also indicated for the management of gastric motility disorders such as diabetic gastric stasis.

BENZQUINAMIDE The agent benzquinamide (Emete-Con) has antiemetic, antihistaminic, anticholinergic, and sedative effects. It is used to treat nausea associated with anesthesia during surgery. Both dry mouth and salivation have been reported with its use. CNS sedation and excitation including drowsiness, fatigue, excitement, and nervousness have been reported. It can potentiate the pressor effects of epinephrine.

CANNABINOIDS Dronabinol [droe-NAB-i-nol] (Marinol) and nabilone [NAB-i-lone] (Cesamet) are psychoactive substances derived from *Cannabis sativa L.* (marijuana). They produce effects similar to those of marijuana. These agents are highly abusable. Tolerance and both physical and psychologic dependence can occur. These agents are indicated to treat the nausea and vomiting associated with cancer chemotherapy in patients who have failed to respond to conventional antiemetic therapy. Close supervision is required when these agents are administered. Side effects include drowsiness and dizziness. Perceptual difficulties, muddled thinking, and elevation of mood can also occur.

Agents Used to Manage Chronic Inflammatory Bowel Disease

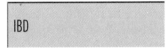

Chronic **inflammatory bowel disease** (IBD) is divided into two subcategories: ulcerative colitis and Crohn's disease. Although probably multifactorial, an autoimmune response is thought to be associated with ulcerative colitis. Crohn's disease extends through all layers of the intestinal wall, whereas ulcerative colitis involves only the mucosa. Crohn's disease can involve the whole intestine, but the colon is most commonly affected. Ulcerative colitis involves the rectum and may involve the distal part of the colon, but does not involve the small intestine. Smoking is protective against ulcerative colitis, and smoking cessation may exacerbate the disease. NSAIAs should be used with caution in patients with IBD.

The drugs used to manage IBD include agents that produce 5-aminosalicylate, steroids, immune modifiers, and antibiotics. Sulfasalazine, an antibacterial agent, has been used for years to manage IBD. This is a combination of sulfapyridine and 5-aminosalicylic acid linked by an azo bond. The intestinal flora break this combination down into its component parts, releasing 5-ASA in the intestines. Because folic acid absorption can be impaired by sulfapyridine, folic acid should be administered concomitantly. Both mesalamine (5-aminosalicylic acid [5-ASA], (Rowasa) suppositories and rectal suspension) and olsalazine (Dipentum), which is converted in the body to 5-aminosalicylic acid, are effective in the treatment of IBD. Depend-

ing on the location of the lesions various routes of administration are used to manage the IBDs.

Because corticosteroids have antiinflammatory action, they are used to manage IBDs, but systemic use can result in many side effects. Immune modulators, such as azathioprine or cyclosporine, reduce the inflammation produced by the disease process.

Review Questions

1. Name the two major types of respiratory diseases and state their differences.
2. Name the autonomic drug group used for bronchodilation and state the most specific agent and route.
3. State the drug group often used for bronchodilation in addition to the one named in question 2. Describe two side effects.
4. State one drug that cannot be used prophylactically for asthma and explain why not.
5. Describe the use of inhalers, including their advantages and types of drugs dispensed in this fashion.
6. State the drug group name for the nasal decongestants.
7. Define the terms *expectorant* and *antitussive* and give one example of each.
8. What drug group is most commonly prescribed for treatment of ulcers and stomach ailments? Describe its mechanism of action.
9. Name a useful laxative for chronic use and a type of laxative for acute use before an x-ray test. Describe one misuse of laxatives.
10. Describe the use of the antidiarrheals and name one.
11. State two antiemetic agents in different groups and describe their mechanism of action. State their appropriate use.
12. Name an agent used for each of these indications: NSAIA-induced ulcers, GERD, reflux esophagitis, and peptic or duodenal ulcers.

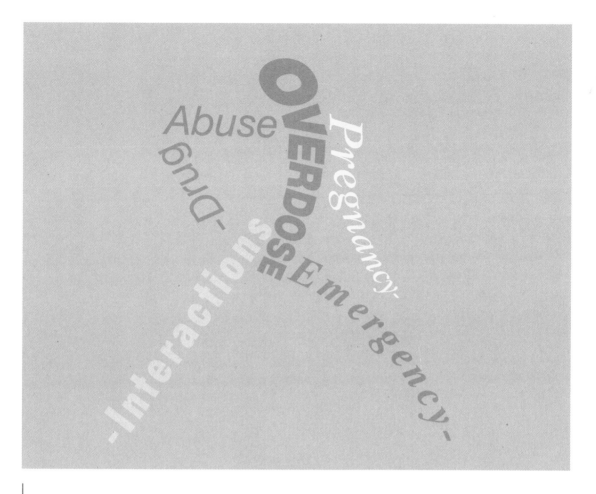

Special Situations

CHAPTER 23

Emergency Drugs

An increasing number of older patients who are taking multiple drugs seek dental treatment each year. The demographics of our population, the use of fluorides, and management of periodontal disease has increased the age of the average dental patient. Dental offices are administering more complicated drug regimens, dental appointments are taking longer, and dental patients are, on average, getting sicker. With these changes, the chance of an emergency occurring in the dental office continues to increase. Both the dentist and the dental hygienist should become familiar with the most common emergency situations, their manage-

ment, and the drugs used to treat these conditions. When an emergency occurs, working together can increase the chance of producing the best outcome. Many emergency situations can be handled correctly with adequate knowledge. Lack of this knowledge during an emergency may cause panic in a dental office. If the dental office and its personnel are prepared for an emergency, handling one will be easier. Before treating patients who might be at risk for an emergency, the treatment of a potential emergency related to their disease should be reviewed. It is the responsibility of each dental health care worker to make sure the members of the team can act in a coordinated manner.

GENERAL MEASURES

To prepare the dental office for an emergency the following steps should be taken:

* **Train.** Train and regularly retrain all office personnel in emergency procedures before an emergency occurs. Practice for an emergency at least once every 6 months.

  Basic Cardiac Life Support (Cardiopulmonary resuscitation [CPR]) training (required)

  Advanced Cardiac Life Support training (ACLS) (optional, unless performing conscious sedation)

* **Phone number.** Post the telephone number of the closest physician, emergency room, and ambulance service (often 911). Program the number(s) into the speed dial function of the phone.

* **Emergency kit.** Select the items for the office's emergency kit, including the drugs and the devices (nondrug items needed). Check every 3 months to make sure that the drugs are not out of date. Some companies have this service by subscription.

To minimize the chances of an office emergency, the procedures listed in Box 23-1 should be performed on each new dental patient. It is easier to prevent rather than treat a dental emergency. If an emergency occurs in the dental office, the steps listed in Box 23-2 should be taken.

PREPARATION FOR TREATMENT

Before any emergency treatment can be administered, investigation of the patient's signs and symptoms must lead to a diagnosis of the

A = Airway
B = Breathing
C = Circulation

Box 23-1   METHODS OF MINIMIZING EMERGENCIES IN THE DENTAL OFFICE

Observe the patient's stature, build, gait, coloring, age, facies, and respiration.

Observe and record the amount of anxiety; use active listening to determine hidden nervousness.

Take the patient's blood pressure and pulse rate, and perform any necessary laboratory examination.

Take a complete patient history, including medication history, past dental and anesthetic experiences, restrictions on physical activity, diseases, and present condition.

Request medical consultations as needed.

Prescribe premedication, if appropriate, and avoid drug interactions.

Box 23-2   TREATMENT OF AN EMERGENCY IN THE DENTAL OFFICE

Recognize the abnormal occurrence.

Make a proper diagnosis.

Call 911 (or appropriate emergency number).

Note the time.

Position the patient properly.

Maintain an airway.

Administer oxygen.

Monitor vital signs.

Provide symptomatic treatment.

Administer cardiopulmonary resuscitation (CPR) if there is no pulse.

problem. In most cases the maintenance of the airway (A), respiration (breathing, B), and circulation (C) are of primary importance. The use of drug therapy in these situations is only ancillary to the primary measures of maintaining adequate circulation and respiration. Remember that drugs are *not* necessary for the proper management of most emergencies. Whenever there is doubt as to whether to give the drug, it should not be given.

Keep up to date

In the dental office, each health care worker should be certified. The legal implications of lack of CPR training could be serious. ACLS training can be helpful in certain rural situations or if the technique of preoperative sedation or conscious sedation is used in the dental office.

The categories of emergencies are discussed. The most commonly used drugs and the choice of drugs and equipment for a dental office emergency kit are addressed.

CATEGORIES OF EMERGENCIES

This chapter discusses the signs, symptoms, and treatment of the most common emergency situations, dividing them into changing consciousness, respiratory, cardiovascular, and other emergencies and drug-related emergencies.

LOST OR ALTERED CONSCIOUSNESS

Many common dental emergencies involve either unconsciousness or altered consciousness. Dental office personnel should be ready to handle these emergencies and determine the best course of treatment.

Syncope—most common

Syncope. The emergency most frequently encountered in the dental office is simple syncope (fainting) or transient unconsciousness. The skin takes on an ashen-gray color and **diaphoresis** occurs. The release of excessive epinephrine results in a pooling of the blood in the peripheral muscles (β-effect, vasodilation), a decrease in total peripheral resistance, and a sudden fall in blood pressure. A reflex tachycardia follows, but soon decompensation results in severe bradycardia. These effects are brought about by anxiety, fear, or apprehension, all of which are common in a dental situation. Treatment involves placing the patient in the Trendelenburg position (head down), causing blood to rush to the head, which has the effect of giving the patient a transfusion of whole blood.

The most important component in the treatment of syncope is for the dental health care worker to exhibit confidence in action and voice. If the hygienist shows control over the situation, the patient will be less anxious and apprehensive and less likely to repeat the syncopal attack.

Spirits of ammonia can be administered by inhalation. The old practice of putting the head between the legs should be avoided because venous return is cut off by the slumped position.

Hypoglycemia. The most common cause of hypoglycemia is an excessive dose of insulin in a patient with diabetes. The medical history in this case is important so the dental health care worker can determine the dose and type of insulin and food intake before the appointment. Often patients inject their usual daily dose of insulin but fail to eat before coming to the dental office. If this is the case, then patients should be asked to eat before any dental procedures are begun. The time of the hypoglycemia can be estimated by knowledge of the peak effect of the particular insulins used (see Chapter 20).

The patient with hypoglycemia has a rapid pulse and decreased respiration and is **loquacious.** Hunger, dizziness, weakness, and occasionally tremor of the hands can occur. Diaphoresis, nausea, and mental confusion are other signs of hypoglycemia. If the signs of hypoglycemia are recognized before they become severe, the patient can be given a sugary drink or oral glucose. If the patient lapses into unconsciousness and has no swallowing reflex, dextrose must be given intravenously.

Diabetic coma. Less common than hypoglycemia, the diabetic coma is caused by elevated blood sugar. Symptoms of frequent urination, loss of appetite, nausea, vomiting, and thirst are seen. Acetone breath; hypercapnia; warm, dry skin; rapid pulse; and a decrease in blood pressure can occur. Treatment is undertaken only in a hospital setting and includes insulin after proper laboratory results are obtained (blood sugar).

Seizures/Epilepsy

Convulsions or seizures. Convulsions are most commonly associated with epilepsy, especially the grand mal type (see Chapter 16), but can also result from a toxic reaction to a local anesthetic agent. Convulsions are abnormal movements of parts of the body in clonic and/or tonic contractions and relaxations. The patient may become unconscious. Generally, convulsions are self-limiting, and treatment should include protecting the patient from self-harm, moving any sharp objects out of the patient's reach, and turning the patient's head to the side to prevent aspiration. In some situations, diazepam may be administered intravenously, but observation of the patient is often sufficient.

RESPIRATORY EMERGENCIES

Respiratory emergencies involve difficulty in breathing and exchange of oxygen. They include hyperventilation, asthma, anaphylactic shock, apnea, and acute airway obstruction.

Hyperventilation. Hyperventilation is one of the most common dental emergency situations. The increased respiratory rate is often brought on by emotional upset associated with dental treatment. Tachypnea, tachycardia, and paresthesia (tingling of the fingers and around the mouth) have been reported. Nausea, faintness, perspiration, acute anxiety, lightheadedness, and shortness of breath can also occur. The treatment is calm reassurance. Encourage patients to hold their breath or "rebreathe" into a paper bag or an unconnected face mask [occasionally portrayed in movies].

Asthma. Normally, patients who have acute asthmatic attacks have a history of previous attacks and carry their own medication. The most common sign of an asthmatic attack is wheezing with prolonged expiration (squeak). The patient's own medication (multiple-dose inhalers containing a β_2-agonist such as albuterol) should be used first. The dose should be repeated several times. If there is no response to these, hospitalization for administration of aminophylline (parenteral or oral) and parenteral corticosteroids and epinephrine should be considered. Oxygen should also be administered.

Anaphylactic shock. The most common cause of anaphylactic shock is an injection of penicillin, although anaphylactic

Anaphylaxis emergency—4 minutes to treat

reactions have also been caused by many other agents. Examples include eating peanuts or being exposed to latex rubber items. The reaction usually begins within 5 to 30 minutes after ingestion or administration of the antigen. Usually, a weak, rapid pulse and a profound decrease in blood pressure occur. There is dyspnea and severe bronchial constriction.

Parenteral epinephrine is the drug of choice and must be administered immediately in cases of severe anaphylactic shock. It may be given in the deltoid or injected under the tongue. If bronchoconstriction is predominant, albuterol administered by inhalation or nebulization may suffice. After the life-threatening symptoms have been controlled, intravenous corticosteroids, intramuscular diphenhydramine, and aminophylline may also be used.

Acute airway obstruction.

Acute airway obstruction or aspiration (such as of vomitus) is usually due to a foreign body (such as a crown preparation) in the pharynx or larynx; laryngospasm may be drug induced. Gasping for breath, coughing, gagging, acute anxiety, and cyanosis are signs and symptoms of acute airway obstruction. Treatment begins by placing the patient in a Trendelenburg position on the right side, and encouraging coughing. Do not allow the patient to sit up. Clearing the pharynx and pulling the tongue forward before performing the Heimlich maneuver (external subdiaphragmatic compression) should be attempted next. Finally, the Heimlich maneuver should be performed and repeated if needed. A cricothyrotomy or tracheotomy, hardly dental office maneuvers, are indicated if the object cannot be dislodged by the other methods.

For aspiration, the use of suction, intubation, and ventilatory assistance is suggested. Steroids, antibiotics, and aminophylline are also administered. When drug-induced laryngospasm is present, succinylcholine, a neuromuscular blocking agent, and positive-pressure oxygen are the agents of choice. The operator must have training and equipment to artificially breathe for the patient before succinylcholine is administered. Prevention of swallowed objects can best be attained by the use of a rubber dam and throat packing, when appropriate.

CARDIOVASCULAR SYSTEM EMERGENCIES

Emergency situations involving the cardiovascular system include angina pectoris, myocardial infarction, cardiac arrest, acute congestive heart failure, arrhythmias, and hypertensive crisis.

The primary concern in any cardiovascular emergency is the maintenance of adequate circulation. Administration of cardiopulmonary resuscitation (CPR), calling emergency personnel, and administration of oxygen are appropriate for most emergencies. The drugs used in cardiovascular emergencies are discussed individually later in the chapter.

Angina pectoris.

Without a previous history of angina, diagnosis of this condition can be difficult. It often begins as substernal chest pain that radiates across the chest, to the left arm, or to the mandible. It may also produce a feeling of heaviness in the chest. The pulse becomes rapid and tachypnea can occur. An anginal attack can be brought on by stress from pain, trauma, or fear, especially in a dental situation.

Premedication with sublingual nitroglycerin before a stressful dental situation may prevent an acute anginal attack. Treatment of an acute anginal attack (see Chapter 15) is with sublingual nitroglycerin. Opioids or diazepam are used in hospitalized patients.

Acute myocardial infarction.

An acute myocardial infarction (heart attack) often begins as severe pain, pressure, or heaviness in the chest that radiates to other parts of the body. Sweating, nausea, and vomiting can occur. The pain is persistent and unrelieved by rest or nitroglycerin (3 doses). In this way a myocardial infarction can be differentiated from an anginal attack. An irregular rapid pulse, shortness of breath, diaphoresis, and indigestion can occur. Treatment includes administration of oxygen, an aspirin tablet, and an opioid analgesic agent and transfer to a hospital. The risk of death is greatest within the first 6 hours.

Hospitalized patients who have suffered a myocardial infarction are given lidocaine for arrhythmias and vasopressor agents to maintain an adequate blood pressure. New drugs that can dissolve clots are administered soon after the event and may reverse the clot.

Cardiac arrest. When cardiac arrest occurs, generally there is sudden circulatory and respiratory collapse. Without immediate therapy, cardiac arrest is fatal. Permanent brain damage occurs in 4 minutes. Pulse is absent and blood pressure is unobtainable. After a few minutes the patient becomes cyanotic and the pupils are fixed and dilated. The first and most important treatment is immediate, adequate CPR. One dentist was sued when his patient had an MI in the office. His first action was to call 9-1-1. His *second* action was to run out to the street and wait for the ambulance. [What's wrong with this picture?]

Other medications used in a hospital setting for cardiac arrest include epinephrine for cardiac stimulation and lidocaine for arrhythmias. Parenteral opioid analgesics are given for the pain. **Defibrillation** is used to treat asystole.

Other cardiovascular emergencies. Arrhythmias, another cardiovascular emergency, depend on an electrocardiogram for diagnosis before treatment. A cerebrovascular accident (CVA, stroke), resulting in weakness on one side of the body or speech defects, is treated with oxygen administration and immediate hospitalization so "clot busters" can be administered. Hypertensive crisis is treated with antihypertensive agents given intravenously (see Chapter 15). Treatment of these cardiovascular emergencies is undertaken in a hospital setting.

OTHER EMERGENCY SITUATIONS

Some emergency situations involve symptoms that do not fit into the other categories.

Extrapyramidal reactions. The antipsychotic agents (see Chapter 17) can produce extrapyramidal reactions. Parkinson-like movements such as uncoordinated tongue and muscular movements and grimacing can occur. Prochlorperazine (Compazine), used for nausea and vomiting, can produce this type of reaction. Intravenous di-

phenhydramine (Benadryl) is the treatment of choice.

Acute adrenocortical insufficiency. Adrenal crisis usually occurs in patients who are taking enough steroids to suppress the adrenal gland. When they are subjected to acute severe stress without increasing their steroid dose a crisis may occur. Unable to respond to the stress, the patient has an adrenal crisis. Nausea, vomiting, abdominal pain, and confusion may result. Cardiovascular collapse and irreversible shock may result in a fatality. The treatment for adrenal crisis is parenteral hydrocortisone and oxygen by inhalation. After hospitalization, patients receive fluid replacement and vasopressor agents if symptoms dictate.

Thyroid storm. Thyroid storm is a condition in which hyperthyroidism is out of control. Signs and symptoms include hyperpyrexia, increased sweating, hyperactivity, mental agitation, shaking, nervousness, and tachycardia. Congestive heart failure and cardiovascular collapse may follow. Temperature is controlled by tepid baths and aspirin. β-Blockers are given to control the cardiovascular symptoms. Another agent that may be used is hydrocortisone. Aspirin should be avoided in these patients (displaces T_4 from binding sites). Sodium iodide and propylthiouracil are given to inhibit the action of the thyroid gland. Untreated severely hyperthyroid patients should not be given atropine or epinephrine because these agents may precipitate a thyroid storm.

Malignant hyperthermia. Malignant hyperthermia is a genetically determined reaction that is triggered by inhalation general anesthetics or neuromuscular blocking agents such as succinylcholine. The most notable symptom is a rapidly rising temperature. Baths and aspirin are used to control the elevated temperature. Prompt treatment with dantrolene (Dantrium) can control acidosis and body temperature by reducing calcium released into the muscles during the contractile response. Before dantrolene, death was a common outcome. Fluid replacement, steroids, and sodium bicarbonate may be used.

DRUG-RELATED EMERGENCIES

Opioid overdose. Opioids, administered in the dental office or prescribed by the dentist, can produce overdose symptoms. Respiration can be depressed or respiratory arrest may occur. Illegitimate use of street drugs (such as heroin) may also produce overdose symptoms. The most common symptoms of overdose from the opioids are shallow and slow respiration and pinpoint pupils. The drug of choice for opioid overdose is naloxone (Narcan), an opioid antagonist. (See Chapter 7.)

Reaction to local anesthetic agents. Toxic reactions to local anesthetic agents usually result from excessive plasma levels of the anesthetic. Both central nervous system (CNS) stimulation and CNS depression can occur. The stimulation is exhibited as excitement or convulsions (see Chapter 10). Following stimulation, depression can occur with symptoms of drowsiness, unconsciousness, or cardiac and respiratory arrest. The treatment of this toxic reaction is symptomatic. If convulsions are a predominant feature, diazepam can be administered. If hypotension is predominant, a pressor agent can be given. In the presence of reflex bradycardia, atropine may be administered. Usually patients who have a toxic reaction to local anesthetics must be watched closely, but drug administration is rarely necessary. This reaction requires a dose of local anesthetic above the maximum dental dose.

Epinephrine. Toxic reactions to epinephrine occur most frequently after the placement of a gingival retraction cord used prior to taking impressions. The symptoms range from nervousness to frank shaking and can also include tachycardia. Because epinephrine is quickly metabolized, the main treatment is to remove the cord and reassure the patient. Becoming panicky will cause the patient to release endogenous epinephrine, and the reaction will continue. Above all else, the dental health care worker must remain *calm!*

EMERGENCY KIT FOR THE DENTAL OFFICE

Although the choice of drugs for a dental office emergency kit will depend on individual circumstances, experience, and personal preference, the dental health care worker should make sure there is an emergency kit in the dental office. Table 23-1 lists some emergency drugs, their therapeutic uses, and their usual adult doses. Other drugs that may be included if the office

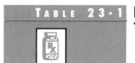

TABLE 23-1 Emergency Drugs and Their Indications

DRUG	AVERAGE ADULT DOSE
LEVEL 1 (CRITICAL DRUGS)	
Albuterol (IH) Ventolin)	2 inhalations
Diphenhydramine	50 mg
Epinephrine	0.5 ml IM, SQ, or IV
Glucose, oral	Titrate to effect
Nitroglycerin	0.4 mg SL (or 1 spray) q5 min × 3 prn
Oxygen	6 L/min
LEVEL 2 (SECONDARY DRUGS)—LEVEL 1 DRUGS PLUS THESE:	
Atropine	0.5 mg IM, IV, or SQ
Beta blockers	Differs by agent
Dextrose 50%	5 mg/min titrate
Diazepam/alprazolam	10 mg IM
Glucagon	1 mg IM or IV
Hydrocortisone	100 mg IV or IM
Methoxamine	10 mg IM
Morphine	3 mg
Spirits of ammonia	One ampule
OTHER DRUGS	
Bretylium	5 mg/kg IV
Calcium chloride	3 mg/kg IV
Flumazenil	0.2 mg IV, may repeat
Lidocaine	1 mg/kg, may follow by 0.5 mg/kg
Naloxone	0.4 mg IV q3 min
Procainamide	100 mg; may follow by 50 mg IV
Verapamil	0.1 mg/kg IV, may repeat

personnel are trained in ACLS include level 2 drugs, atropine, and lidocaine, and calcium chloride.

DRUGS

Table 23-1 lists the drugs that should be considered for inclusion in a simple emergency dental kit. These may vary, depending on the preference and experience of the practitioner. Some equipment and drugs that are not used by dental office personnel are kept in the emergency kit for use by a physician or for those with ACLS training in an emergency.

Obtaining small quantities of these medications may be difficult because they are often sold in packages of 12. A hospital pharmacy may be able to help the practitioner because the pharmacy buys in large quantities and could sell the few ampules that are needed for the dental office emergency kit. The security of the kit should be ensured by the use of a "breakable" lock that can be used to determine whether tampering has occurred. The kit should be stored in a prominent place in the dental office, but control of the agents such as the diazepam or an opioid, if included, should be ensured.

Level 1 (critical) drugs

EPINEPHRINE Epinephrine must be included in the dental office emergency kit for treatment of cardiac arrest, anaphylaxis, or acute asthmatic attack. It should not be used in treatment of shock because it can cause decreased venous return with increased ischemia and can precipitate ventricular fibrillation. The rationale for the use of epinephrine for cardiac arrest is β-stimulation of the myocardium. In the treatment of severe anaphylaxis and acute asthmatic attacks, it acts as a physiologic antagonist to the massive release of mediators that occurs in these conditions. Without epinephrine, these chemicals lead to bronchoconstriction and decreased oxygen exchange. Because epinephrine's cardiac effects are diminished in the presence of acidosis, adequate mechanical resuscitation and external cardiac massage accompany its administration. Epinephrine may be administered by intravenous or intracardiac routes (by trained personnel). Dental personnel may find injection into the frenulum under the tongue more convenient.

DIPHENHYDRAMINE Diphenhydramine (Benadryl), an antihistamine, is used in the treatment of some allergic reactions. Because antihistamines compete with histamine for tissue receptor sites, a rapid reversal of allergic symptoms cannot be expected. For this reason epinephrine and diphenhydramine are used together in severe allergic reactions or anaphylaxis.

OXYGEN Oxygen is indicated in most emergencies, especially if respiratory difficulty is a problem. Patients with COPD should be given oxygen with caution because apnea may result. All dental office personnel should know the procedure for administering inhalation oxygen. All potential members of the dental team should review the procedure on a regular basis.

NITROGLYCERIN Sublingual nitroglycerin tablets or nitroglycerin spray (see Chapter 15) should be kept in the dental office emergency kit to manage an acute anginal attack. The sublingual spray may be used in place of the tablets.

GLUCOSE Oral glucose, or any available liquid carbohydrate, is used to manage hypoglycemia in the conscious or semiconscious patient with diabetes. If the patient can swallow, then the oral route is preferable. A small amount may be placed in the buccal pouch, where it can be slowly swallowed. Tubes of glucose for this purpose are available, or cake frosting in tubes may be used.

ALBUTEROL Albuterol is a β_2-adrenergic agonist that produces bronchodilation. It is used in the management of an acute attack of asthma or respiratory distress accompanying anaphylaxis.

If used properly, albuterol can produce bronchodilation in a few seconds.

Level 2 drugs

BENZODIAZEPINES Diazepam (Valium) and midazolam (Versed) are the drugs of choice for the treatment of most convulsions if a drug is needed. However, in the majority of cases, convulsive episodes are self-limiting and require only supportive care in the form of protecting the patient from physical harm and administering oxygen.

One cause of convulsions in the dental office is a toxic reaction to a local anesthetic from an overdose or an idiosyncrasy (see Chapter 10). Anticonvulsant drugs should be used conservatively because they may enhance CNS depression of the local anesthetic.

AROMATIC AMMONIA SPIRITS Containers of aromatic ammonia spirits, designed to be crushed, can be used to treat syncope. Aromatic ammonia acts by irritating the membranes of the upper respiratory tract, resulting in stimulation of respiration and blood pressure. A dental office should have one (unexpired) container near each dental chair for easy access.

MORPHINE Morphine and meperidine are opioid analgesics administered to a patient who has suffered an acute myocardial infarction. These agents relieve pain and allay apprehension. They are used for cases of pulmonary embolism and angina for the same reasons.

METHOXAMINE Methoxamine, which is an α-adrenergic agonist, may be included in the emergency kit. By peripheral vasoconstriction, it produces a mild increase in blood pressure. There is no concomitant stimulation of the myocardium; in fact, a reflex bradycardia results. Methoxamine is indicated in the treatment of hypotension. The product contains bisulfite, a compound to which some patients exhibit hypersensitivity reactions. Patients with asthma

are more likely to exhibit a reaction to sulfites. Phenylephrine (Neo-Synephrine), also an α-adrenergic agonist, is used like methoxamine. Dopamine, an α- and β-adrenergic agonist, is used for certain kinds of shock. One advantage of dopamine is that it increases renal and splanchnic blood flow and cardiac output.

HYDROCORTISONE A corticosteroid used for allergic reactions, anaphylaxis, and adrenal crisis is hydrocortisone sodium. Even given intravenously, hydrocortisone has a slow onset of action. Epinephrine is still the drug of choice for anaphylaxis and serious allergic reactions because it acts immediately as a physiologic antagonist. Administration of hydrocortisone should follow the use of epinephrine, and it may be given intramuscularly or intravenously.

DEXTROSE Intravenous dextrose is used to manage hypoglycemic episodes when a patient with diabetes is unconscious and cannot swallow. Hypoglycemia occurs most commonly when the patient's insulin, exercise, and food intake are out of balance. In the dental office, all patients with hypoglycemia should be recognized before unconsciousness occurs.

GLUCAGON Glucagon is used for the management of severe hypoglycemic reactions. It can be given intramuscularly, intravenously, or subcutaneously. If patient does not respond to the glucagon, intravenous glucose should be considered.

ATROPINE Atropine is used as a preoperative antisialogogue and to increase the cardiac rate when it has been slowed by vagal stimulation. It is administered intramuscularly, intravenously, and subcutaneously.

β-BLOCKERS β-Blockers, such as esmolol or labetalol, are administered by intravenous infusion to manage intraoperative or postoperative tachycardia or hypertension.

Other drugs

NALOXONE Naloxone (Narcan), a pure opioid antagonist, is the drug of choice for opioid-induced apnea. Its use is extremely safe, but more than one administration may be needed because of its short duration of action. The initial dose is 0.4 mg (1 ml) intravenously, but it can also be given subcutaneously or intramuscularly. The onset of action is approximately 2 minutes by the intravenous route. This dose should be repeated several times in case the dose of opioid was high, (sometimes a combination of self-administered plus dentist-administered opioids.)

Another potential problem with giving naloxone is precipitating withdrawal in an addict (see Chapter 7). Naloxone is effective in reversing the respiratory depression caused by opioid drugs; if no response occurs, other causes for the respiratory depression must be considered. Naloxone should be in a dental emergency kit if patients are given opioids preoperatively or intraoperatively.

FLUMAZENIL Flumazenil (Mazicon) is a benzodiazepine antagonist used for reversing most of the effects of the benzodiazepines. It may be used after conscious sedation with diazepam or lorazepam. It should be in the emergency kit only if parenteral benzodiazepines are administered in the dental office.

ANTIARRHYTHMICS Procainamide, lidocaine, verapamil, and bretylium are used for their antiarrhythmic effect. The specific arrhythmia should be identified before an antiarrhythmic agent is selected. Arrhythmias are not something that most dental offices are equipped to treat.

EQUIPMENT

An oxygen mask, a manual resuscitation bag, and an oxygen tank with a flow gauge are needed to administer positive pressure oxygen. A **sphygmomanometer** and stethoscope are used to take a patient's blood pressure. Disposable syringes,

---

BOX 23-3 EMERGENCY DEVICES

Level 1 (critical devices)

Syringes/needles
Tourniquets
System to give oxygen*

Level 2 (secondary devices)

Cricothyrotomy device
Endotracheal tube
Laryngoscope
System to give IV infusions

---

*Oxygen and system (e.g., Ambu bag).

---

needles, and a tourniquet are used to administer medications. A laryngeal suction cannula is used to suction the throat if aspiration occurs. Box 23-3 lists essential equipment for a dental office emergency.

With ACLS training a more advanced emergency kit can be prepared. Nasal and oral airways are used to maintain an unobstructed airway. Endotracheal tubes and a laryngoscope are required for intubation. Intravenous solutions, tubing, butterfly needles, and adhesive tape are used for intravenously administering drugs. A cricothyrotomy (incision through skin and cricothyroid membrane before performing a tracheotomy) kit can be used for acute airway obstruction when other measures fail.

Many dental offices will not have staff trained to use the more advanced equipment. Without training, attempts to use this equipment may be more harmful than using simple measures. If untrained, stick to CPR.

REVIEW QUESTIONS

1. State what general measures the dental health care worker should be familiar with

in order to respond to any emergency situation.

2. For each of the following common emergencies, state the signs, symptoms, and treatment (including drugs):
   a. cardiac arrest
   b. angina pectoris
   c. acute myocardial infarction
   d. convulsions
   e. syncope
   f. asthma
   g. anaphylactic shock
   h. apnea
   i. hypoglycemia

3. List the equipment required to treat the emergencies in question 2 and explain the rationale for the inclusion of each item.

4. Give the names and potential uses of the drugs required in an emergency kit for the dental office.

5. Plan an imaginary emergency kit for the office in which you will work.

Pregnancy and Breast Feeding

Dental treatment of the pregnant or nursing woman is always of special concern to dental health care workers. Pregnant women often need additional dental treatment during their pregnancies, and, in addition, that treatment must be carefully planned. Many questions about drug therapy for the pregnant or breast-feeding woman arise. The literature, unfortunately, does not provide all the answers. This chapter attempts to offer guidelines for determining the relative risk when prescribing drugs for the pregnant woman or nursing mother. No unnecessary drug should be administered to the pregnant woman. If a drug is to be administered, the risk to the fetus must be weighed against the benefit to the woman. An adequate health history, including whether a woman might be pregnant (ages 11 to 63), should be taken at each dental appointment. Close coordination with the patient's obstetric health care professional is recommended when questions about her potential use of drugs arise. Consultations should be documented in the patient's chart. Box 24-1 lists the dental implications involved in managing a pregnant dental patient.

Box 24-1 MANAGEMENT OF THE PREGNANT DENTAL PATIENT

- Avoid elective dental treatment except in the second trimester.
- Avoid any unnecessary drugs, especially during the first trimester.
- If drugs are needed, check the FDA categories to choose the safest.
- Minimize periodontal problems—perform oral prophylaxis before pregnancy or during second trimester; monitor for periodontal conditions.
- Avoid radiographs unless absolutely necessary; use lead apron.
- Pay particular attention to periodontal disease because it has been associated with low-birth-weight newborns.
- Position patient in recumbent position in last trimester with right hip elevated (not Trendelenburg).
- If morning sickness is a problem, schedule an afternoon appointment.
- Give frequent breaks for urination, especially during the first trimester.

GENERAL PRINCIPLES

> Teratogenic = produces abnormal fetus

Two main concerns must be addressed when considering whether to give a drug to a pregnant woman. The first is that the drug may be teratogenic. The term *teratogen* is derived from the Greek prefix *terato-*, meaning "monster," and the suffix *-gen*, meaning "producing." These two combine to give rise to the meaning of teratogen: "producing a monster." The second is that the drug can affect the near-term fetus, causing the newborn infant to have an adverse reaction, such as respiratory depression or jaundice. A relatively new concern is the long-term (physiologic and psychologic) consequences of in utero exposure to agents not evident at birth.

HISTORY

In 1941, a relationship between getting German measles during pregnancy and blindness, deafness, and death of the offspring was noted. Scientists recognized that exogenous agents could affect the unborn fetus, producing congenital abnormalities. Again in 1961, this lesson was still being taught. A "harmless" sedative, thalidomide, available over the counter (OTC) in Europe, was taken by pregnant women. An increase in the rare birth defect phocomelia (short or absent limbs) occurred shortly thereafter. Thalidomide was later implicated in these birth defects.

Environmental factors are also thought to contribute to birth defects. The factory owners operating in Matamoros have been accused of having released many toxic chemicals and hazardous waste products. The incidence of fetal birth defects during this time was much greater than in other populations. Still, identifying a correlation between toxic materials and birth defects takes financial assistance. Who would give that money?

PREGNANCY

PREGNANCY TRIMESTERS

Pregnancy involves three trimesters, each 3 months long. During the first trimester, the organs in the fetus are forming. This is considered the most critical time for teratogenicity. If abnormalities occur very early in development, spontaneous abortion is the usual outcome. With later exposure, abnormalities occur in the fetus. Often a woman is unaware that she is pregnant for at least one half of this trimester.

Dental prophylaxis with detailed instructions and a visual examination of the oral cavity without x-rays should be performed if the patient is pregnant. Because this is the time when the woman may feel nauseated in the morning (morning sickness), other elective dental treatment should be avoided during this time.

The second trimester is an excellent time for the patient to receive both oral health instructions and another dental prophylaxis, if needed. The patient's periodontal status should be carefully evaluated during this time. The patient is most comfortable during this trimester.

The third trimester is closest to delivery. The woman is beginning to feel uncomfortable, and it is difficult for her to lie prone for any length of time. If dental treatment is needed, she may feel more comfortable sitting or with the right hip elevated. Also, this is the time when premature labor is most likely to begin. Drugs that may affect the newborn child should not be given during this trimester.

TERATOGENICITY

Teratogenicity—difficult to identify

It is very difficult to prove that a drug is teratogenic in humans. Some of the reasons include the following:

- Different animal species and humans vary among themselves in their responses to drugs.
- Timing of the drug exposure varies with each drug.
- One drug can produce a variety of abnormalities, and different drugs can produce the same abnormality.
- Drugs that are teratogenic are not uniformly so.
- A drug's effect on the fetus may be different from its effect on the mother.
- The teratogenic effects of a certain drug on the fetus may not be evident for many years.

Before a drug can be easily proved to be teratogenic, it must be highly teratogenic. Drugs that are known teratogens include drugs such as thalidomide, certain vitamin A analogues (isotretinoin), antineoplastic agents (busulfan, cyclophosphamide), oral anticoagulants (warfarin), lithium, methimazole, penicillamine, some antiepileptic agents (phenytoin, trimethadione, valproic acid), the tetracyclines, certain steroids (diethylstilbestrol, androgens) and ethyl alcohol. Table 24-1 lists selected drugs with adverse effects on the fetus.

FOOD AND DRUG ADMINISTRATION PREGNANCY CATEGORIES

The U.S. Food and Drug Administration (FDA) has developed pregnancy categories A, B, C,

FDA pregnancy "grades"

D, and X. Each drug that is the subject of FDA regulation for pregnancy labeling is given a category based on its known potential for risk. Table 24-2 gives a summary of the criteria for the different categories. Note that the availability of animal or human studies is a criterion. Category A is the safest, and category X should not be used in pregnant women. Categories B, C, and D fall in between these two criteria.

BREAST FEEDING

Questions about the safety of a certain drug given to a nursing mother are appearing more frequently because nursing is becoming more popular. As during pregnancy, the risk-to-benefit ratio should be carefully considered before drugs are given to the nursing mother. Drugs without strong indications for use should not be taken. Almost all drugs given to the mother can pass into the breast milk in varying concentrations. While nursing, the baby ingests

▮ᴛ ᴀʙʟᴇ 24-1   Selected Drugs with Adverse Effects on the Fetus

Dʀᴜɢ	Tʀɪᴍᴇsᴛᴇʀ	Eꜰꜰᴇᴄᴛ
ACE inhibitors	All	Renal damage
Amphetamines	All	Abnormal developmental patterns
Androgens	2nd, 3rd	Masculinization of female fetus
Antidepressants, tricyclic	3rd	Neonatal withdrawal symptoms
Antineoplastics	1st, all	Congenital malformations
Barbiturates	All	Neonatal dependence
Carbamazepine	1st	Neural tube defects
Chlorpropamide	All	Neonatal hypoglycemia, prolonged
Clomipramine	3rd	Neonatal lethargy, hypotonia, cyanosis, hypothermia
Cocaine	All	Increased spontaneous abortion, abruptio placentae, premature labor, abnormal development, decreased school performance
Diazepam	All	Neonatal dependence
Diethylstilbestrol	All	Vaginal adenosis, vaginal adenocarcinoma
Ethanol	All	Fetal alcohol syndrome
Etretinate	All	Multiple congenital malformations
Heroin	All	Neonatal dependence
Iodide	All	Congenital goiter, hypothyroidism
Isotretinoin	All	Extremely high risk of congenital anomalies
Lithium	1st	Ebstein's anomaly
Methadone	All	Neonatal dependence
Methylthiouracil	All	Hypothyroidism
Metronidazole	1st	May be mutagenic
Penicillamine	1st	Cutis laxa, other congenital malformations
Phencyclidine	All	Abnormal neurologic examination, poor suck reflex and feeding
Phenytoin	All	Abnormal neurologic examination, poor suck reflex and feeding
Propylthiouracil	All	Fetal hydantoin syndrome
Smoking	All	Intrauterine growth retardation, sudden infant death syndrome
Streptomycin	All	Eighth nerve toxicity
Tamoxifen	All	Increased spontaneous abortion and fetal damage
Tetracycline	All	Discolored teeth/altered bone
Thalidomide	1st	Phocomelia
Valproic acid	All	Neural tube defects
Warfarin	1st 2nd 3rd	Hypoplastic nasal bridge, chondrodysplasia CNS malformations Risk of bleeding, D/C 1 month before delivery

Modified from Katzung BG: *Basic & clinical pharmacology*, ed 7, Stamford, Conn, 1988, Appleton & Lange.
Boldface indicates dental drug.

TABLE 24-2 FDA Pregnancy Categories for Drugs[a]

	DESCRIPTION	EXAMPLES
A	Adequate studies have failed to demonstrate a risk to fetus (in first trimester) and no evidence of risk in later trimesters; possibility of fetal harm appears remote.	Thyroid supplements (levothyroxine), vitamins (folic acid, riboflavin; vitamins A, D, and C[b])
B	Animal studies have failed to demonstrate a risk to the fetus, and there are no adequate studies in pregnant women; **or** animal studies show an adverse effect on the fetus but well-controlled studies in pregnant women have failed to demonstrate a risk to the fetus.	Acetaminophen, opioids,[c] penicillins, cephalosporins, erythromycin,[d] prednisone, caffeine, sulfonamides,[e] cimetidine, fluoxetine, insulin, NSAIAs[f]
C	Animal studies have shown an adverse effect on the fetus and there are no adequate studies in humans, **or** no studies are available in either animals or women. Potential benefits may warrant its use.	Epinephrine, phenylpropanolamine, trimethobenzamide, aspirin,[f] atropine, promethazine, theophylline, lisinopril, potassium chloride, disulfiram, acyclovir, propranolol
D	Positive evidence of human fetal risk based on adverse reaction data, but potential benefits in serious situations may warrant its use.	Warfarin, tetracycline, phenytoin, diazepam, trimethadione, lorazepam, amitriptyline
X	Studies in animals or humans have demonstrated fetal abnormalities and/or there is positive evidence of human fetal risk, and the risks clearly outweigh any potential benefits.	Isotretinoin, diethylstilbesterol, phencyclidine (PCP), triazolam

[a]Any unnecessary medication should be avoided in pregnant women. [b]When used at RDA levels. [c] In usual therapeutic doses. [d] Except erythromycin estolate. [e] Except near-term, when kernicterus can be produced. [f] Except near-term, when dystocia and delayed parturition can be produced and then categorized as D.

the drug, which may produce an effect in the infant. The amount of drug that appears in the milk depends on the plasma concentration of the drug, lipid solubility, degree of ionization, and binding to plasma proteins.

For a few drugs, nursing is clearly contraindicated. If these drugs must be given, breast feeding should be discontinued or the milk expressed and discarded until the mother stops taking the contraindicated drug. For drugs that are not contraindicated, the timing of nursing can further reduce the dose to which an infant is exposed. Table 24-3 summarizes the available data on the use of dental drugs for nursing mothers.

DENTAL DRUGS

Questions relating to drug administration in conjunction with dental treatment refer to whether a specific drug may be safely given to

the pregnant woman. In general, a drug should be used in a pregnant woman only if the benefits to the pregnant woman outweigh the risks to the fetus and a definite indication exists. Table 24-3 summarizes the information about which dental drugs can be used in pregnant women.

LOCAL ANESTHETIC AGENTS

No drug is used more frequently in the dental office than local anesthetic agents. Local anesthetic amides have been reported to produce fetal bradycardia and neonatal depression when given in very large doses near to term. High doses may produce uterine vascular constriction leading to fetal heart rate changes. Lidocaine, prilocaine, and etidocaine have been tested in animals without teratogenic effects (category B). Bupivacaine has been shown to be teratogenic in rats and rabbits (category C), whereas mepivacaine and procaine have not been tested (cat-

T A B L E 2 4 - 3   Dental Drug Use During Pregnancy,[a] FDA[b] Categories, and Nursing Safety

Dental Drug	Trimester 1st	Trimester 2nd/3rd	FDA Category	Comments	Nursing OK?	Nursing Comments
LOCAL ANESTHETICS						
Lidocaine	Yes	Yes	C	First choice anesthetic; fetal bradycardia near term	Yes	Central nervous system changes
Mepivacaine	Yes	Yes	C	Fetal bradycardia near term; no animal testing	Yes	Central nervous system changes
Bupivacaine	No	No	C	Embryocidal in rabbits; high lipid solubility	No	Central nervous system changes
VASOCONSTRICTORS						
Epinephrine	Yes	Yes	C	Vasoconstriction can produce hypoxia; limit to cardiac dose	Yes	Hyperactivity or irritability
ANALGESICS						
Aspirin	No	No	C/D	Bleeding; near-term dystocia and prolonged gestation, delayed parturition, premature closure of patent ductus arteriosis; treatment of certain pregnancy problems	Yes, caution	Occasional low dose poses minimal hazard; chronic high dose may present problems; infant may have inhibition of prostaglandins
Nonsteroidal antiinflammatory agents (NSAIAs)	No	No	B-C/D[c]	See aspirin B = ibuprofen, naproxen, ketoprofen C = etodolac, tolmetin, diflunisal, mefenamic acid, nabumetone, oxaprozin	No	Avoid NSAIAs; ibuprofen may be used when more information is available
Acetaminophen	Yes	Yes	B	Teratogenic at overdose levels	Yes	Present in milk in small amounts (peak 1-2 hr); no documented problems
Opioids	Yes	Yes	B[d]/C[e]	Respiratory depression near term; use low-dose, short duration; high doses contraindicated	Yes	Small doses, no problem; large doses (addict), sedation, poor feeding, constipation
PENICILLINS/CEPHALOSPORINS						
Penicillin V	Yes	Yes	B	Safe, especially penicillin V	Yes	Allergy, diarrhea
Amoxicillin, ampicillin	Yes	Yes	B	Safe	Yes	Allergy, diarrhea
Augmentin[f]	Yes	Yes	B	Safe	Yes	Allergy, diarrhea
Cephalosporins	Yes	Yes	B	Safe	Yes	Allergy, diarrhea
MACROLIDES						
Erythromycin	Yes	Yes	B	Safe, except estolate form (cholestatic jaundice)	Yes[g]	Present in milk; diarrhea
Clarithromycin	Avoid		C	Teratogenic in mice and monkeys		Insufficient information
Azithromycin	Probably OK		B	Unlikely to need in dentistry		Insufficient information

Drug	Safe During Pregnancy	FDA Category[b]	Comments	Safe During Breast-Feeding	Comments
TETRACYCLINES					
Tetracycline	No	D	Stains teeth; affects bones	No	Tooth staining questionable
Doxycycline	No	D	Stains teeth; affects bones	No	Tooth staining questionable
Minocycline	No	D	Stains teeth; affects bones	No	Tooth staining questionable
OTHERS					
Clindamycin	Yes	B	Very low risk of pseudomembranous colitis	Yes/No[g]	Diarrhea; pseudomembranous colitis
Metronidazole	Yes, caution	B	Only if alternatives do not exist	No	Express and discard milk
ANTIFUNGALS					
Nystatin	Yes	B	Not absorbed into systemic circulation from gastrointestinal tract	Yes	Not absorbed into systemic circulation from mouth or gastrointestinal tract
Clotrimazole, topical	No?	B	Poorly absorbed topically; abnormal liver function	Yes, caution	No proof of problems
Miconazole, topical	No	B	No link with fetal abnormalities	Yes	No proof of problems
Ketoconazole, systemic	No	C	Embryotoxic in rats	Yes	No proof of problems
ANTIVIRALS					
Acyclovir	No	B	Limited experience	No	Concentrated in milk
Penciclovir	Probably	B	Topical	No	Inadequate information
ANTIANXIETY AGENTS					
Nitrous oxide (with oxygen)	No	D	Ensure adequate oxygen intake; female operators should avoid chronic exposure[h]	Yes	Nitrous oxide excreted via the lungs; amount in milk is negligable
Benzodiazepines[i]		D/X	Floppy infant syndrome; cleft lip; neural tube defects; do not use in dentistry		Chronic use by nursing mother can lead to infant lethargy and weight loss; slower metabolism may get accumulation of drug and its metabolites
Alprazolam	No	D		No	
Diazepam	No	D		No	
Halazepam	No	D		No	
Lorazepam	No	D		No	
Midazolam	No	D		No	
Estazolam	No	X		No	
Quazepam	No	X		No	
Temazepam	No	X		No	
Triazolam	No	X		No	

[a]Do not administer any drug that is not absolutely necessary; potential risk to the fetus must be weighed against the benefit to the woman; consult the patient's health care provider before using drugs.
[b]See Table 24-2 for definition of FDA categories.
[c]D in 3rd trimester of pregnancy.
[d]Oxycodone, meperidine, hydrocodone.
[e]Codeine.
[f]Augmentin = amoxicillin + clavulanic acid.
[g]References differ.
[h]Check levels in the dental operatory; minimize risk, increase ventilation exchanges.
[i]Clorazepate, flurazepam, oxazepam—no category.

egory C). Small doses used by careful, slow injection have not been associated with any problems in the fetus. Lidocaine is the local anesthetic of choice for the pregnant woman because it is a category B drug and is not associated with methemoglobinemia (as is prilocaine) and not highly lipid soluble (as is etidocaine), prolonging its effect.

Epinephrine. Small doses of epinephrine, administered with appropriate care, are similar to those produced endogenously. Large doses could produce adverse effects in the fetus, including anoxia from vasoconstriction. If procedures are to be short, then local anesthetics without epinephrine are preferred. These comments also apply to other vasoconstrictor substances contained in local anesthetic solutions.

ANALGESICS

Analgesics should be given in the lowest possible dose and for the shortest duration possible to control pain. In dentistry, adjunctive therapy (incision, drainage, and curettage) should be used first.

ASA—No

Aspirin. Studies in animals have shown that aspirin can cause a variety of birth defects involving the eyes, central nervous system (CNS), gastrointestinal tract, and skeleton. In humans, controlled studies have not been able to demonstrate that aspirin use during pregnancy increases the incidence of birth defects. During the third trimester, aspirin can prolong gestation, complicate delivery, decrease placental function, or increase the risk of maternal or fetal hemorrhage. Premature closure of the patent ductus arteriosus may occur. (See Chapter 6.) These effects have been reported with chronic high-dose aspirin use. Abuse of aspirin may increase stillbirths or neonatal death.

Nonsteroidal antiinflammatory agents. The nonsteroidal antiinflammatory agents (NSAIAs) produce effects similar to aspirin; therefore if they are given near, the outcome on the fetus term would be expected to be the same. They can delay delivery and make it more difficult, as well as constrict the ductus arteriosus. NSAIAs also potentiate vasoconstriction if hypoxia exists. All NSAIAs carry a warning to avoid use during pregnancy. For ibuprofen and naproxen, studies in animals have not shown adverse effects on the fetus. Diflunisal (category C), but not naproxen (category B), has been shown to be teratogenic in rabbits in large doses. Ibuprofen is the NSAIA of choice for the nursing mother.

NSAIAs—No

Acetaminophen. Although no controlled studies in humans have been done, acetaminophen (APAP) is generally considered to be safe in pregnancy. In large doses, it may be associated with fetal renal changes similar to those that occur in adults.

APAP—Yes

Opioids. Doses used by addicts have been demonstrated to produce problems. The opioids, with the exception of codeine, have not been associated with teratogenicity. Retrospective studies have associated the use of codeine during the first trimester with fetal abnormalities involving the respiratory, gastrointestinal, cardiac, and circulatory systems, as well as causing inguinal hernia and cleft lip and palate. These studies suggest that codeine or other opioids should not be used indiscriminately during the first trimester. Whether the birth defects associated with codeine are related to its ubiquitous use or to some difference it possesses is not known. Near-term administration can produce respiratory depression in the infant. If the mother is addicted, the infant will experience withdrawal symptoms after birth. The use of codeine in limited quantities for a limited duration of time is common in clinical practice. Although opioids appear in breast milk when analgesic doses are administered, the small amounts appear to be insignificant. By properly timing the doses of analgesic, the dose the infant receives is reduced further. The infant should be observed for signs of sedation and constipation.

ANTIINFECTIVE AGENTS

Antiinfective agents should only be used when a definite indication for their use exists. Prophylactic use, use when no indication exists, and use when an infection can be locally treated are inappropriate.

Penicillin. The most common antiinfective agent used in dentistry is penicillin. It is generally agreed that the penicillins are safe to use during pregnancy. Using penicillin VK for a dental infection that is not controlled by local measures would be acceptable. Penicillins appear in breast milk, and infants should be observed for signs of diarrhea, candidiasis, and allergic reactions.

Erythromycin. Erythromycins, other than the estolate form, also appear to be safe for use during pregnancy. The estolate form (Ilosone) should not be used in pregnant women because it has been associated with reversible hepatic toxicity in the mother. Erythromycin is concentrated in breast milk but has not been documented to produce problems.

Cephalosporins. The first- and second-generation cephalosporins have not been associated with teratogenicity. These cephalosporins should be used in dentistry only if a specific indication exists.

Tetracyclines. All tetracyclines, including tetracycline and doxycycline, are contraindicated during pregnancy because of the potential for adversely affecting the fetus. They cross the placenta and are deposited in the fetal teeth and bones. Deciduous teeth may become stained and fetal bone growth inhibited. Hepatotoxicity can occur in the pregnant woman treated with large doses of tetracycline. Whether the amount excreted in milk, after it is complexed with the calcium in milk, can produce problems in the nursing infant is not known.

Clindamycin. Clindamycin should be used for dental infections during pregnancy for susceptible anaerobic infections not sensitive to penicillin. It is also indicated for prophylaxis of endocarditis in penicillin-allergic patients. No adverse fetal problems have been reported. Because clindamycin is excreted in breast milk if it is given to nursing mothers, the infant should be monitored for diarrhea.

Metronidazole. In animals, metronidazole can produce birth defects. Metronidazole should be used carefully during the first trimester. It would be difficult to encounter a dental situation in which the risk to the fetus would not be greater than the benefit to the mother. Because animal studies have shown metronidazole to be carcinogenic, the nursing mother should only be given metronidazole if the breast milk is expressed and discarded during treatment and for 48 hours after the last dose.

Nystatin. Nystatin is safe to use during pregnancy to treat oral candida infections. When applied topically or taken orally it is not absorbed into the systemic circulation. It may also be used by either the pregnant woman or the nursing infant to treat thrush.

Clotrimazole. Small amounts of clotrimazole are absorbed from topical administration of this agent. No occurrences of abnormality have been reported, but nystatin is safer.

Ketoconazole. Ketoconazole is classified by the FDA as a category C drug. It has been shown to be teratogenic in rats, producing an abnormal number of digits (syndactyly and oligodactyly). Dystocia during delivery has been demonstrated in animals. Ketoconazole appears in breast milk and may increase the chance of kernicterus (jaundice) occurring in the nursing infant. If ketoconazole must be used, breast milk must be expressed and discarded during therapy and for 72 hours after cessation of therapy.

Fluconazole, like ketoconazole, is also scheduled as category C.

ANTIANXIETY AGENTS

Nitrous oxide–oxygen mixture. Operating room personnel exposed to trace amounts of nitrous oxide have a significantly higher incidence of spontaneous abortion and birth defects in their children, regardless of whether the man or woman was exposed. These data suggest that methods for reducing the environmental exposure, especially chronically, should be explored and implemented. Pregnant dental health care workers should have knowledge of the levels of nitrous oxide that are present in the dental offices in which they practice.

Benzodiazepines. First-trimester use of the benzodiazepines (chlordiazepoxide and diazepam) has been reported to increase the risk of congenital malformations. Cleft palate and lip and neural tube defects have been seen. Other benzodiazepines may be associated with this increase in risk also. Temazepam and triazolam are FDA pregnancy category X drugs, and alprazolam, halazepam, and lorazepam are category D drugs. Benzodiazepines are indicated during pregnancy only for the treatment of status epilepticus (no dental use).

Chronic ingestion of the benzodiazepines can produce physical dependence in the infant. Floppy infant syndrome, or neonatal flaccidity, has been seen at birth, with inadequate sucking reflex or apnea. Use of benzodiazepines in the nursing mother, which may accumulate in the **neonate** because of slower metabolism, may cause sedation and feeding difficulties. Therefore if they are needed the infant should be monitored for sedation.

Alcohol. Although alcohol is not a dental drug, it is mentioned here because the evidence for the teratogenicity of alcohol is very strong. **Fetal alcohol syndrome (FAS)** is the name associated with the changes that occur in an infant exposed to excessive alcohol intake by the mother. FAS involves abnormalities in these three areas: growth retardation (prenatal or postnatal), CNS abnormalities (neurologic or intellectual), and facial dysmorphology (such as microcephaly, microphthalmia or short palpebral fissures, and flat maxillary area or a thin lip). Infants born to those mothers who drank throughout pregnancy show more tremors, hypertonia, restlessness, crying, and abnormal reflexes compared with control groups after birth.

> PG + alcohol = FAS

Pregnant dental patients should be encouraged to abstain from the ingestion of alcohol. No threshold level that is safe for the pregnant woman is known. Well-documented studies show that adverse effects on the fetus are dose related and can extend for years after the birth of the baby. The dental health care worker, as a health care professional, is in a position to remind the pregnant woman to care for her oral cavity and also her baby's development.

REVIEW QUESTIONS

1. Describe the proper method for the dental hygienist to obtain information about possible pregnancy or breast-feeding patients. State the information to be obtained.
2. Explain the three trimesters and the special risks for each one.

3. Define *teratogenicity* and describe why identifying drugs that produce it is so difficult.
4. Explain the FDA pregnancy categories and state their significance.
5. Determine the factors that are important when a breast-feeding woman is to receive drugs.

6. For the commonly used dental drugs, such as local anesthetics, antibiotics, and analgesics, state the agents in each group that are the least safe.
7. Describe two activities that the dental health care worker should perform before giving a pregnant woman any medications, to minimize future legal problems.

CHAPTER 25

Drug Interactions

> Drug interactions—good or bad

A drug interaction is defined as the action of an administered drug on either the effectiveness or the toxicity of another drug that is administered earlier, simultaneously, or later. This phenomenon often, but not always, results in undesired drug effects. Not every potential drug interaction occurs in all patients. For every drug interaction that is identified, the clinician must ask the question, "Is the interaction clinically significant?" This is one of the most difficult questions to answer because the availability of complete evidence is frequently absent. It is a problem of growing concern to the health professions and is directly related to an increase in multiple drug therapy. Many dental patients regularly use more drugs than in the past; therefore the possibility of encountering or producing drug interactions has increased. As more studies are done, which of these drug interactions is of greatest concern will be elucidated [one hopes, at least].

Dental health care workers may encounter drug interactions in several situations. First, a patient may already be taking drugs that interact with each other. Often the drug interactions have been taken into account and the doses of the drugs altered to account for the interaction. Second, drugs prescribed, suggested for use, or used in the dental office may interact with the drugs the patient is taking prescribed by the patient's physician. It is important to remember that many patients who seek dental treatment are already taking medication, either self-prescribed in the form of over-the-counter (OTC) medication or prescribed by their physicians.

A complete medical and drug history is necessary to minimize the problems of drug interactions. Obtaining information about both prescription and OTC medications is important. This chapter discusses some of the possible mechanisms for drug interactions and discusses the more common drug interactions encountered in dental practice. In many instances these drug interactions are discussed in the chapters on individual drug groups and so are only briefly mentioned here. The proliferation of CD ROMs, Internet sites, and books assist the dental health care worker in determining whether drug interactions may be present.

MECHANISMS OF INTERACTIONS

When two or more drugs interact, the result may be an increased effect (potentiation or enhancement of the pharmacologic effects) or a decreased effect (antagonism between the agents). By understanding the mechanisms by which drug interactions occur, one can more accurately predict the outcome of the interaction of two drugs.

Although the mechanism of many drug interactions is presently poorly understood, the more commonly known mechanisms are discussed here. Drug interactions may be divided into two groups: pharmacokinetic interactions (alteration in absorption, distribution, metabolism, or excretion) or pharmacodynamic interactions (acts at receptor site). The drug that causes the interaction is referred to as the **precipitant drug,** and the drug whose effect is altered is referred to as the **object drug.**

PHARMACOKINETIC

Most drug interactions are the pharmacokinetic type. The pharmacokinetic type of interac-

Affects ADME

tion involves an alteration in the pharmacokinetics (absorption, distribution, metabolism, excretion) of a drug.

Absorption Drug interactions related to absorption may have two outcomes. The onset of action of the drug can be delayed or the amount of drug that is absorbed can be altered (increased or decreased). The absorption of a drug may be altered in several ways, including inactivation by chelation, binding with another drug, ionizing more or less (which indirectly changes absorption), and changing the motility of the gastrointestinal tract.

It is important to distinguish between the rate and the extent of absorption. With treatment for an acute problem (e.g., pain in a tooth), the onset of action is important. The extent of absorption is less important. With chronic ingestion, the rate of absorption is less important but the extent of absorption (percent absorbed of total dose taken) is important because it will have an impact on the level of the drug in the blood after reaching a plateau (leveling out with chronic use). The absorption of a drug will be decreased if an inactive or insoluble derivative is formed in the intestinal tract. For example, calcium chelates with tetracycline, resulting in a decrease in antimicrobial effectiveness. If gastrointestinal tract motility is slowed (e.g., by anticholinergic agents), the rate of absorption of certain drugs may be decreased because they are not carried into the small intestine (where most absorption occurs) as soon and the onset of action is delayed. With increased gastrointestinal motility, slowly absorbed drugs may pass through the gastrointestinal tract before absorption is complete. Disintegration and dissolution are the rate-limiting steps for the absorption of some drugs. If the pH of the gastrointestinal tract is altered, the dissolution may be reduced, thereby reducing the absorption. Because the ionization of weak acids and bases is pH dependent, altering the pH may alter the proportion of drug in the ionized form, which leads to a change in absorption.

Interfering with enterohepatic circulation is another mechanism by which a drug interaction can occur. When the object drug is excreted into the gastrointestinal tract, the precipitant drug can bind with it. The bound drug is then excreted through the feces. Another interaction with enterohepatic circulation involves antibiotics altering the flora, which affects the breakup of the conjugated form of some drugs.

Distribution. Distribution is the travel of drugs throughout the body and to its site at which the drugs act. It is affected by the degree of plasma protein binding. Drugs that are highly protein bound can be displaced from their binding sites by other drugs that are also highly protein bound (only so many available sites, so it is like bumper cars). Drugs in the body are reversibly bound to the plasma proteins. The amount of this binding varies with the particular drug. Only the free drug exerts the drug's pharmacologic effect; the bound portion is biologically inactive but serves as a reservoir for the drug.

Because many weak acids are bound to the same site on the plasma proteins, one acidic drug can displace another acidic drug from its plasma protein–binding sites. This results in an increase in the plasma concentration of the free drug (first drug) that has been displaced and indirectly increases its pharmacologic effect and toxicity (in an acute situation). For example, warfarin (Coumadin) is 97% protein bound. If aspirin, another acidic drug that is protein bound, displaces even 1% of the bound warfarin from its plasma protein binding sites, then the concentration of free warfarin is increased by 33% (3% increases to 4%). This increase in free warfarin increases its pharmacologic effect and toxicity,

which can lead to hemorrhage. Because warfarin is highly bound to plasma proteins, it can interact with many drugs. Another group of drugs that is highly protein bound is the sulfonylureas (oral hypoglycemic agents). This group of drugs also interacts with many other drugs.

The drug interaction involving displacement from plasma protein–binding sites can be called "self correcting" because there is an immediate effect (first week) followed by a delayed effect. Over several days, the displacement of drugs from their plasma protein–binding sites increases the amount of free drug in the blood stream. With more free drug available the metabolism and excretion of the drug is increased.

In summary, the early effect of displacement increases the drug's pharmacologic effect, and the late effect (depending on the mechanism of excretion) decreases its pharmacologic effect (more is being metabolized and excreted).

Metabolism. The metabolism of one drug may be stimulated or inhibited by another drug. Before drugs can be excreted by the kidney, they must be metabolized in the liver to more water-soluble derivatives. Certain drugs induce hepatic microsomal enzymes whose function is to metabolize many drugs. If there is an increase (induce) in these enzymes, then drugs that are metabolized by these enzymes will be metabolized faster and will have less effect. Common enzyme inducers include phenobarbital, carbamazepine, phenytoin, primidone, and rifampin. Enzyme induction is usually a slow process, taking at least 7 days for the maximum effect to occur, because time is needed for synthesis of new enzymes. Returning the enzymes to prestimulated levels also takes a similar amount of time. Based on the time course, the interaction between enzyme inducers and other drugs does not occur within a few hours or days.

Interference with the metabolism (several different, often unknown, mechanisms) of a drug increases its pharmacologic effect. This effect is usually faster and can occur as soon as the level of the inhibiting drug builds up in the liver, often within 24 hours. For example, cimetidine inhibits the metabolism of other drugs, enhancing the action of these drugs. Agents that inhibit the metabolism of other drugs include erythromycin, allopurinol, disulfiram, INH, metronidazole, propoxyphene, and sulfonamides.

Excretion. Drug interactions involving excretion can affect the amount of drug that is either secreted or reabsorbed. As the amount of free drug rises (could occur with protein binding displacement), then the amount presented to the kidney is larger and the amount excreted rises. With active tubular secretion, two or more drugs may compete for the same site of excretion. Administering one drug, probenecid, interferes with the excretion of another drug, penicillin, because they are excreted by the same mechanism. The mechanism becomes saturated. Tubular reabsorption is another method by which the body retains some drugs. The pH of the urine determines the amount of a drug that is ionized as it passes through the urine and therefore the amount of tubular reabsorption. In this way, changes in the pH may produce changes in the excretion of either weak acids or bases.

PHARMACODYNAMIC

> Drug interactions involving receptors

The pharmacodynamic drug interactions usually occur at the receptor site. The potential outcomes may be divided into antagonism, synergism, or an additive effect. The adrenergic (sympathetic) nervous system, the cholinergic (parasympathetic) nervous system, and the central nervous system (CNS) possess sites for these drug interactions to occur.

The enzyme monoamine oxidase (MAO) has no effect on epinephrine (EPI) levels and only a small effect on endogenous norepinephrine (NE) released at the synapse. Therefore it is unlikely that a drug interaction between EPI or NE and the monoamine oxidase inhibitors (MAOIs) would occur. But, the sympathomimetics with either a central (e.g., amphetamine) or mixed (both direct and indirect actions; e.g., ephedrine and phenylpropanolamine) mechanism of action release larger quantities of norepinephrine. MAO is responsible for inactivation of the NE released by indirect action. For the indirect-acting adrenergics, the MAOIs can potentiate their hypertensive effects. Therefore indirect-acting sympathomimetics should not be given to patients taking MAOIs, because they can result in severe hypertension. Epinephrine can be used.

If the MAOIs are combined with the serotonin-specific reuptake inhibitors or with tryptophan from foods such as cheese and wines, serotonin syndrome can occur (see Chapter 17).

The tricyclic antidepressants block the reuptake of norepinephrine, and the antihypertensive agent guanethidine must be taken up to exert its effect. Therefore, because the tricyclic antidepressants prevent the uptake of guanethidine, they antagonize its effect.

In the parasympathetic nervous system the anticholinergic drugs block the action of the cholinergic nervous system. Other agents, including phenothiazines and tricyclic antidepressants, also possess anticholinergic activity. Used concomitantly, agents with anticholinergic action can produce excessive anticholinergic activity. This can result in dry mouth, constipation, tachycardia, urinary retention, and mydriasis.

DENTAL DRUG INTERACTIONS

Although many drug interactions are documented in the literature, this discussion centers on those most likely to be encountered in dentistry. The drugs included in this section are analgesics, antiinfectives (antibiotics), benzodiazepines, and epinephrine. These are the agents most frequently used in dentistry. Tables 25-1 through 25-5 list the most common interactions and should be available in the dental office for easy reference. This list is only a guide; the actual clinical effect can be determined only by considering the individual patient's disease, medications, and other contributing factors. Just because a drug interaction is listed does not mean the two drugs cannot be used together. What it does mean is that caution should be exercised if two interacting drugs are used concomitantly.

ANALGESICS

Aspirin. The drug interactions associated with aspirin are listed in Table 25-1. The most important drug interaction between a dental drug and a medical drug occurs between aspirin and the anticoagulant warfarin. If a patient is taking aspirin every day for clot prevention, the patient should continue taking that aspirin.

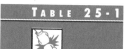

When they are given alone, the salicylate agents can produce hypoprothrombinemia and a decrease in platelet adhesiveness, thereby prolonging the bleeding time. The salicylates and the oral anticoagulants are bound to the same plasma protein–binding sites. When salicylates are given to patients taking warfarin, the salicylates displace the warfarin from the binding sites and increase the level of free (unbound) warfarin. When the unbound warfarin concentration is increased, the therapeutic effect is also increased and severe hemorrhage can occur. Patients taking orally administered anticoagulants should not be given aspirin or aspirin-containing products, such as Percodan or Empirin #3.

The salicylates also interact with probenecid (Benemid). Probenecid, used alone, increases the excretion of uric acid and is employed in the treatment of gout. When salicylates are administered to patients taking probenecid, the uricosuric effect of the probenecid is blocked. This can result in either increased uric acid concentrations in the blood or precipitation of an acute attack of gout. An occasional analgesic dose of

TABLE 25-1 Drug Interactions of Aspirin (ASA)	
MEDICAL DRUG	POTENTIAL EFFECT
ALTER SALICYLATE LEVELS	
Vitamin C	↑Salicylate levels
Nizatidine	
Steroids	↓Salicylate levels
Antacids	
↑EFFECT OF MEDICAL DRUG	
Oral anticoagulants—warfarin (Coumadin)	Bleeding/hemorrhage
Valproic acid (VA) (Depakene)	ASA displaces bound VA → ↑risk VA toxicity; bleeding/hemorrhage
Methotrexate	ASA ↑level → ↑toxicity
Acetazolamide (Diamox)	ASA ↑level → ↑toxicity
Phenytoin (Dilantin)	>2 gm ASA → ↑toxicity
Sulfonylureas/insulin; chlorpropamide	>2 gm ASA → enhanced hypoglycemic response
Ethyl alcohol	↑ASA-induced gastric damage; ↑ASA-induced bleeding time
↓EFFECT OF MEDICAL DRUG	
ACE inhibitors	↓Antihypertensive effect
β-Blockers	
Loop diuretics	
Nonsteroidal antiinflammatory agents	↓NSAIA blood levels
Probenecid (Benemid)	↓Uricosuric effect
Sulfinpyrazone (Anturane)	

salicylate may be insufficient to interact with probenecid, but large doses can inhibit probenecid's uricosuria. An alternative analgesic should be prescribed for patients taking probenecid.

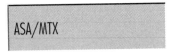

The excretion of methotrexate appears to be blocked by the salicylates. Methotrexate, an antimetabolite, is used to treat cancer, arthritis, and severe psoriasis. Patients who are taking methotrexate and are given aspirin can exhibit severe methotrexate toxicity.

The salicylates interact with corticosteroids and alcohol to cause an additive ulcerogenic effect. Because all of these agents can cause gastrointestinal irritation and exacerbate ulcers, their concomitant use should be avoided. Occasional use of small doses may be used.

In patients with diabetes the salicylates tend to produce hypoglycemia. In patients taking oral hypoglycemic agents (sulfonylureas), salicylates may contribute to hypoglycemic coma. In these patients, caution should be used if moderate to large doses of the salicylates are given. An occasional small dose of salicylate does not seem to be a problem. The effect of salicylates on patients taking insulin is unpredictable, but hypoglycemia is more common.

Aspirin also interferes with the blood levels of ibuprofen, potentially reducing its effectiveness. They also have similar side effects and would offer no advantage taken together.

Nonsteroidal antiinflammatory agents.

Nonsteroidal antiinflammatory agents (NSAIAs) such as ibuprofen can reduce the antihypertensive effects of the β-adrenergic blockers, furosemide, thiazide diuretics, triamterene, and the ACE inhibitors like captopril. The mechanism of interaction involves both retention of fluids by the NSAIAs and possibly by inhibition of prostaglandins. The NSAIAs have been reported to increase the effects of phenytoin, lithium, warfarin, and digoxin. Toxicity of methotrexate and

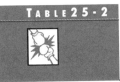

Drug Interactions of the Nonsteroidal Antiinflammatory Agents [NSAIAs]

TABLE 25-2

Medical Drug	Potential Outcome
ACE inhibitors— Captopril (Catapres) **β-Blockers Diuretics-** Thiazide eg HCTZ Furosemide (Lasix) Triamterene	↓Antihypertensive effect
Warfarin (Coumadin) **Lithium** Digoxin Phenytoin Sympathomimetics	↑Effect of medical drug
Cyclosporin	Nephrotoxicity
Methotrexate	Increase methotrexate toxicity; less problem with rheumatoid arthritis doses
Probenecid	↑NSAIAs level, okay with caution
Salicylates (aspirin)	↓NSAIAs blood level, OK to continue 1/d for anticlotting effect
Corticosteroids	↑Ulcerogenic risk
Antidiabetics	↑Serum concentration of hypoglycemic drugs

Bold, More important.

cyclosporin is increased in the presence of the NSAIAs. Table 25-2 lists the drug interactions of the NSAIAs.

Opioids. The most important drug interaction associated with the opioids occurs with other CNS depressants (Table 25-3). The primary outcome of this interaction is additive CNS depression leading to respiratory depression. Other CNS depressants include the sedative-hypnotic agents, minor tranquilizers, major tranquilizers (phenothiazines), antihistamines, and alcohol.

In patients taking MAOIs the administration of meperidine (Demerol) has produced a severe reaction including sweating, hypertension, exci-

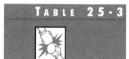

TABLE 25-3 Drug Interactions of the Opioids

OPIOIDS	MEDICAL DRUG	POTENTIAL OUTCOME
GENERAL OPIOIDS		
	Alcohol	Additive CNS depression
	Barbiturates	
SPECIFIC OPIOIDS		
Propoxyphene	Carbamazepine	Carbamazepine toxicity
Meperidine	Barbiturates	↑Toxicity of meperidine
	Chlorpromazine, neuroleptics	↓ BP → CNS depression
	Monoamine oxidase inhibitors	Severe reactions; excitation, rigidity, ↑ BP
Methadone	Barbiturates	↓ Methadone levels
	Phenytoin	↓ Methadone levels; withdrawal
	Rifampin	

tation, and rigidity. In some patients, hypotension and coma have also developed. Meperidine should not be given to patients receiving MAOIs. Other opioids may be given with caution, preferably in a decreased dosage.

By stimulation of liver microsomal enzymes, barbiturates, phenytoin, and rifampin can reduce methadone levels. As used in "methadone maintenance," lowering of the methadone levels could precipitate a withdrawal syndrome. Stimulation of these enzymes takes several doses.

Acetaminophen. Recent evidence has determined that patients taking normal doses of acetaminophen are much more likely to have a prolonged INR (International Normalized Ratio). The etiology is unknown, but the two should be used concomitantly with caution.

ANTIINFECTIVES

Antiinfective drug interactions are listed in Table 25-4. Some antibiotics, when used in combination, may have an additive, synergistic, or antagonistic effect. The concentration of each antibiotic, the order in which the antibiotics are administered, the particular pathogen being treated, and the number of microorganisms affect the outcome.

Typically, bacteriostatic and bactericidal antibiotics, such as penicillin and tetracycline, would demonstrate antagonism. An example of synergism is the combination of sulfonamides and trimethoprim. Because these two agents act at different steps in the production of folic acid, resistance to the combination would require resistance at two different steps.

Oral contraceptives. The drug interaction between the antiinfective agents and the oral contraceptives has been discussed in the lay press. Rifampin is the most frequently documented antiinfective agent to interact with oral contraceptives. Amoxicillin and tetracyclines have been said to reduce the effectiveness of the oral contraceptives, but a recent literature review has not been able to document this effect. Although extremely uncommon considering the widespread use of oral contraceptives, the seriousness of the interaction means that every woman taking oral contraceptives (birth control pills) must be informed of the remote possibility of this occurrence. This notification should be documented (even if there is no association between antibiotics and birth control pills).

Warfarin. The action of warfarin may be increased by giving antibiotics. The antibiotics in-

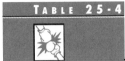

TABLE 25-4 **Drug Interactions of Antibiotics**

ANTIBIOTICS	POTENTIAL OUTCOME
GENERAL ANTIBIOTICS	
Bacteriostatic + bactericidal antibiotics	Activity of -cidal antibiotic inhibited by -static antibiotic
Oral anticoagulants (OA)	↑ Effectiveness of OA
Oral contraceptives (OC)	↓ Effectiveness of OC
PENICILLIN	
Erythromycin	May interact
β-Blockers	If anaphylactic reaction occurs, more difficult to treat
Probenecid (Benemid)	Prolongs action of penicillin; inhibits active secretion
ERYTHROMYCIN ↓CYTOCHROME P-450 ENZYMES	
Benzodiazepines, triazolam	↑Benzodiazepine effect
Carbamazepine	↑Carbamazepine level
Cyclosporine	Potential nephrotoxicity
Lovastatin	Rhabdomyolysis
Theophylline (Slo-Bid)	Erythromycin ↑ theophylline effect; theophylline ↓ erythromycin effect
CLINDAMYCIN	
Kaolin-pectin	↓Absorption of clindamycin
TETRACYCLINE (TCN)	
Divalent and trivalent cations (Ca, Mg, Zn, Al, Fe); bismuth subsalicylate (Pepto-Bismol); food, dairy products	Chelation of cation by TCN; ↓ effectiveness of TCN; avoid administration within 2 hours
DOXYCYCLINE (DOXY)	
Divalent trivalent cations (Ca, Mg, Zn, Al, Fe); bismuth subsalicylate (Pepto-Bismol)	Chelation of cation by DOXY; ↓ effectiveness of DOXY; food and dairy products OK
Anticonvulsants	↓ Effectiveness of DOXY
Barbiturates	↓ Effectiveness of DOXY
Carbamazepine	↓ Effectiveness of DOXY
Phenytoin	
METRONIDAZOLE	
Disulfiram (Antabuse)	CNS toxicity, psychosis, confusion
Ethyl alcohol	Disulfiram-like reaction
5-Fluorouracil	↓ Clearance of 5-FU; ↑ toxicity of 5-FU

hibit the bacterial flora in the intestine responsible for the synthesis of vitamin K. If the concentration of vitamin K available to be absorbed is decreased, fewer coagulation factors will be produced in the liver. The oral anticoagulant's (vitamin K antagonist) action will be amplified. Antibiotics differ in their interaction with warfarin (see Table 15-1).

Penicillin. The bactericidal penicillin and the bacteriostatic tetracycline antagonize the action of each other. Probenecid can prolong the action of the penicillins by interfering with its absorption. This can be used to therapeutic advantage for difficult infections.

Erythromycin. Erythromycin inhibits the P-450 cytochrome oxidase hepatic enzymes and therefore the metabolism of drugs metabolized by these enzymes is decreased. Examples of these drugs include theophylline, warfarin, digoxin, and carbamazepine. The outcome of this interaction may be enhancement of these drugs' effects or even toxicity of these drugs.

| TABLE 25-5 | Drug Interactions of the Benzodiazepines* |

MEDICAL DRUG	POTENTIAL OUTCOME
Alcohol; CNS depressants	Additive or ↑ CNS depression
Digoxin	↑ Digoxin effect
Levodopa	↑ Parkinsonism; ↓levodopa effect
Phenytoin	Clonazepam → ↑phenytoin effect
Probenecid	↑ Lorazepam effect
Inhibitors of oxidative metabolism; e.g., cimetidine, oral contraceptives, disulfiram, erythromycin, fluoxetine, INH, ketoconazole, metoprolol, omeprazole, propoxyphene, propranolol, valproic acid	↓ Effect of oxidized (phase I) benzodiazepines (↓ metabolism), e.g., chlordiazepoxide (Librium), diazepam (Valium), alprazolam (Xanax), triazolam (Halcion)
Oral contraceptives	↑ Effect of conjugated (phase II) benzodiazepines (↑ metabolism), e.g., lorazepam (Ativan), oxazepam (Serax), temazepam (Restoril)
Enzyme stimulators, e.g., rifampin, smoking	Enhances hepatic metabolism; ↓ effect of diazepam

INH, Isoniazid.
*These interactions have not been verified for all the benzodiazepines; several have only been reported with one benzodiazepine.

Tetracycline. The absorption of tetracycline itself is inhibited by divalent and trivalent cations. It should be given at least 1 hour before or 2 hours after the use of dairy products, oral antacids, or sucralfate. Doxycycline can be taken with dairy products or food, but large doses of antacids, iron, or calcium will impair absorption of doxycycline. The effectiveness of doxycycline is reduced by agents that stimulate the metabolism of doxycycline, such as barbiturates.

Metronidazole. The possibility of a disulfiram-like reaction with metronidazole makes it important for the patient to be warned against drinking alcohol while taking this medication. Alcohol-containing mouthwashes should also be avoided. Patients taking disulfiram for alcoholism may have a drug interaction with metronidazole.

| Metronidazole/alcohol |

BENZODIAZEPINES

The benzodiazepines, CNS depressants themselves, are additive with other CNS depressants (Table 25-5). With chronic use, such as for muscular relaxation to treat temporomandibular joint problems, the oxidized benzodiazepines may accumulate if their metabolism is blocked by cimetidine, oral contraceptives, or valproic acid (inhibitors of oxidative metabolism). Enzyme stimulators reduce the effect of diazepam. The small doses used as preoperative anxiolytics will not have significant drug interactions except for acute use of CNS depressants (e.g., a patient gets drunk before his dental appointment because of fear).

EPINEPHRINE

Epinephrine, a vasoconstrictor, is commonly added to local anesthetic agents to reduce systemic toxicity and prolong duration of action. The two epinephrine drug interactions that are

TABLE 25-6 Drug Interactions of Epinephrine (EPI)

Medical Drug Group	Examples	Potential Outcome
Tricyclic antidepressants	Amitriptyline (Elavil), Imipramine (Tofranil)	Pressor response to IV EPI markedly enhanced
β-blockers, nonselective	Pindolol (Visken) Propranolol (Inderal) Timolol (Blocadren)	Hypertension and bradycardia
Antidiabetics	Tolbutamide (Orinase), Chlorpropamide (Diabinese)	↑ Blood glucose
INTERACTIONS *NOT* SIGNIFICANT IN DENTISTRY		
Phenothiazines	Chlorpromazine (Thorazine)	Reverse pressor response of EPI, avoid EPI to raise BP
Monoamine oxidase (MAO) inhibitors	Phenelzine Tranylcypromine	EPI not inactivated by MAO; small effect because of "denervation supersensitivity"

BP, Blood pressure; *IV,* intravenous; *MAO,* monoamine oxidase.

TABLE 25-7 Selected Cytochrome CYP-450 Isoenzymes: Substrates, Inhibitors, and Inducers

Isoenzyme	Substrate	Inhibitors	Inducers
CYP 1A2	Antidepressants, tricyclic Haloperidol Theophylline Verapamil	Fluoroquinolones Cimetidine Disulfram Estrogens	Barbiturates Carbamazepine
CYP 2C8/9/10	Anticonvulsants Estrogen NSAIAs Omeprazole s-Warfarin	Anticonvulsants Antidepressants, SSRI Cimetidine Omeprazole	Barbituates Rifampin
CYP 2C18/19	Antidepressants Naproxen Propranolol Proton pump inhibitors	Antidepressants, SSRI Imidazoles Omeprazole	
CYP 2D6	Antiarrhythmics Antidepressants Antipsychotics Opioids	Antidepressants, SSRI Antipsychotics Cimetidine	Not susceptible Rifampin
CYP 2E1	Alcohol	INH	Alcohol, INH
CYP 3A3	Erythromycin	Cimetidine	
CYP 3A4	Antidepressants Benzodiazepines Calcium channel blockers Cimetidine Estrogens Carbamazepine HMG-Co-A reductase inhibitors Imidazoles Macrolides	Antidepressants Cimetidine Corticosteroids Grapefruit juice Imidazoles Macrolides Omeprazole	Anticonvulsants Corticosteroids
CYP 3A5	HMG-CoA reductase inhibitors Midazolam Steroids Nifedipine Testosterone		

most carefully documented are those that occur with nonselective β-adrenergic blocking agents and tricyclic antidepressants (Table 25-6). Both can produce hypertension, and the β-blockers also produce reflex bradycardia (unopposed α-agonist action). Patients with diabetes who

Epinephrine + nonspecific β-blockers

are given epinephrine may need an increase in either sulfonylurea or insulin. Short-term administration of epinephrine should have little effect unless the patient is a very brittle (has difficulty obtaining appropriate blood glucose concentration) diabetic or in poor control. Epinephrine virtually does not react with MAOIs, although this interaction is much publicized (check advertisements for local anesthetics containing levonordefrin).

Cytochrome P-450 isoenzymes. With more information available, the enzyme inducers and inhibitors have been found to act on some isoenzymes of the P-450 mixed function oxidases. Table 25-7 lists some isoenzymes such as 2D6 and 3A4. It includes both inhibitors and induc-

ers. The drugs in the substrate column are metabolized by those isoenzymes. One example is as follows: Look at the row labeled 1A2 and note that theophylline is metabolized by (substrate) 1A2 isoenzyme. In the same row note that the barbiturates are inducers of 1A2 isoenzyme. Therefore, could one conclude that the blood level of theophylline would go up or down if a barbiturate were added?

With knowledge of the action of isoenzymes, potential drug interactions can be predicted. Drugs with a major action on these enzymes will become drugs with a greater potential for drug interactions.

SUMMARY

The recognition of the possibility of drug interactions is the first step toward preventing problems from these interactions. The dentist and the hygienist should make sure that an adequate drug interaction chart is posted in the dental office for easy reference. Many reference books are available on the subject of drug interactions. Table 25-8 lists some "red flag" drugs and gives general drug interactions that are likely to be most significant. Only with a high level of suspicion and availability of adequate reference material can the dental health care team give patients the complete care they deserve. The most important dental-related drug interactions are listed in Box 25-1.

TABLE 25-8 "Red Flag" Drugs

DRUG (GROUP)	COMMENTS
Alcohol	Especially with benzodiazepines
Inhibits metabolism—↑ other drug's effect	Cimetidine (Tagamet) Erythromycin Disulfiram Allopurinol
Digoxin	Cardiac drug; narrow therapeutic index
Enzymes inducers—↓ other drug's effect	Phenobarbital, isoniazid, phenytoin, carbamazepine, rifampin, griseofulvin
Sulfonylureas (oral hypoglycemic agents)	First generation is highly protein bound; e.g., tolbutamide
Oral contraceptives	With antibiotics—risk for event small; if event occurs, large liability incurred
Warfarin (Coumadin)	Narrow therapeutic index, influenced by many drugs

REVIEW QUESTIONS

1. Describe the mechanism by which tetracycline and calcium interact. Explain how to minimize this interaction.
2. Explain the mechanism(s) of action by which warfarin and aspirin interact to produce hemorrhage.
3. Describe the mechanism of a drug interaction that involves enzyme induction, and give two examples of drugs that act in this fashion.

BOX 25-1 THE MOST IMPORTANT DENTAL-RELATED DRUG INTERACTIONS

The criteria for this list includes the liklihood of occurring, potential severity, and frequency of use in practice. Omitted are interactions that require several days or would be unlikely to occur with outpatient dentistry.

1. ASA or NSAIAs + warfarin
2. Metronidazole + alcohol
3. Ibuprofen + lithium
4. Epinephrine + β-blockers (non-selective)
5. Tetracycline and cations (++ or +++)
6. Epinephrine + TCA
7. ASA or NSAIAs + acetaminophen
8. Acetaminophen + alcohol
9. ASA or NSAIAs + MTX
10. Epinephrine + cocaine
11. Probenecid − ASA, NSAIAs
12. Penicillin + probenecid
13. Ketoconazole [-azoles] + miscellaneous
14. BCP & antibiotics
15. NS + EtOH
16. NS + BP medications
17. Erythromycin + stuff (theophylline)
18. Epinephrine + halothane

ASA, Aspirin; *BCP,* birth control pills; *BP,* blood pressure; *EtOH,* alcohol; *MTX,* methotrexate, *NSAIAs,* nonsteroidal antiinflammatory agents; *TCA,* tricyclic antidepressants.

4. Name four common medical drugs with which the salicylates interact. For each of these drug interactions, state the potential outcome.

5. Describe one drug group (with several subgroups) with which ibuprofen may interact. State the potential outcome. Describe the relationship between the mechanism of the NSAIAs and their drug interaction. State another individual drug whose blood level can be increased by the NSAIAs.

6. Explain the interaction between two different CNS depressants, and state specific groups of drugs that would be classified as CNS depressants.

7. Describe the interaction between the barbiturates and the oral anticoagulants and the potential outcome. State two other drugs that act by the same mechanism as the barbiturates.

8. Explain the mechanism of the interactions between epinephrine and both the β-adrenergic blocking agents and the tricyclic antidepressants. State how these potential interactions can be managed in clinical practice.

9. Describe the mechanism of drug interactions between epinephrine and both the MAOIs and the phenothiazines. Explain the importance of these compared with those in question 8.

10. State the item(s) dental health care workers should have in the dental office to keep alert about drug interactions.

11. Discuss cytochrome P-450 isoenzymes. Include the terms *substrate*, *precipitant*, *inhibitor*, and *inducer*. State how the knowledge of these isoenzymes can assist in the prediction of future drug interactions.

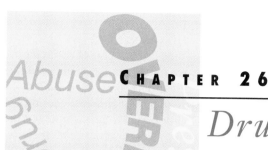

Drug Abuse

Dental health care workers may become involved with drug abuse in a variety of ways. Drugs that can be abused include both legal and illegal drugs. Patients seen in the dental office may be abusing drugs. Another interaction with the abusing patient involves the "potential" patient. "Potential" patients call the dental office, complain of pain, and request a prescription. Employees working in the dental office, including the dentist, dental hygienist, dental assistant, receptionist, bookkeeper, or other employees, may abuse drugs. Friends and relatives, as well as their friends and relatives, may abuse drugs. In our society, drug abuse, especially in adolescents, is epidemic. Wherever there are people, drug abuse can occur. Therefore the dental health care worker should become familiar with the various types of drugs commonly abused and their patterns of abuse. It is important to be able to recognize the problem in others. Because drug abuse is also a community issue, the dental health care worker should have a heightened awareness of the potential for patients to present with abuse problems (a high index of suspicion, but not unrealistically high). The proper awareness is only learned with experience.

Alcohol and tobacco—worst public health problems

Alcohol and tobacco are two drugs whose abuse causes more medical problems than all the other drugs of abuse combined. If no one in the United States used tobacco or drank alcohol, half of the filled hospital beds would be empty.

The idea of using drugs to produce profound effects on mood, thought, and feeling is as old as civilization. Only the kinds of substances used for this purpose have changed. Abuse has assumed a much bigger role in society because the forms of drugs used today are much stronger and have a much faster onset of action. This quick reinforcement produces abuse more quickly. For example, natives in Columbia have chewed cocoa leaves for many years as part of their culture, with little inappropriate use. Purifying cocaine and making it into a powder form to be "snorted" increased its abuse. When cocaine was **"free-based,"** it became easier to abuse, but the chemical reaction was dangerous. The most recent adaptation of cocaine, making it into "rocks," has increased abuse of the drug even more by making it available to smoke in convenient, small, reasonably priced doses. As is common with drugs of abuse, the potential for abuse is greatly increased when a drug is very potent, has a quick onset of action, is inexpensive, and is easy to distribute—making it the perfect drug of abuse.

Agents used for their psychoactive properties (capable of changing behavior or inducing psychosis-like reactions or both) can be divided into those that also have therapeutic value (opioids and sedative-hypnotics) and those that have no proven therapeutic value (psychedelics). Some agents may move from one category to the other. For example, marijuana, an agent previously considered to be worthless, is now claimed to be useful in the treatment of the nausea associated with cancer chemotherapy and for glaucoma. However, more controlled studies are needed to determine whether this claim is true.

DARE—not effective

The preventive approach to drug abuse now begins in elementary school. One program—the DARE (Drug Abuse Resistance Education) program—uses police officers in elementary schools to teach about drug abuse and develop a rapport with students in each grade. By helping the students develop self-esteem and by discussing different situations in which students may find themselves, it is hoped that substance abuse will be reduced. Unfortunately, studies to determine the value of the DARE program have shown the program to have either no benefit or to have a negative effect (more drug abuse).

GENERAL CONSIDERATIONS

Abuse of a drug is defined as the use of a drug for nonmedical purposes, almost always for altering consciousness. Both legitimate and illegitimate drugs may be abused. Whether a drug has an abuse potential is determined by the drug's pharmacologic effect. In contrast, the *misuse* of a drug means using the drug in the wrong dose or for a longer period than prescribed. The difference between these two usages is subtle.

DEFINITIONS

Terms relating to abuse that are used in this chapter are defined as follows:

- *abstinence syndrome:* A state of being free of drugs that is the goal of any treatment program.
- *addiction:* This vague term, although still used, should be replaced with *dependence*. *Addiction* is the pattern of abuse that includes compulsive use despite complications (medical or social) and frequent relapses after "quitting."
- *dependence:* A combination of either physical or psychologic manifestations (withdrawal) occurring in a drug-dependent person when the drug is removed.
- *drug abuse:* Self-administration of a drug in a socially unacceptable manner, resulting in negative consequences. A component of abuse is that harm is being produced from using the drug.
- *drug dependence:* A state, that may be either physical or psychologic, or both, that occurs as a consequence of the interaction between a drug and a patient. It is characterized by a compulsion to take the drug to obtain its effects or to prevent the abstinence syndrome. Tolerance may occur.
- *enabling:* The behavior of family or friends that associate with the addict that results in continued drug abuse. An example of enabling behavior is when a wife lies to others

about why her alcoholic husband is not at a gathering or calls into his work and says he is sick. This inappropriate coping mechanism requires family therapy.
- *misuse:* Use of the drug for a disease state in a way considered inappropriate.
- *physical/physiologic dependence:* The state in which the drug is necessary for continued functioning of certain body processes. In a dependent person, discontinuing the drug produces the abstinence syndrome sometimes called withdrawal (physiologic reactions).
- *psychologic dependence:* The state in which, following withdrawal of the drug, there are manifestations of emotional abnormalities and drug-seeking behavior. Craving is present, but there is no physiologic dependence.
- *tolerance:* With repeated dosing, the dose of a drug must be increased to produce the same effect. Or, the same dose of a drug, with consecutive dosing, produces less effect.
- *withdrawal:* The constellation of symptoms that occurs when a physically dependent person stops taking the drug.

PSYCHOLOGIC DEPENDENCE

Psychologic dependence is a state of mind in which a person believes that he or she is unable to maintain optimum performance without having taken a drug. Psychologic dependence can vary in severity from mild desire (such as for a morning cup of coffee) to compulsive obsession (such as for the next dose of cocaine). Even though some highly abused drugs have only psychologic dependence, the "need" to use these drugs can be as strong or stronger than drugs with a physical dependence.

PHYSICAL DEPENDENCE

Physical dependence refers to the altered physiologic state that results from constantly increasing drug concentrations. The presence of physical dependence is established by the withdrawal or abstinence syndrome, a combination of many drug-specific symptoms that occur on abrupt discontinuation of drug administration. Withdrawal symptoms are often the opposite of the symptoms of use of the drug, for example, excessive parasympathetic action (such as diarrhea, lacrimation, and piloerection ("cold turkey") when withdrawing from the opioids. Although sources differ, a measure of the degree of physical and psychologic dependence and tolerance is listed in Table 26-1.

TOLERANCE

Tolerance—body "gets used to" drug

Tolerance is characterized by the need to increase the dose continually in order to achieve the desired effect or the giving of the same dose, which produces a diminishing effect. The type of tolerance referred to in this discussion of abuse of psychoactive drugs is *central* (functional or behavioral) *tolerance*, that is, a definite decrease in the response of brain tissue to constantly increasing amounts of a drug. (Think of the brain becoming "stronger" [less responsive] to "withstand" the large doses it must tolerate.) In terminal patients, this tolerance requires ever-increasing doses of opioids even if the pain remains constant. The doses reached over time with the terminally ill would be fatal to a patient without tolerance.

Tolerance of metabolic origin (dispositional or metabolic tolerance) is caused by an accelerated rate of metabolism of the drug and is excluded in this discussion. Metabolic tolerance is an insignificant factor in the tolerance observed in humans to most of the psychoactive drugs.

ADDICTION, HABITUATION, AND DEPENDENCE

Addiction and habituation are terms that have been misused almost as much as the drugs they attempt to characterize. Any use of these terms must be preceded by an adequate definition. In both addiction and habituation the desire to continue using the drug is present, but in addiction, dependence is also present. Habituation and addiction are really only degrees of misuse or abuse of drugs. It has been recommended that these terms be replaced by the term **dependence**, a state of psychologic or physical desire to use a drug.

Terminology not clear . . .

Drugs that produce tolerance and physical dependence are grouped according to their abil-

▮ TABLE 26-1 Comparison of Substances of Abuse

DRUG GROUP	TOLERANCE	WITHDRAWAL	PHYSICAL ADDICTION	PSYCHOLOGIC ADDICTION
Opioids	High	High	High	High
Sedative-hypnotics, alcohol	Medium-high	Medium-high	High	Medium-high
STIMULANTS				
Cocaine	Low	Low	Medium low	Medium high
Amphetamines	Medium-high		Medium low	Medium high
HALLUCINOGENS				
LSD	Some	No	Low	Low
PCP	Low	No	Low	Low
Marijuana	Low	Low	Low	Low
Nicotine	Yes	Yes	Yes	Yes

ity to be substituted for one another. For example, if a person is addicted to heroin, an opioid, then other opioids, such as morphine, can prevent withdrawal. However, a barbiturate cannot be substituted for an opioid and vice versa. Therefore the opioids and barbiturates are separate groups of dependence-producing drugs. The phenomenon of substitution to suppress withdrawal between different drugs is called *cross-tolerance* or *cross-dependence*. It is observed among members of the same drug group but not among different drug groups. Cross-tolerance may be either partial or complete and is determined more by the pharmacologic effect of the drug than by its chemical structure.

Most characteristics of drug abuse are determined by the individual drug involved, but the following generalizations can be made:

* When comparing drugs in the same group, the time required to produce physical dependence is shortest with a rapidly metabolized drug and longest with a slowly metabolized drug.
* The time course of withdrawal reactions is related to the half-life of the drug. The shorter the half-life, the quicker the withdrawal is.

> Eighty percent of incarcerated (jailed) individuals are there because of drug abuse problems.

Many drugs have been abused extensively, and whether abuse can occur is a function of a particular drug's effects on neurotransmitters (combined with some genetic component within the user). At various times, airplane glue sniffing, propellant inhalation, smoking banana peels, smoking peyote (contains mescaline), and ingesting morning glory seeds have been attempted. The problems and treatment of drug abuse are less related to the drugs themselves, although they can cause definite problems, than to the "inner person" of the patient involved in this type of behavior and his or her genetic predisposition.

To treat abuse, a multifactorial approach is needed: counseling, education, self-help groups, and an intense desire to stop.

Propellant that is included in paint cans (especially the aluminum color) is preferred. The procedure is called *"huffing"* because the contents are sprayed into a plastic bag and fumes are repeatedly inhaled. Abuse of paint can easily produce irreversible damage to the liver and brain.

> "Huffing" volatile substances

This chapter discusses the properties of the specific groups of agents abused and the differences among the groups. The abusable drugs are divided into the following groups: central nervous system (CNS) depressants ("downers"), CNS stimulants ("uppers"), and hallucinogens. Some drugs, depending on the dose, may fall in more than one group. For example, marijuana may be classified as either a CNS depressant or a hallucinogen. Table 26-2 lists the common drugs of abuse by categories.

TABLE 26-2 Drugs of Abuse by Category

Drug Group	Most Common Examples	Other Examples
Opioids	Heroin	Morphine Codeine Meperidine Hydromorphone
Stimulants	Cocaine Methamphetamine	Amphetamines Methylphenidate Nicotine
Depressants (sedative-hypnotics)	Ethanol Benzodiazepines Inhalants Nitrous oxide*	Barbiturates Nonbarbiturate sedatives
Hallucinogens	D-Lysergic acid diethylamide (LSD)	Mescaline Phencyclidine (PCP)
Other	Marijuana	Caffeine

*In dentistry because of availability.

CENTRAL NERVOUS SYSTEM DEPRESSANTS

Central nervous system depressants include alcohol, opioids, barbiturates, benzodiazepines, volatile solvents (glue and gasoline), and nitrous oxide (abused mainly in dentistry).

ETHYL ALCOHOL

Alcoholism affects 1:10

Ethyl alcohol, or ethanol [ETH-an-ol], is a sedative agent used socially. Because it is legal, its availability makes it the most frequently abused drug. Abuse of alcohol, called *alcoholism*, is the number one public health problem in the United States and is associated with many major medical problems. The incidence of alcoholism in the United States is about 10% (i.e., 1 in 10). Many "accidental" deaths are associated with the use of alcohol. Two-fifths of traffic fatalities involve alcohol. Over 50% of gunshot wounds in teenagers are preceded by alcohol. Probably more pregnancies, bar fights, and police calls for domestic violence also are preceded by alcohol use than other causes. The best use of resources for addiction would be to deal with alcoholism as soon as it can be identified.

Pharmacokinetics. Ethyl alcohol is rapidly and completely absorbed from the gastrointestinal tract. Peak levels while fasting occur in less than 40 minutes. Food delays absorption and reduces the peak levels. Alcohol is oxidized in the liver to acetaldehyde, which is then metabolized to CO_2 (carbon dioxide) and H_2O (water).

$$Ch_3\text{-}CH_2\text{-}OH \rightarrow CO_2 + H_2O$$

Its metabolism follows zero-order kinetics, so a constant amount of alcohol is metabolized per unit of time regardless of the amount ingested. Because of its zero-order kinetics, excessive intake of alcohol can produce a prolonged effect. It is also excreted from the lungs (alcohol breath) and in urine.

Acute intoxication. With mild intoxication, impairment of judgment, emotional lability, and nystagmus occur. When intoxication is moderate, dilated pupils, slurred speech, **ataxia,** and a staggering gait are noted. If intoxication is severe, seizures, coma, and death can occur. Treatment includes ventilation support, fluids and electrolytes, thiamine (B_6), glucose, sodium bicarbonate, and magnesium.

Withdrawal. Withdrawal from alcohol use occurs after the use of alcohol. The more alcohol con-

Delirium tremens = DTs

sumed, and the more time spent consuming, the more violent is the withdrawal syndrome. Stage 1 usually begins 6 to 8 hours after drinking has stopped and includes withdrawal, psychomotor agitation, and autonomic nervous system hyperactivity. Stage 2 withdrawal includes hallucinations, paranoid behavior, and amnesia. Stage 3 includes disorientation, delusions, and grand mal seizures. It takes 3 to 5 days after cessation of drinking alcohol for stage 3 to occur. A cross-tolerant benzodiazepine (e.g., chlordiazepoxide; see Chapter 11) may be used to prevent withdrawal symptoms. Withdrawal from alcohol is termed *delirium tremens (DTs)* because the patient will often experience shaky (tremor) movements. Alcohol withdrawal can be life threatening if not properly treated.

Chronic effects. The chronic medical effects of alcoholism can include deficiency of proteins, minerals, and water-soluble vitamins. Impotence, gastritis, esophageal varices, arrhythmias, and hypertension have been reported. If a pregnant woman is using ethanol chronically, fetal alcohol syndrome can occur. The infant is retarded in body growth and has a small head (microencephaly), poor coordination, underdevelopment of the midface, and joint anomalies. More severe cases include cardiac abnormalities and mental retardation. Chronic alcohol use increases the risk of cancer of the mouth, pharynx, larynx, esophagus, and liver. This may work with tobacco to make the risk higher than with alcohol alone. The liver can be affected with alcoholic hepatitis and amnesic syndrome (Wernicke-Korsakoff syndrome), and peripheral neuropathy can occur.

Alcoholism. Alcoholism is a disease in which the alcoholic continues to drink despite the knowledge that drinking is producing a variety of problems. There is a genetic link for alcoholism; children of alcoholics are at a much greater risk for becoming alcoholics. In the future, genetic testing may be able to identify at-risk children and target that population for intense educational and social intervention for prevention.

"Red flags" for alcohol abuse include drinking at an inappropriately early time, shaking when not drinking, blackouts when drinking, and being told that you drink too much. Missing work and problems in personal relationships are also strong warning signs.

A self-test for alcoholism involves asking questions that can be remembered with the acronym CAGE.*

- Have you ever felt you ought to **C**ut down on your drinking?

---

*More information on CAGE can be obtained by reading Ewing: Detecting alcoholism: the CAGE, *JAMA* 252:1905-1907, 1984.

- Have people **A**nnoyed you by criticizing your drinking?
- Have you ever felt bad or **G**uilty about your drinking?
- Have you ever had a drink first thing in the morning to steady your nerves or get rid of a hangover (**E**ye-opener)?

Treatment. Alcoholics Anonymous is the most successful group for treating alcoholism. This is a self-help organization that is made up of recovering alcoholics. The members (who are recovering alcoholics) give support to alcoholics who are attempting recovery. In most alcoholics, inpatient detoxification is usually not required. In fact, inpatient treatment does not give the alcoholic any experience in recovery in the "real world." It is not surprising that inpatient treatment is often followed by relapse (insurance companies often will pay for 30 days of inpatient treatment before they will pay for additional outpatient counseling). Outpatient psychiatric treatment can help provide some insight for alcoholics.

> Alcoholics Anonymous gives best results

DRUG TREATMENT Older alcoholics who are motivated and socially stable can be given disulfiram [dye-SUL-fi-ram] (Antabuse). Occasionally, employers will observe the ingestion of disulfiram as a condition of employment. Alcohol is metabolized to water and carbon dioxide (see figure below):

Because disulfiram inhibits the metabolism of aldehyde dehydrogenase, a buildup of ac-

This builds up

Disulfiram

$\ominus$

CH_3-CH_2-OH (Alcohol) → Acetaldehyde → (Acid aldehyde dehydroxygenase) → $CO_2 + H_2O$

etaldehyde occurs. Acetaldehyde produces significant side effects if alcohol is ingested. These include vasodilation, flushing, tachycardia, **dyspnea,** throbbing headache, vomiting, and thirst. The reaction may last from 30 minutes to several hours. Certain drugs that produce the disulfiram-like reaction (e.g., metronidazole) may cause a minor version of these symptoms with alcohol intake.

Naltrexone (ReVia), an oral opioid antagonist, is an old drug with a new use. Originally it was indicated to prevent relapse in the opioid-dependent patient. Its new use is to reduce alcohol craving. Because naltrexone is partially effective in decreasing craving from alcohol, the logical conclusion is that alcohol stimulates some of the opioid receptors (among other receptors). More detailed knowledge of the receptors affected by alcohol may increase the chance of developing other agents to manage this disease. Other agents that might be useful are related to other neurotransmitters, such as dopamine or serotonin.

Dental treatment of the alcoholic patient. The dental health care worker must have an index of suspicion for alcoholism in patients treated in the dental office. The great majority of alcoholics look exactly like our neighbors, not like those characterized in old movies (e.g., unshaven, shaky). All health care workers have been given the charge to identify and assist patients in obtaining treatment.

The dental treatment of the alcoholic patient includes some modifications, depending on the severity of the disease process. Most alcoholic patients have poor oral hygiene primarily because of neglect rather than poor hygiene (or maybe neglect of oral hygiene). Check for the sweet musty breath and painless bilateral hypertrophy of parotid glands characteristic of alcoholism. Cirrhosis of the liver can occur when alcoholics continue to abuse alcohol. The major problem in these patients is a failure of the liver to perform adequately. Because of hepatic failure, the liver is able to store less vitamin K and the conversion of vitamin K to the coagulation factors is reduced. The outcome of these effects is a deficiency in coagulation factors II, VII, IX, and X (vitamin K–dependent factors) with resulting bleeding tendencies. Thrombocytopenia secondary to portal hypertension and bone marrow depression magnifies the hemostatic deficiency, sometimes resulting in spontaneous gingival bleeding. With the presence of esophageal varices, spontaneous bleeding can occur. Later in liver failure, the abdomen becomes distended with fluid (the patient appears 9 months pregnant).

Box 26-1 SIGNS OF ADVANCED ALCOHOLIC LIVER DISEASE*

Head area

Edema/puffy face
Parotid gland enlargement
Advanced periodontal disease
Sweet, musty breath odor
Ecchymoses, petechiae, bleeding

Rest of the body

Memory deficit
A lot of injuries
Spider angiomas
Jaundice
Ankle edema
Ascites
Palmar erythema
White nails
Transverse pale band on nails

*Modified from Little JW et al: *Dental management of the medically compromised patient*, ed 5, St Louis, 1997, Mosby.

Oral complications of alcoholism include glossitis, loss of tongue papillae, angular/labial cheilosis, and candida infection. Healing after surgery may be slow and bleeding difficult to stop.

Because alcohol and tobacco use and abuse predispose a patient to oral squamous cell carcinoma, the dental health care worker should check any oral lesions carefully. Special attention should be paid to leukoplakia and ulceration (especially on the lateral border of the tongue or the floor of the mouth).

With reduced liver function, the liver has difficulty metabolizing drugs usually metabolized in the liver. The levels of drugs metabolized by the liver, such as amide local anesthetics and oxidized benzodiazepines, will not fall as rapidly as in normal patients. With a single dose of drug, the dose does not have to be altered. With re-peated doses, the dose must be reduced or the interval between doses prolonged to prevent excessive blood levels of drugs metabolized by the liver. The signs of potential advanced alcoholic liver disease are listed in Box 26-1.

DENTAL CONSIDERATIONS The dental health care worker should have an index of suspicion so that alcoholics can be identified. The dental worker should smell the patient's breath, palpate the parotid glands, expect poor oral hygiene, and evaluate the patient's bleeding tendency. Those with cirrhosis and severe hepatic disease will have greatly prolonged prothrombin times and may require vitamin K a few days before a surgical procedure in which bleeding is expected. Table 26-3 lists the dental management of the alcoholic patient.

TABLE 26-3   Dental Management of the Alcoholic Patient

CONDITION	COMMENTS	MANAGEMENT
Bleeding abnormalities		Platelets—during and after chronic Thrombocytopenia—secondary to congestive splenomegaly, folate deficience, bone marrow EtOH toxicity; quickly reverse if stop drinking; begins up to 2-3 days & increase 20-60,000/day Impaired aggregation—decreased TX $_2$, increased bleeding time (like ASA or NSAIDs); improves 2-3 weeks after stopping Decreased hemostasis—vitamin K-dependent clotting factors missing
If cirrhosis and decreased liver function, clotting factors not being made (vitamin K dependent)	LFT test-AST,	Give vitamin K, give whole blood (fresh clotting factors) PT prolonged
GASTROINTESTINAL TRACT PROBLEMS		Use local hemostatic procedure
Stomach bleeding varices	Avoid NS, ASA	Topical
DRUG INTERACTIONS		??Acute intake—high levels Chronic intake—increased metabolism
Acute alcohol use		Chronic alcoholism
Enzyme-induced drugs metabolized by liver are metabolized faster, leading to lower blood levels of drugs metabolized by the liver	Raise drug level	Liver does not function properly, therefore drugs metabolized by liver are not metabolized as fast and levels increase Metabolism decreased
DI—Tylenol levels 4 gm; ASA, NS	4 gm usual	Less with some EtOH, none with more

From *JADA*, 128:68, 1997.
ASA, Aspirin; *EtOH,* alcohol; *NSAIDs,* nonsteroidal antiinflammatory drugs; *TX,* thromboxane.

NITROUS OXIDE

Typical nitrous abuser = dentist, 40s, male, poly-substance abuser

Nitrous oxide (N_2O) is an incomplete general anesthetic readily available in many dental offices (see Chapter 12). It is abused primarily by dental personnel—dentists, dental hygienists, and dental assistants. Food service employees sometimes become nitrous oxide abusers because it is available in the aerosol in canned whipping cream products. Misuse often begins as "therapeutic" use only, progressing to abusive or "recreational" use at a later stage.

Abuse pattern. Nitrous oxide is available in the dental office (tanks), as propellant for whipping cream, as "funny car" fuel (less pure), and by initiating a chemical reaction (impure, contains nitrogen dioxide). The availability of this gas to dental office personnel probably accounts for its unique abuse pattern.

Abuse of nitrous oxide can result in psychologic but not physical abuse. Inhalation of 50% to 75% produces a "high" for 30 seconds followed by a sense of euphoria and detachment for 2 to 3 minutes. Tingling or warmth around the face, auditory illusions, slurred speech, and a stumbling gait can occur. The typical chemical-dependent dentist (with nitrous oxide as his drug of choice) is a 40-year-old white male who has often abused illicit drugs and primarily uses alone.

Adverse reactions. Adverse reactions include dizziness, headache, tachycardia, syncope, and hypotension. Nitrous oxide impairs the ability to drive or operate heavy machinery. Other effects of nitrous oxide use include hallucinations and religious experiences. Equilibrium, balance, and gait are affected. With chronic use it can produce chronic mental dysfunction and infertility.

If 100% nitrous oxide is inhaled, nausea, cyanosis, and falling may occur. Without oxygen, nitrous oxide (pure) can produce hypoxia that results in death. Dentists who have self-administered nitrous oxide have been found dead in their dental chairs with the mask still attached to their face.

MYELONEUROPATHIC Chronic use or abuse can lead to myelopathy (sensory and motor) resulting in a combination of symptoms pathognomonic for nitrous oxide abuse. Initial symptoms include loss of finger dexterity and numbness or paresthesia of the extremities. Position and vibration sensory neurons are lost. Other sensations, such as to pain, light touch, and temperature, may be lost. Later, Lhermitte's sign (feels like electricity up and down spine), clumsiness, and weakness can be demonstrated. Neurologic deficiencies include extensor plantar reflex and polyneuropathy (slow conduction velocity in nerves). The neurologic deficiency is similar to that of spinal cord degeneration in pernicious anemia. The neurologic problems from vitamin B_{12} are improved by parenteral vitamin B_{12}. Whether B_{12} improves nitrous oxide myelopathy is controversial. If the abuse of nitrous oxide is discontinued soon enough, clinical improvement can occur. However, with an increase in abuse the myelopathy is often irreversible.

Myelopathy with abuse may be irreversible

OPIOID ANALGESICS

Heroin, methadone (Dolophine), morphine, hydromorphone (Dilaudid), meperidine (Demerol), oxycodone (Percodan), and pentazocine (Talwin) are currently the most popular abused opioids. Opioids used as analgesics are discussed in Chapter 7, which focuses on the pharmacology of the opioids themselves. It should be noted that opioids sold illegally on the street may be adulterated. They may contain other unknown agents or diluters and often contain inactive filler so the doses can be more easily divided.

In addition to being analgesics, opioids produce a state described as complete satiation of all drives. The opioids elevate the user's mood, cause euphoria, relieve fear and apprehension, and produce a feeling of peace and tranquility. They also suppress hunger, reduce sexual desire, and diminish the response to provocation. Undoubtedly, initial abuse is reinforced by this "positive" experience. Other effects include slowed respiration, constipation, urinary retention, and peripheral vasodilation.

With the development of physical dependence, however, the driving motivation to obtain the drug becomes more and more negative. Fear of the withdrawal syndrome begins to override other motivation. At this point the addict may resort to criminal activity and violence to support the drug habit. These activities are not direct actions of the drug, but are related to opioid dependence.

Pattern of abuse. Heroin is the opioid most commonly administered parenterally. The signs and symptoms of an acute overdose are fixed, pinpoint pupils, depressed respiration, hypotension and shock, slow or absent reflexes, and drowsiness or coma. Tolerance develops to most of the pharmacologic effects of the opioids, including the euphoric, analgesic, sedative, and respiratory depressant actions. However, tolerance does not develop to miosis or constipation.

The symptoms and time course of the withdrawal syndrome are determined by the specific drug abused and the dose of drug used. Withdrawal usually begins at the time of the abuser's next scheduled dose. The first signs of withdrawal from heroin are yawning, lacrimation, rhinorrhea, and diaphoresis, followed by a restless sleep. With further abstinence, anorexia, tremors, irritability, weakness, and excessive gastrointestinal activity occur. The heart rate is rapid, the blood pressure is elevated, and chills alternate with excessive sweating. Without treatment, symptoms disappear by about the eighth day after the last dose of heroin.

Management of acute overdose and withdrawal. If the triad of narcotic overdose (respiratory depression, pinpoint pupils, and coma) is

> Triad = respiratory depression, pin point pupils (P³), and coma

present, naloxone (Narcan) should be administered immediately. If there is no response, it is unlikely that the depressed respiration is caused by opioid overdose.

In the past, immediate withdrawal reaction from an opioid sold on the street was only moderately distressing to the patient because of the poor quality and dilution of these drugs. Recently, very-high-quality heroin has reached the streets, and overdoses are more common and the withdrawal more intense. Some addicts go "cold turkey" because the daily cost of their habit has risen too high. After withdrawal they begin using, but a smaller dose (therefore less expensive) is needed to produce the desired effect.

Patients in withdrawal can be made comfortable with methadone, a long-acting opioid that can replace heroin and then be gradually withdrawn. A phenothiazine or benzodiazepine is often administered for relief of tension. Long-term rehabilitation programs use several treatment approaches. These include substitution of a physiologically equivalent drug (e.g., methadone) in high doses, gradual weaning from methadone, or use of a long-acting opioid antagonist (e.g., naltrexone) (see Chapter 7). Other psychotropic agents may be helpful in managing the alcoholic patient because of the high incidence of comorbidity of psychiatric conditions.

Dental implications. The following should be considered when treating a dental patient who abuses opioids (narcotics):

PAIN CONTROL Because an opioid abuser develops tolerance to the analgesic effects of any opioid, treating pain with opioids is ineffective and can cause a recovering addict to begin using opioids again. It is best to alleviate the cause of the pain first (I&D or O&R) and prescribe non-steroidal antiinflammatory agents (NSAIAs) for analgesia.

Be alert for "shoppers!"

PRESCRIPTIONS FOR OPIOIDS Opioid abusers often come to the dental office requesting an opioid for severe pain ("shopping"). Frequently the drug abuser suggests the name or partial name of a specific opioid or states allergies to several less potent agents.

INCREASED INCIDENCE OF DISEASE Certain diseases that can be transmitted by use of needles for injections have a higher incidence in opioid abusers. These include hepatitis B, human immunodeficiency virus (HIV) producing acquired immune deficiency syndrome (AIDS), and sexually transmitted diseases. Infections caused by the use of nonsterile solutions and instruments can produce osteomyelitis and abscesses in the kidneys and heart valves. Intravenous drug abusers have about a 30% chance of developing cardiac valve damage over a 3-year period.

Unlike as in rheumatic heart disease, the valve most often damaged is the tricuspid. As in rheumatic heart disease, prophylactic antibiotics should be given before dental treatment if a murmur or valvular damage is present (see Chapter 8).

CHRONIC PAIN The dental health care worker will occasionally encounter dental patients with chronic pain. There are two ways in which these patients present to the dental office: a patient with symptoms of chronic dental-related pain (temporomandibular joint disorder or trigeminal neuralgia) or a patient reporting an elongation of the period of pain related to normal dental treatment (e.g., patient gets several refills of opioids for a root canal and no pathology can be identified). Patients who have pain for a much longer time than normal deserve a workup for chronic pain. Opioids are usually not effective in the management of chronic pain. If the dentist begins providing prescriptions for opioids to some patients, it is very difficult to stop writing these prescriptions for the patient. The patient may state, "I hurt real bad!" Another subtle lever that may increase the chance that the dentist would prescribe more opioids is the unsettling feeling that he or she has not performed some dental treatment correctly. Sometimes mild references to malpractice can magnify this worry. Do not be "blackmailed" into prescribing opioids if you feel uncomfortable. Just state your policy, for example, "The policy of this office is that no refills for an opioid (narcotic) analgesic are given without an additional office visit. It is important to identify the cause of the pain so that it can be alleviated."

Opioid street drugs. Opioids available on the street change with time and are different in different parts of the country. The dental health care worker should be aware of the fact that most drug abusers misuse more than one substance and that street drugs are often adulterated. An illicitly produced meperidine derivative that produced classic opioid effects contained MPTP. MPTP, a powerful neurotoxic agent, has a toxicity unrelated to its opioid effects. It produces classic and permanent (irreversible) Parkinson's disease by destroying the cells in the substantia nigra (they make dopamine) within a very short period. This contaminant has become a valuable research tool because it can induce Parkinson's disease in animals, providing an animal model for research of drugs for treatment of Parkinson's disease.

SEDATIVE-HYPNOTICS

Sedative-hypnotics includes barbiturates; alcohol; meprobamate (Miltown); methaqualone (Quaalude; not made legally now, called "ludes"); chloral hydrate; benzodiazepines, such as chlordiazepoxide (Librium) and diazepam

(Valium); and nitrous oxide. Although their chemical structures vary greatly, their pharmacologic actions and pattern of abuse are similar.

Initial symptoms resemble the well-known symptoms of alcohol intoxication: loss of inhibition, euphoria, emotional instability, quarrelsomeness, difficulty in thinking, poor memory and judgment, slurred speech, and ataxia. With increasing doses, drowsiness and sleep occur, respiration is depressed, cardiac output is decreased, and gastrointestinal activity and urine output are diminished. Paradoxical reactions can range from elation to excessive stimulation. The mechanism of excitement with a CNS depressant is related to an increased sensitivity to blocking of the inhibitor fibers, leaving the excitatory fibers unopposed. With additional CNS depression, the excitatory fibers are also depressed, resulting in sedation.

> Addict's usual dose becomes closer to fatal dose with increasing tolerance.

Pattern of abuse. The CNS depressant drugs are generally taken orally, often in a combination with some of the other drugs of abuse. With an acute overdose, respiratory and cardiovascular depression occur, leading to coma and hypotension. The pupils may be unchanged or small, and lateral nystagmus is seen. Confusion, slurred speech, and ataxia are always present. Compared with opioids, the CNS depressants have a slower onset of tolerance and physical dependence. Tolerance to the sedative effect is *not* accompanied by a comparable tolerance to the lethal dose. With prolonged misuse, emotional instability, hostile and paranoid ideations, and suicidal tendencies are common.

Although the withdrawal syndrome for all CNS depressants is similar, its time course depends on the half-life of the drug abused. The first signs of withdrawal are insomnia, weakness, tremulousness, restlessness, and perspiration. Often nausea and vomiting together with hyper-

thermia and agitation occur. Delirium and convulsions may culminate in cardiovascular collapse and loss of the temperature-regulating mechanism.

Another troubling abuse of the sedative-hypnotics involves administering them to other people in order to control them. Old movies have demonstrated the "slipping of a Mickey Finn" (chloral hydrate) to knock a person out ("knock-out drops"). A recent similar practice involves using a short-acting benzodiazepine, flunitrazepam or rohypanol (nickname is "Ruffies"), to make an unsuspecting young woman excessively sedated. After the woman becomes semiconscious, certain males perform "date rape" on the woman. Because of excessive sedation and the amnesia produced by the flunitrazepam, recounting or even remembering what happened is difficult. Therefore prosecution would be unlikely because it would be difficult to prove whether the action was or was not consensual.

Management of acute overdose and withdrawal. The most important consideration with an acute overdose of a CNS depressant is support of the cardiovascular and respiratory systems. An airway must always be established and maintained. Early gastric lavage after intubation and dialysis can assist in removal of some drugs. CNS stimulants are harmful and should not be given.

In contrast to withdrawal from opioids, withdrawal from CNS depressants can be life threatening and the patient should be hospitalized. The treatment of withdrawal from any CNS depressant includes (1) replacement of the abused drug with an equivalent drug and (2) gradual withdrawal of the equivalent drug.

The drug usually substituted for the abused drug is a long-acting benzodiazepine such as chlordiazepoxide or diazepam. The substitute drug is then gradually withdrawn over a period of weeks; during this time the patient receives psychotherapy.

CENTRAL NERVOUS SYSTEM STIMULANTS

The CNS stimulants include cocaine, the amphetamines, caffeine, and nicotine.

COCAINE

Cocaine is a CNS stimulant with local anesthetic properties when applied topically. It is used primarily for its stimulant action by "sniffing," "snorting," or intravenous injection. The most recent variant is a free-base form that is smoked and goes by the street name of "crack" or "rock." It is more pure and potent, and the resultant intoxication is far more intense than that of snorted cocaine. It acts much quicker and is much more euphoric and addicting. Cocaine induces intense euphoria, a sense of total self-confidence, and anorexia. Because of its short duration of action, the effects of cocaine last only a few minutes. Feeling of paranoia and extreme excitability cause some cocaine users to perform violent acts while under its influence. The paranoia produced by cocaine causes people to be unpredictable. The senseless violent acts sometimes committed by cocaine users cause society to fear cocaine abusers. Unpredictable actions are feared the most. Psychologic dependence becomes intense, but neither tolerance nor withdrawal has been shown. Cocaine's medical use is on mucous membranes (the inside of the nose), where it produces local anesthesia and vasoconstriction to reduce hemorrhage. There is *no* appropriate dental use of cocaine. Although cocaine abuse is greatly publicized, the proportion of the population using cocaine is relatively small (compared with alcohol and tobacco).

AMPHETAMINES

Drugs in the amphetamine class include methamphetamine (Desoxyn), dextroamphetamine (Dexedrine), diethylpropion (Tenuate), methylphenidate (Ritalin), and phenmetrazine (Prelu-

din). Another member of this group is phentermine (Fastin), the *phen* in Phen-Fen (diet drug combination removed from the market). Because methamphetamine produces a much longer duration of effect than cocaine, "meth" use is spreading across the nation. Kansas City, at this time, is the axel on which the wheel of distribution turns. Many meth labs have been raided, but more pop up immediately. The manufacture of methamphetamine can be carried out with common chemistry lab equipment and the precursor drug that can be bought over the counter. Unfortunately, these meth labs are quite explosive, smell bad (distinctive odor), and have been found in many residential neighborhoods.

The sympathomimetic CNS stimulants are abused for their ability to produce a euphoric mood, a sense of increased energy and alertness, and a feeling of omnipotence and self-confidence. Other effects include mydriasis, increased blood pressure and heart rate, anorexia, and increased sweating.

CNS stimulants are taken orally, parenterally (intravenously or "skin popping"), intranasally, or by inhalation (smoking). With prolonged use, tolerance develops to the euphorigenic effect and toxic symptoms appear, including anxiety, aggressiveness, stereotyped behavior, hallucinations, and paranoid fears.

Signs and symptoms of an acute overdose include dilated pupils (sympathetic autonomic nervous system stimulation), elevated blood pressure, rapid pulse, and cardiac arrhythmias. The patient may exhibit diaphoresis, hyperthermia, fine tremors, and hyperactive behavior. Oral adverse reactions include xerostomia and bruxism.

Although tolerance develops to the central sympathomimetic effect, no tolerance develops to the tendency to induce toxic psychoses at higher doses. Modest levels of abuse over a long period do not produce withdrawal reactions except fatigue and prolonged sleep, but very large doses can precipitate a withdrawal syndrome consisting of aching muscles, ravenous appetite with abdominal pain, and long periods of sleep. This is followed by profound psychologic depression and sometimes even suicide. During this period, abnormal electroencephalographic results have been recorded.

Management of acute overdose and withdrawal.

Treatment of an overdose of a CNS stimulant is symptomatic. It may include a phenothiazine for psychotic symptoms, a short-acting sympathomimetic-blocking agent if hypertension is severe, and a tricyclic antidepressant if severe depression occurs.

The most serious sociologic problem with stimulant abuse is the induction of mental abnormalities, especially in young abusers. Experimental evidence suggests that amphetamine psychoses can be induced in previously unaffected volunteer subjects. The psychoses are dose-related, and repeated dosing can reproduce the psychoses.

CAFFEINE

Caffeine, the most widely used social drug in the world, is contained in coffee, tea, cola drinks, and other drinks named to reflect the effect of their contents. Its action on the CNS is stimulation—that's why many people use these beverages. Caffeine toxicity can occur with as little as 300 mg of caffeine (contained in two to three cups of coffee). With five cups or more of caffeine daily, physical dependence can occur. Although many people do not consider it a drug, a withdrawal syndrome can be identified that begins around 24 hours after the last cup of coffee. It consists of headache, lethargy, irritability, and anxiety. Tolerance develops to the effects of caffeine, and some persons continue to use caffeine even when it produces harm. Table 26-4 lists the caffeine content of several beverages.

TOBACCO

Nicotine.
Awareness of the toxicity from chronic smoking and chewing of tobacco has increased

TABLE 26-4 **Caffeine Content of Selected Caffeine-Containing Beverages**

BEVERAGE	CAFFEINE
Cup of coffee—brewed	100-150/5 oz
Decaffeinated coffee	2-4/5 oz
Cup of tea—brewed	60-75/5 oz
Cola drink	60-105/12 oz
Mountain Dew	55/12 oz (0)*
Jolt	71/12 oz
Chocolate, milk	3-6/oz
Chocolate, bittersweet	25/oz
No Doze	100 mg/tablet

*In Canada.

dramatically over the last two decades. The CNS-active component of tobacco is nicotine, but a large number of components of the gaseous phase of tobacco smoke contribute to its undesirable effects: carbon monoxide, nitrogen oxides, volatile nitrosamines, hydrogen cyanide, volatile hydrocarbons, and many others.

Pattern of abuse.
Approximately twenty five percent of the adult American population smokes. Children commonly

> Cigars are the new "dumb craze!"

begin smoking between 11 and 14 years of age. In some geographic areas, more teenage girls than teenage boys smoke. The newest "craze" is cigar smoking; it is portrayed as glamorous, and famous movie stars are observed smoking cigars. Smokers claim that the most desirable effects of smoking are increased alertness, muscle relaxation, facilitation of concentration and memory, and decreases in appetite and irritability. These are consistent with the effect of nicotine on the CNS. In addition, nicotine produces an increase in blood pressure and pulse rate and induces nausea, vomiting, and dizziness as a result of stimulation of the chemoreceptor trigger zone. Smokers are tolerant to these latter effects, but such tolerance is not of long duration. The first cigarette of the day may induce a certain degree of dizziness and nausea. Chronic use of tobacco is causally related to many serious diseases, including coronary artery disease and oral and lung cancers.

Smokeless tobacco. In some communities, more than one fourth of high school boys use chewing tobacco. Oral mucosal changes include chronic gingivitis, leukoplakia, and precancerous lesions. In these patients, an extremely thorough oral examination should be done at each prophylaxis. Education concerning the oral health hazards that smokeless tobacco poses should also be included.

Management and withdrawal. The withdrawal syndrome that occurs after cessation of chronic tobacco smoking varies greatly from person to person. The most consistent symptoms are anxiety, irritability, difficulty in concentrating, and cravings for cigarettes. Drowsiness, headaches, increased appetite, and sleep disturbances are also common. The syndrome is rapid in onset (within 24 hours after the last cigarette) and can persist for months.

The syndrome of withdrawal from tobacco can be suppressed to some extent by administration of nicotine chewing gum (Nicorette, Nicorette DS) or nicotine patches (Nicoderm, Nico-

TABLE 26-5 Nicotine-Containing Products

Vehicle	Product
Patch	Habitrol, Nicoderm, Nicotrol, ProStep
Gum	Nicorette (DS)
Nasal spray	Nicotrol NS

trol, and Habitrol) (Table 26-5). These products do reduce the irritability and difficulty in concentrating, but appear to be less effective in controlling insomnia, hunger, and the craving for tobacco. The most important dental side effect of the use of nicotine gum is dislodging dental fillings. Another form of nicotine replacement is a nasal spray (Nicotrol NS). A potential problem with the nasal spray is that the rapid rise in blood level more closely mimics the effect of using tobacco.

Bupropion. Another approach to treating tobacco cessation involves the use of bupropion (Wellbutrin, Zyban), an antidepressant to reduce craving. Dentists can prescribe bupropion, but should encourage concomitant treatment modalities (e.g., behavior modification). The recommended dosage schedule is 150 mg qd for 3 days, followed by 150 mg bid for an additional 2 to 3 months if the patient is experiencing success. Refills should not be indicated on the original prescription because the dental health care worker should talk with the patient by phone before authorizing a refill (see discussion in Chapter 17).

The dental health care worker's role in tobacco cessation. Dental health care workers are in a special situation to be helpful in promoting tobacco cessation because of their role in encouraging patients to change habits (e.g., floss, brush teeth, use fluoride). Smoking cessation is another habit change [think behavior modification]. The dental health care worker is in a position to point out some of the oral manifestations of nicotine and tobacco abuse first hand—in the patient's own mouth. The National Cancer Institute currently has a program for dental personnel that includes a variety of patient education devices.* Every dental office should offer its patients help in smoking cessation.

---

*National Cancer Institute: 800-4-CANCER.

PSYCHEDELICS (HALLUCINOGENS)

The psychedelic agents are capable of inducing states of altered perception and generally do not have any medically acceptable therapeutic use. The drugs in this section include lysergic acid diethylamide (LSD) and phencyclidine (PCP), but many other agents, including psilocybin, dimethyltryptamine (DMT), 2,5-dimethoxy-4-methylamphetamine (STP), methylene dioxyamphetamine (MDMA), and mescaline (peyote), also fall into this class. Clearly, the agents discussed in this section represent only a fraction of those released on the illicit drug market. These hallucinogens are often mislabeled or adulterated with substances such as strychnine.

Psychedelics affect perceptions in such a way that all sensory input is perceived with heightened awareness; sounds are brighter and clearer, colors are more brilliant, and taste, smell, and touch are more acute. Psychedelic-induced dependence is psychologic, and tolerance develops within a short time. These two characteristics combined with the unpredictable nature of the response favor periodic rather than continuous abuse of psychedelic drugs. Prolonged use can cause long-lasting mental disturbances varying from panic reactions to depression to schizophrenic reactions.

LYSERGIC ACID DIETHYLAMIDE

Lysergic acid diethylamide (LSD) is the most potent hallucinogen; only micrograms are required for an effect. In addition to its psychogenic actions, LSD has sympathomimetic effects including tachycardia, rise in blood pressure, hyperreflexia, nausea, and increased body temperature.

An overdose of LSD produces symptoms that include widely dilated pupils, flushed face, elevated blood pressure, visual and temporal distortions, hallucinations, derealization, panic reaction, and paranoia. Because the user does not lose consciousness and is highly suggestible,

treatment is to provide reassurance ("talking the user down"). Rarely, chlorpromazine has been used to treat the situation in an emergency. Flashbacks, commonly precipitated by marijuana, can occur years after ingesting LSD. LSD is currently making another comeback.

PHENCYCLIDINE

Phencyclidine (PCP, or angel dust), originally developed as an animal tranquilizer, was very popular in the 1970s. It inhibits the reuptake of dopamine, serotonin, and norepinephrine. Although it has anticholinergic properties, hypersalivation is produced. It is a powerful CNS stimulant with dissociative properties. Users may exhibit sweating and a blank stare. Changes in body image and disorganized thought have led to bizarre behavior. Elevation of blood pressure and pulse and muscle movement and rigidity occur. It is abused alone or as an adulterant to other street drugs.

MARIJUANA

Marijuana (marihuana, cannabis) is derived from the hemp plant, and its active ingredient is tetrahydrocannabinol [tet-ra-hi-dro-can-NAB-i-nol] (THC). Marijuana can be administered orally or by inhalation (smoking), and its effects include an increase in pulse rate, reddening of the conjunctivae (bloodshot eyes), and behavioral changes. Slight changes in blood pressure and pupil size, as well as hand tremors, have been noted. With normal doses, euphoria and enhanced sensory perception occur. This is followed by sedation and altered consciousness (a dreamlike state).

Studies of the influence of marijuana on driving have concluded that the drug impairs motor and mental abilities required for safe driving. For example, the perception of time and distance is distorted and reflexes are decreased. A more common adverse reaction is apprehensive, nervous, and panic-stricken feelings that the user is losing his or her mind. This reaction responds to friendly reassurance. Psychologic dependence on marijuana is determined by the frequency of use. Physical dependence, tolerance, and withdrawal symptoms are very rare.

Of particular interest to the dental health care worker is the fact that a high level of marijuana abuse may cause xerostomia. It has been noted anecdotally that some marijuana users develop gingivitis. In these patients the gingival tissue was inflamed, and various leukoplakias with hyperkeratosis and parakeratosis with pseudoepitheliomatous hyperplasia were identified. Heavy marijuana smoking can lead to chronic bronchitis and precancerous changes in the bronchioles. THC is known to reduce intraocular pressure and has been used in the treatment of resistant glaucoma. It is also effective as an antiemetic to treat the nausea associated with cancer therapy.

IDENTIFYING THE DRUG ABUSER

"Shoppers" interact with many health care workers in an attempt to obtain controlled substances for illegitimate uses. Some references suggest that "shoppers" can be identified by the presence of poor hygiene, long-sleeved shirts, scars along veins, sunglasses, abrupt changes in behavior, moodiness, and behaving as though they were under the influence of an intoxicant. Usually this is not the case.

Most "shoppers" are excellent story tellers and actors with convincing histories and the presence of a pathologic dental condition. They look and behave like a typical patient. They may suggest specific drugs or give a history of allergy to analgesics they do not want. Notice the patient's response to your mentioning of drugs you are going to prescribe. This can be a tip off that the patient is hoping for a more potent drug.

Intravenous drug abusers are more likely to contract sexually transmitted diseases and are

> Abusers have more STDs—blood-borne infections

more likely to have hepatitis or be a carrier (HVB and HVC), be HIV positive, or have AIDS and to be infected with MDR tuberculosis and to have altered valves.

The dental office should not stock many controlled substances because it can become the target of robberies and burglaries. Addicts searching for drugs can be violent. The location of the supply of controlled substances must be under lock and key and in an inconspicuous place.

THE IMPAIRED DENTAL HEALTH CARE WORKER

When dental health care workers abuse drugs, they can present a danger to the patients being treated. A professional who is abusing drugs, like most abusers, is in denial, and confrontation by staff, relatives, and friends is often ineffective. The dentist's dental practice deteriorates and mood swings, including depression, occur. Often suicide is thought to be the only recourse.

Any dental health care worker who observes or suspects that another worker is abusing drugs should report the person to the appropriate "impaired professional committee" for their profession. Most state boards currently have committees to work with any impaired dental professional (those that have abused alcohol or drugs). The committee's goal is to assist the dental health care worker in becoming a functioning practitioner again. The objective of these committees is not to punish the worker to make the person lose his or her license. These committees can also investigate a suspicion of abuse. The difficulty in self-regulation is the silent practitioners who do not want to get involved.

REVIEW QUESTIONS

1. Define the following terms:
   a. psychologic dependence
   b. tolerance
   c. physical dependence
   d. withdrawal syndrome

e. addiction

f. enabling

g. abstinence

h. abuse

2. Explain the difference between abuse and addiction.

3. Describe the symptoms of withdrawal from an opioid analgesic agent such as heroin. Include the time course, depending on the specific opioid.

4. State the treatment for the withdrawal syndrome and for an overdose of an opioid analgesic agent.

5. Explain the rationale for the different methods of treating opioid addiction.

a. methadone maintenance program

b. naltrexone use

c. clonidine use

6. State diseases that are more common in intravenous drug abusers. Clarify the importance of these diseases to the dental health care worker.

7. Explain the rationale for the inclusion of alcohol in the discussion of the sedative-hypnotics.

8. Describe the withdrawal syndrome from the sedative-hypnotic agents and explain its potential severity.

9. Define *delirium tremens* and discuss its treatment.

10. State the best method to treat an alcoholic, and state two potential drugs used in managing alcoholism.

11. Describe the dental health care worker's responsibility, if any, in identifying a patient who is a drug addict.

12. Describe the symptoms of an overdose of a CNS stimulant.

13. State the current therapeutic use(s) of the amphetamines.

14. Name three psychedelic or hallucinogenic agents.

15. State the danger(s), if any, of phencyclidine (PCP).

16. Discuss the adverse reactions associated with marijuana use.

17. Describe a therapeutic use of marijuana.

18. Describe the long-term problems associated with cigarette smoking. Mention several organs that are affected.

19. Discuss the use of smokeless tobacco in adolescents and their idols [think baseball].

20. Describe the increased use of cigars and hypothesize about probable causes.

21. Explain the agreement, if any, between the government and the tobacco industry.

22. Describe the dental health care worker's role, if any, in a dental office tobacco cessation program. Could a community role for the dental health care worker be planned?

23. Compare and contrast the terms *addiction* and *habituation*.

24. State the major adverse effects associated with the use of cocaine. Explain the difference in problems produced by powdered cocaine and crack cocaine (alkaloid).

25. State oral changes that can occur with smokeless tobacco. Discuss some influences on the use of smokeless tobacco.

26. Describe the characteristics of a "shopper," and explain the importance of the "index of suspicion." Can a dental health care worker become too suspicious?

ONSET

Potency

Efficacy

Distribution-

-PRESCRIPTION

APPENDIXES

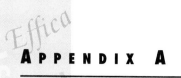

A P P E N D I X **A**

Top 200 Drugs

Top 200 Drugs, 1998—Ranked by Dispensed Total Prescriptions

Rank*	Brand Name†	Generic Name	Pharm Group‡	Indication‖	Introduced
193	Accolate	Zafirlukast	Leukotriene receptor antagonist	Asthma	9/96
41	Accupril	Quinapril	ACE inhibitor	HTN	12/91
24	Acetaminophen/Codeine (Teva)	Acetaminophen Codeine	Nonopioid Opioid	Pain	11/81
95	Acetaminophen/Codeine (Purepac)	Acetaminophen Codeine	Nonopioid Opioid	Pain	08/82
77	Adalat CC	Nifedipine	CCB	HTN	07/93
198	Adderall	Amphetamine mixed salts	Adrenergic agonists	ADD	2/96
13	Albuterol IH (Warrick Pharm)	Albuterol	β_2-Adrenergic agonist	Asthma	12/89
185	Albuterol IH (Zenith)	Albuterol	β_2-Adrenergic agonist	Asthma	08/93
82	Albuterol nebulizer solution (Warrick)	Albuterol	β_2-Adrenergic agonist	Asthma	N/A
184	Alesse	Levonorgestrel Ethinyl estradiol	Progestin Estrogen	Birth control	3/97
56	Allegra	Fexofenadine	Antihistamine, nonsedating	Allergy	08/96
160	Allopurinol (Mylan)	Allopurinol	Xanthine oxidase inhibitor	Gout	10/86
155	Alprazolam (Mylan)	Alprazolam	Benzodiazepine	Antianxiety	03/94
38	Alprazolam (Greenstone)	Alprazolam	Benzodiazepine	Antianxiety	09/93
73	Alprazolam (Geneva)	Alprazolam	Benzodiazepine	Antianxiety	09/93
171	Altace	Ramipril	ACE inhibitor	HTN	05/91
189	Amaryl	Glimepiride	Antidiabetic	Diabetes	11/95
39	Ambien	Zolpidem	Sedative-hypnotic	Insomnia	03/93
66	Amitriptyline (Mylan)	Amitriptyline	Antidepressant, TCA	Depression, chronic pain	05/81
199	Amitriptyline (Sidmark)	Amitriptyline	Antidepressant, TCA	Depression, chronic pain	9/84
15	Amoxicillin (Teva)	Amoxicillin	Antibiotic	Infection	11/81
40	Amoxil	Amoxicillin	Antibiotic	Infection	12/74
79	Atenolol (Lederle)	Atenolol	β_1-Adrenergic blocker	HTN	01/92
62	Atenolol (Geneva)	Atenolol	β_1-Adrenergic blocker	HTN	09/91

Rank*	Brand Name†	Generic Name	Pharm Group‡	Indication‖	Introduced
75	Atenolol (Mylan)	Atenolol	β_1-Adrenergic blocker	HTN	01/92
97	Atrovent IH	Ipratropium	Anticholinergic	Asthma	03/87
19	Augmentin	Amoxicillin Clavulanate	Antibiotic	Infection	08/84
126	Axid	Nizatidine	H_2-RA receptor antagonist	GERD, PUD	05/88
119	Azmacort IH	Triamcinolone	Corticosteroid	Asthma	05/84
128	Bactroban	Mupirocin	Antiinfective, topical	Skin infection	03/88
31	Biaxin	Clarithromycin	Antibiotic, macrolide	Infection	11/91
142	BuSpar	Buspirone	Antianxiety	Antianxiety	11/86
29	Cardizem CD	Diltiazem	CCB	HTN	01/92
54	Cardura	Doxazocin	α_1-Adrenergic blocker	HTN, BPH	01/91
89	Carisoprodol (Schein)	Carisoprodol	Muscle relaxant	Muscle spasms	11/87
92	Ceftin	Cefuroxime	Antibiotic, cephalosporin	Infection	02/88
67	Cefzil	Cefprozil	Antibiotic, cephalosporin	Infection	02/92
20	Cephalexin (Teva)	Cephalexin	Antibiotic, cephalosporin	Infection	05/87
136	Cephalexin (Apthecon)	Cephalexin	Antibiotic, cephalosporin	Infection	06/87
182	Cimetidine (Mylan)	Cimetidine	H_2-RA (receptor antagonist)	GERD, PUD	05/94
27	Cipro	Ciprofloxacin	Antibiotic (quinolone)	Infection	10/87
10	Claritin	Loratadine	Antihistamine, nonsedating	Allergy	04/93
55	Claritin-D 12 HR	Pseudoephedrine Loratadine	Decongestant Antihistamine, nonsedating	Allergy	11/94
93	Claritin-D 24 HR	Pseudoephedrine Loratadine	Decongestant Antihistamine, nonsedating	Allergy	09/96
180	Climara transdermal	Estradiol	Estrogen	Menopause	12/94
87	Clonazepam (Teva)	Clonazepam	Benzodiazepine	Anxiety, epilepsy	09/96
135	Clonidine (Mylan)	Clonidine	α_2-Adrenergic agonist	HTN	07/86
23	Coumadin	Warfarin	Anticoagulant	Prevent thrombosis	11/75
78	Cozaar	Losartan	Angiotensin II RA receptor antagonist	HTN	05/95
130	Cyclobenzaprine (Mylan)	Cyclobenzaprine	Muscle relaxant	Muscle spasms	07/91
121	Cyclobenzaprine (Schein)	Cyclobenzaprine	Muscle relaxant	Muscle spasms	05/89
104	Cycrin	Medroxyprogesterone	Progestin	Hormones	12/87
90	Daypro	Oxaprozin	NSAIA	Pain	01/93
177	Deltasone	Prednisone	Corticosteroid, oral	Inflammation	04/72
68	Depakote	Valproate	Anticonvulsant	Seizures	04/83
115	Desogen	Ethinyl estradiol Desogestrel	Estrogen Progestin	Oral contraceptive	01/93
107	Diazepam (Mylan)	Diazepam	Benzodiazepine	Antianxiety	08/85

Rank*	Brand Name†	Generic Name	Pharm Group‡	Indication‖	Introduced
71	Diflucan	Fluconazole	Antifungal	Fungal infection	02/90
60	Dilantin	Phenytoin	Anticonvulsant	Seizures	09/76
174	Diovan	Valsartan	Angiotensin II RA (receptor antagonist)	HTN	12/96
197	Dyazide	Triamterene Hydrochlorothiazide	Diuretic, K-sparing Diuretics, thiazide	HTN	02/68
172	Effexor	Venlafaxine	Antidepressant	Depression	03/94
165	Elocon	Mometasone	Corticosteroid, topical	Inflammation	08/87
170	Endocet	Oxycodone Acetaminophen	Opioid Nonopioid	Pain	N/A
116	Ery-Tab	Erythromycin	Antibiotic, macrolide	Infection	10/81
159	Estrace	Estradiol	Estrogen	Replacement	12/75
158	Estraderm	Estradiol	Estrogen	Replacement	09/86
149	Estradiol (Watson)	Estradiol	Estrogen	Replacement	04/96
64	Flonase	Fluticasone	Corticosteroid, nasal	Allergy	12/94
139	Flovent	Fluticasone	Corticosteroid, oral	Asthma	3/96
76	Fosamax	Alendronate	Biphosphonate, bone resorption inhibitor	Osteoporosis	10/95
113	Furosemide (Watson)	Furosemide	Diuretic, loop	Edema, CHF	11/85
143	Furosemide (Zenith)	Furosemide	Diuretic, loop	Edema, CHF	11/87
26	Furosemide (Mylan)	Furosemide	Diuretic, loop	Edema, CHF	N/A
167	Gemfibrozil (Teva)	Gemfibrozil	Antihyperlipidemic	Hyperlipidemia	12/93
183	Glipizide (Mylan)	Glipizide	Antidiabetic	Diabetes, type II	05/94
22	Glucophage	Metformin	Antidiabetic	Diabetes, type II	04/95
43	Glucotrol XL	Glipizide	Antidiabetic	Diabetes, type II	05/94
83	Glyburide (Copley)	Glyburide	Antidiabetic	Diabetes, type II	04/94
140	Glyburide (Greenstone)	Glyburide	Antidiabetic	Diabetes, type II	04/94
138	Guaifenesin/PPA (Duramed)	Guaifenesin Phenylpropanolamine	Expectorant Decongestant	Cough/cold combinations	02/87
98	Humulin 70/30	Insulin, 70/30	Insulin	Diabetes	07/89
59	Humulin N	Insulin, NPH	Insulin	Diabetes	07/83
164	Humulin R	Insulin, regular	Insulin	Diabetes	07/83
94	Hydrochlorothiazide (Purepac)	Hydrochlorothiazide	Diuretic, thiazide	HTN, edema	01/78
103	Hydrochlorothiazide (ESI Lederle)	Hydrochlorothiazide	Diuretic, thiazide	HTN, edema	8/63
129	Hydrochlorothiazide (Zenith)	Hydrochlorothiazide	Diuretic, thiazide	HTN, edema	8/63
44	Hydrocodone w/APAP (Mallinckrodt)	Hydrocodone Acetaminophen	Opioid Nonopioid	Pain	01/95

Rank*	Brand Name†	Generic Name	Pharm Group‡	Indication‖	Introduced
4	Hydrocodone/APAP (Watson)	Hydrocodone Acetaminophen	Opioid Nonopioid	Opioid Nonopioid	07/90
49	Hytrin	Terazosin	α_1-Adrenergic blocker	HTN, BPH	09/87
147	Hyzaar	Losartan HCTZ	Angiotensin II RA Diuretic, thiazide	HTN	4/95
25	Ibuprofen (Greenstone)	Ibuprofen	NSAIA	Pain	11/85
105	Ibuprofen (Par Pharm)	Ibuprofen	NSAIA	Pain/inflammation	03/95
69	Imdur	Isosorbide mononitrate	Nitrate	Angina	09/93
109	Imitrex	Sumatriptan	Serotonin agonist	Migraine headache	03/93
42	K-Dur	Potassium	Electrolyte	Hypokalemia	09/86
120	Klor-Con	Potassium	Electrolyte	Hypokalemia	09/86
11	Lanoxin	Digoxin	Digitalis glycoside	CHF	08/67
168	Lasix	Furosemide	Diuretic, loop	Edema, CHF	03/68
80	Lescol	Lovastatin	HMG-CoA reductase inhibitor	Hyperlipidemia	04/94
144	Levaquin	Levofloxacin	Antibiotic (quinolone)	Infection	12/96
33	Levoxyl	Levothyroxine	Thyroid	Hypothyroidism	06/87
8	Lipitor	Atorvastatin	HMG-CoA reductase inhibitor	Hyperlipidemia	01/97
106	Lo-Ovral	Ethinyl estradiol Norethindrone	Estrogen Progestin	Oral contraceptive	04/76
150	Loestrin Fe 1.5/30	Ethinyl estradiol Norethindrone Iron	Estrogen Progestin Iron	Oral contraceptive	09/76
163	Loestrin Fe 1/20	Ethinyl estradiol Norethindrone Iron	Estrogen Progestin	Oral contraceptive	09/76
192	Lorabid	Loracarbef	Antibiotic	Infection	08/92
65	Lorazepam (Mylan)	Lorazepam	Benzodiazepine	Anxiety	2/88
125	Lorazepam (Purepac)	Lorazepam	Benzodiazepine	Anxiety	11/85
47	Lotensin	Benazepril	ACE inhibitor	HTN	07/91
179	Lotrel	Amlodipine Benazepril	CCB ACE inhibitor	HTN	3/95
100	Lotrisone	Betamethasone Clotrimazole	Corticosteroid, topical Antifungal, topical	Fungal infection	7/84
132	Macrobid	Nitrofurantoin	Antiinfective, urinary	UTI	02/92
114	Medroxyprogesterone (Greenstone)	Medroxyprogesterone	Progestin	Hormone	07/93
151	Methylprednisolone (Duramed)	Methylprednisolone	Corticosteroid, oral	Inflammation	08/86
111	Metoprolol (Mylan)	Metoprolol	β_1-Adrenergic blocker	HTN	01/94

Rank*	Brand Name†	Generic Name	Pharm Group‡	Indication‖	Introduced
191	Metoprolol (Geneva)	Metoprolol	β_1-Adrenergic blocker	HTN	10/93
117	Mevacor	Lovastatin	HMG-CoA reductase inhibitor	Hyperlipidemia	09/87
187	Miacalcin nasal	Calcitonin salmon	Hypercalcemia antidote	Osteoporosis	8/95
91	Monopril	Fosinopril	ACE inhibitor	HTN	5/91
88	Naproxen (Teva)	Naproxen	NSAIA	Pain	6/98
141	Naproxen (Mylan)	Naproxen	NSAIA	Pain	10/93
188	Necon 1/35	Ethinyl estradiol Norethindrone	Estrogen Progestin	Birth control	12/89
148	Neomycin/polymyxin/HC	Neomycin Polymyxin B Hydrocortisone	Antibiotic Antibiotic Corticosteroid, topical	Ear infection	05/84
122	Neurontin	Gabapentin	Anticonvulsant	Epilepsy	02/94
96	Nitrostat SL	Nitroglycerin	Nitroglycerin	Angina	05/75
9	Norvasc	Amlodipine	CCB	HTN	09/92
153	Ortho-Cept	Ethinyl estradiol Desogestrel	Estrogen Progestin	Oral contraceptive	10/92
118	Ortho-Cyclen	Ethinyl estradiol Norgestimate	Estrogen Progestin	Oral contraceptive	12/89
61	Ortho-Novum 7/7/7	Ethinyl estradiol Norethindrone	Estrogen Progestin	Oral contraceptive	02/84
46	Ortho-Tri-Cyclen	Ethinyl estradiol Norgestimate	Estrogen Progestin	Oral contraceptive	10/92
14	Paxil	Paroxetine	Antidepressant, SSRI	Depression	01/93
124	Penicillin VK (Teva)	Penicillin VK	Antibiotic	Infection	9/57
57	Pepcid	Famotidine	H_2-RA (receptor antagonist)	GERD, PUD	11/86
157	Phenergan supp	Promethazine	Antihistamine (H_1-RA)	Nausea, sedation	5/55
181	Plendil	Felodipine SR	CCB	HTN	7/91
161	Potassium chloride (Ethex)	Potassium	Electrolyte	Hypokalemia	07/90
30	Pravachol	Pravastatin	HMG-CoA reductase inhibitor	Hyperlipidemia	11/91
35	Prednisone (Schein)	Prednisone	Corticosteroid, oral	Inflammation	11/87
1	Premarin	Estrogen, conjugated	Estrogen	Menopause	05/64
16	Prempro	Estrogen, conjugated Medroxyprogesterone	Estrogen Progestin	Menopause	02/95
36	Prevacid	Lansoprazole	Proton pump inhibitor	GERD, PUD	05/95
6	Prilosec	Omeprazole	Proton pump inhibitor	GERD, PUD	10/89
48	Prinivil	Lisinopril	ACE inhibitor	HTN	12/87
34	Procardia XL	Nifedipine	CCB	HTN	09/89
196	Promethazine (ESI Lederle)	Promethazine	Antihistamine H_1-RA	Nausea, sedation	5/55

Rank*	Brand Name†	Generic Name	Pharm Group‡	Indication‖	Introduced
190	Propacet N 100	Propoxyphene N Acetaminophen	Opioid Nonopioid	Pain	07/85
32	Propoxyphene N APAP (Mylan)	Propoxyphene N Acetaminophen	Opioid Nonopioid	Pain	8/57
81	Propoxyphene w/APAP (Qualitest)	Hydrocodone Acetaminophen	Opioid Nonopioid	Pain	04/76
51	Propoxyphene-N/APAP (Teva)	Propoxyphene N Acetaminophen	Opioid Nonopioid	Pain	12/85
162	Propranolol LA (ESI Lederle)	Propranolol LA	β-Adrenergic blocker	HTN	11/67
72	Propulsid	Cisapride	Cholinergic, GI emptying	Nausea, GERD	08/93
152	Provera	Medroxyprogesterone	Progestin	Hormone	04/76
5	Prozac	Fluoxetine	Antidepressant, SSRI	Depression	01/88
169	Ranitidine (Geneva)	Ranitidine	H_2-RA	GERD, PUD	8/97
123	Ranitidine (Novapharm)	Ranitidine	H_2-RA	GERD, PUD	07/97
154	Ranitidine (Mylan)	Ranitidine	H_2-RA	GERD, PUD	7/98
52	Relafen	Nabumetone	NSAIA	Pain/inflammation	02/92
200	Retin-A	Tretinoin	Retinoid	Acne	04/73
99	Rezulin	Troglitazone	Antidiabetic	Diabetes	1/97
175	Rhinocort	Budesonide	Corticosteroid, nasal	Nasal stuffiness	06/94
127	Risperdal	Risperidone	Antipsychotic	Schizophrenia	01/94
110	Roxicet	Oxycodone Acetaminophen	Analgesic, opioid Analgesic, nonopioid	Pain	12/81
101	Serevent	Salmeterol	$β_2$-Adrenergic agonist	Asthma	03/94
133	Serzone	Nefazodone	Antidepressant	Depression	01/95
194	Sumycin	Tetracycline	Antibiotic	Infection	11/53
2	Synthroid	Levothyroxine	Thyroid	Hypothyroidism	12/63
166	Tamoxifen (Barr)	Tamoxifen	Antiestrogen	Breast cancer	11/93
134	Temazepam (Mylan)	Temazepam	Benzodiazepine	Antianxiety	03/87
173	Timoptic-XE	Timolol	$β_1$-Adrenergic blocker	Glaucoma	01/94
156	TobraDex, ophth	Tobramycin Dexamethasone	Antibiotic, topical Corticosteroid, topical	Eye infection	05/88
63	Toprol-XL, ophth	Metoprolol	$β_1$-Adrenergic blocker, ophth	Glaucoma	02/92
186	Trazodone (Sidmak)	Trazodone	Antidepressant	Depression	12/87
145	Tri-Levlen	Ethinyl estradiol Levonorgestrel	Estrogen Progestin	Oral contraceptive	01/86
45	Triamterene/HCTZ (Geneva)	Triamterene HCTZ	Diuretic, K-sparing Diuretic, thiazide	HTN	10/87
74	Triamterene/HCTZ (Mylan)	Triamterene HCTZ	Diuretic, K-sparing Diuretic, thiazide	HTN	06/96

Rank*	Brand Name†	Generic Name	Pharm Group‡	Indication‖	Introduced
28	Trimethoprim/sulfa (Teva)	Trimethoprim Sulfamethoxazole	Antiinfective Antiinfective	Infection	01/83
3	Trimox	Amoxicillin	Antibiotic (penicillin)	Infection	11/77
58	Triphasil	Ethinyl estradiol Levonorgestrel	Estrogen Progestin	Oral contraceptive	11/84
37	Ultram	Tramadol	Opioid	Pain	03/95
85	Vancenase AQ 84 DS	Beclomethasone	Corticosteroid, nasal	Nasal stuffiness	07/96
18	Vasotec	Enalapril	ACE inhibitor	HTN	01/86
50	Veetids	Penicillin VK	Antibiotic	Infection	07/75
137	Verapamil SR (Mylan)	Verapamil	CCB	HTN	4/99
112	Verapamil SR (Zenith)	Verapamil	CCB	HTN	10/86
70	Viagra	Sildenafil	Enhances NO action, (inhibits phosphodiesterase type 5)	ED	3/98
178	Warfarin (Barr)	Warfarin	Anticoagulant	MI, thrombophlebitis	3/97
84	Wellbutrin SR	Bupropion	Antidepressant	Depression	10/96
108	Xalatan	Latanoprost	Prostaglandin, ophth	Glaucoma	08/96
176	Xanax	Alprazolam	Benzodiazepine	Antianxiety	11/81
131	Zantac	Ranitidine	H₂-RA (receptor antagonist)	GERD, PUD	06/83
146	Zestoretic	Lisinopril Hydrochlorothiazide	ACE inhibitor Diuretic, thiazide	HTN	03/89
17	Zestril	Lisinopril	ACE inhibitor	HTN	01/88
102	Ziac	Bisoprolol Hydrochlorothiazide	β-Adrenergic blocker Diuretic, thiazide	HTN	11/93
86	Zithromax susp	Azithromycin	Antibiotic, macrolide	Infection	03/92
7	Zithromax Z-Pak	Azithromycin	Antibiotic, macrolide	Infection	03/93
21	Zocor	Simvastatin	HMG-CoA reductase inhibitor	Hyperlipidemia	01/92
12	Zoloft	Sertraline	Antidepressant, SSRI	Depression	02/92
195	Zyban	Bupropion	Antidepressant	Tobacco cessation	5/97
53	Zyrtec	Cetirizine	Antihistamine, nonsedating	Allergy	01/96

Modified from Top 200 drugs of 1998, *Am Druggist*, Feb 1999, pg 42-43.
*Drugs are ranked from number 1, the most prescribed drug in 1997, to number 200, the least prescribed drug.
†Name by which prescribed; if prescribed by generic name that is listed in this column.
‡Acronyms: *ACE*, angiotensin converting enzyme inhibitor; H₂RA, histamine₂ receptor antagonist (H₂-blockers); *NSAIA*, nonsteroidal antiinflammatory agent; *ophth*, ophthalmic; *SSRI*, serotonin specific reuptake inhibitor; *TCA*, tricyclic antidepressant.
‖One indication listed; many other indications. Acronyms: *ADD*, attention deficit disorder; *BPH*, benign prostatic hypertrophy; *CCB*, calcium channel blocker; *CHF*, congestive heart failure; *ED*, erectile dysfunction; *GERD*, gastrointestinal esophageal reflux disease; *GI*, gastrointestinal; H₁-*RA*, H₁-receptor antagonist; H₂-*RA*, H₂ receptor antagonist; *HTN*, hypertension; *MI*, myocardial infarction; *PUD*, peptic ulcer disease; *UTI*, urinary tract infection.

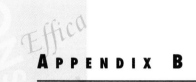
The Latest Drugs on the Market

The Latest Drugs on the Market

TRADE	GENERIC	DRUG GROUP	INDICATION
Accolate	Zafirlukast	Leukotriene LT_{D4} + LT_{E4} receptor antagonist (LTRA)	Asthma
Actiq	Fentanyl, oral transmucosal	Analgesic, opioid	Pain
Actonel	Risedronate	Bisphosphonate	Osteoporosis, Paget's
Agenerase	Amprenavir	Protease inhibitor	HIV
Aggrastat	Tirofiban	Antiplatelet	Unstable angina
Alora	Estradiol	Estrogen, transdermal	Estrogen replacement
Alrex	Loteprednol	Corticosteroid, ophth	Inflammation
Amerge	Naratriptan	5-Hydroxytryptamine $(5\text{-HT})_{1D+1B}$ agonist	Migraine
Aphthasol	Amlexanox	Antiinflammatory, topical	Aphthous stomatitis
Arava	Leflunomide	Antimetabolite, RA	RA
Aricept	Donepezil	AChE inhibitor	Alzheimer's
Arthrotec	Cytotec + diclofenac	Prostaglandin (PGE_2) + NSAIA	Arthritis, protect stomach
Atacand	Candesartan	Angiotensin II receptor antagonist	Antihypertensive
Atridox	Doxycycline	Tetracycline	Periodontal disease
Avapro	Irbesartan	Angiotensin II receptor antagonist	Antihypertensive
Azopt	Brinzolamide	Carbonic anhydrase inhibitor, ophth	Glaucoma
BactoShield	Chlorhexidine	Antibacterial	Infection
Bactroban	Mupirocin	Antibacterial	Skin infection (impetigo)
Betasept	Chlorhexidine	Antibacterial	Infection
Casodex	Bicalutamide	Antiandrogen, nonsteroidal	Prostate cancer
Celebrex	Celecoxib	NSAIA, COX II specific inhibitor	Arthritis
Celexa	Citalopram	Antidepressant, SSRI	Depression
Cerebryx	Fosphenytoin	Anticonvulsant	Seizures
Climara	Estradiol	Estrogen, transdermal	Estrogen replacement
Coreg	Carvedilol	α- + β-Blocker	Hypertension

TRADE	GENERIC	DRUG GROUP	INDICATION
Covera-HS	Verapamil SR	CCB	Hypertension
Cozaar	Losartan	Angiotensin II receptor antagonist (AIIRA)	Hypertension
Cytotec	Prostaglandin E_2	Prostaglandin	NSAIA-Induced GI problems
Cytovene	Ganciclovir	Antiviral, systemic	HIV-associated CMV
Daypro	Oxaprozin	NSAIA	Pain, inflammation
Dermatop	Prednicarbate	Corticosteroid, topical	Inflammation
Detrol	Tolterodine	Antimuscarinic	Urinary overaction
Doryx	Doxycycline	Tetracycline	Infection
Doxy	Doxycycline	Tetracycline	Infection
Doxychel	Doxycycline	Tetracycline	Infection
Droxia	Hydroxyurea	Antineoplastic	Cancer
Dyna-Hex topical	Chlorhexadine	Antibacterial	Infection
Emadine	Emedastine	Levocabastine (Livostin)	Ophth
Enbrel	Etanercept	Disease modifing antiflammatory (DMARDs)	Arthritis
Estraderm	Estradiol	Estrogen, transdermal	Estrogen replacement
Evista	Raloxifene	Selective estrogen receptor modulator (SERM)	Osteoporosis, postmenopausal
Exelon	Rivastigmine		Alzheimer's
Exidine	Chlorhexidine	Antibacterial	Infection
Ferrlecit	Ferric gluconate	Iron salt	Iron deficiency
Glucophage	Metformin	Antidiabetic	NIDDM
Havrix	Hepatitis A vaccine, inactivated	Vaccine	Hepatitis A prevention
Herceptin	Trastuzumab	Antineoplastic; monoclonal antibody	Breast cancer
Hibiclens	Chlorhexidine	Antibacterial	Infection
Hibistat	Chlorhexidine	Antibacterial	Infection
Hydrea	Hydroxycarbamide	Antineoplastic	
Infasurf	Calfactant	Surfactant, lung	RDS
Integrilin	Eptifibatide	Antiplatelet	
Lamictal	Lamotrigine	Anticonvulsant	Partial seizures (65% of epilepsy)
Lipitor	Atorvastatin	HMG-CoA reductase inhibitor	Hyperlipidemia
Lotemax	Loteprednol	Corticosteroid, ophth	Inflammation, eyes
Lovenox	Enoxaparin	Heparin, low molecular weight	Deep vein thrombosis (hip replacement)
Lymerix	Lyme disease vaccine	Vaccine	Lyme disease prevention
Marvelon	Desogestrel Eethinyl estradiol	Progestin Estrogen	Birth control

TRADE	GENERIC	DRUG GROUP	INDICATION
Maxalt	Rizatriptan	5-Hydroxytryptamine (5-HT$_{1D}$) agonist	Migraine
Meridia	Sibutramine	Inhibits reuptake of NE, 5-HT, and DA (less)	Obesity
Micardis	Telmisartan	AIIRA	
Migranal nasal spray	Dihydroergotamine	Ergot alkaloids	Migraine HA
Mirapex	Pramipexole	Dopamine D$_2$-agonist	Parkinsonism
Mircette	Ethinyl estradiol Desogestrel	Estrogen Progestin	Pregnancy prevention
Nicorette mint	Nicotine	Nicotine replacement	Tobacco cessation
Norvasc	Amlodipine	CCB	Hypertension
Ortho-Cept	Desogestrel Ethinyl estradiol	Progestin Estrogen	Birth control
Panretin	Alitretinoin	Antineoplastic, retinoid	AIDS, Kaposi's
Peridex oral rinse	Chlorhexidine	Antibacterial	Infection
PeriChip	Chlorhexidine	Antibacterial	Infection
PerioGard	Chlorhexidine	Antibacterial	Infection
Periostat	Doxycyline	Antibiotic, tetracycline	Periodontal disease
Pletal	Cilostazol	Inhibits platelet aggregation	Clotting
Prandin	Repaglinide	Oral hypoglycemic	NIDDM
Pravachol	Pravastatin	HMG-CoA reductase inhibitor	Hypercholesteremia
Preveon	Adefovir	RTI	HIV
PrevPac	Lansoprazole Amoxicillin Clarithromycin	PPI Antibiotic (penicillin) Antibiotic (macrolide)	Helicobacter pylori–associated ulcers
Priftin	Rifapentine	Antitubercular	Tuberculosis
Propulsid	Cisapride	Cholinergic enhancer	GERD, antiemetic
Provigil	Modafinil	CNS stimulants, nonamphetamine	Narcolepsy
Pulmicort Turbuhaler	Budesonide	Corticosteroid, topical, powder	Asthma
Rebetron	Intron A and rebetol	Immune stimulants	Hepatitis C
Refludan	Lepirudin	Anticoagulant	Heparin-induced ITTP
RenaGel	Sevelamer	Phosphate binder	ESRD
Remicade	Infliximab	GI, MCA	Crohn's
Requip	Ropinirole	DOPA agonist	Parkinsonism
Revasc		Antithrombotic	Thrombosis
Rezulin	Troglitazone	Decreases insulin resistance	NIDDM
RotaShield	Rotavirus vaccine	Vaccine	Rotavirus prevention
Simulect	Basiliximab	Iimmunosuppressive, renal; MCA	Renal transplant

TRADE	GENERIC	DRUG GROUP	INDICATION
SingulAir	Montelukast	Leukotriene antagonist	Bronchospasm
Sonata	Zaleplon	Antianxiety agent (like Ambien)	Insomnia
Sucraid	Sacrosidase	GI enzyme	Sucrose, isomaltose malabsorption, congenital
Sustiva	Efavirenz	NNRTI	HIV
Synagis	Palivizumab	MCA	RSV
Tasmar	Tolcapone	COMT inhibitor, prolongs levodopa's effect	Parkinsonism
Teczem	Enalapril + diltiazem	Vaso**tec** + Cardi**zem**	Hypertension
Thalomid	Thalidomide	Immunomodulator	Leprosy, aphthous
Tiazac	Diltiazem	CCB	Hypertension
Trovan	Trovafloxacin	Antibiotic, fluoroquinolones	Infection, anaerobic
Ultram	Tramadol	μ-Opioid agonist + inhibit reuptake NE and 5-HT	Analgesic, central
Valstar	Valrubicin	Antineoplastic, bladder	Bladder cancer
Viagra	Sildenafil	Phosphodiesterase type 5 (PDE5) inhibitor	ED
Vibramycin	Doxycycline	Tetracycline	Infection
Vibra-Tabs	Doxycycline	Tetracycline	Infection
Vioxx	Rofecoxib	NSAIA, COX II–specific inhibitor	Arthritis
Vitrasert	Ganciclovir	Antiviral, intraocular	HIV-associated CMV
Vitravene	Fomiversen	CMV retinitis	HIV-associated CMV
Vivelle	Estradiol	Estrogen, transdermal	Estrogen replacement
Xeloda	Capecitabine	Antineoplastic, antimetabolite	Cancer
Xopane	Oxaproxin K	NSAIA	Pain
Zemplar	Paricalcitol	Vitamin D analogue	Hyperparathyroidism caused by ESRD
Ziagen	Abacavir	RTI	HIV
Zyrtec	Cetirizine	Antihistamine, nonsedating	Allergies

AIIRA, Angiotensin II receptor antagonist; *CCB*, calcium channel blocker; *CMV*, cytomegalic virus; *CNS*, central nervous systems; *COMT*, catechol-O-methyl-transferase; *COX*, cyclooxygenase; *DA*, dopamine; *ED*, erectile dysfunction; *ESRD*, end-stage renal disease; *5-HT*, 5-hydroxytryptamine (serotonin); *GERD*, gastroesophageal reflux disease; *GI*, gastrointestinal; *HA*, headache; *HIV*, human immunodeficiency virus; *LT*, leukotriene; *MCA*, monoclonal antibody; *NE*, norepinephrine; *NIDDM*, non–insulin-dependent diabetes mellitus; *NNRTI*, nonnucleotide reverse transcriptase inhibitor; *NSAIA*, nonsteroidal antiinflammatory agents; *PDE5*, phosphodiesterase type 5 inhibitor; *PPI*, proton pump inhibitor; *RA*, rheumatoid arthritis; *RDS*, respiratory distress syndrome; *RSV*, respiratory syncytial virus; *RTI*, reverse transcriptase inhibitor; *SERM*, selective estrogen receptor modulator; *SSRI*, serotonin-specific reuptake inhibitor; *TNF*, tumor necrosis factor.

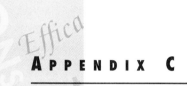

APPENDIX C

Commonly Prescribed Dental Drugs*

ANALGESICS

NONOPIOIDS

OTC

- Acetaminophen 500-650 mg q 4-6 h prn
    Regular = 325 mg
    Extra-strength = 500 mg
- Ibuprofen 400-600 mg q 4-6 h prn
    OTC = 200 mg
- Naproxen sodium (Aleve)
    220-440 mg q 8-12 h prn
    OTC = 220 mg

R︭

Jane Doe, DDS 1234 Main Ave. City, ST 12345	(111) 555-1234

Name _____ Date _____

Address _____ Age _____

R︭

   Ibuprofen 400 mg tabs
   Disp: #24
   Sig: 1-2 tabs qid prn pain

Substitution Permitted _____ _____ Dispense as written

DEA# _____ Print name

Jane Doe, DDS 1234 Main Ave. City, ST 12345	(111) 555-1234

Name _____ Date _____

Address _____ Age _____

R︭

   Naproxen 500 mg tabs
   Disp: #8
   Sig: 1 tab bid prn for pain

Substitution Permitted _____ _____ Dispense as written

DEA# _____ Print name

OPIOIDS

Weak—some pain

Jane Doe, DDS 1234 Main Ave. City, ST 12345	(111) 555-1234

Name _____ Date _____

Address _____ Age _____

R︭

   APAP/codeine 300/30 mg [Tylenol #3]
   Disp: #24
   Sig: 1-2 tabs q 4-6 h prn pain

Substitution Permitted _____ _____ Dispense as written

DEA# _____ Print name

---

*Prescription blanks used as samples are in the format legal
for Missouri. Other states may have different requirements.

545

Intermediate to moderate pain

Jane Doe, DDS 1234 Main Ave. City, ST 12345   (111) 555-1234

Name _____ Date _____

Address _____ Age _____

Rx

Hydrocodone/APAP 5/500 mg tab [Vicodin]
Disp: #24
Sig: 1-2 tabs q 4-6 h prn pain

Substitution Permitted _____ _____ Dispense as written

DEA# _____   Print name

Strong to severe pain

Jane Doe, DDS 1234 Main Ave. City, ST 12345   (111) 555-1234

Name _____ Date _____

Address _____ Age _____

Rx

APAP/Oxycodone 325/5 mg [Percocet]
Disp: #16
Sig: 1-2 tabs q 4-6 h prn pain

Substitution Permitted _____ _____ Dispense as written

DEA# _____   Print name

Very weak—codeine allergy

Jane Doe, DDS 1234 Main Ave. City, ST 12345   (111) 555-1234

Name _____ Date _____

Address _____ Age _____

Rx

Propoxyphene N/APAP 100/650 mg tab [Darvocet N 100]
Disp: #12
*Sig: 1 tab q 4-6 h prn pa [Do not exceed 6 tabs/24 hrs]**

Substitution Permitted _____ _____ Dispense as written

DEA# _____   Print name

*Acetaminophen overdose if more is used.

ANALGESICS/ANESTHETICS, TOPICAL

Jane Doe, DDS 1234 Main Ave. City, ST 12345   (111) 555-1234

Name _____ Date _____

Address _____ Age _____

Rx

Lidocaine viscous 2%
Disp: 100 ml
Sig: ✔ If generalized lesions: Swish & swirl in mouth and spit 1 tsp q 4 h prn discomfort
✔ If few localized lesions: Dry and apply to oral lesions with Q-tip q 4 h prn discomfort [may use more frequently if areas small]

Substitution Permitted _____ _____ Dispense as written

DEA# _____   Print name

OTC

- Diphenhydramine 12.5 mg/5 ml (syrup or elixir)
  OTC—1 bottle
  Swish, swirl, and spit 1 tsp q 4 h prn discomfort
- Orabase B (has benzocaine 20%) 5 gm
  Dry and apply to oral lesions with Q-tip q 4 h prn discomfort

ANTIINFECTIVE AGENTS

Duration: For as long as the symptoms persist plus 2 to 3 days

TREATMENT OF INFECTION, GENERAL

Jane Doe, DDS 1234 Main Ave. City, ST 12345   (111) 555-1234

Name _____ Date _____

Address _____ Age _____

R℞

Penicillin VK 500 mg tabs
Disp: #28
Sig: 1 tab qid (q6h) until gone

Substitution Permitted   Dispense as written

DEA#   Print name

Jane Doe, DDS 1234 Main Ave. City, ST 12345   (111) 555-1234

Name _____ Date _____

Address _____ Age _____

R℞

Amoxicillin 500 mg caps
Disp: #28
Sig: 1 cap tid (q8h) until gone

Substitution Permitted   Dispense as written

DEA#   Print name

Jane Doe, DDS 1234 Main Ave. City, ST 12345   (111) 555-1234

Name _____ Date _____

Address _____ Age _____

R℞

Erythromycin 250 or 500 mg tabs
Disp: #14
Sig: 1 tab qid until gone, with food

Substitution Permitted   Dispense as written

DEA#   Print name

Jane Doe, DDS 1234 Main Ave. City, ST 12345   (111) 555-1234

Name _____ Date _____

Address _____ Age _____

R℞

Clindamycin 150 mg caps
Disp: #28
Sig: 1 cap tid (q8h) until gone
Note: higher doses used in severe
infections

Substitution Permitted   Dispense as written

DEA#   Print name

---

or

Jane Doe, DDS 1234 Main Ave. City, ST 12345   (111) 555-1234

Name _____ Date _____

Address _____ Age _____

R℞

Erythromycin estolate 400-800 mg tabs
Disp: #14
Sig: 1 tab qid until gone, with food

Substitution Permitted   Dispense as written

DEA#   Print name

Jane Doe, DDS 1234 Main Ave. City, ST 12345   (111) 555-1234

Name _____ Date _____

Address _____ Age _____

R℞

Metronidazole 250 mg
Disp: #28 tabs
Sig: 1 tab q6h (qid) until gone;
with food, no alcohol

Substitution Permitted   Dispense as written

DEA#   Print name

Jane Doe, DDS 1234 Main Ave. City, ST 12345   (111) 555-1234

Name _____   Date _____

Address _____   Age _____

℞

Metronidazole 500 mg
Disp: #14 tabs
Sig: 1 tab q12h (bid) until gone;
with food, no alcohol

Substitution Permitted _____   Dispense as written

DEA# _____   Print name

ANTIBIOTIC PROPHYLAXIS

Jane Doe, DDS 1234 Main Ave. City, ST 12345   (111) 555-1234

Name _____   Date _____

Address _____   Age _____

℞

Amoxicillin 500 mg
Disp: #4 caps
Sig: Tk 4 cap 1 h b/f dental appt.

Substitution Permitted _____   Dispense as written

DEA# _____   Print name

INFECTIONS, PERIODONTAL-RELATED

Jane Doe, DDS 1234 Main Ave. City, ST 12345   (111) 555-1234

Name _____   Date _____

Address _____   Age _____

℞

Doxycycline 100 mg caps
Disp: #14 [28]
Sig: 1 cap bid until gone

Substitution Permitted _____   Dispense as written

DEA# _____   Print name

Jane Doe, DDS 1234 Main Ave. City, ST 12345   (111) 555-1234

Name _____   Date _____

Address _____   Age _____

℞

Clindamycin 150 mg
Disp: #4 caps
Sig: 4 cap 1 h b/f dental appt.

Substitution Permitted _____   Dispense as written

DEA# _____   Print name

Jane Doe, DDS 1234 Main Ave. City, ST 12345   (111) 555-1234

Name _____   Date _____

Address _____   Age _____

℞

Tetracycline 500 mg caps
Disp: #28
Sig: 1 cap qid until gone, no dairy

Substitution Permitted _____   Dispense as written

DEA# _____   Print name

Jane Doe, DDS 1234 Main Ave. City, ST 12345   (111) 555-1234

Name _____   Date _____

Address _____   Age _____

℞

Biaxin 500 mg caps tabs
Disp: #2
Sig: 2 cap 1 h b/f dental appt.

Substitution Permitted _____   Dispense as written

DEA# _____   Print name

Jane Doe, DDS 1234 Main Ave. City, ST 12345   (111) 555-1234

Name _____ Date _____

Address _____ Age _____

℞

Zithromax 500 mg caps tabs
Disp: #2
Sig: 2 cap 1 h b/f dental appt.

Substitution Permitted _____ Dispense as written

DEA# _____

Print name

Jane Doe, DDS 1234 Main Ave. City, ST 12345   (111) 555-1234

Name _____ Date _____

Address _____ Age _____

℞

Cephalexin 500 mg caps
Disp: #2
Sig: 2 cap 1 h b/f dental appt.

Substitution Permitted _____ Dispense as written

DEA# _____

Print name

Impetigo

Jane Doe, DDS 1234 Main Ave. City, ST 12345   (111) 555-1234

Name _____ Date _____

Address _____ Age _____

℞

Mupirocin 2% ung [Bactroban]
Disp: 15 Gm
Sig: Ap & rub in tid for 5 days

Substitution Permitted _____ Dispense as written

DEA# _____

Print name

ANTIFUNGAL AGENTS

Duration: Usually 2 weeks needed, may require continuous therapy with immune suppression

TOPICAL

OTC

* Clotrimazole [generic, Mycelex] ointment 15 gm
* Miconazole [generic, Micatin] ointment 15 gm

    [location in store: check athletes' foot and vaginal cream aisles]

℞

Jane Doe, DDS 1234 Main Ave. City, ST 12345   (111) 555-1234

Name _____ Date _____

Address _____ Age _____

℞

Nystatin aqueous susp 100,000
Units/ml
Disp: 280 mls
Sig: Swish, swirl [hold for 2 min], &
spit 1 tsp (500,000 units) in mouth
qid until gone; do not eat or drink for
30 min after use
Note: [50% sucrose]

Substitution Permitted _____ Dispense as written

DEA# _____

Print name

Jane Doe, DDS 1234 Main Ave. City, ST 12345   (111) 555-1234

Name _____ Date _____

Address _____ Age _____

℞

Nystatin lozenges 200,000 units
[Mycostatin pastilles]
Disp: #70
Sig: Slowly dissolve 1-2 [200-400
units] lozenges in mouth 4-5 x/day
for up to 14 days until gone

Substitution Permitted _____ Dispense as written

DEA# _____

Print name

Jane Doe, DDS 1234 Main Ave. City, ST 12345   (111) 555-1234

Name _____ Date _____

Address _____ Age _____

R

Nystatin vag supp 100,000 units
Disp: #14 to 70
Sig: Slowly dissolve 1 in mouth qid ud

Substitution Permitted _____ Dispense as written

DEA# _____ Print name

Not FDA approved for oral use.

Jane Doe, DDS 1234 Main Ave. City, ST 12345   (111) 555-1234

Name _____ Date _____

Address _____ Age _____

R

Clotrimazole 10 mg vag supp
Disp: 14 to 70
Sig: Slowly dissolve 1 in mouth 5x/d
until gone

Substitution Permitted _____ Dispense as written

DEA# _____ Print name

Not FDA approved for oral use.

SYSTEMIC

Jane Doe, DDS 1234 Main Ave. City, ST 12345   (111) 555-1234

Name _____ Date _____

Address _____ Age _____

R

Ketoconazole 200 mg
Disp: 14 tabs
Sig: 1 tab qd until gone

Substitution Permitted _____ Dispense as written

DEA# _____ Print name

Jane Doe, DDS 1234 Main Ave. City, ST 12345   (111) 555-1234

Name _____ Date _____

Address _____ Age _____

R

Nystatin 100,000 units/gm
Disp: 15 gm cream
Sig: Dry and ap to lesions and
inside denture q8h prn

Substitution Permitted _____ Dispense as written

DEA# _____ Print name

ANTIVIRAL AGENTS (HERPES LABIALIS)

TREATMENT

Only one agent approved for use in recurrent lesions.

Jane Doe, DDS 1234 Main Ave. City, ST 12345   (111) 555-1234

Name _____ Date _____

Address _____ Age _____

R

Penciclovir 1% oint [Denavir]
Disp: 2 gm
Sig: Ap q 2 h w/a for 4 days

Substitution Permitted _____ Dispense as written

DEA# _____ Print name

Jane Doe, DDS 1234 Main Ave. City, ST 12345   (111) 555-1234

Name _____ Date _____

Address _____ Age _____

R

Clotrimazole 10 mg [Mycelex]
Disp: #70 troches
Sig: Slowly dissolve 1 troche in
mouth 5 x per day until gone

Substitution Permitted _____ Dispense as written

DEA# _____ Print name

Acyclovir topical and systemic—no studies to show positive effect with recurrent episodes in immunocompetent patients.

PREVENTION

Recurrent infections, chronic suppressive therapy (≥6 episodes/yr):

Jane Doe, DDS 1234 Main Ave. City, ST 12345   (111) 555-1234

Name _____ Date _____

Address _____ Age _____

Rx

Acyclovir 400 mg tab
Disp: #60
Sig: 1 tab bid

_____ _____

Substitution Permitted   Dispense as written

_____ _____

DEA#   Print name

CORTICOSTEROIDS

TOPICAL

WEAK

OTC

Hydrocortisone 1% cream

Jane Doe, DDS 1234 Main Ave. City, ST 12345   (111) 555-1234

Name _____ Date _____

Address _____ Age _____

Rx

Hydrocortisone 2.5% cream
Disp: 15 gm
Sig: Dry and ap to oral lesions qid ud

_____ _____

Substitution Permitted   Dispense as written

_____ _____

DEA#   Print name

Jane Doe, DDS 1234 Main Ave. City, ST 12345   (111) 555-1234

Name _____ Date _____

Address _____ Age _____

Rx

Orabase HCA
Disp: 5 gm
Sig: Dry and ap to oral lesions qid ud

_____ _____

Substitution Permitted   Dispense as written

_____ _____

DEA#   Print name

INTERMEDIATE

Jane Doe, DDS 1234 Main Ave. City, ST 12345   (111) 555-1234

Name _____ Date _____

Address _____ Age _____

Rx

Triamcinolone cream 0.025%
Disp: 15 gm
Sig: Dry and ap to oral lesions qid ud

_____ _____

Substitution Permitted   Dispense as written

_____ _____

DEA#   Print name

Jane Doe, DDS 1234 Main Ave. City, ST 12345   (111) 555-1234

Name _____ Date _____

Address _____ Age _____

Rx

Triamcinolone cream 0.1%
Disp: 15 gm
Sig: Dry and ap to oral lesions qid ud

_____ _____

Substitution Permitted   Dispense as written

_____ _____

DEA#   Print name

Jane Doe, DDS 1234 Main Ave. City, ST 12345   (111) 555-1234

Name _____ Date _____

Address _____ Age _____

Rx

TAC in Orabase 0.1%
Disp: 5 gm
Sig: Dry and ap to oral lesions qid ud

_____ _____
Substitution Permitted   Dispense as written

_____ _____
DEA#   Print name

Jane Doe, DDS 1234 Main Ave. City, ST 12345   (111) 555-1234

Name _____ Date _____

Address _____ Age _____

Rx

Fluocinonide 0.05% gel
Disp: 15 gm
Sig: Dry and ap to oral lesions qid ud

_____ _____
Substitution Permitted   Dispense as written

_____ _____
DEA#   Print name

STRONG

VERY STRONG—CAUTION

Jane Doe, DDS 1234 Main Ave. City, ST 12345   (111) 555-1234

Name _____ Date _____

Address _____ Age _____

Rx

Fluocinonide 0.05% cream [Lidex]
Disp: 15 gm
Sig: Dry and ap to oral lesions qid ud

_____ _____
Substitution Permitted   Dispense as written

_____ _____
DEA#   Print name

Jane Doe, DDS 1234 Main Ave. City, ST 12345   (111) 555-1234

Name _____ Date _____

Address _____ Age _____

Rx

Clobetasol cr 0.05% [Temovate]
Disp: 15 gm
Sig: Dry and ap to oral lesions qid ud

_____ _____
Substitution Permitted   Dispense as written

_____ _____
DEA#   Print name

Jane Doe, DDS 1234 Main Ave. City, ST 12345   (111) 555-1234

Name _____ Date _____

Address _____ Age _____

Rx

Fluocinonide elixir 0.05%
Disp: 180 ml
Sig: Swish, swirl and spit 1 tsp in mouth qid prn discomfort

_____ _____
Substitution Permitted   Dispense as written

_____ _____
DEA#   Print name

Jane Doe, DDS 1234 Main Ave. City, ST 12345   (111) 555-1234

Name _____ Date _____

Address _____ Age _____

Rx

Clobetasol oint 0.05%
Disp: 15 gm
Sig: Dry and ap to oral lesions qid ud

_____ _____
Substitution Permitted   Dispense as written

_____ _____
DEA#   Print name

SYSTEMIC

Jane Doe, DDS 1234 Main Ave. City, ST 12345   (111) 555-1234

Name _____ Date _____
Address _____ Age _____

℞

Prednisone 40 mg taper:
Prednisone 10 mg
Disp: #29 tabs
Sig: 40 mg x 3 d, 30 mg x 3 d,
20 mg x 3 d, 10 mg x 2 d

Substitution Permitted

_____ _____
DEA#   Dispense as written

           Print name

Jane Doe, DDS 1234 Main Ave. City, ST 12345   (111) 555-1234

Name _____ Date _____
Address _____ Age _____

℞

Prednisone 60 mg taper:
Prednisone 10 mg
Disp: 48 tabs
Sig: 60 mg x 2 d, 50 mg x 2 d,
40 mg x 2 d, 30 mg x 2 d,
20 mg x 2 d, 10 mg x 2 d

Substitution Permitted   Dispense as written

DEA#   Print name

Jane Doe, DDS 1234 Main Ave. City, ST 12345   (111) 555-1234

Name _____ Date _____
Address _____ Age _____

℞

Methylprednisolone 4 mg dosepak
Disp: 21 tabs
Sig: Tk ud on package

Substitution Permitted   Dispense as written

DEA#   Print name

MISCELLANEOUS AGENTS

IMMUNOSUPPRESSIVES—DOSAGE INDIVIDUALIZED

- Azathioprine 50 mg tabs [Imuran]
- Cyclophosphamide 50 mg [Cytoxan]
- Methotrexate (MTX) [Rheumatrex]

Saliva-altering

DECREASE

Jane Doe, DDS 1234 Main Ave. City, ST 12345   (111) 555-1234

Name _____ Date _____
Address _____ Age _____

℞

Atropine 0.4 mg tabs
Disp: #4
Sig: Tk 1-2 tabs 2 hr b/f dental appt.

Substitution Permitted   Dispense as written

DEA#   Print name

INCREASE

℞ price >$100

Jane Doe, DDS 1234 Main Ave. City, ST 12345   (111) 555-1234

Name _____ Date _____
Address _____ Age _____

℞

Pilocarpine 5 mg tabs
Disp: #90
Sig: 1 tab tid prn for xerostomia —
may increase gradually until side
effects occur

Substitution Permitted   Dispense as written

DEA#   Print name

℞ price <$10-15

Jane Doe, DDS 1234 Main Ave. City, ST 12345   (111) 555-1234
Name _____   Date _____
Address _____   Age _____
℞

Pilocarpine 2% opth drops
Disp: 30 ml (2 bottles)
Sig: Jk 5 drops (5 mg) po tid prn
for xerostomia, may increase
gradually prn

Substitution Permitted   Dispense as written

DEA#   Print name

Aphthous Stomatitis

Jane Doe, DDS 1234 Main Ave. City, ST 12345   (111) 555-1234
Name _____   Date _____
Address _____   Age _____
℞

Aphthasol 5% paste
Disp: 5 gm
Sig: Ap to oral ulcers pc & hs

Substitution Permitted   Dispense as written

DEA#   Print name

TMD Use

MUSCLE RELAXANTS

Note: stronger relaxant, significant sedation.

Jane Doe, DDS 1234 Main Ave. City, ST 12345   (111) 555-1234
Name _____   Date _____
Address _____   Age _____
℞

Cyclobenzaprine 10 mg [Flexeril]
Disp: 20 tabs
Sig: 1 bid or 1 hs

Substitution Permitted   Dispense as written

DEA#   Print name

Jane Doe, DDS 1234 Main Ave. City, ST 12345   (111) 555-1234
Name _____   Date _____
Address _____   Age _____
℞

Carisoprodol 350 mg [Soma]
Disp: 20 tabs
Sig: 1 bid

Substitution Permitted   Dispense as written

DEA#   Print name

ANTIDEPRESSANTS

Jane Doe, DDS 1234 Main Ave. City, ST 12345   (111) 555-1234
Name _____   Date _____
Address _____   Age _____
℞

Amitriptyline 10 mg
Disp: #30 tabs
Sig: Jk 1 tab hs

Substitution Permitted   Dispense as written

DEA#   Print name

Oral Rinses

Jane Doe, DDS 1234 Main Ave. City, ST 12345   (111) 555-1234

Name _____   Date _____

Address _____   Age _____

℞

Chlorhexidine 0.12% [Peridex, Periogard]

Disp: 480 mls

Sig: Brush teeth and rinse with topful of solution bid, don't rinse mouth after use

Substitution Permitted   Dispense as written

DEA#   Print name

Tobacco Use Cessation

Nicotine replacement dosage forms—majority are available OTC

Jane Doe, DDS 1234 Main Ave. City, ST 12345   (111) 555-1234

Name _____   Date _____

Address _____   Age _____

℞

Zyban SR 150 mg

Disp: #60

Sig: Tk 1 tab for 3 days, then tk 1 tab bid thereafter

Duration: 6 weeks

Substitution Permitted   Dispense as written

DEA#   Print name

SAMPLE PRESCRIPTIONS FOR CHILDREN

Children's dosages of medication are most frequently expressed in mg/kg/day. This number must be changed to lbs and to amount of drug **per dose.**

ANALGESICS, CHILDREN

OTC:

- Acetaminophen 2.5-5 mg/lb q 4-6 h prn pain
- Ibuprofen 2.5 mg/lb q 4-6 h prn pain

℞

- Acetaminophen 120 mg and codeine 12.5 mg/5 ml elixir [has alcohol] or suspension 5 mg/lb q 4-6h prn pain

ANTIBIOTICS

- Penicillin VK, < 12 years old 15-25 mg/lb/day q 8h (5-8 mg/lb tid)
- IE proph
     Amoxicillin 50 mg/kg
     Clindamycin 20 mg/kg

SEDATION

- N_2O-oxygen sedation
- Benzodiazepine—depends on agent (e.g., diazepam 0.15 mg/kg)

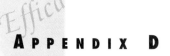

APPENDIX D

Medical Acronyms

Term	Meaning
5-FU	5-Fluorouracil
5-HT	serotonin (5-hydroxy-tryptamine)
AAC	antibiotic associated colitis
ACE	angiotensin-converting enzyme
ACEI	angiotensin-converting enzyme inhibitor
ACTH	adrenocorticotropic hormone
AD(H)D	attention deficit (hyperactivity) disorder
ADA	American Dental Association
ADHA	American Dental Hygiene Association
ADP	adenosine diphosphate
AHA	American Heart Association
AHF	antihemophilic factor
AIDS	acquired immunodeficiency syndrome
AII	angiotensin II
ALG	antilymphocyte globulin
ALL	acute lymphocytic leukemia
ALT	alanine aminotransferase (formerly called SGPT)
APAP	*N*-acetyl *para*-aminophenol
APTT	activated partial thromboplastin time
ARA	angiotensin receptor antagonist
ARB	angiotensin receptor blocker
ASA	aspirin
ASA I, II, III, IV	American Society of Anesthesiology

Term	Meaning
ASCVD	atherosclerotic cardiovascular disease
AST	aspartate aminotransferase (formerly called SGOT)
ATG	antithymocyte globulin
ATP	adenosine triphosphate
AV	atrioventricular
AZT	zidovudine, azidothymidine
BCG	Bacillus Calmette-Guérin vaccine
BCP	birth control pill
BE	bacterial endocarditis
BMS	bone marrow suppression
BMT	bone marrow transplant
BNDD	Bureau of Narcotic Dangerous Drugs Department
BP	blood pressure
BPH	benign prostatic hypertrophy
BT	bleeding time
BUN	blood urea nitrogen
CAT	computed axial tomography
CAD	coronary artery disease
CABG	coronary artery bypass graft
C & S	culture and sensitivity
CBC	complete blood count
CDC	Centers for Disease Control
c-GMP	cyclic guanosine monophosphate
CHF	congestive heart failure
CIS	carcinoma in-situ
CK	creatine phosphokinase
CLL	chronic lymphocytic leukemia

Term	Meaning
CML	chronic myelocytic leukemia
CNS	central nervous system
COMT	catecholamine-*O*-methyl transferase
COPD	chronic obstructive pulmonary disease
CRH	corticotropin-releasing hormone
CSF	corticotropin-stimulating factor
CVA	cerebral vascular accident
CVS	cardiovascular system
D/C	discontinue
DDAVP	1-deamino-8-*d*-arginine vasopressin, desmopressin
ddC	zalcitabine
ddI	didanosine
DEA	Drug Enforcement Administration
DIC	disseminated intravascular coagulation
DIP	distal interphalangeal joints
DM	diabetes mellitus, dextromethorphan
DMARD	disease-modifying antirheumatic drug
DNA	deoxyribonucleic acid
DTs	delirium tremens
EACA	epsilon aminocaproic acid
EBV	Epstein-Barr virus
ECG	electrocardiogram
ED$_{50}$	effective dose 50%
EEG	electroencephalogram
ENL	erythema nodosum leprosum
EPA	Environmental Protection Agency
EPS	extrapyramidal syndrome
ESRD	end-stage renal disease
EtOH	ethanol (alcohol)
FAD	flavin adenine dinucleotide
FDA	Food and Drug Administration
FMN	flavin mononucleotide
FTA	fluorescent treponema antibodies

Term	Meaning
G6PD	glucose-6-phosphate dehydrogenase [NADP+]
GABA	γ-aminobutyric acid
GBV	hepatitis G virus
GCF	gingival crevicular fluid
GI(T)	gastrointestinal (tract)
GU	genitourinary
GVHD	graph verses host disease
HAV	hepatitis A virus
HB$_c$Ag	hepatitis core antigen
HB$_c$Ab	hepatitis B core antigen
HBIG	hepatitis B immune globulin
HBP	high blood pressure
HB$_s$Ag	hepatitis B surface antigen
HBV	hepatitis B virus
HCTZ	hydrochlorothiazide
HCV	hepatitis C virus, parenteral non-A, non-B hepatitis]
HDL	high-density lipoprotein
HDV	hepatitis D virus, delta hepatitis virus
HER2	human epidermal growth factor receptor 2 protein
HEV	hepatitis E virus, epidemic non-A, non-B hepatitis
HGBV-C	hepatitis GB virus—C
HGV	hepatitis G virus
HIV	human immunodeficiency virus
HPA	hypothalamic—pituitary adrenal [axis]
HPV	human papilloma virus
HR	heart rate
HRT	hormone replacement therapy
HSV	herpes simplex virus
HSV-1	herpes simplex virus, type I
HSV-2	herpes simplex virus, type II
HTN	hypertension
HZV	herpes zoster virus
I & D	incision and drainage
IBD	inflammatory bowel disease
IBS	irritable bowel syndrome
ID	intradermal

Term	Meaning
IDDM	insulin dependent diabetes mellitus
IDU	idoxuridine
IE	infective endocarditis
IgE	immune globulin E
IgG	immune globulin G
IgM	immune globulin M
IM	intramuscular
IND	investigational new drug
INH	isoniazid
INR	International Normalized Ratio
ISI	International Sensitivity Index
IV	intravenous
IVF	in vitro fertilization
IUD	intrauterine device
LD$_{50}$	lethal dose 50%
LDH	lactic acid dehydrogenase
LDL	low-density lipoprotein
LH	leutinizing hormone
LFT	liver function test
LJP	localized juvenile periodontitis
LSD	lysergic acid diethylamide
MAC	*Mycobacterium avium* [intracellulare] complex
MAO	monoamine oxidase
MAOI	monoamine oxidase inhibitor
MCA	monoclonal antibody
MD	multiple dystrophy
MDM	minor determinate mixture
MDR	multidrug resistant
MHC	major histocompatibility complex
MI	myocardial infarction
MRI	magnetic resonance imaging
MS	multiple sclerosis, morphine sulfate
MTX	methotrexate
N$_2$O	nitrous oxide
NDA	new drug application
NHL	non-Hodgkin's lymphoma
NIDDM	non–insulin-dependent diabetes mellitus

Term	Meaning
NMS	neuromalignant syndrome
NNRTI	nonnucleoside reverse transcriptase inhibitor
NPH	neutral protein Hagedorn (insulin)
NPO	nil per os (nothing by mouth)
NREM	nonrapid eye movement
NS	normal saline
NSALAs	nonsteroidal antiinflammatory *agents*
NSAIDs	nonsteroidal antiinflammatory *drugs* [IN-seds]
NTG	nitroglycerin
NTX	naltrexone
N&V	nausea and vomiting
O$_2$	oxygen
OA	osteoarthritis
OB	obstetrics
OCs	oral contraceptives
OCD	obsessive-compulsive disorder
OD	overdose
O&E	observation and examination
OGTT	oral glucose tolerance test
OPV	oral poliovirus vaccine
OSHA	Occupational Safety Health Administration
OTC	over-the-counter
PABA	*para*-amino benzoic acid
2-PAM	pralidoxime
PANS	parasympathetic autonomic nervous system
para1	unipara (1 child)
PAS	*para*-aminosalicylic acid
PAT	paroxysmal atrial tachycardia
PBP	penicillin binding proteins
PCN	penicillin
PCP	*Pneumocystis carinii*, phencyclidine
PCR	polymerase chain reaction
PD	Parkinson's disease
P/D	packs per day
PDE5	phosphodiesterase type 5
PDT	photodynamic therapy

Term	Meaning
PG	pregnant
PG(s)	prostaglandins
pH	function of amount of hydrogen ion (log $1/[H^+]$)
PID	pelvic inflammatory disease
PMC	pseudomembranous colitis
PMS	premenstrual syndrome
PO	per os (by mouth)
PPD	purified protein derivative
PPL	penicilloyl polylysine
PT	prothrombin time
PTCA	percutaneous transluminal coronary angioplasty
PTH	parathyroid hormone
PTT	partial thromboplastin time
PTU	propylthiouracil
PUD	peptic ulcer disease
PVD	peripheral vascular disease
PVT	paroxysmal ventricular tachycardia
QRS	EKG effects of cardiac muscle depolarization
RA	rheumatoid arthritis
RAS	recurrent aphthous stomatitis
RBC	red blood cell
RHD	rheumatic heart disease
RNA	ribonucleic acid
R/O	rule out
RPR	rapid plasma reagin
RSV	respiratory syncytial virus
SA	sinoatrial [node]
SANS	sympathetic autonomic nervous system
SAR	structure-activity relationship
SC	subcutaneous
SGOT	serum glutamic-oxaloacetate transferase (AST)
SGPT	serum glutamic-pyruvate transferase (ALT)

Term	Meaning
SL	sublingual
SLE	systemic lupus erythematosus
SMP-TMX	sulfamethoxazole-trimethoprim
SOB	shortness of breath
SQ	subcutaneous
SSRI	serotonin specific reuptake inhibitor
STD	sexually transmitted disease
STS	serologic test syphilis
SVT	supraventricular tachycardia
T_3	triiodothyronine
T_4	levothyroxine
TB	tuberculosis
TBG	thyroid binding globulin
TCA	tricyclic antidepressants
TCN	tetracycline
THC	tetrahydrocannabinol
TI	therapeutic index
TIA	transient ischemic attacks
TMD	temporomandibular disease
TMJ	temporomandibular joint
TNF	tumor necrosis factor
TNM	tumor node metastasis
TPA	tissue plasminogen activator
TPP	thiamine pyrophosphate
TPR	total peripheral resistance
TRH	thyroid-releasing hormone
TSH	thyroid-stimulating hormone
TT	thrombin time
Tx	treatment
TXA	thromboxane(s)
VLDL	very-low-density lipoproteins
VZV	varicella-zoster virus
WBC	white blood cells

Medical Terminology

This appendix does not attempt to provide a course in medical terminology. To cover that subject completely would require an entire book. But there are many new medical vocabulary words in pharmacology needed to discuss drugs and their effects. In fact, many that sound strange now will seem familiar later. Without this vocabulary, you will find it difficult to comprehend drug reference sources. Because some of the words will be unfamiliar, you have an opportunity to learn these and other new terms.

When you see a medical terminology word that you do not know, approach the word like a puzzle and attempt to identify any pieces that you know. Consider whether you have seen a piece before and what it might mean. Guess what those few letters might mean. Then "look up" the drug in a database, medical dictionary, or even the glossary in the appendix. Write the word on a small card (⅓ of 3×5 card), and write the definition on the other side. After you have written the definition on the card, consider the word parts and identify the little pieces that make up the word. These pieces may be beginning pieces (prefixes), middle pieces (word roots [=core]) or end pieces (suffixes). There are also pieces that mean *no* or *not* or that reverse the word's meaning. These little pieces come from Greek and/or Latin word parts. Now let's look at a couple of words.

Hypertension: (Hyper-) have you heard someone say "that person is 'hyper-'?" It means a lot of, or more of, or too much of. So we know that the piece of the word *hyper-* means excessive. *Tension* refers to tension or blood pressure. So *hypertension* means excessive blood pressure. What would be the definition of *hypotension?*

Dysmenorrhea: Dys- means bad, difficult, or abnormal; for example, teenagers use the phrase to "dys you." *Men-* is a root word meaning monthly and is associated with menstruation. The suffix *-rhea* refers to flowing. From these parts the definition of this word is the painful flowing menstruation.

The prefix *a-* refers to less or lack of. Can you define amenorrhea?

If the prefix for the nose is *rhin-* (as in *rhinoceros*—**nose** horns, wild animal, charge) then what does *rhinorrhea* mean?

If the suffix *-itis* means inflammation, then what does *rhinitis* mean?

Thyroidectomy: Thyroid refers to the thyroid gland, whereas *-ectomy* means surgical removal. So the word means surgically removing the thyroid gland. How about *tonsilectomy?*

Box 1 lists a few prefixes. Box 2 lists a few core words. Box 3 lists a few suffixes. Add new word parts as you learn them.

When a new drug group is named, a generic name and a trade name are given. The generic name is longer, and the trade name is short and easier to remember. *Sometimes*, when more members of a drug group are discovered and marketed, the subsequent drugs in the group are given the same suffix. A few drug suffixes—drug names ending in the same letters that belong to the same group are listed in Box 4.

Box 1 A Few Prefixes

a- without, absent
brady- slow
hemi- one-half
hyper- above, excessive
intra- within
lith- stone, calculus
pan- all
qua- four; quarter (¼ of a dollar), *qid* means 4 times a day
sub- under (submarine?)
tachy- fast
tri- tricycle (3-wheeled), tid (3 times a day)

Box 2 A Few Root Words

bronch- bronchus
cardi- heart
cephal- head
chol- gall, bile
col- colon
cyan- blue
derm- skin
epitheli- epithelium (outside of skin)
gast- stomach
hem- blood
hepat- liver
leuk- white
lingu- tongue
lip- fat
my- for muscle
neph- kidney
neur- nerve
path- disease
pneum- lungs, air
poster- back, behind
proct- rectum
prostat- prostate
stenosis- narrowing
stomat- mouth
thrombo- blood clot
vertebr- spine

Box 3 A Few Suffixes

-algia pain
-dynia pain
-ectomy surgical removal
-itis inflammation
-lysis destruction, loosening
-malacia softening
-megaly enlargement
-ologist specialist
-oma tumor
-otomy incision into
-penia fewer (abnormal)
-plasty surgical repair
-ptosis droopy or falling down
-rrhea flow
-scopy visual examination ("scope it out")
-thorax chest

Box 4 Suffixes For Drugs

Suffix	Drug group
-azolam	benzodiazepines
-clovir	antiviral agent
-cycline	antibiotic
-dipine	calcium channel blockers
-ecoxib	COX II–specific antiinflammatory
-floxacin	antiinfective, quinolones
-glinide	hypoglycemic, oral
-glitazone	thiazolidinediones (antidiabetic)
-ifene	antiestrogen
-lukast	leukotriene inhibitor
-mycin	antibiotic
-olol	β-blockers
-prazole	proton pump inhibitor
-pril	ACE inhibitors
-sartan	angiotensin II receptor antagonist
-stigmine	cholinergic agent
-triptan	serotonin agonist, migraine
-tron	serotonin antagonist
-[con]azole	antifungal, azoles
-[va]statin	HMG-Co reductase inhibitors

Internet Searches

World Wide Web (WWW) is a term applied to a large number of computers interconnected around the world. If we view the WWW using an astronomy analogy, the Web would be represented by the universe, large groups of computers would be represented as the solar system (e.g., the University of Missouri), and each planet would represent each academic unit (e.g., School of Dentistry). With this set up, a message from a faculty member's computer could be sent via the WWW to Alpha Centauri, the star closest to earth.

HOW CAN YOU LEARN ABOUT THE WEB?

You can learn about the Web the same way you learn to ride a bicycle. Do it! Don't be afraid to push buttons or click or double click anything—you will never know where you might end up, but it can be an adventure! Additional search strategies are available with each search engine and from the Web.

The WWW can be used to obtain information about almost everything, but drugs and diseases and their treatment is the target here. Caution: information on the Web cannot be taken as gospel: it must be judged. There is a plethora of incorrect information so please don't rely on one source.

1. The first method is to go to any browser and type in the words of a subject in which you are interested. The more specific you can get, the narrower the search. But, don't make the search so narrow that nothing appears. You can change the search at any time. The browsers are also called *search engines.* Common search engines are listed on p 564.

2. Another way to obtain information about drugs is to go to a single browser and begin there. Each browser has a list of topics available on that browser, sort of like a table of contents. You might look under diseases, drugs, medicine, or therapy. When you get to this section, search only that section, as you did above. If you find a site that you might want to return to, bookmark it and its location will remain in your computer for future use. These bookmarks can also be arranged for easy retrieval.

3. Another method to find information is to look at groups of Web sites. Other sections that can be useful include government sites (e.g., nlm.gov, cdc.gov); other media such as newspapers (e.g., kcstar.com); drug and dental company sites (company name.com); drug-specific sites (e.g., viagra.com); professional associations (e.g., ADA.org); organizations based on a disease (e.g., disease name.org); and university sites (e.g., umkc.edu). Travel sites and sports sites are numerous, but these sites are do it yourself. URLs are listed in professional journals, on TV (e.g., PBS.org), and in magazines on the Web (called *infozines*).

4. To identify good URLs on specific topics use any of the above directions. The URLs found often have hot links to other web

sites, and so forth. One drug site I found contained over 1000 hot links to other sites. It is very easy to get a bunch of URLs, and after using them you will determine which are useful to you. Web sites vary greatly, from just a company's address to a full complete learning resource on a topic (some of the drug and financial sites). Some books even give "grades" or stars to URL sites (just like movie ratings). Individuals may also have their own website. At some colleges, each student can make his or her own web page. Individual web pages can be for family (with pictures of the kids), professional (dental office, communication with peers about patients—I saw this patient and you won't believe. . . . What should I do?), or provide information (individual web pages often have information not found elsewhere). Individuals prepare some informative, awesome web sites. You can too!

5. The Web is the perfect place to identify scientific literature. Government sites provide availability of Medline (as well as lots of others). You can search scientific topics, such as herpes, and look at specific information about the topic (treatment). Medline is much more reliable than the rest of the Web.

6. Other stuff to explore. Bulletin Boards list information for lots of people to read (or provide stuff for the others to read). A few caveats, if you sign up for a bulletin board make sure you remember how to unsubscribe because the volume of mail can be overwhelming. Chat rooms involve people chatting (typing on a keyboard back and forth) about anything. Some rooms are topic related and some are free-for-all. (It is not a good idea to plan to meet someone that you met on the Web. Many chat rooms are sexual in nature.)

URL sites are in Transition—they stop, change, move, and die. These sites are *not* picked as the best sites. They are just a few of the many sites available, and you will identify your favorite sites.

Search Engines

http://altavista.cigital.com/
hppt://www.lycos.com
http://wc3.webcrawler.com
hppt://www.fastsearch.com
http://www.infoseek.com
http://www.yahoo.com
http://www.hotbot.com
http://www.dogpile.com

All Sites Except as Otherwise Noted: http://www.

Government sites

cdc.gov
whitehouse.gov
nlm.nih.gov (for Medline searches)
healthfinder.gov
http://pharminfo.com
niddk.nih.gov

Drug related

helix.com
medce.com
rxmed.com
rxlist.com
medicinenet.com
medscape.com
pharminfo.com

Disease related

oncolink.upenn.edu
Oncoweb.com
achoo.com
healthatoz.com
cancer.org
healthcg.com
mentalwellness.com
childbirth.org
lungusa.org
psych.org

Disease related—cont'd

aan.com
headlice.org
psycom.net/depression.central.html
mentalhealth.com
allergy.mcg.edu
healthguide.com
immunet.org
pharmacy.org
drugstore.com

Dental hygiene

cabrillo.cc.ca.us
Pennwell.com/
cdha.org
dmha.org
dentalsite.com
ADHA.org

Educational institutions

umkc.edu
iowa.edu
ucla.edu

Professional organizations

apa.org
ada.org
amhrt.org
ama.org

Drug manufacturers

merck/com/home.htm
abbott.com
sb.com
dentalcare.com

Publishers

mosby.com
lexicomp.com
mghmedical.com

TV/radio

kmbc.com
kcmo.com
nbc.com
pbs.com

Newspapers/magazines

nytimes.com
time.com

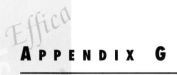

APPENDIX G

What If. . . .

This **"What if" Appendix** addresses a number of patient-related questions that are among the most common you will encounter in daily practice. The "decision trees" help guide you through the steps involved in assessing clinical situations quickly and making related treatment decisions.

Topics covered in **"What if?"** include drugs safe to use in pregnancy, allergy management, infective endocarditis prophylaxis, and a summary of the relationship of dental treatment, warfarin, and the International Normalized Ratio.

Allergies discussed include codeine, aspirin, penicillin, sulfites, and latex.

What if. . . . the patient is pregnant?

Drug Use in Pregnancy.* KC Quickie† Format.

Drug Group	Drug Name	OK to Use
Local anesthetics	Lidocaine with epinephrine	Yes
Analgesics	Aspirin	No
	Acetaminophen	Yes
	NSAIAs	No
	Opioids	Yes
Antiinfective agents/Antibiotics	Penicillin	Yes
	Erythromycin	Yes‡
	Tetractcycline	No
	Doxycycline	No
	Clindamycin	Yes
	Metronidazole	No

*For more details see Chapter 24, p. 492.
†Copyright 2000.
‡Avoid erythromycin estolate in pregnancy.

What if. . . . the patient is allergic to aspirin?

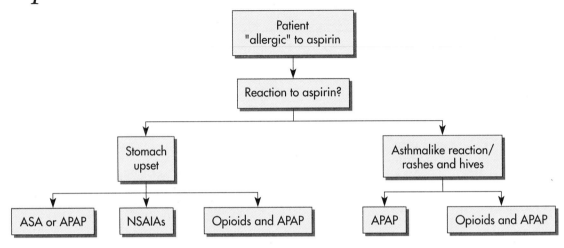

What if. . . . the patient is allergic to penicillin?

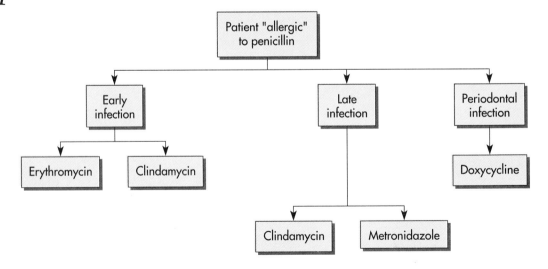

What if. . . . the patient is allergic to sulfites?

Lack of cross-hypersensitivity among the following: "sulfa" drugs, sulfites, sulfar, sulfate, or sulfide. "Sulfa drugs" are used to treat urinary tract infections, and their allergic reaction is usually rash. Dental patients allergic to "sulfa" drugs may safely be given local anesthetics or a vasoconstrictor that contains sulfites.

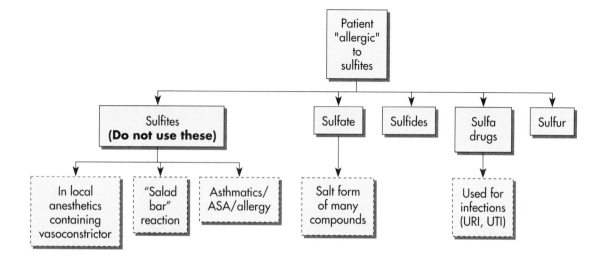

What if. . . . the patient is allergic to codeine?

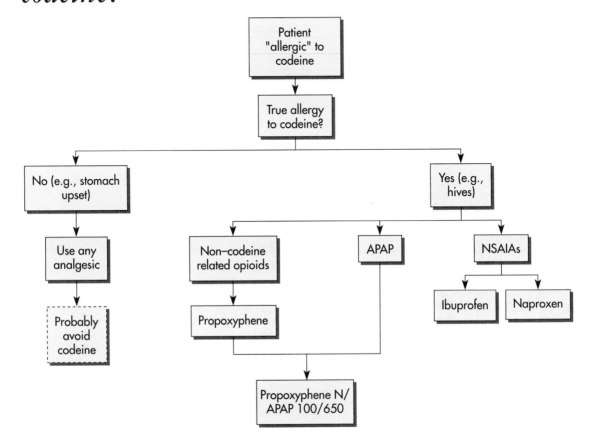

What if. . . . the patient is allergic to latex?

The increased use of latex-containing products has exposed more people with increasing frequency to latex allergens. Latex comes from the rubber tree and contains natural latex. Patients who are frequently exposed to latex-containing products (e.g., patients with spina bifida) and health care workers who use latex products (e.g., dental professionals) have a greater likelihood of developing allergies.

The extent of the reactions to latex range

from contact dermatitis to severe anaphylactic reaction with death within a few minutes. If a dental practitioner uses any latex materials in his or her office, then parenteral epinephrine should be readily available.

There is also a cross-hypersensitivity between the foods listed below and latex allergy. If a patient is allergic to the listed fruits then the dental health care worker should carefully question the patient regarding any reactions to latex-containing products (e.g., balloons, condoms). The patient should also be informed about cross-hypersensitivity that may occur between these fruits and latex. When powdered gloves are used, the latex can be absorbed into the powder and circulated around the room. This airborne latex can float around rooms and can even be stirred up with cleaning. Airborne latex can produce respiratory reactions such as asthma and anaphylaxis.

If a patient has an allergy to latex he or she should be given the first appointment so that the latex particles have not contaminated the operatory air. The ventilation should be checked and measured for turnovers to make sure that the particles are removed overnight. Be aware of the occupants of the building because use of latex in another office could inject latex particles into the central heating or cooling.

Manufactured latex products may contain a small amount of natural latex proteins, or a very large amount, or somewhere in between. Asking for more information on the latex gloves used in the dental office may reduce the exposure to allergenic proteins.

When treating a latex-allergic patient, non-latex equipment should be substituted for any products that contains latex. Newer catalogues contain a wide range of dental-related products (e.g., nonlatex bite blocks, dams, and adhesives for bandages). Books that contain additional information about latex allergy may contain infection control topics.

FOODS WITH POTENTIAL FOR CROSS-HYPERSENSITIVITY WITH LATEX HYPERSENSITIVITY

apples	papayas
avocados	peaches
bananas	pears
carrots	pineapples
celery	potatoes
cherries	rye
chestnuts	strawberries
hazelnuts	tomatoes
kiwis	wheat
melons	

DENTAL OBJECTS COMPOSED OF LATEX

All commonly used brands contain latex

Gloves
Rubber dam
Local anesthetic cartridges (stopper)
Syringes (black rubber inside)
Bite block

Some many contain latex

Strings that hold mask on
Strings that hold gown on
Glasses bridges

*What if . . . the cardiac patient needs antibiotics?**

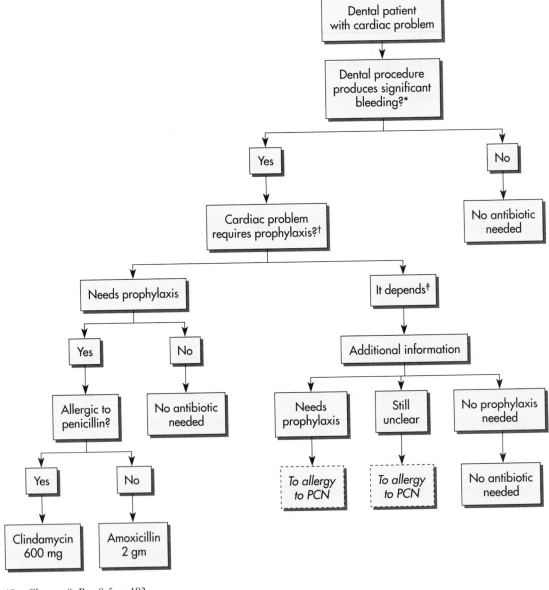

*See Chapter 8, Box 8-5, p. 192.
†See Chapter 8, Box 8-6, p. 192.
‡Includes rheumatic heart disease, mitral valve prolapse, and unspecified murmur.

What if . . . the patient with joint prosthesis needs antibiotics?

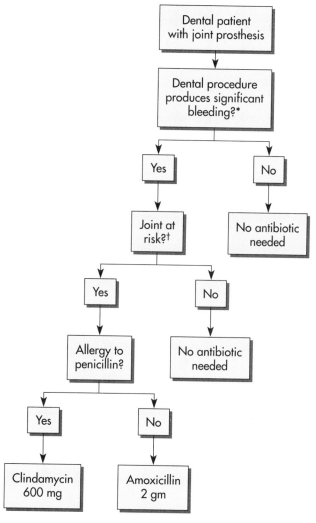

*See Chapter 8, Box 8-5, p. 192.
†See Chapter 8, Box 8-7, p. 194.

What if . . . the patient is taking warfarin (Coumadin)?

Summary* Dental Procedures and INR† Acceptable (Safe) KC Quickie* Format

DENTAL PROCEDURE	OK TO TREAT IF INR <
Periodontal probing	~4
Restorative, simple scaling/root planning endodontics	3.5
Extraction, simple	2.5-3.5‡
Extraction, multiple	2-3.5
Periodontal surgery	2.5

*See Chapter 15, Table 15-15, p. 362.
†Copyright 2000.

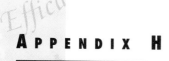
Oral Manifestations—Xerostomia and Taste Changes*

Agents That Produce Xerostomia (Dry Mouth)

DRUG GROUP	EXAMPLES
Adrenergic agents (decongestants, anoretics)†	Albuterol (Proventil, Ventolin) Dextroamphetamine (Dexedrine) Dopamine (Intropin) Ephedrine Epinephrine (Adrenalin) Isoproterenol (Isuprel) Metaproterenol (Alupent) Methylphenidate (Ritalin) "Phen-fen" = phentermine + fenfluramine† Phentermine (Adipex-P, Fastin, Ionamin, Zantryl) Phenylephrine (Neo-Synephrine) Phenylpropanolamine (PPA, Dexatrim [in Entex-LA]) Pseudoephedrine (Sudafed)
Serotonin amplifiers†	Dexfenfluramine (Redux)† Fenfluramine (Pondimin)†
Antiarrhythmics	Disopyramide Procainamide Quinidine
Anticholinergics‡	Anisotropine (Valpin) Atropine Belladonna Belladonna alkaloids with phenobarbital (Donnatal) Buclizine (Bucladin-S) Clidinium (in Librax, in Clindex) Dicyclomine (Bentyl) Flavoxate (Urispas) Glycopyrrolate (Robinul [Forte]) Homatropine (Isopto-Homatropine) Ipratropium (IH) (Atrovent) L-Hyoscyamine (Anaspaz, Levsin) Mepenzolate (Cantil) Methantheline (Banthine) Methscopolamine (Pamine) Oxybutynin (Ditropan) Propantheline (Pro-Banthine) Scopolamine (hyoscine)

DRUG GROUP	EXAMPLES
Antiparkinsonian	Amantadine (Symmetrel) Benztropine (Cogentin) Biperiden (Akineton) Ethopropazine (Parsidol) Levodopa + carbidopa (Sinemet) Pergolide (Permax) Procyclidine (Kemadrin) Selegiline (Eldepryl) [AKA deprenil and deprenyl] Trihexyphenidyl (Artane)
Anticonvulsants	Carbamazepine (Tegretol) Gabapentin (Neurontin)
Antidepressants, tricyclic	Amitriptyline (Elavil) Amoxapine (Asendin) Clomipramine (Anafranil) Desipramine (Norpramin, Pertofrane) Doxepin (Sinequan, Adapin) Imipramine (Tofranil) Nortriptyline (Aventyl) Protriptyline (Vivactil) Trimipramine (Surmontil)
Antidepressants, other	Bupropion (Wellbutrin, Zyban) Maprotiline (Ludiomil) Mirtazapine (Remeron) Nefazodone (Serzone)‖ Sibutramine (Meridia) Trazodone (Desyrel) Venlafaxine (Effexor)‖
Antidepressants, SSRI	Fluoxetine (Prozac) Fluvoxamine (Luvox)] Paroxetine (Paxil) Sertraline (Zoloft)
Antidepressants, MAO inhibitor	Isocarboxazid (Marplan) Phenelzine (Nardil) Tranylcypromine (Parnate)

Drug Group	Examples
Antihistamines	Acrivastine (in Semprex-D) Azatadine (Optimine) (ophthalmic) Brompheniramine (Dimetane) Carbinoxamine (Clistin) Chlorpheniramine (Chlor-Trimeton) Clemastine (Tavist) Cyclizine Cyproheptadine (Periactin) Dexchlorpheniramine (Polaramine) Dimenhydrinate (Dramamine) Diphenhydramine (Benadryl) Hydroxyzine (Atarax, Vistaril) Levocabastine (Livostin) (ophthalmic) Meclizine (Antivert) Methdilazine Olopatadine (Patanol) (ophthalmic) Phenindamine Promethazine (Phenergan) Tripelennamine (PBZ) Triprolidine (Actidil)
Antihistamines, nonsedating	Astemizole (Hismanal) Cetirizine (Zyrtec) Fexofenadine (Allegra) Loratadine (Claritin)

Antihypertensives	Calcium channel blockers
	  Bepridil (Vascor)
	α_1-antagonist
	  Prazosin (Minipress)
	  Doxazocin (Cardura)
	  Terazosin (Hytrin)
	α_2-agonist
	  Clonidine (Catapres)§
	  Guanabenz (Wytensin)
	  Guanfacine (Tenex)
	  Methyldopa (Aldomet)
	Peripheral α antagonists
	  Guanethidine (Ismelin)
	  Guanadrel (Hylorel)
	  Reserpine

Antipsychotics,‡ phenothiazines	Acetophenazine (Tindal) Chlorpromazine (Thorazine) Clozapine (Clozaril) Droperidol (Inapsine) Fluphenazine (Prolixin) Haloperidol (Haldol) Loxapine (Loxitane) Mesoridazine (Serentil) Methdilazine (Tacaryl) Molindone (Moban) Pimozide (Orap) Piperacetazine (Quide) Prochlorperazine (Compazine) Promazine (Sparine)

Drug Group	Examples
	Promethazine (Phenergan) Quetiapine (Seroquel) Risperidone (Risperdal)‖ Thiethylperazine Thioridazine (Mellaril) Thioxanthenes Trifluoperazine (Stelazine) Triflupromazine (Vesprin) Trimeprazine (Temaril)

Benzodiazepines/ sedative-hypnotics	*Benzodiazepines*
	  Alprazolam (Xanax)
	  Chlordiazepoxide (Librium)
	  Clonazepam (Klonopin)
	  Clorazepate (Tranxene)
	  Diazepam (Valium)
	  Estazolam (ProSom)
	  Flunitrazepam
	  Flurazepam (Dalmane)
	  Halazepam (Paxipam)
	  Lorazepam (Ativan)
	  Midazolam (Versed)
	  Oxazepam (Serax)
	  Prazepam (Centrax)
	  Quazepam (Doral)
	  Temazepam (Restoril)
	  Triazolam (Halcion)
	Others
	  Phenobarbital
	  Zolpidem (Ambien)

Cardiac glycoside	Digoxin

Diuretics	*Thiazides*
	  Hydrochlorothiazide (HCTZ)
	Loop
	  Bumetanide (Bumex)
	  Furosemide (Lasix)
	Combinations
	  Dyazide
	  Maxzide

Antiemetics	Metoclopramide (Reglan) Cisapride (Propulsid) Dronabinol (Marinol) Nabilone (Cesamet) Ondansetron (Zofran) Oxybutynin (Ditropan)
Miscellaneous	Caffeine Cromolyn (Intal), Ergotamine (Ergostat, in Cafergot) Nicotine (smoking cessation) *Vitamin A analogues* Isotrenition (Accutane)

Drug Group	Examples
Muscle relaxants	Carisoprodol (Soma), Chlorzoxazone (Parafon Forte) Cyclobenzaprine (Flexeril)† Methocarbamol (Robaxin) Orphenadrine (Norflex)
Opioids	Codeine Meperidine Morphine Oxycodone Pentazocine Propoxyphene Tramadol

*See Box 14-1, p. 313, and Box 14-2, p. 315 for other oral effects of drugs.
†Taken off market 1998.
‡More likely than others to produce xerostomia.
‖Less likely to cause xerostomia.
§Most likely to produce xerostomia.

Agents That Alter Taste

Drug	Taste Effects
ACE inhibitors	
Aceon	
Acetazolamide	M
Adenosine	M
Albuterol	C
Allopurinol	N
Al(OH)$_3$	Chalky
Amiodarone	U
Amoxapine	U, A
Ampicillin	N
Antineoplastics	N
Antithrombin III	F
Aspirin	N
Auranofin	M
Aurothioglucose	M
Aztreonam	A
Benazepril	C

Drug	Taste Effects
Benzocaine	N
Bepridil	A
Bitolterol	A
Budesonide	B, L
Calcifediol	M
Calcitriol	M
Carboprost tromethamine	A
Ceftriaxone	A
Chlorhexidine	C, L
Cidofovir	A
Clarithromycin	A
Clofazimine	A
Clofibrate	N
Clomipramine	U
Cyclophosphamide	N
Gold salts	N
Griseofulvin	N
Interferon alfa-2a	M, C
Interferon alfa-n3	M, C
Iodinated glycerol	M
Iron dextran complex	M
Potassium iodide	M
Labetalol	A
Levamisole	P
Lithium	A
Lomefloxacin	A
Losartan	A
Lovastatin	A
Mechlorethamine	M
Mesna	B
Metaproterenol	B
Methazolamide	M
Methimazole	A
Methylergonovine	F
Metronidazole	M, C
Moexipril (ACE inhibitor)	A
Moricizine	B

Taste changes: *A*, abnormal; *B*, bad; *C*, change; *D*, disturbance; *F*, foul; *L*, loss; *M*, metallic; *N*, not specified; *P*, perversion; *T*, bitter; *U*, unpleasant.

Drug	Taste Effects
Nedocromil	U
Norfloxacin	B
Nortriptyline	U
Ofloxacin	A
Omeprazole	A
Pamidronate	L
Penicillamine	N
Pentamidine	B, M
Perindopril	D
Perindopril erbumine	A
Phytonadione	C
Pirbuterol (Maxair)	C
Pravastatin	A
Praziquante	B
Propafenone	L
Protirelin	B
Protriptyline	U
PTU	L
Quinapril	C
Quinid	B

Drug	Taste Effects
Quinidine	B
Quinine	B
Ramipril	A
Ranitidine/ bismuth	D
Rifabutin	P
Ritonavir	A
Simvastatin	U
Sodium phenylbutyrate	A
Succimer	B
Terbinafine	A
Terbutaline	B
Tetracycline	N
Trazodone	B
Triazolam	A
Tricyclic antidepressants	N
Ursodiol	U
Ursodiol	M
Valsartan	A
Vinblastine	M
Vinorelbine	M

APPENDIX I

Altered Pharmacokinetics

Dental Drug Use in Patients with Altered Renal Function, ESRD* or Hepatic Dysfunction

Drug	$T_{1/2}$ (hr) Normal/ESRD (= means both sides equal)	(%) Unchanged; Metabolism and Excretion	Protein Binding (%)	Normal (N) Dose (mg); Dosing Interval	Dose (mg) Renal Failure: CrCl > 50 (ml/min)	CrCl 10-50 (ml/min)	CrCl < 10 (ml/min)	Normal Dose in Hepatic Dysfunction
Analgesics								
Acetaminophen	2/3	Hepatic conjugation	20-30	650 q4h	q4h	q6h	q8h	Don't use
Aspirin	2-3/=	Hepatic metabolism (renal)	80-90	650 q4h	q4h	q4-6	Don't use	Don't use
NSAIDs								
Ibuprofen	2-3/=	1%; hepatic metabolism	99	800 q8h	N†	N	N	?, AR‡ = hepatic
Naproxen	10-18/=	1%, hepatic metabolism	99	500 q12h	N	N	N	Lower, AR = hepatic
Opioids								
Morphine	2-3/=	20%; hepatic metabolism	20-30	20-25 q4h	N	¾ N	½ N	Lower
Codeine	2.5-3.5/?	10%; hepatic metabolism	7	30-60 mg q6h	N	¾ N	½ N	Lower
Meperidine	2-7/7-32	Hepatic metabolism to active	70	50-100 q3-4h	N	¾ N, or N q6h	½ N, or N q8h	Lower
Propoxyphene	9-15/12-20	<10%; 50% first-pass, hepatic metabolism	78	65-100 q6h	N	Don't use	Don't use	Lower
Antibiotics								
Penicillin VK	0.5-1/4.1	60-90%; rest hepatic metabolism	50-80	250 q6h	N	N	N	Yes
Amoxicillin	1-2/5-20	50-70%; rest hepatic metabolism	15-25	250-500 q8h	q8h	q8-12h	q12-24h	Yes
Augmentin	1-2/5-20	50%; 25% in feces	15-25	250-500 q8h	q8h	q8-12h	q12-24h	Yes
Dicloxacillin	0.5-0.7/1-2	35-70 renal	95	250-500 q6h	N	N	N	
Erythromycin	2/6	15%; hepatic metabolism	70	250-500 q6h	N	N	½ N	Don't use; AR-jaundice
Clarithromycin	3-7/?	15%-25%, renal	70	500-1000 q12h	N	¾ N	½ N	Don't use
Azithromycin	11-14; 68	Hepatic, bile	7-50	500 qd × 1d; 250 qd × 4d	N	?	?	Don't use
Cephalexin [1st]‖	1-2/3	Most excreted unchanged	6-15	250-500 q6h	N	q12h	q24h	Yes
Cefaclor [2nd]	1/3	70%	25	250-500 q8h	N	¾ N	½ N	AR—jaundice
Cefixime [3rd]	3-6/12	50%-70%	50	200 q12h	N	¾ N	½ N	AR—jaundice
Tetracycline	6-15/57-108	48%-60%; 30% feces (via bile)	55-90	250-500 q6h	q8-12h	q12-24h	q24h	Avoid
Doxycycline	15-20/18-25	35%-45%; 20% hepatic metabolism, 30% intestinal wall, 20% unchanged in urine, 30% in feces	80-90	100 q24h	N	N	N	Lower
Minocycline	11-16/12-26	10%; 75% hepatic metabolism, 25% in feces	70	100 q12h	N	N	N	Lower
Ciprofloxacin	3-6/6-9	50%-70% renal	20-40	500-750 q12h	N	¾ N	½ N	
Clindamycin	2-4/3-5	10%; rest hepatic metabolism	60-95	150-300 q6h	N	N	N	Lower
Metronidazole	8/7-21	20%; hepatic oxidation and glucuronide conjugation; renal: 80% metabolite, 20% unchanged	20	7.5/kg q6-8h	q8h	q8-12h	q12-24h	Lower
Antifungal/Antiviral								
Miconazole								
Ketoconazole	3-8; 1.5-3.3/3.3	13%; hepatic metabolism	99	200 q24h	N	N	N	Decrease
Itraconazole	21/25	35%	99	100-200 q12h	N	N	½ N	Decrease?
Acyclovir	1.5-3.3	80% (renal), hepatic metabolism		q6h	q6h	q8h	q12h	Yes
Local Anesthetic								
Lidocaine	1-2; 2-2.2/1.3-3	10%; hepatic metabolism	60-66	50 mg over 2 min (antiarrhythmic dose)	N	N	N	Smaller local anesthetic doses OK
Benzodiazepines								
Alprazolam	12-15; 9.5-19/=	Hepatic metabolism, inactive	70-80	0.25-5 q8h	N	N	N	Lower
Chlordiazepoxide	5-30/=	Hepatic metabolism, active	94-97	15-60 q24h	N	N	½ N	Don't use
Lorazepam	5-10/32-70	Hepatic glucuronide	87	1-2 q8-12h	N	N	N	Lower
Diazepam	50-100; 20-90/=	Hepatic metabolism, active metabolite	94-98	1.5 q24h	N	N	N	Lower
Midazolam	1.2-12.3/=	Hepatic metabolism	93-96		N	N	½ N	Lower?
Triazolam	2-4/=	Hepatic glucuronide; in feces	85-95	0.25-0.5 qhs	N	N	N	Yes

Modified from Aronoff GR et al: *Drug prescribing in renal failure*, 4 ed, Philadelphia, 1999, American College of Physicians.

*ESRD = End stage renal disease.

†*N*, Use normal dose; fraction and *N*, use that fraction of the normal dose; q4h, every 4 hours; q6h, every 6 hours. With drugs that may have more effect with renal dysfunction there are two ways to lower the amount of drug given: (1) lower the dose of the drug given, (2) increase the interval between doses; some drugs are changed by each mechanism, some drugs can be dosed by either mechanism.

‡*AR*, Adverse reaction.

‖Cephalosporin generation.

Dosing Changes in Renal and Hepatic Disease

NO CHANGE	DOSE CHANGE IN RENAL DISEASE	CONTRAINDICATED IN RENAL DISEASE	DOSE CHANGE NEEDED IN HEPATIC DISEASE
Diazepam	Acyclovir	Aspirin—with severe	Codeine
Doxycycline	Amoxicillin	Propoxyphene—if severe	Doxycycline
Erythromycin	Cephalosporins	Tetracycline	Diazepam
Ibuprofen	Clarithromycin		Clindamycin
Ketoconazole	Codeine		Erythromycin
Lorazepam	Meperidine		Metronidazole
Minocycline	Metronidazole		Erythromycin
Naproxen	Morphine		Propoxyphene
Oxazepam	Penicillin VK		Naproxen
Temazepam			Morphine
Triazolam			Minocycline
			Metronidazole
			Meperidine
			Lorazepam

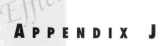

APPENDIX J

Natural/Herbal Products

The use of natural products began many years ago. The witch doctor gathered and prepared parts of plants and used the resulting products to treat illnesses. Even then, proper incantations and confidence-instilling activities were administered along with the herbs. As modern society developed, the use of natural produces in the United States declined. Prescription drugs were "king"—they were strong, they were science in action!

The next technology involved advances in scientific discoveries and the abrupt increase in knowledge at the molecular level. The medical health system costs rose, and the time providers spent with their patients decreased. The provider-patient rapport suffered, and the patients became skeptical, and even distrustful, of the health care workers and system. They turned elsewhere for alleviation of their medical conditions. Products with many claims for "cures" became more popular. People listened and acted on suggestions from their neighbors. People wanted something to make them healthy without any effort. They would ask, "What pill can be taken to make up for no exercise?" Or, how do you lose 20 lb in 2 weeks? Cut off your head is the only answer that makes sense. No one asked if these easy answers would cause problems.

The recent trend in the use of natural or herbal substances has been an exponential rise in the use of these products and the number of people using them. In the minds of the public, natural substances have been given a special place—they work and they won't hurt you. Natural is imagined as:

a beautiful woman with long flowing blonde hair wearing a trailing diaphanous gown, skipping across a meadow strewn with wild flowers in bloom (of course, there is a breeze).

With this view in mind, one can see why some believe that all herbs have a useful place in curing human illnesses.

But, take a look at nature on the African savanna. Birth, growth, and death follow in suit and are inevitable. Creatures eat grass and are then eaten by other creatures who are in turn eaten by others at the top of the food chain. On the savanna, many animals produce a great abundance of dung. The dung beetles eat dung—a very useful function. An antelope is killed and eaten by a lion, and it requires more thorough cleaning. Vultures take the bigger pieces that are left, and then maggots continue the job. Finally, fungi and bacteria invade the carcass to finish it off. Nature is a circle. The natural products from this savanna would include dung pills and maggot capsules.

To answer any questions about a substance used in or on the body, certain scientific evidence must be available. The scientific method requires that the studies to be conducted meet certain criteria. Studies should use herbs with known and reliable contents, be designed using the double-blind study, contain a sufficient number of patients, produce a measurable outcome, and stand up to statistical testing for significance (a difference really exists). Of course, the quantity of scientific facts about each natural substance varies, but in many cases no studies that meet the acceptable criteria have been performed.

These inadequate published "studies" may contain the following deficiencies: no double-blind design, dose used was too low (subtherapeutic), no appropriate control group, no statistical analysis, and the duration of the study was not long enough. Other questions that the dental health care worker should ask before reaching a conclusion include these: What is the potential bias of the people conducting the study? Who sponsored the study (gave money)? What is the potential economic impact of the conclusions reached? Just be skeptical! (Think of the herbs as similar to a new roof job being proposed to elderly homeowners [after a hurricane]) by people who "want to help you."

The biggest hurdle in gaining adequate information has to do with patent laws. Because these natural products have been around for many years, they cannot be patented by the pharmaceutical companies. Patents give a company 17 years to exclusively market a drug and charge prices in line with recovery of economic outlays for testing. Therefore the companies determine that the large studies needed to prove scientific facts about these herbs are not economically warranted. Because generic herbs are readily available, the companies cannot recoup their investment in research. It is interesting that some herbs are beginning to be advertised as "standardized." One wonders what that means.

WHAT ARE IN THESE PRODUCTS?

We are able to identify some of the constituents contained in the available herbal products. The amount of each ingredient varies with each plant, each batch, each season, and each geographic location. The "strength" of the ingredients in each plant vary with the type of soil, amount and timing of watering, temperature, sunlight, humidity, genetics, and other unknown factors (music). Consider a marijuana plant. One plant may have a high concentration of THC, a centrally acting substance that produces a "high" while another plant may have little if any THC. But, the latter plant matter could be used to produce a strong rope or clothing (hemp).

When herbal products that were on the market (taken off shelves) were tested, no relationship existed between the dose stated on the bottle and the actual amount of the constituent contained in the product. Some products had much more than listed, some had much less, and some had none. This fact held across all brands tested. For several products, the actual active ingredient is not known, so the "strength" of the herb cannot be determined. What could you measure? Other products are processed in such a way as to produce an end product that does not contain the active ingredient. How can a product whose constituents are unknown and variable be tested? Properly designed clinical trials are difficult [impossible] to design and economically unfeasible.

CAN THESE PRODUCTS CAUSE HARM (SAFETY)?

Just like drugs, all herbs have a potential to produce adverse effects. It may be due to the active ingredient, an overdose, or contaminates in the product. Some herbs or natural products have been removed from the market after several deaths were reported and determined to be produced by the product. One product, tryptophan, was found to contain a contaminate that produced fatal hepatotoxicity. A product made from ground-up rocks for calcium supplementation also contained the contaminant arsenic.

DIETARY SUPPLEMENTS

In 1994, the Dietary Supplement Health and Education Act (DSHEA) was put into law. This put the herbal and natural substances into a class of substances termed "dietary supplements." The requirements for these dietary supplements in terms of proof of claims is much less than that for drugs available on prescription or over-the-counter in the United States.

Several components of this Act make finding the answers to previously posed questions even more difficult. First, these supplements are considered safe unless proved unsafe by government. (Prescription drugs have to be tested to determine the range of adverse reactions.) This law placed the burden of proof of toxicity with the Food and Drug Administrations (FDA). With the FDA already stretched to its limit evaluating and overseeing drug studies for efficacy and safety, the chance of testing all the available herbs currently on the market would be impossible. Would you like to be given a prescription drug that had no proof of efficacy and/or safety? This evidence is required for prescription drugs, not for herbal products.

Other aspects of this Act prevent the use of therapeutic claims on the label. This means that these products cannot have labels such as "for treatment of hypertension." But, the labels can contain claims of effects on the structure/function of body. So a natural product could be said to "increase immunity" without a comment about what that might mean to the person's health. Another rule is that information may be provided (not necessarily scientific) but cannot be false/misleading. Again, the responsibility for proof of misleading labeling is in the hands of the FDA.

The Act required that the following phrase must be included on each natural product's label:

This product is not intended to diagnose, treat, cure, or prevent any disease."

This phrase is also required in the advertising of these herbal products (They say it really fast in TV ads). Another requirement is that this "information" must be physically separate from the natural product. The product would be on one shelf and the information would be placed in another aisle. It is unclear what benefit separating the information from the product would serve other than getting the Act passed. Health food store employees help customers obtain the literature and associate it with the products to determine their purchase choices.

WHY DO DENTAL HEALTH CARE WORKERS NEED TO KNOW ABOUT THESE PRODUCTS?

1. To be able to make personal choices in the use of herbal products based on evidence.
2. To find out about medical conditions previously unstated by the patient. By knowing the indication(s) for the herb, the dental health care worker can be alerted to the presence of unreported diseases. For example, if a patient is taking St. John's Wort, they may be treating depression.
3. To be able to identify drug interactions with dental drugs that might affect the patient.
4. To identify sources of oral manifestations.

The following table lists some natural or herbal products, their "alleged" indications, and some potential adverse effects. This table does not attempt to indicate which herbs may work. Before use of any herbal substance it is important to accurately evaluate available evidence.

Natural Herbs: Their Source, Indications, and Adverse Effects

Agent	Plant	Alleged Indications*/Properties	Adverse Effects
Alfalfa	*Medicago sativa*	Laxative, diuretic, kidney stones, urinary infections, antifungal, vitamins/mineral	Pancytopenia, induces systemic lupus erythrmatosus
Aloe vera	*Aloe vera*	Cure everything, acne, wound healing, peptic ulcers, laxative, burns, abrasions, demulcent	
Billberry	*Vaccinium myrtillus*	Varicose veins, thrombosis, angina, diarrhea; opthalmologic effects	
Basil		**Gum disease**	
Black cohosh	*Cimicifuga racemosa*	Menstrual cramps (estrogen-like), allergic reaction to bee stings, hypercholesteremia, morning sickness, hot flashes, poisonous bites	Nausea, vomiting, increased perspiration, dizziness, visual and central nervous system disturbances, miscarriage, seizures
Dong quai	*Angelica sinensis*	Menstrual cramps, menopausal symptoms; blood tonic; strengthening heart, spleen, liver, kidneys; antispasmodic	Dermatitis and photosensitization
Dung ho†	*From dung*	What ails you	Psychologic
Echinacea	*Echinacea augustifolia, E. purpurea*	Antiseptic, vasodilator, nasal decongestant, antimicrobial, immunostimulant, AIDS, radiation poisoning	
Feverfew	*Chrysanthemum parthenium*	Antiinflammatory, migraine headache, worms, muscle tension, stimulates appetite, helps menstruation, fever, stomachache, arthritis, insect bites (2/3 of tested marketed products had no active ingredient)	Lowers pain threshold, nervousness, insomnia, dizziness, flushing, anxiety, restlessness, psychoses
Garlic	*Allium sativum alliin → allicin (smelly)*	Antibiotic, strengthens blood vessels, reduces cholesterol, bronchitis, antibacterial, immune effect, antispasmodic, lower blood pressure	Bleeding (via platelets), allergies, heartburn, flatulence
Ginkgo	*Ginkgo biloba*	Stimulates circulation (prevention of peripheral vascular disease), increases mental alertness, antiallergy, antioxidant, antiasthmatic, Alzheimer's disease (little bioequivalence)	Allergic, bleeding (via platelets)

*Alleged means that claims have been made about product (not one product has enough information to meet the requirements for a prescription drug of the F.D.A.).
†This would be a possible product, natural and from the African savannah.

Agent	Plant	Alleged Indications/Properties	Adverse Effects
Ginseng	*Panax ginseng* *P. quinquefolius*	Stress, diabetes, immunostimulant, stimulates appetite, cocaine withdrawal, impotence	
Goldenseal	*Hydrastis canadensis*	**Gum disease, canker sores,** liver problems, skin diseases, antiinflammatory, indigestion, bladder infections	
Kava kava	*Piper methylsticum*	Nervousness, anxiety, insomnia, antiinflammatory, analgesic, diuretic, analgesic, gout, rheumatism	Potentiate CNS depressants, Additive with alcohol
Slippery elm	*Ulmus rubra*	Immunostimulant, diarrhea	
Ma Huang/ephedra	*Ephedra sinica, intermedia, equisetina, distachya*	Asthma, elevates blood pressure, vascular stimulant, hay fever, emphysema, weight loss, nasal decongestant	Misuse by adolescents leading to death, use pseudoephedrine (OTC)
Red raspberry		Sore throat, **canker sores;** hot flashes, menstrual cramps, morning sickness; intestinal tonic; relaxes uterus	
Saw palmetto	*Serenoa repens*	Prostatic hypertrophy, antiseptic, diuretic, antiandrogenic, antiinflammatory	Gastrointestinal; diarrhea
St. John's wort (klamath weed, amber touch-and-heal, goatweed, rosin rose wort)	*Hypericum perforatum L.*	Depression, headache, antiinflammatory, arthritis, astringent, antibacterial, antifungal, AIDS, anxiety, irregular menstruation, anticancer, antiviral	Photodermatitis, orthostatic hypotension
Valerian	*Valeriana officinalis*	Insomnia, anxiety, antispasmodic	No interaction with benzodiazepines or alcohol; drowsiness
White willow	*Salix purpurea, S. Fragilis, daphnoides, (alba)*	Antispasmodic, analgesic (aspirin comes from this plant), antiseptic, astringent, fever	No platelet effects
Yohimbe	*Pausinytalia yohimbe*	Impotence, angina, aphrodisiac	Orthostatic hypotension

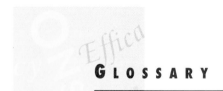

GLOSSARY

Term	Meaning
Abscess	accumulation of pus in a body tissue, usually caused by a bacterial infection
ACE inhibitor	drug group used to treat high blood pressure (angiotensin-converting enzyme inhibitor)
Acetic acid	substance produced when acetylcholine is broken down
Acetylcholinesterase	enzyme that destroys acetylcholine; inactivates effect
Acromegaly	enlargement of peripheral body parts such as head, face, hands, feet; secondary to metabolic disorder
Active transport	movement of ions or molecules across cell membrane; uses energy to accomplish; can be against a gradient
Addiction	dependence on a substance (such as alcohol or other drugs) or an activity, to the point that stopping is very difficult and causes severe physical and mental reactions
Adrenal medulla	center portion of the adrenal gland, secretes epinephrine
Adverse effect	unwanted effects of a drug
Adverse reaction	unwanted effects of a drug
Affective disorder	mental disorder involving abnormal moods and emotions, includes depression and bipolar affective disorder (manic-depressive disorder)
Afferent	coming back to center, for example, nerves from periphery to CNS
Afterload	load against which the heart beats
Akathisia	motor restlessness, muscular quivering
Akinesia	loss (or difficulty) of voluntary movement
Allergy	hypersensitivity reaction caused by an antigen-antibody reaction
Alopecia	baldness or loss of hair, mainly on the head
Ampules	sterile sealed glass containers, broken before use
Anabolic steroid	drug similar to testosterone that builds muscles and strengthens bones
Anaphylactic shock	serious allergic reaction resulting in difficulty breathing, low blood pressure and death
Anaphylaxis	hypersensitivity reaction that produces difficulty breathing; life threatening
Anesthesia	loss of sensation in a certain part of the body (local/general)
Anorexia	reduced appetite, not hungry, food aversion
Anorgasmia	no orgasm
Antacid	drug that neutralizes stomach acids; used to treat indigestion, heartburn, and acid reflux
Anticoagulant	prevents blood coagulation
Antiemetic	prevents vomiting
Antithyroglobulin	antibodies to thyroglobulin
Anxiolytic	action of antianxiety agents, reduces anxiety
Apnea	breathing stops, for either a short or long period; drug or disease induced

Term	Meaning
Arachidonic acid	precursor of prostaglandins and leukotrienes
Arrhythmia	loss of rhythm; refers to irregular heartbeat
Arteriosclerosis	thickening and hardening of artery walls; atherosclerosis
Artery	a large blood vessel that carries oxygen in the blood from the heart to tissues and organs in the body
Arthralgia	pain in joint
Arthritis	osteoarthritis: inflamed joints with pain and stiffness; rheumatoid arthritis: autoimmune disease of joints characterized by inflammation, pain, stiffness, and redness
Arthus	type of immediate hypersensitivity produced when an antigen is administered to a previously sensitized rabbit
Ascorbic acid	chemical term for vitamin C
Asthma	disorder characterized by bronchial constriction and inflamed airways; difficulty breathing
Ataxia	cannot coordinate voluntary muscle activity; caused by disorders in the brain or drugs such as alcohol or CNS depressants
Atherosclerosis	lipid deposits inside arteries, location of clogging of blood vessels
Atony	lack of tone, relaxation
Atrial fibrillation	the atria beat rapidly and inconsistently; irregular heartbeat
Atrial flutter	atria beat rapidly but consistently; an irregular heartbeat
Attention deficit disorder (ADD)	a disorder present in children and adults, characterized by learning and behavior problems, inability to pay attention, and sometimes hyperactivity
Aura	a sensation that sometimes comes before a migraine headache or seizure; may include sensations of movement or discomfort or emotions
Autocoids	substances produced by some cells that change the function of other cells, (e.g., histamine)
Autoimmune	reaction that consists of destruction that occurs as a result of the immune response of the body to itself
Bacillus	any bacteria that is rod shaped; responsible for many diseases, such as diphtheria, tetanus, and tuberculosis
Bacteremia	condition in which bacteria are present in the bloodstream; may occur after minor surgery or infection and may be dangerous for people with a weakened immune system or abnormal heart valves
Bacteriostatic	term used to describe a substance that stops the growth of bacteria, such as an antibiotic
Barbiturates	group of sedative-hypnotic drugs that reduce activity in the brain; are habit-forming and are possibly fatal when taken with alcohol
Bacillus Calmette-Guérin vaccine	vaccine used to protect against tuberculosis
Bile	fluid made in the liver, and stored in the gallbladder; aids in digestion
Bipolar disorder	illness in which the patient goes back and forth between opposite extremes; the most notable bipolar disorder is manic-depressive disorder, which is characterized by extreme highs and lows in mood
Bladder	organ to collect and store urine until it is expelled
Blood clot	semisolid mass of blood that forms to help seal and prevent bleeding from a damaged vessel
Bradycardia	slow heart rate, usually below 60 beats per minute in adults

Term	Meaning
Bronchodilator	drug that increases the diameter of the bronchioles, improves breathing, and relieves muscle contraction or buildup of mucus
Bronchospasm	temporary narrowing of the airways in the lungs, either as a result of muscle contraction or inflammation; may be caused by asthma, infection, lung disease, or an allergic reaction
Bundle of His	bundle of conduction tissue located between the atrium and the ventricles
Calcium	mineral in the body that is the basic component of teeth and bones; essential for cell function, muscle contraction, transmission of nerve impulses, and blood clotting
Calcium channel blocker	drug used to treat chest pain, high blood pressure, and irregular heartbeat by preventing the movement of calcium into the muscle
Cancer	group of diseases in which cells grow unrestrained in an organ or tissue in the body; can spread to tissues around it and destroy them or be transported through blood or lymph pathways to other parts of the body
Candidiasis	yeast infection caused by the fungus *Candida albicans*; occurs vaginally and orally
Canker sore	small, painful sore, usually occurs on the inside of the lip or cheek or sometimes under the tongue; most likely an autoimmune reaction, many triggers; aphthous stomatitis
Cardiac arrest	cessation of the heart beat; results from a heart attack, respiratory arrest, electrical shock, drug overdose, or a severe allergic reaction
Cardiopulmonary resuscitation (CPR)	administration of heart compression and artificial respiration to restore circulation and breathing
Cardiovascular system	the heart and blood vessels that are responsible for circulating blood throughout the body
Cellulitis	skin infection caused by bacteria (usually streptococci); characterized by fever, chills, heat, tenderness, and redness; if dental, treat agressively
Cerebrospinal fluid	clear, watery fluid circulating in and around the brain and spinal column
Cerebrovascular disease	disease affecting any artery supplying blood to the brain; may cause blockage or rupture of a blood vessel, leading to a stroke
Chemotherapy	treatment of infections or cancer with drugs that act on disease-producing organisms or cancerous tissue; may also affect normal cells; antibiotics or antineoplastics
Cholesterol	substance in body cells that plays a role in the production of hormones and bile salts and in the transport of fats in the bloodstream
Cholinergic	stimulated, activated, or transmitted by choline
Chronic obstructive pulmonary disease	combination of the lung diseases emphysema and bronchitis, characterized by blockage of airflow in and out of the lungs
Cleft lip	birth defect in which the upper lip is split vertically, often associated with cleft palate
Cleft palate	birth defect in which the roof of the mouth is split, extending from behind the teeth to the nasal cavity; often occurs with other birth defects such as cleft lip and partial deafness
Colitis	inflammation of the large intestine (the colon), which usually leads to abdominal pain, fever, and diarrhea with blood and mucus
Congenital	present or existing at the time of birth
Contraindication	an aspect of a patient's condition that makes the use of a certain drug or therapy an unwise or dangerous decision

Term	Meaning
Cycloplegia	spasm of accommodation
Defibrillation	short electric shock to the chest to normalize an irregular heartbeat
Delusions	false belief; remains even when evidence to the contrary exists
Dependence	relies on drug to feel "normal"
Depolarization	change in polarity (e.g., positive to negative)
Depression	feelings of hopelessness, sadness, and a general disinterest in life; in most cases there is no known cause; may be due to neurotransmitter abnormality
Dermatitis	inflammation of skin
Diabetes insipidus	output of large amounts of dilute urine; results from lack of antidiuretic hormone
Diabetes mellitus	disease with abnormal glucose use; insulin lacking or does not work properly; many complications (e.g., periodontal disease)
Diaphoresis	perspiration (sweating)
Diffusion	random movement of molecules in solution or suspension, distributes molecules to different compartments (parts of body); moves from a higher concentration to a lower concentration
Direct-acting	acts by stimulation of the receptor
Distribution	how drug moves around the body (where it goes)
Diuretic	drug that increases the amount of water in the urine, removing excess water from the body; used in treating high blood pressure and fluid retention
DNA (deoxyribonucleic acid)	responsible for passing genetic information in nearly all organisms
Drug	substances that affect the body; used to treat diseases
Duration	the time it takes for a drug's effect to cease
Dwarfism	undersized, abnormal; body parts not in proportion
Dynorphins	endogenous opioid ligand, stimulates kappa receptor
Dysgeusia	impairment and/or perversion of taste
Dysmorphology	study of abnormal tissue development
Dyspepsia	"upset stomach"
Dysphoria	unpleasant feeling
Dyspnea	difficulty breathing
Dysrhythmia	abnormal rhythm
Dystocia	difficult childbirth
Dystonia	abnormal tone of tissue; can be hyper- or hypo-
Dysuria	difficult or painful urination
Ectopic	out of place, (e.g., heart beats from outside the conduction tissues)
Ectopic foci	location where ectopic events occur
Edematous	edema (fluid retention) present
Efficacy	maximal amount of beneficial effect resulting from a treatment
Electrocardiogram	graphic record of heart's nerve action potential
Electroconvulsive therapy	sending electricity through patient's brain; treatment of depressed patient, neuromuscular blockers prevent convulsions (formerly did not use when treating depression)
Embolism	blockage of a blood vessel by an embolus- something previously circulating in the blood (such as a blood clot, gas bubble, tissue, bacteria, bone marrow, cholesterol, fat, etc.)
Embryotoxicity	toxicity to embryo; may produce abnormality

Term	Meaning
Emphysema	chronic disease in which the small air sacs in the lungs (the alveoli) become damaged; characterized by difficulty breathing
Endocarditis	inflammation of the inner lining of the heart, usually the heart valves; typically caused by an infection
Endocrine gland	gland that secretes hormones into the bloodstream
Endorphin	group of chemicals produced in the brain; reduce pain and positively affect mood
Endothelium	smooth muscle lining blood vessels and heart
Enkephalins	endogenous opioid ligand, stimulates delta receptor
Enteral	by way of the gastrointestinal tract
Enuresis	involuntary urine release
Enzyme	chemical, originating in a cell, that regulates reactions in the body
Enzyme-linked receptors	receptors that, when stimulated, alter the body's function via enzymes
Epilepsy	disorder of the nervous system in which abnormal electrical activity in the brain causes involuntary effects (e.g., seizures)
Epinephrine	hormone produced by the adrenal glands in response to stress, exercise, or fear; increases heart rate and opens airways to improve breathing; also called *adrenaline*
Epinephrine reversal	with high doses of epinephrine the α effect predominates and leads to an increase in blood pressure and a reflex decrease in heart rate (like norepinephrine); when the dose is lower, effects predominate (α receptors are less sensitive), β_1 increases heart rate, β_2 produces vasodilation and reflex tachycardia
Erythema	redness of skin
Estrogen	a group of hormones (produced mainly in the ovaries) that are necessary for female sexual development and reproductive functioning
Estrogen replacement therapy	treatment with synthetic estrogen drugs to relieve symptoms of menopause and to help protect women against osteoporosis and heart disease
Ethanol	ethyl alcohol
Ethyl alcohol	alcohol with two carbons (ethyl); form of alcohol in alcoholic beverages
Euthyroid	normal thyroid
Excretion	removal of wastes from the body
Exophthalmos	eyeballs that protrude, caused by hyperthyroidism
Expectorant	medication used to promote the coughing up of phlegm from the respiratory tract
Extrapyramidal	refers to part of brain outside the nerve tracks (shaped like pyramids); related to adverse reactions of the antipsychotics; Parkinsonian-like
Facilitated diffusion	movement of agent across cell membranes mediated via a protein
Fetal alcohol syndrome	combination of defects in a fetus as a result of the mother drinking of alcohol during pregnancy
Fiber	constituent of plants that cannot be digested, which helps maintain healthy functioning of the bowels (e.g., bran flakes)
Fibrillation	rapid, inefficient contraction of muscle fibers of the heart caused by disruption of nerve impulses
Fight or flight	effects that occur when the sympathic autonomic nervous system is stimulated
Fluoride	halogen added to municipal water to decrease caries; mineral that helps protect teeth against decay
Flushing	transient erythema
Food and Drug Administration (FDA)	government organization responsible for approval of prescription drugs

Term	Meaning
Free base	releasing base from salt form, used to change one from of cocaine into another more desirable form (before rock cocaine)
Fungus	group of organisms that include yeasts and molds, toadstools, and candidiasis
Gagging reflex	gagging that occurs when a foreign body touches the mucous membranes in the back of mouth; sometimes occurs with alginate impressions or fluoride trays
Gastritis	inflammation of the mucous membrane lining of the stomach; causes include viruses, bacteria, and use of alcohol and other drugs
Gastroparesis	some paralysis of stomach muscles, common with diabetes
Generic drug	nonproprietary name (not trade name)
Genital herpes	an infection caused by the herpes simplex virus, which causes a painful rash of fluid-filled blisters on the genitals; transmitted through sexual contact
Geographic tongue	disorder of tongue, different colored patches visible, lesions move; lesions look like continents on a world map
Gestation	period between fertilization of an egg by a sperm and birth of a baby
Gigantism (giant-ism)	abnormal growth of body or its parts
Gingivitis	inflammation of the gums, typically caused by a buildup of plaque resulting from poor oral hygiene
Gland	group of cells or an organ that produces substances that are secreted or excreted
Glaucoma (wide angle)	disease with elevated pressure in eye, treated with ophthalmic drops, 95% of cases
Glaucoma (narrow-angle)	disease with elevated pressure in eye, due to narrow angle, treated with emergency surgery in 5% of glaucoma cases
Glossitis	tongue inflammation
Glossodynia	painful (or burning) tongue
Glossopyrosis	same as glossodynia
Gluconeogenesis	hydrolysis of glycogen to glucose (make glucose)
Glucose	sugar that is the main source of energy for the body
Glucuronide (dation)	(process of) combining a drug with glucuronic acid, product is more water soluble, more easily excreted
Glutamate	form produced by adding glutamic acid; inhibitor neurotransmitter in central nervous system
Glycogenolysis	breaking down glycogen
Glycoside	structure produced when sugar condenses with other radicals
Goiter	enlargement of the thyroid gland, which produces a swelling on the neck
Gout	disorder marked by high levels of uric acid in the blood; usually experienced as arthritis in one joint
Gradient	rate of change of variable, especially concentration of drug in two different places
Grand mal	type of seizure occurring with epilepsy, producing loss of consciousness, involuntary jerking movements
Graves' disease	hyperplasia of thyroid gland, exophthalmos common
Gynecomastia	swelling of male breasts, can be side effect of drug
H_2 (histamine) blocker	blocks acid production produced by histamine, used to treat acid reflux and ulcers
Hallucination	perception that occurs when there is actually nothing there to cause it (such as hearing voices when there are none)

Term	Meaning
Hapten	substance that cannot cause antibody production alone; combines with larger molecule that acts as a carrier to stimulate formation of antibodies
Hashimoto's (disease) thyroiditis	lymphocytes enter thyroid, diffuse goiter, hypothyroidism produced
Heart valve	structure at each exit of the four chambers of the heart that allows blood to exit but not to flow back in
Heart block	disorder of the heart caused by a blockage of the nerve impulses throughout the heart that alters heartbeat; may lead to dizziness, fainting, or stroke
Heart attack	see Myocardial infarction
Heart rate	rate at which the heart pumps blood; units = heartbeats per minute
Heart failure	the heart cannot pump effectively
Heartburn	burning sensation experienced in the center of the chest up to the throat; caused by gastrointestinal esophageal reflux disease (GERD)
Heimlich maneuver	maneuver in which fist of treating person is placed on abdomen of choking person above navel and is forcefully pushed; used to remove object lodged in throat
Hematocrit	percentage of total blood volume that consists of red blood cells, which is determined by laboratory testing; can be an indicator of disease or injury
Hematuria	blood in the urine, can be caused by kidney infection
Hemoglobin	pigment in red blood cells that is responsible for carrying oxygen; hemoglobin bound to oxygen gives blood its red color
Hemolysis	breakdown of red blood cells in the spleen, can cause jaundice and anemia if the red blood cells are broken down too quickly
Hemolytic	destruction of blood cells; liberates hemoglobin
Hemophilia	inherited disorder, blood lacks a protein needed to form blood clots, leads to excessive bleeding
Hemorrhage	blood loss through broken vessel wall
Hemorrhoid	bulging vein near the anus, often caused by childbirth or straining during bowel movements
Hemostasis	stop bleeding
Hepatic microsomal enzymes	enzymes in the liver that are responsible for metabolizing drugs, mixed function oxidases
Hepatic	related to the liver
Hepatitis	inflammation of the liver, which may or may not be caused by a viral infection; can be caused by poisons, drugs, or alcohol
Hepatitis B	caused by the hepatitis B virus, transmitted through sexual contact or contact with infected blood or body fluids
Hepatitis A	caused by the hepatitis A virus, usually transmitted by contact with contaminated food or water
Hepatitis D	causes symptoms when hepatitis B is present
Hepatitis C	transmitted through sexual contact or contact with infected blood or body fluids
Hernia	bulging of an organ or tissue through a weakened area in the muscle wall
Herpes simplex	infection that causes blister-like sores on the face, lips, mouth, or genitals
Hiatal hernia	part of the stomach bulges up into the chest cavity through the diaphragm
High-density lipoprotein (HDL)	protein found in the blood that removes cholesterol from tissues, "good cholesterol"
Histamine	chemical released during allergic reactions, causing inflammation; causes production of acid in the stomach and narrowing of the bronchioles

Term	Meaning
Hives	common term for urticaria, an itchy, inflamed rash that results from an allergic reaction
Hormone replacement therapy [HRT]	use of natural or artificial hormones to treat hormone deficiencies
Hormone	produced by a gland or tissue that is released into the bloodstream; controls body functions such as growth and sexual development (e.g., insulin)
Huffing	illegal use of hydrocarbon inhalants (e.g., paint, gasoline); inhalant is deposited in a plastic bag and the user breathes in and out
Human immunodeficiency virus (HIV)	a retrovirus that attacks helper T cells of the immune system and causes acquired immunodeficiency syndrome (AIDS); transmitted through sexual intercourse or contact with infected blood
Hydrogen bond	bond between the H^+ and other atoms
Hypercalcemia	abnormally high levels of calcium in the blood; can lead to disturbance of cell function in the nerves and muscles
Hypercapnia	increase in the arterial level of carbon dioxide, abnormal
Hypercholesterolemia	an abnormally high level of cholesterol in the blood, which can be the result of an inherited disorder or a diet that is high in fat
Hyperglycemia	abnormally high levels of blood glucose, usually as a result of untreated or improperly controlled diabetes mellitus
Hyperlipidemia	lipid levels in the blood are abnormally high, including hypercholesterolemia
Hyperlipoproteinemia	elevation of the lipoproteins in the blood
Hyperplasia	increase in the number of cells in an organ or tissue
Hyperprolactinemia	increased level of prolactin in blood, abnormal
Hyperpyrexia	elevated body temperature, side effect of aspirin overdose
Hypertension	abnormally high blood pressure, even when at rest
Hyperthermia	elevated body temperature
Hyperthyroidism	overactivity of the thyroid gland, causing nervousness, weight loss, hair changes
Hyperuricemia	elevated blood level of uric acid, associated with gout
Hypoglycemia	lower blood sugar
Hypoprothrombinemia	lower level of prothrombin in blood
Hypotension	abnormally low blood pressure
Hypothyroidism	underactivity of the thyroid gland, causing tiredness, cramps, a slowed heart rate, and possibly weight gain
Hypoxia	reduced level of oxygen in tissues or body
Iatrogenic	term used to describe a disease, disorder, or medical condition that is a direct result of medical treatment
Idiopathic	something that occurs of an unknown cause
Idiosyncratic	peculiar characteristic; may be caused by a drug
Ileum	lowest section of the small intestine, which attaches to the large intestine
Immune system	cells, substances, and structures in the body that protect against infection and illness
Immunity	resistance to a specific disease because of the responses of the immune system
Immunosuppressant	inhibits the activity of the immune system; used to prevent transplant organ rejection and for disorders where the body's immune system attacks its own tissues (rheumatoid arthritis, psoriasis)

Term	Meaning
Impetigo	contagious skin infection caused by bacteria, usually occurring around the nose and mouth; commonly occurring in children, common causative organisms include streptococci and staphylococci
Implant	organ, tissue, or device surgically inserted and left in the body
Impotence	inability to acquire or maintain an erection of the penis
Incontinence	cannot hold urine or feces
Incubation period	period from when an infectious organism enters the body to when symptoms occur
Indirect-acting	acts either before or after the receptor; (e.g., cause release of neurotransmitter, blocks metabolism of neurotransmitter)
Induction	increase in production (e.g., enzymes in the liver); time from the start of general anesthesia until surgical anesthesia occurs
Infection	disease-causing microorganisms that enter the body, multiply, and damage cells or release toxins
Inflammation	redness, pain, and swelling in an injured or infected tissue
Inflammatory bowel disease (IBD)	general term for two inflammatory disorders affecting the intestines; also known as *Crohn's disease* and *ulcerative colitis*
Influenza	viral infection, characterized by headaches, muscle aches, fever, weakness, and cough; commonly called the "flu"
Infusion	introduction of a substance, such as a drug or nutrient, into the bloodstream or a body cavity
Inhaler	device used to introduce a powdered or misted drug into the lungs through the mouth, usually to treat respiratory disorders such as asthma
Inhibition	reduces an effect (e.g., liver enzymes)
Injection	use of a syringe and needle to insert a drug into a vein, muscle, or joint or under the skin
Innervation	nerves that are connected to tissue
Inotropic	influencing contraction of muscle (especially cardiac)
Insomnia	inability to sleep, difficulty falling or remaining asleep
Insulin shock	reaction that occurs when blood sugar is too low; excessive insulin is one factor
Insulin	hormone made in the pancreas that plays an important role in the absorption of glucose (the body's main source of energy) into muscle cells
Interferon	protein produced by body cells that fights viral infections and certain cancers
International Normalized Ratio (INR).	lab value that adjusts the prothrombin time ratio to take into account the difference in the potency of prothrombin used in different labs; used to monitor warfarin usage, calculated by taking the PT ratio to the power of the International Sensitivity Index (ISI); $ISI = [PT_r]^{[ISI]}$
International Sensitivity Index (ISI)	factor that is used to convert an individual's PT to an INR; corrects for variability in sensitivity of prothrombin used in different laboratories
Intestine	long, tubular organ extending from the stomach to the anus; absorbs food and water, passes the waste as feces
Intrauterine device	plastic device inserted into the uterus that helps to prevent pregnancy
Intravascular	within blood vessels
Intrinsic	term used to describe something originating from or located in a tissue or organ
Intubation	passage of a tube into an organ or structure; used to refer to the passage down esophagus for artificial respiration (e.g., during general anesthesia)

Term	Meaning
Invasive	describes something that spreads throughout body tissues, such as a tumor or microorganism; also describes a medical procedure in which body tissues are penetrated
Iodine	element for the formation of thyroid hormones
Iodine-131	radioactive iodine, used to treat hyperthyroidism
Ion channel receptors	receptors that are activated by a change in the amount of ions flowing through the channels
Ionic bond	combining of molecules in which one ion becomes negatively charged and the other ion becomes positively charged
Iron	mineral necessary for the formation of important biological substances such as hemoglobin, myoglobin, and certain enzymes
Iron-deficiency anemia	type of anemia caused by a greater-than-normal loss of iron resulting from bleeding, problems absorbing iron, or a lack of iron in the diet
Ischemia	condition in which a tissue or organ does not receive a sufficient supply of blood
Jaundice	yellowing of the skin and whites of the eyes because of the presence of excess bilirubin in the blood; usually a sign of a disorder of the liver
Jock itch	fungal infection in the groin area
Kaposi's sarcoma	skin cancer that is characterized by purple-red tumors that start at the feet and spread upward on the body; commonly occurs in people who have AIDS
Kidney	one of two organs that are part of the urinary tract; responsible for filtering the blood and removing waste products and excess water as urine
Lacrimation	secretion of tears
Larynx	the voice box, the organ in the throat that produces voice and also prevents food from entering the airway
Leukocyte	white blood cell
Lipid-lowering drugs	drugs taken to lower the levels of specific fats called *lipids* inthe blood in order to reduce the risk of narrowing of the arteries
Lipids	group of fats stored in the body and used for energy
Lipolysis	breakdown of fats
Lipoproteins	substances containing lipids and proteins, comprising most fats in the blood
Liver failure	final stage of liver disease, in which liver function becomes so impaired that other areas of the body are affected, most commonly the brain
Liver	largest organ in the body, producing many essential chemicals and regulating the levels of most vital substances in the blood
Loquacious	talkative
Low-density lipoprotein	type of lipoprotein that is the major carrier of cholesterol in the blood, with high levels associated with narrowing of the arteries and heart disease
Lumbar spine	lower part of the spine between the lowest pair of ribs and the pelvis; made up of five vertebrae
Lungs	two organs in the chest that take in oxygen from the air and release carbon dioxide
Luteinizing hormone	hormone produced by the pituitary gland that causes the ovaries and testicles to release sex hormones and plays a role in the development of eggs and sperm
Lyme disease	disease caused by bacteria transmitted through the bite of a tick; characterized by fever, rash, and inflammation of the heart and joints
Lymph	milky fluid containing white blood cells, proteins, and fats; plays an important role in absorbing fats from the intestine and in the functioning of the immune system

Term	Meaning
Lymphadenopathy	disease that affects lymph nodes; often refers to swelling of lymph nodes; associated with infection
Lymphocyte	white blood cell that is an important part of the body's immune system, helping to destroy invading microorganisms
Lymphokines	substances that are released by lymphocytes, involved in immune response
Lymphomas	group of cancers of the lymph nodes and spleen that can spread to other parts of the body
Lysis	destruction of blood cells, bacteria; caused by immune reaction
Macroangiopathy	disease of larger blood vessels
Macrophages	mononuclear cells with phagocytic action
Magnesium	mineral that is essential for many body functions, including nerve impulse transmission, formation of bones and teeth, and muscle contraction
Malignant hyper-thermia	acute rise in body temperature, muscle rigidity; caused by change in body's muscle metabolism; can be fatal
Malignant	cells that exhibit uncontrolled growth, such as a cancerous tumor
Mandible	lower jaw
Mania	mental disorder characterized by extreme excitement, happiness, overactivity, and agitation; usually refers to the high of the highs and lows experienced in manic-depressive disorder
Manic-depressive disorder	mental disorder characterized by extreme mood swings, including mania and depression, or a continuing shift between the two extremes
Marijuana	plant containing the active ingredient tetrahydrocannabinol; hallucinogen, sedative
Mast cell	cell present in most body tissues that releases substances in response to an allergen, which causes symptoms such as inflammation
Mastectomy	surgical procedure in which all or part of the breast is removed to prevent the spread of cancer
Measles	illness caused by a viral infection, causing a characteristic rash and a fever; primarily affects children
Medulla	the soft center part of an organ or body structure (e.g., medulla oblongata, renal medulla (e.g., renal medulla)
Megaloblastic anemia	anemia resulting from the lack of vitamin B_{12} or folic acid
Melanoma	skin tumor composed of cells called *melanocytes*
Meniere's disease	disorder of the inner ear, causing ringing in the ear and the sensation that one's surroundings are spinning
Meningitis	inflammation of the protective membranes that covers the brain, called the *meninges;* usually caused by infection by a microorganism (meningitis caused by bacteria is life-threatening; viral meningitis is more mild)
Menopause	the period in a woman's life when menstruation stops, resulting in a reduced production of estrogen and cessation of egg production
Menstrual cycle	periodic discharge of blood and mucosal tissue from the uterus, occurring from puberty to menopause in a woman who is not pregnant
Menstruation	shedding of the lining of the uterus during the menstrual cycle
Mescaline	active ingredient in peyote (cactus); a hallucinogen
Metabolic tolerance	with chronic use drug produces less effect because of metabolic change
Metabolism	process by which the body changes a drug chemically to make it easier to excrete
Metabolite	compound that is produced when a drug is metabolized

Term	Meaning
Metastasis	spreading of a cancerous tumor to another part of the body; through the lymph, blood, or across a cavity; also sometimes refers to a tumor that has been produced in this way
Metered-dose inhaler (MDI)	inhaler that gives a specific amount of medication with each use
Methadone maintenance	program to treat opioid addicts (heroin) by administering a high dose of oral methadone, usual doses of heroin then cannot produce euphoria
Microangiopathy	disease of small capillaries
Microcephaly	small head; abnormal
Microorganism	any tiny, single-cell organism (e.g., bacterium, virus, or fungus)
Microphthalmia	small eyes; abnormal
Migraine	severe headache, usually accompanied by vision problems and/or nausea and vomiting, and that typically recurs
Mineral	substance that is a necessary part of a healthy diet (e.g., potassium, calcium, sodium, phosphorus, and magnesium)
Minipill	oral contraceptive containing only progesterone (no estrogen)
Miosis	constriction of pupil
Mitral valve prolapse	common condition in which the mitral valve in the heart is deformed, may cause blood to leak back across the valve; may be characterized by a heart murmur and sometimes chest pain and disturbed heart rhythm
Mitral valve	valve in the heart that allows blood to flow from the left atrium to the left ventricle, but prevents blood from flowing back in
Mitral insufficiency	problem with the ability of the mitral valve in the heart to prevent backflow of blood from heart chambers
Molecule	smallest unit of a substance that possesses its characteristics
Monoamine oxidase	enzyme that destroys single amines
Monoamine oxidase inhibitor	substance that works by blocking an enzyme that breaks down stimulating chemicals in the brain; used to treat depression
Morbidity	state of being ill or having a disease
Mortality	death rate, measured as the number of deaths per a certain population; may describe the population as a whole, or a specific group within a population (e.g., infant mortality)
Mucous membrane	soft, pink cells that produce mucus; found in respiratory tract (including mouth), eyelids, and urinary tract
Mucus	slippery fluid produced by mucous membranes that lubricates and protects the internal surfaces of the body
Multiple sclerosis	disease in which the protective coverings (myelin) of nerve fibers in the brain are gradually destroyed; symptoms varying from numbness to paralysis and loss of control of bodily function
Murmur	characteristic sound (heard through a stethoscope) of blood flowing irregularly through the heart; can be harmless or may be an indication of disease
Muscarinic	receptors that are activated by muscarine, contained in certain mushrooms; anticholinergics block this action
Muscle relaxants	group of drugs used to relieve muscle spasm and to treat conditions such as arthritis, back pain, and nervous system disorders such as stroke and cerebral palsy
Myalgia	muscle pain

Term	Meaning
Myasthenia gravis	disease in which the muscles, mainly those in the face, eyes, throat, and limbs, become weak and tire quickly; caused by the body's immune system attacking the receptors in the muscles that pick up nerve impulses
Mycobacterium	genus of slow-growing bacterium; resistant to the body's defense mechanisms and responsible for diseases such as tuberculosis and leprosy
Mydriasis	dilation of the pupils
Myeloma	cancerous cells in the bone marrow
Myocardial infarction (MI)	heart attack, heart vessel becomes clogged, severe pain in the chest experienced, can be fatal
Myocardium	heart muscle
Myopathy	a muscle disease
Myositis	inflammation of muscle
Narcolepsy	frequent and uncontrollable episodes of falling asleep, excessive sleepiness
Narcotic analgesics	pain relievers that bind to opioid receptors in the brain; inhibit ascending pain fibers, alter response to pain; often causes tolerance and dependence
Narcotic	addictive substance that blunts the senses; with increased dosages causes sedation, coma, and death; called *opioids*
Nausea	feeling the need to vomit
Necrosis	death of tissue cells
Negative feedback	secretion of hormone 1 inhibits the release of hormones 2 and 3 that stimulate the secretion of hormone 1, (e.g., give prednisone (1), inhibits CRF (2), and ACTH (3), both of which stimulate release of hydrocortisone)
Neonate	newborn infant from birth to 1 month of age
Neoplasm	tumor
Nephritis	inflammation of kidney(s), caused by an infection, an abnormal immune system response; a metabolic disorder
Nerve action potential	changes in voltage (via ions) that transmits the nerve impulse along the nerve fiber
Nerve	fibers that transmit electrical messages between the brain and most body areas, convey information both ways
Nerve block	preventing transmission of pain from an area of the body by injecting a local anesthetic near a nerve
Neuralgia	pain along the course of a nerve
Neuromuscular junction	synapse between the nervous innervation and the somatic (voluntary) muscles
Neuropathy	disease, inflammation, or damage to the nerves connecting the brain and spinal cord to the rest of the body
Neurosis	mental illness with anxiety; stimulates useless action (e.g., counting things); relatively mild emotional disorders (such as mild depression and phobias)
Neurotransmitters	chemicals that are released after excitation of the presynaptic neuron, cross synapse to excite the postsynaptic neuron
Neutropenia	deficiency of white blood cells
Neutrophil	white blood cell in granulocyte group
Nicotinic	receptors that are activated by nicotine, contained in cigarettes
Nitrates	drugs that produce wide-spread vasodilation, used to treat angina pectoris and heart failure, reduce preload and afterload
Nocturnal enuresis	bedwetting at night

Term	Meaning
Non–insulin-dependent diabetes	occurs mainly in over 40, overweight persons; treated with diet changes and oral drugs that reduce glucose levels in the blood, known as type II diabetes, insulin may be needed in some patients
Nonsteroidal antiinflammatory drug	drug group that relieves pain and reduce inflammation, they are not corticosteroids, (e.g., ibuprofen)
Norepinephrine	hormone that regulates blood pressure by causing blood vessels
NSAID	see Nonsteroidal antiinflammatory drug, pronounced *in-sed*
Nystagmus	persistent, rapid, rhythmic, involuntary movement of the eyes; used by police to check for the effect of drugs
Obesity	condition in which there is an excess of body fat; used to describe those who weigh at least 20 percent more than the maximum amount considered normal for their age, sex, and height
Object drug	in drug interactions, drug already present upon which the second drug acts
Obsessive compulsive disorder	action that must be repeated to make person comfortable, (e.g., hand washing)
Occlusion	blocking of an opening or passageway in the body
Oligodactyly	fewer than five digits
Onset	time it takes for a drug's effect to begin
Opacities	not transparent
Opportunistic infections	infection by organisms that would be harmless to a healthy person, but cause infection in those with a weakened immune system (e.g., persons with AIDS or chemotherapy patients)
Optic	pertaining to the eyes
Oral contraceptives	pills that prevent pregnancy; contain a progesterone and an estrogen
Organophosphate	organic compounds that combine with acetylcholinesterase, in activating it, called irreversible cholinesterase inhibitors; used as insecticides and war gases
Orgasm	involuntary contraction of genital muscles experienced at the peak of sexual excitement
Orphan drugs	drugs used to treat rare diseases; difficult to get marketed because potential sales are small; new rules allow these drugs to be approved with fewer studies
Orthopnea	breathing difficulty experienced while lying flat; can be a symptom of heart failure or asthma
Orthostatic hypotension	when a person stands up from the supine position, and the blood pools in the lower extremities and the blood flow to the brain is greatly reduced, causing dizziness and potential fainting; common side effect of some antihypertensives
Osteoarthritis	disease that breaks down the cartilage that lines joints, especially weight-bearing or malaligned joints; leads to inflammation, pain, and stiffness
Osteomalacia	loss of minerals and softening of bones because of a lack of vitamin D; called *rickets* in children
Osteoporosis	condition in which bones become less dense and more brittle and fracture more easily
Otitis media	inflammation of the middle ear caused by infection from the nose, sinuses, or throat
Ototoxicity	harmful effect that some drugs have on the organs or nerves in the ears, which can lead to hearing and balance problems
Outpatient treatment	medical attention that does not include an overnight stay at a hospital

Term	Meaning
Ovaries	two almond-shaped glands located at the opening of the fallopian tubes on both sides of the uterus; produce eggs and the sex hormones estrogen and progesterone
Over-the-counter	medication that can be purchased without a provider's prescription
Overdose	excessively large dose of a drug, can lead to coma and death, used to commit suicide
Ovulation	development and release of the egg from the ovary, which usually occurs halfway through a woman's menstrual cycle
Oxidation	chemical reaction that adds oxygen; can damage cells (free radicals)
Oxygen	gas that is colorless, odorless, and tasteless; essential to almost all forms of life
Oxytocin	hormone from the pituitary gland; causes contraction of the uterus and stimulation of milk flow
Pacemaker	small electronic device that is surgically implanted to stimulate the heart muscle to produce a normal heartbeat
Palate	roof of the mouth
Palliative treatment	treatment that relieves the symptoms of a disorder without curing it
Pallor	abnormally pale skin; usually refers to the skin of the face
Palpebral fissures	eyelid folds
Palpitation	abnormally rapid and strong heartbeat
Pancreas	gland that produces enzymes that breaks down food and hormones (insulin and glucagon) that help to regulate blood glucose levels
Pancreatitis	inflammation of the pancreas; one cause is alcohol abuse
Panic disorder	attacks of anxiety, made worse by stress; patient focuses on avoiding situations in which it occurs
Paralysis	inability to move a muscle
Paralytic ileus	ilium motility reduced or absent, often caused by general anesthetics
Paranoia	mental disorder involving delusions (e.g., "the FBI is following me")
Parathyroid glands	small glands located in the neck that produce a hormone that regulates the levels of calcium in the blood
Parenteral	introduction of a substance into the body by any route other than the digestive tract; often used to mean an injection
Parkinson's disease, Parkinsonism	lack of brain dopamine; leads to muscle stiffness, weakness, and trembling; symptoms include restlessness, tremors, rigidity, and lack of facial expression
Paroxysmal	sudden onset of symptoms (e.g., paroxysmal tachycardia
Partial seizure	abnormal electrical discharge in the cortex of the brain, affecting certain functions
Pathogen	substance capable of causing a disease; usually refers to a disease-causing microorganism
Pedal	relates to feet (check for pitting edema in feet for congestive heart failure)
Peptic ulcer disease (PUD)	erosion in the lining of the esophagus, stomach, or small intestine, most related to the presence of *Helicobacter pylori*
Perception	nerve impulse going to central nervous system
Peripheral resistance	opposition to flow of blood through the vessels, varies with vessel diameter; total peripheral resistance
Peripheral vascular disease (PVD)	narrowing of blood vessels in the legs or arms, causing pain and possibly tissue death (gangrene) as a result of a reduced flow of blood to areas supplied by the narrowed vessels

Term	Meaning
Peritoneum	membrane that lines the abdominal cavity and covers the abdominal organs
Pernicious anemia	anemia resulting from deficiency (failure to absorb) of vitamin B_{12} caused by a deficiency of intrinsic factor (IF) (autoimmune disease); abnormal red blood cells are produced (macrocytic, megaloblastic)
Perversion	different from normal
Petit mal	complete seizure characterized by loss of consciousness for brief periods, posture retained (do not fall)
Peyote	cactus that contains mescaline, a hallucinogen
Phagocytic	relating to cells that ingest bacteria, foreign particles, and other cells
Pharmacokinetic	movement of a drug within the body
Pharmacologist	specialist in pharmacology
Pharmacology	science of drugs and their properties
Pharyngitis	inflammation of the throat (the pharynx), causing sore throat, fever, earache, and swollen glands
Pharynx	throat; the tube connecting the back of the mouth and nose to the esophagus and windpipe
Pheochromocytoma	tumor that secretes epinephrine
Phobia	persisting fear of and desire to avoid something
Phocomelia	defective development of arms and/or legs; foot or hand connected to body (flipperlike)
Photophobia	abnormal sensitivity of the eyes to light
Photosensitivity	abnormal sensitivity to light
Pigmentation	coloration of the skin, hair, and eyes by melanin
Piloerection	hair on body standing up
Pituitary gland	gland located at the base of the brain, releases hormones that control other glands and body processes
Placebo	inactive substance given in place of a drug, required to adequately test drugs (total effect of the drug equals the effect that a patient taking the drug gets—the effect that the placebo produces)
Placebo effect	the positive or negative response to a drug that is caused by a person's expectations of a drug rather than the drug itself
Placenta	organ formed in the uterus during pregnancy that links the blood of the mother to the blood of the fetus; provides the fetus with nutrients and removes waste
Plaque	patch of differentiated tissue on body; fatty deposits in an artery cause narrowing of the artery and heart disease; dental plaque: coating on the teeth, consisting of saliva, bacteria, and food debris, which causes tooth decay; demyelinated patch, (e.g., multiple sclerosis)
Plasma	fluid part of the blood (no cells), contains nutrients, salts, and proteins
Platelet adhesiveness	stickiness of platelets; if reduced, retards clotting
Platelet	megakaryocyte fragment shed into blood, plays an important role in blood clotting, contains no nucleus; adhesiveness affected by aspirin
Plummer's disease	hyperthyroidism from nodular toxic goiter
Pneumonia	inflammation of the lungs, alveoli filled with exudate, most cases are caused by a bacterial or viral infection; symptoms include fever, shortness of breath, and the coughing up of phlegm

Term	Meaning
Polyp	mass of tissue that bulges outward from the surface, growth occurs on mucous membranes such as the nose and intestine; bleeds easily and can become cancerous
Polyuria	excessive production of urine; can be a symptom of a disease, commonly diabetes
Posterior	describes something that is located in or relates to the back of the body
Postural hypotension	unusually low blood pressure that occurs after suddenly standing or sitting up
Potassium	a mineral that plays an important role in the body, helping to maintain water balance, normal heart rhythm, conduction of nerve impulses, and muscle contraction
Precipitant drug	in drug interactions, drug added that interacts with original drug
Precocity	development occurs early, used to refer to early puberty
Preganglionic fibers	nerve fibers that precede the ganglia, especially in autonomic nervous system
Preload	force pushing into the heart
Premenopausal	period of time from beginning of menstruation until hormones begin to decrease
Priapism	penile erection; painful and persistent
Progesterone	female sex hormone; plays role in reproduction, thickens uterine lining
Prostate gland	organ located under the bladder that produces a large part of the seminal fluid
Prostatic hypertrophy	enlarged prostate gland, common in older men
Proteins	large molecules made up of amino acids that play many major roles in the body, including forming the basis of body structures such as skin and hair, and important chemicals such as enzymes and hormones
Prothrombin time	time in seconds that it takes for the patient's blood to clot when combined with thromboplastin and calcium
Prothrombin	agent involved in clotting
Pruritus	itching
Psoriasis	skin disorder characterized by patches of thick, red skin often covered by silvery scales
Psychoactive	has effect on mood
Psychosis	mental disorder in which a serious inability to think, perceive, and judge clearly causes loss of touch with reality
Pulse	changes in diameter of blood vessel caused by the heart beat; synonymous with the heart rate
Purkinje fibers	part of the conduction system of the heart located in the ventricles
Quinidine-like	has effects on cardiac muscle similar to quinidine
Raynaud's syndrome	disease involving constriction of blood vessels of extremities
Reaction	effect of brain on interpretation of nerve impulse received to central nervous system
Rebound congestion	vasoconstrictor given, vasoconstriction; repeat; stop vasoconstrictor, vasodilation (stuffy nose)
Receptor	structural protein molecule that binds with specific agents (ligands)
Retraction cord	cord used around tooth to separate tissue from tooth, improves accuracy of impression, many contain epinephrine
Rodenticide	kill rodents
Sacral	part of the vertebral column near the pelvis, includes the coccyx
Salicylism	reaction to an overdose of aspirin
Salivation	secretion of saliva

Term	Meaning
Schizophrenia	category of psychosis
Semen	fluid containing secretions from the prostate gland and sperm, which is expelled upon ejaculation
Sialadenitis	inflammation of salivary gland
Side effect	unwanted effects of a drug
Silage	fodder for winter use, contained in silo
Silent killer	refers to lack of symptoms, hypertension
Sinus	channels that carry fluid
Somatic	relating to body or trunk of body
Sphygmomanometer	instrument that inflates with a gauge to measure blood pressure
Starling's law	cardiac output and stroke volume increases with an increase in end-diastolic pressure, up to a point; then the heart fails
Subdiaphragmatic	below the diaphragm
Sublingual gland	salivary gland located below the tongue
Sublingually	under the tongue
Submaxillary gland	salivary gland in lower jaw
Supraventricular	referring to the atrium (part of heart above ventricles)
Synaptic cleft	space between nerve cells or between nerve cells and effector organ (space between)
Syncope	fainting, loss of consciousness
Syndactyly	fusion or webbing of fingers or toes; fewer digits
Tachycardia	increase in heart rate
Tachyphylaxis	with repeated administration, the body quickly has a decrease in response
Tardive dyskinesia	voluntary muscle performance; irreversible; side effect of antipsychotics
Temporomandibular joint	joint of the lower jaw
Teratogenicity	abnormal fetus, *terato* means "monster-producing"
Tetraiodothyronine	thyroid hormone, T_4
Therapeutic effect	desired effect of a drug
Therapeutic index	LD_{50}/ED_{50}; used to compare safety of drugs
Thrombophlebitis	inflammation of the venous vessels
Thromboplastin	substance present in tissues and platelets that is necessary for blood coagulation
Thyroidectomy	thyroid removal
Thyrotoxicosis	produced by excessive thyroid hormone
Tinnitus	ringing of the ears
Tolerance	process of becoming less responsive to a drug over time; the need for larger amounts of a drug to produce the same effect
Tracheotomy	surgical opening of trachea; emergency procedure for choking
Transferases	enzymes that move one-carbon groups from one substance to another
Tremors	muscle movement producing shaking, involuntary
Trigeminal neuralgia	pain in the trigeminal (side of face) nerve
Triglycerides	type of fat found in blood; risk factor for atherosclerosis
Triiodothyronine	thyroid hormone, T_3
Unipolar depression	mental disorder with only depression as a component (in contrast to bipolar where there is depression and elation alternating)
Urethral	refers to urethra, canal between bladder and outside of body
Urinary retention	retain urine in bladder, associated with prostatic hypertrophy
Urination	excretion of urine

Term	Meaning
Urticaria	itching wheals, hypersensitivity reaction caused by foods, drugs, emotions, or physical agents
Vagovagal reflex	bradycardia with arterial hypotension; associated with stimulation of the vagus
Vagus	vagal nerve, parasympathetic autonomic nervous system stimulates vagus (produces bradycardia)
Van der Walls forces	induced dipoles bond
Vasoconstriction	blood vessels narrow
Vasodilation	blood vessels wider
Vasomotor collapse	fainting
Ventricular arrhythmia	abnormal rhythms originating from ventricles
Vesicles	sac containing something, in autonomic nervous system they store neurotransmitters
Viscous	thick
Volume depleted	amount of water in body (a lot in blood) too low
von Willebrand's disease	disease with tendency to bleed, prolonged bleeding time; inherited
Xerostomia	reduced saliva (dry mouth)

Index

Drug Index

Inoculum, 153
insulin
    allergic reaction to, 432
    and Autonomic Nervous System (ANS),
        19
    and DCCT, 429
    and dental office emergency, 477
    and diabetes, 426, 430
    and diabetes mellitus, 420
    for diabetic coma, 478
    and drug interactions, 504, 509
    and glucagon, 435-436
    and hypoglycemia, 113, 477, 483
    inactivation of, 28
    managing dental patient taking, 431*b*
    preparations of, 431*t*
    serum levels, *431*
    and sulfonylureas, 432
    and troglitazone, 435
Intal, respiratory drug, 463
interferon, for RAS, 309
Intralipid, and propofol for general
        anesthesia, 275
Intropin, 97
iodide, 424
iodine, radioactive, 424
Ipecac, emetic, 471
Ipratropium, 87-88, 459, 464
Iron, 469, 506
Itraconazole, for chronic candidiasis, 307
Ismelin, antihypertensive agent, 354
Isocaine, 224-225
Isoflurane
    adverse effects from, 272
    MAC for, 272
isoniazid (INH); *see* INH
    and Centers for Disease Control, 187-188
    glucocorticoids and, 410
    and tuberculosis treatment, 187, 188
isoproterenol, 91, 94, 97
    respiratory drug, 458
Isoptin, 335, 348
Isuprel, 91, 94, 97, 458
Itraconazole, 203, 307, 468

K

Kabikinase, anticoagulant, 363
kaolin, 306
Kaopectate, 306, 470
Kenalog, for angular cheilitis/cheilosis, 307
kanamycin, for nondental use, 182
Ketalar, 275
ketamine, 267, 275
ketoconazole, 198, 198*t*
    and adverse reactions, 202-203
    for chronic candidiasis, 307
    and cimetidine interaction, 468
    dosage forms, 203
    drug interactions of, 203
    hydrochloride acid and, 202
    mechanisms of action, 202
    and nonsedating antihistamines, 401
    pharmacokinetics, 202
    in pregnancy and nursing, 202, 496
ketorolac, 122
Klonopin, anticonvulsant, 375

L

labetalol, 99
    α- and β-blocking agent, 348
    selectivity, 99
    for surgical cardiac problem, 483
Laniazid, and tuberculosis treatment, 188
Lanoxin, digitalis glycosides, 325
Lasix, loop diuretic, 346
leukotrienes
    autocoids and antihistamines, 404
    for bronchoconstriction, 404
leuprolide, 442
    GnRH, 421
levodopa, 89, 469
levonordefrin, 96, 96-97
    and drug interactions, 509
    vasoconstrictor with local anesthetic,
        224-225
levonorgestrel, 438
Levoprome, 91, 126, 127
levothyroxine, and hypothyroidism, 420,
        423
Librium
    antianxiety agent, 241
    and drug abuse, 522
Lidex, for oral lesions, 316
lidocaine, 54, 91, 225, 233, 306, 479
    and adverse reactions, *224*
    allergic reactions to, 222
    amide local anesthetic, 233, 233*t*
    antiarrhythmic, 484
    and CNS depression, 223-*224*
    comparison of names, *12*
    drug interaction and, 99
    with epinephrine, 223, 224
    for HSV-1, 305
    local anesthetic, 11, 12
    mixed with tetracycline, 174
    names of, 11-12
    origin of, 214
    and pregnant or nursing patient, 493-494
    topical anesthetic, 233, 233*t*
Lioresal, antianxiety agent, 257
Lipitor, antihyperlipidemic agent, 356
lisinopril, antihypertensive agent, 350
Lispro, 430-431
lithium, 119, 121-122, 173
    antipsychotic agent, 393
    for bipolar disorder, 381
    and drug interactions, 504
    effects of, 173
    potency and efficacy, *122*
    toxicity and, 119
    used with anticonvulsants, 393
Lithobid, antipsychotic agent, 393
LOCAL ANESTHETIC AGENTS,
        212-235
    benzonatate, 226
    bupivacaine, 225
    Carbocaine, 224
    Citanest, 225
    Citanest Forte, 225
    combinations, 223*t*
    Dyclone, 226
    dyclonine, 226
    Isocaine, 224
    lidocaine, 223, 232, 233

LOCAL ANESTHETIC
        AGENTS—cont'd
    Marcaine, 225
    mepivacaine, 224
    Novocain, 226
    Octocaine, 223
    Polocaine, 224
    Pontocaine, 226
    prilocaine, 225, 232, 233
    propoxycaine, 226
    Ravocaine, 226
    ropivacaine, 226
    Tessalon Perles, 226
    tetracaine, 226
    and vasoconstrictors, 227-229, 229 104*t*
    Xylocaine, 223, 233
Lomotil, 175, 470
Lonamin, 98
Loperamide, antidiarrheal drug, 470
Lopid, antihyperlipidemic agent, 357
Lopressor, β-adrenergic blocking agent,
        336
Loratadine
    antihistamine, 397, 399-400
    nonsedating antihistamine, 401
    xerostomia and, 401
Lorazepam
    antianxiety agent, 241
    anticonvulsant, 375
    for conscious sedation, 251
    in pregnancy and nursing, 496
    and preoperative dental anxiety, 250
losartan, and CHF, 327
lovastatin, antihyperlipidemic agent, 356*t*
Lozol, antihypertensive agent, 344
LSD; *see* Lysergic acid diethylamide
Ludes, and drug abuse, 522
Lupron, 442
Luvox, 391
Lypressin, 422
lysergic acid diethylamide (LSD), and drug
        abuse, 527

M

Maalox, 306
malathion, 87
Marcaine
    origin of, 214
    and prolonged duration of action, 225
marijuana
    adverse reactions to, 527-528
    antiemetic, 471, 512
    and drug abuse, 512, 527, 527-528
    effects of, 527-528
    federal control of, 13
Marinol
    antiemetic, 471
    for gastrointestinal reactions, 451
Maxzide, potassium-sparing diuretic, 346
Mazicon, to reverse benzodiazepines, 484
Mebaral, as anticonvulsant, 372
Meclizine, antihistamine, 399
Medrol, 413*t*
medroxyprogesterone, 438
    progestins, 437
mefenamic acid, 118
Mellaril, antipsychotic agent, 382